Minimally Invasive Neurosurgery

Minimally Invasive Neurosurgery

Edited by

Mark R. Proctor, MD
Department of Neurosurgery
Children's Hospital, Boston, MA

Peter M. Black, MD, PhD
Children's Hospital and
Brigham and Women's Hospital, Boston, MA

HUMANA PRESS ✶ TOTOWA, NEW JERSEY

© 2005 Humana Press Inc.
999 Riverview Drive, Suite 208
Totowa, New Jersey 07512

www.humanapress.com

All rights reserved.

No part of this book may be reproduced, stored in a retrieval system, or transmitted in any form or by any means, electronic, mechanical, photocopying, microfilming, recording, or otherwise without written permission from the Publisher.

All papers, comments, opinions, conclusions, or recommendations are those of the author(s), and do not necessarily reflect the views of the publisher.

Due diligence has been taken by the publishers, editors, and authors of this book to assure the accuracy of the information published and to describe generally accepted practices. The contributors herein have carefully checked to ensure that the drug selections and dosages set forth in this text are accurate and in accord with the standards accepted at the time of publication. Notwithstanding, since new research, changes in government regulations, and knowledge from clinical experience relating to drug therapy and drug reactions constantly occur, the reader is advised to check the product information provided by the manufacturer of each drug for any change in dosages or for additional warnings and contraindications. This is of utmost importance when the recommended drug herein is a new or infrequently used drug. It is the responsibility of the treating physician to determine dosages and treatment strategies for individual patients. Further, it is the responsibility of the health care provider to ascertain the Food and Drug Administration status of each drug or device used in their clinical practice. The publishers, editors, and authors are not responsible for errors or omissions or for any consequences from the application of the information presented in this book and make no warranty, express or implied, with respect to the contents in this publication.

This publication is printed on acid-free paper. ∞

ANSI Z39.48-1984 (American Standards Institute) Permanence of Paper for Printed Library Materials.

Cover design by Patricia F. Cleary

Cover illustrations: BACKGROUND: Color Plate 5 and Chapter 5, Fig. 5 (computer model showing magnetoencephalography), see complete caption and discussion on pp. 123, 124. FOREGROUND: *(From top)* Chapter 14, Fig. 1 (delivery of gene therapy to a malignant glioma via direct parenchymal injection under stereotactic guidance), see complete caption and discussion on pp. 299, 300; Chapter 19, Fig. 2 (endoscopic approach to the carpal tunnel, operating room setup), see complete caption and discussion on p. 389; Chapter 6, Fig. 2 (surgery with NC4 microscope guidance), see complete caption and discussion on pp. 132, 133; Color Plate 6 and Chapter 15, Fig. 1D (endoscopic image of wide fenestration of a ventricular cyst), see complete caption and discussion on pp. 323, 324.

For additional copies, pricing for bulk purchases, and/or information about other Humana titles, contact Humana at the above address or at any of the following numbers: Tel.: 973-256-1699; Fax: 973-256-8341; E-mail: orders@humanapr.com; or visit our Website: www.humanapress.com

Photocopy Authorization Policy:

Authorization to photocopy items for internal or personal use, or the internal or personal use of specific clients, is granted by Humana Press Inc., provided that the base fee of US $30.00 per copy is paid directly to the Copyright Clearance Center at 222 Rosewood Drive, Danvers, MA 01923. For those organizations that have been granted a photocopy license from the CCC, a separate system of payment has been arranged and is acceptable to Humana Press Inc. The fee code for users of the Transactional Reporting Service is: [1-58829-147-2/05 $30.00].

Printed in the United States of America. 10 9 8 7 6 5 4 3 2 1

eISBN: 1-59259-899-4

Library of Congress Cataloging-in-Publication Data

Minimally invasive neurosurgery / edited by Mark R. Proctor, Peter M. Black.
  p. cm.
 Includes bibliographical references and index.
 ISBN 1-58829-147-2 (alk. paper)
 1. Brain--Endoscopic surgery. I. Proctor, Mark R. II. Black, Peter McL.
RD594.M555 2005
617.4'810597--dc22
                                                                 2005003214

To our colleagues and trainees at Children's Hospital Boston and Brigham and Women's Hospital

Preface

The rapid technological advances of the last quarter of a century have dramatically changed surgery. Advances in imaging and technology have made it safer, less invasive, and more effective. In neurosurgery, these advances have been driven by the delicate and complex nature of the nervous system and the need to perform surgical procedures with sufficient precision to leave surrounding neural tissue unharmed. They have culminated in the concept of "minimally invasive neurosurgery." Colloquially, many have referred to these newer surgical techniques as "bloodless surgery," but no conventional surgery is truly bloodless and the term is really a misnomer. Minimally invasive surgery attempts to deal with complex problems in a way that minimizes both blood loss and trauma to the normal tissues, including the skull and spine, muscular elements supporting the nervous system, and of course nerves themselves. Minimally invasive techniques are defined by two fundamental prerequisites: a precise definition of the operative anatomy, and a minimally invasive surgical corridor to the target. Minimally invasive techniques are now being used to treat tumors, vascular lesions, hydrocephalus, craniosynostosis, spinal disorders, and many other neurosurgical disorders.

Advances in imaging of the central nervous system have been crucial, and the widespread use of computed tomography (CT) and magnetic resonance imaging (MRI) is one of the primary innovations that allow the application of minimally invasive techniques to neurosurgery. With precise definition of anatomy in the brain and spine, the surgeon can now have more confidence in approaching lesions in the central nervous system while avoiding the normal tissue in the vicinity. Advances in both anatomical and functional MRI permit reliable presurgical and intraoperative brain mapping to resect lesions accurately while sparing eloquent areas. These achievements have made surgery safer and less traumatic and hospital stays shorter. They have also opened the door to novel strategies; for instance, MRI techniques such as spectroscopy offer the possibility of replacing surgery with imaging in the diagnosis of certain brain lesions, and CT and MRI angiography has often replaced intravascular angiograms in the diagnosis of vascular lesions.

Minimally invasive therapy of the brain embodies techniques that achieve results comparable to traditional surgical procedures via small access incisions, penetrating beams, or catheters navigated through the blood stream. The term "minimally invasive surgery" became popular in general surgery with the development of modern endoscopic techniques that allowed procedures such as cholecystectomy to be performed through small access incisions. Endoscopy continues to change our approach to many neurosurgical disorders; however, in neurosurgery there has been a development of many other minimally invasive techniques as well. Image-guided surgery including intraoperative imaging has revolutionized the way we approach many lesions. Conformal radiation, laser hyperthermia, and focused ultrasound are leading to a rethinking of techniques for addressing brain lesions. Interventional radiology often allows an "insider's" approach to vascular lesions via the arterial or venous system as opposed to a standard craniotomy approach.

In *Minimally Invasive Neurosurgery* we review the impact of these new technologies in creating the contemporary revolution in minimally invasive neurosurgery. We feel honored to have the participation of many of the world's experts in their fields in completing this project. Part I is dedicated to the cutting edge techniques and technology available to neurosurgeons today. This includes a thorough discussion of neurosurgical endoscopic equipment, one of the mainstays of minimally invasive surgery. Experts in the field of radiology discuss magnetic resonance imaging with an emphasis on MR principles, as well as advanced techniques including spectroscopy, functional imaging, and brain mapping. Significant emphasis is also placed on the application of image navigation directly in the operating room, using both preoperative and intraoperative systems. Endovascular approaches to vascular disease, including arteriovenous malformations, aneurysms, and atherosclerotic disease, are extensively reviewed. Next, novel approaches, including radiofrequency, radiosurgery, and thermal therapy, are discussed. Finally, the minimally invasive techniques that allow "molecular neurosurgery," including gene and viral vectors and local delivery systems, are reviewed.

In Part II experts in the neurosurgical fields of pediatrics, vasculature, tumors, spine, peripheral nerves, and trauma discuss how they use minimally invasive techniques in their practice. This two part approach is meant to give both in-depth familiarity with the technologies and then a practical "how to" approach to their uses.

We hope that you will find *Minimally Invasive Neurosurgery* informative, cutting edge, and applicable to your practice as minimally invasive techniques continue to revolutionize neurosurgery. We are grateful to all those who have contributed to this book, in their writing or in other less tangible ways.

Mark R. Proctor, MD
Peter M. Black, MD, PhD

Contents

Preface .... *vii*
Contributors .... *xi*
Color Plates .... *xv*

PART I. TECHNIQUES

1. Endoscopic Techniques, Equipment, and Optics
   Liliana C. Goumnerova 3

2. MR Imaging of the Central Nervous System
   Liangge Hsu 13

3. Proton MR Spectroscopy
   Amir A. Zamani 75

4. Functional Brain Mapping Options
   for Minimally Invasive Neurosurgery
   Alexandra J. Golby and Kathleen A. McConnell 87

5. Image Guidance in Minimally Invasive Neurosurgery
   Richard D. Bucholz and Lee McDurmont 113

6. Intraoperative Imaging Using the Siemens 0.2- and 1.5-Tesla
   MR Systems
   Christopher Nimsky and Rudolf Fahlbusch 129

7. Endovascular Treatment of Intracranial Aneurysms
   *Christos Gkogkas, John Baker, Alexander M. Norbash,
   and Kai U. Frerichs* 151

8. Stent Angioplasty for Treatment of Intracranial
   Cerebrovascular Disease
   Adel M. Malek and Clemens M. Schirmer 175

9. The Role of Embolic Agents in Endovascular Treatment
   of Intracranial Arteriovenous Malformations and Tumors
   *Ricardo A. Hanel, Bernard R. Bendok, Jay U. Howington,
   Elad I. Levy, Lee R. Guterman, and L. Nelson Hopkins* 187

10. Radiofrequency Lesioning
    Michael Petr and John M. Tew, Jr. 209

11. Radiosurgery: *Techniques and Applications*
    William A. Friedman 225

12 MRI-Guided Thermal Therapy for Brain Tumors
Ferenc A. Jolesz and Ion-Florin Talos 261

13 Gene-Based and Viral-Based Therapies
Manish Aghi and E. Antonio Chiocca 269

14 Local Delivery Methods Into the CNS
Timothy W. Vogel and Jeffrey N. Bruce 297

PART II. SPECIALTIES

15 Minimally Invasive Pediatric Neurosurgery
Michael Weaver and Mark R. Proctor 319

16 Minimally Invasive Techniques in Vascular Neurosurgery
Prithvi Narayan and Daniel L. Barrow 331

17 Minimally Invasive Treatment for Brain Tumors
Dennis S. Oh and Peter M. Black 345

18 New Directions in Spinal Surgery
Ian F. Dunn and Marc E. Eichler 355

19 Endoscopic Techniques in the Management
of Carpal Tunnel Syndrome
David F. Jimenez 385

20 Minimally Invasive Procedures in Traumatic Brain Injury
*Edward Ahn, William C. Chiu, Max Wintermark, Bizhan Aarabi,
and Howard Eisenberg* 401

Index 423

Contributors

BIZHAN AARABI, MD • *Department of Neurosurgery, University of Maryland School of Medicine, Baltimore, MD*
MANISH AGHI, MD, PhD • *Department of Neurosurgery, Massachusetts General Hospital and Harvard Medical School, Boston, MA*
EDWARD AHN, MD • *Department of Neurosurgery, University of Maryland School of Medicine, Baltimore, MD*
JOHN BAKER, MD • *Department of Radiology, Brigham and Women's Hospital, Harvard Medical School, Boston, MA*
DANIEL L. BARROW, MD • *Department of Neurosurgery, Emory University School of Medicine, Atlanta, GA*
BERNARD R. BENDOK, MD • *Departments of Neurological Surgery and Radiology, Northwestern University Feinberg School of Medicine, Chicago, IL*
PETER M. BLACK, MD, PhD • *Department of Neurosurgery, Brigham and Women's Hospital and The Children's Hospital, Harvard Medical School, Boston, MA*
JEFFREY N. BRUCE, MD • *Department of Neurological Surgery, Columbia University College of Physicians and Surgeons, New York, NY*
RICHARD D. BUCHOLZ, MD, FACS • *Division of Neurological Surgery, St. Louis University School of Medicine, St. Louis, MO*
E. ANTONIO CHIOCCA, MD, PhD • *Department of Neurological Surgery, James Cancer Hospital and Solove Research Institute, The Ohio State University Medical Center, Columbus, OH*
WILLIAM C. CHIU, MD • *Department of Surgery, University of Maryland School of Medicine, Baltimore, MD*
IAN F. DUNN, MD • *Department of Neurosurgery, Brigham and Women's Hospital and The Children's Hospital, Harvard Medical School, Boston, MA*
MARC E. EICHLER, MD • *Department of Neurosurgery, Brigham and Women's Hospital and The Children's Hospital, Harvard Medical School, Boston, MA*
HOWARD EISENBERG, MD • *Department of Neurosurgery, University of Maryland School of Medicine, Baltimore, MD*
RUDOLF FAHLBUSCH, MD • *Department of Neurosurgery, University of Erlangen-Nuremberg, Erlangen, Germany*
KAI U. FRERICHS, MD • *Department of Radiology, Brigham and Women's Hospital, Harvard Medical School, Boston, MA*
WILLIAM A. FRIEDMAN, MD • *Department of Neurological Surgery, University of Florida College of Medicine, Gainesville, FL*
CHRISTOS GKOGKAS, MD • *Department of Radiology, Brigham and Women's Hospital, Harvard Medical School, Boston, MA*
ALEXANDRA J. GOLBY, MD • *Department of Neurosurgery, Brigham and Women's Hospital, Harvard Medical School, Boston, MA*

LILIANA C. GOUMNEROVA, MD • *Department of Neurosurgery, The Children's Hospital, Harvard Medical School, Boston, MA*

LEE R. GUTERMAN, PhD, MD • *Department of Neurosurgery and Toshiba Stroke Research Center, School of Medicine and Biomedical Sciences, University at Buffalo, State University of New York, Buffalo, NY*

RICARDO A. HANEL, MD • *Department of Neurosurgery and Toshiba Stroke Research Center, School of Medicine and Biomedical Sciences, University at Buffalo, State University of New York, Buffalo, NY*

L. NELSON HOPKINS, MD • *Department of Neurosurgery and Toshiba Stroke Research Center, School of Medicine and Biomedical Sciences, University at Buffalo, State University of New York, Buffalo, NY*

JAY U. HOWINGTON, MD • *Neurological Institute of Savannah, Savannah, GA*

LIANGGE HSU, MD • *Department of Neuroradiology, Brigham and Women's Hospital, Harvard Medical School, Boston, MA*

DAVID F. JIMENEZ, MD, FACS • *Division of Neurological Surgery, University of Texas Health Sciences Center at San Antonio, San Antonio, TX*

FERENC A. JOLESZ, MD • *Department of Radiology, Brigham and Women's Hospital, Harvard Medical School, Boston, MA*

ELAD I. LEVY, MD • *Department of Neurosurgery and Toshiba Stroke Research Center, School of Medicine and Biomedical Sciences, University at Buffalo, State University of New York, Buffalo, NY*

ADEL M. MALEK, MD, PhD • *Cerebrovascular and Endovascular Program, Division of Neurosurgery, Beth Israel Deaconess Medical Center, Harvard Medical School, Boston, MA*

KATHLEEN A. MCCONNELL, MD • *Department of Radiology, New York University, New York, NY*

LEE MCDURMONT, BS • *Department of Surgery, St. Louis University School of Medicine, St. Louis, MO*

PRITHVI NARAYAN, MD • *Department of Neurosurgery, The Mount Sinai Hospital, Mount Sinai School of Medicine, New York, NY*

CHRISTOPHER NIMSKY, MD • *Department of Neurosurgery, University of Erlangen-Nuremberg, Erlangen, Germany*

ALEXANDER M. NORBASH, MD • *Department of Radiology, Boston Medical Center, Boston University School of Medicine, Boston, MA*

DENNIS S. OH, MD • *Department of Neurosurgery, Brigham and Women's Hospital, Harvard Medical School, Boston, MA*

MICHAEL PETR, MD, PhD • *Department of Neurosurgery, University of Cincinnati College of Medicine, Cincinnati, OH*

MARK R. PROCTOR, MD • *Department of Neurosurgery, The Children's Hospital, Harvard Medical School, Boston, MA*

CLEMENS M. SCHIRMER, MD • *Division of Neurosurgery, Beth Israel Deaconess Medical Center, Harvard Medical School, Boston, MA*

ION-FLORIN TALOS, MD • *Department of Radiology, Brigham and Women's Hospital, Harvard Medical School, Boston, MA*

JOHN M. TEW, JR., MD • *The Neuroscience Institute, Department of Neurosurgery, University of Cincinnati College of Medicine and Mayfield Clinic, Cincinnati, OH*

TIMOTHY W. VOGEL, MD • *Department of Neurological Surgery, Columbia University College of Physicians and Surgeons, New York, NY*
MICHAEL WEAVER, MD • *Department of Neurosurgery, Temple University School of Medicine, Philadelphia, PA*
MAX WINTERMARK, MD • *Department of Radiology, University of Maryland School of Medicine, Baltimore, MD*
AMIR A. ZAMANI, MD • *Department of Radiology, Brigham and Women's Hospital, Harvard Medical School, Boston, MA*

Color Plates

Color Plates follow p. 112.

Color Plate 1. *Fig.1, Chapter 4:* Statistical maps of fMRI activation demonstrate effect of varying the threshold. (*See* full caption on p. 99 and discussion on p. 98.)

Color Plate 2. *Fig. 2, Chapter 4:* Validation of fMRI as a clinical tool for assessing language lateralization and localization. (*See* full caption on p. 102 and discussion on pp. 101–102. By permission of Oxford University Press.)

Color Plate 3. *Fig. 3, Chapter 4:* fMRI studies of patients with left and right MTLE encoding various stimuli. (*See* full caption on p. 104 and discussion on p. 103.)

Color Plate 4. *Fig. 4, Chapter 4:* Diffusion tensor imaging of white matter tracts in low-grade glioma. (*See* full caption and discussion on p. 105. Courtesy of Dr. Ian-Florin Talos.)

Color Plate 5. *Fig. 5, Chapter 5:* Computer model showing magnetoencephalography. (*See* full caption on p. 124 and discussion on p. 123.)

Color Plate 6. *Fig. 1, Chapter 15*: MRI series of fenestration of large suprasellar cyst. (*See* full caption on p. 324 and discussion on p. 323. Courtesy of Dr. Liliana Goumnerova.)

Color Plate 7. *Fig. 5, Chapter 20:* Comparison of perfusion-CT and conventional studies of patient with Glasgow Coma Scale score of 9. (*See* complete caption and discussion on pp. 409, 410.)

Part I

Techniques

1
Endoscopic Techniques, Equipment, and Optics

Liliana C. Goumnerova, MD

INTRODUCTION

Neuroendoscopy has rapidly established itself as an important field of neurosurgery. This became possible with technical developments in the field of endoscopy allowing the application of this technique to neurosurgery. In addition, the minimally invasive nature of endoscopy and the associated overall minimal morbidity have made neuroendoscopy an accepted and rapidly developing modality in neurosurgery with many potential areas of application. However, as with any new field, it requires skills that are not always intuitive to the neurosurgeon who is not trained in endoscopic techniques. It also relies on the development of new technology specifically designed for neurosurgical applications and procedures. Therefore, in addition to technology development, neurosurgeons need to be specially trained in endoscopy to apply it correctly and with the minimal morbidity it allows. This chapter reviews some of the issues regarding neuroendoscopic equipment, its appropriate selection, and the different applications of Neuroendoscopy.

HISTORY

The first endoscopic neurosurgical procedure was performed by Lespinasse in 1910. Although not a neurosurgeon but a urologist, he successfully performed endoscopy via burr holes with choroid plexus coagulation in two children with hydrocephalus. He never published this procedure, although he reported on it at a local surgical society meeting (1).

The first neurosurgeon to perform a third ventriculostomy was Mixter (2), who combined ventriculoscopy with that procedure in 1923 in an attempt to treat hydrocephalus. However, this procedure was abandoned mainly because of the lack of adequate diagnostic techniques and also because of technical issues related to the endoscopes.

Not until the development of better endoscopes, improved imaging techniques in neuroradiology, better understanding of neurophysiology, and knowledge of microsurgical anatomy did neuroendoscopy reestablish itself in neurosurgery.

From: *Minimally Invasive Neurosurgery*, edited by: M.R. Proctor and P.M. Black © Humana Press Inc., Totowa, NJ

The reintroduction of endoscopy in Neurosurgery occurred in the second half of the 20th century *(3,4)* and consisted of the use of flexible endoscopes as assistive devices in microsurgery, primarily to improve visualization and also to perform a biopsy of an intraventricular tumor.

Currently, endoscopy is performed for spinal disease (disc removal and exploration of the spinal subarachnoid spaces), for peripheral nerve surgery (carpal tunnel syndrome), for craniosynostosis (endoscope-assisted strip craniectomy), and in the treatment of a variety of intracranial disorders (e.g., hydrocephalus, cysts, intraventricular brain tumors, intraparenchymal hemorrhage, aneurysm clipping). This list of diseases and neurosurgical conditions treated by endoscopy will most certainly expand with the growing experience of neurosurgeons and with the refinement of the current endoscopic equipment for specific applications.

EQUIPMENT

Endoscopes can be divided into two groups: flexible/steerable endoscopes or ventriculoscopes and rigid endoscopes. A number of systems are on the market, and this review is not intended to serve as an endorsement of any specific system. In addition to the actual endoscope, light sources, cameras and monitors for viewing while the procedure is performed, instruments for use with the endoscope, and a number of holding devices to immobilize the endoscopes are integral parts of the system. The procedures can be recorded with some of the newer digital imaging technologies available for neurosurgical procedures, as well as with VHS tapes; recording is advisable for most procedures.

Flexible Endoscopes

These endoscopes are similar to the standard bronchoscopes and rely on flexible fiberoptic illumination. The endoscopes are comprised of a number of glass fibers that are incorporated into a plastic sheath. The size of the fiber bundle determines the resolution of images. The endoscopes have up to 180° of freedom of movement at the distal tip of the endoscope, depending on the manufacturer. This occurs at the last 3–5 cm of length of the endoscope. The endoscopes are fitted with at least one working channel, which can also serve as a site for fluid egress and irrigation throughout the procedure. Working instruments, consisting of biopsy forceps, graspers, and scissors, are available and are also flexible in their design and construction. The available steerable endoscopes range in size from 1 to 15 mm outer diameter depending on the number of fibers within them. The main disadvantage of flexible endoscopes is that their optics are worse than those of the rigid endoscopes. They cannot be autoclaved and must be gas-sterilized, which limits their longevity. In addition, frequent use can damage the fiber bundle, which further decreases image resolution. Their advantage is that they can be used to navigate in the ventricular system and around corners when used as an assist-device during microsurgical operations.

Rigid Endoscopes

Rigid endoscopes utilize rod lens telescopes and therefore have superior optics in comparison with the flexible endoscopes; as a result, they have become the most frequently utilized endoscopes in neurosurgery. The endoscopes consist of a lens, an illumination glass fiber, and a metal shaft that houses the lens and light fiber. There are two main designs: a sheath with a single channel for the endoscope and an endoscopic sheath with multiple separate channels for instruments in addition to the lens and light fiber. The rod lens system that is utilized in neuroendoscopy was invented by Hopkins and therefore is also referred to as the Hopkins system.

Rigid endoscopes come in a variety of sizes and lengths of shafts. The design of the lens can also allow for viewing angles of 0°, 30°, 70°, or 110°, thus allowing one to look straight forward, to the side, and also to the back. Rigid endoscopes can be autoclaved, are reusable, and are less fragile than flexible endoscopes. Their disadvantage is their rigidity; one cannot maneuver them in the intraventricular or intracranial spaces as freely as the flexible endoscopes. Therefore, with rigid endoscopy, it is crucial to plan the entry burr hole in such a location as to allow for the greatest freedom of movement without endangering any neurovascular structures.

Both flexible and rigid systems require immobilization of the endoscope so that the surgeons' hands are free to use instruments throughout the procedure. There are systems that allow fixation of any endoscope to the operating room table via mechanical or pneumatic devices. Some may be fitted or attached to the head holder or the stereotactic head frame with specially designed adapters. In addition, with the newly developed frameless navigation systems, the rigid endoscopes can also be registered and the images can be merged *(5–8)*. These fixation devices are of crucial importance: the endoscope must be rigidly immobilized throughout the procedure without endangering the patient. They also need to be minimally intrusive and not restrict the surgeon's ability to manipulate instruments and the actual endoscope.

Flexible endoscopes require an introducer/trocar with a shaft, and a number of sizes are available for the different sizes of endoscopes. Usually, one utilizes a shaft that is slightly larger than the outer diameter of the endoscope so that there is some cerebrospinal fluid (CSF) egress around the endoscope, providing an additional outlet in case the working channel is occupied by an instrument. Frequently, these introducers have peel-away shafts that allow endoscopically guided placement of catheters, in either the ventricles or the cysts.

Rigid endoscopes may have a trocar as part of their system or are designed with a blunt tip to the shaft to allow for introduction without a trocar. Again, their sizes vary to allow for the different sizes of endoscopes. Most rigid endoscopes have at least two working channels, and some of the newer designs incorporate up to four channels (both for rigid instruments and for irrigation). The choice of an endoscope with one common channel or multiple channels depends to some extent on the procedure to be performed; a recent review by Kehler et al. *(9)* summarizes the advantages and disadvantages of both designs.

A number of instruments have been developed for use in endoscopy and consist of trocars, biopsy forceps (different sizes), grasping forceps, scissors, and both monopolar and bipolar coagulation tips. These instruments also have different angled tips allowing for more flexibility and for specialized applications. Balloon catheters are also utilized for dilation of the various fenestrations performed endoscopically; the most commonly used catheters are the Fogarty balloon catheters. Some lasers are also used with endoscopes (Nd-Yag), although with limited application *(10,11)*.

Visualization with an endoscope requires fluid-filled spaces; any bleeding or spillage of tumor or cyst content may obscure the view. Therefore, irrigation is very important for clearing of the CSF spaces and can also be used to dilate the ventricular spaces so as to allow more movement of the endoscope within them.

Irrigation can be performed either continuously or via pulse/bolus injection throughout the procedure. This is the most helpful maneuver if bleeding is encountered during endoscopy; usually irrigation is continued until the bleeding is stopped and the CSF is clear. The solution utilized can be either lactated Ringer's solution or normal saline. It is important to monitor the amount of fluid injected/irrigated and the amount of fluid that has drained out so as to avoid a potential increase in intracranial pressure or pressure on the floor of the third ventricle. In addition, continuous confirmation of the anatomy and position by visualization of the endoscope and the landmarks can be accomplished in this manner and can avoid potentially serious complications *(12)*. New methods of orientation within the ventricular system are being developed in case bleeding is encountered and the normal anatomic landmarks are lost. One new approach is connection of an optical position measurement system to the endoscope that allows for coupling of digitized endoscopic images to the accurate endoscopic position. In cases of bleeding, the previously set landmarks and the overlay of the images allows the surgeon to navigate within the operative field based on virtual images and to perform a procedure. This is still an experimental technique but clearly has the potential to be a helpful tool in neuroendoscopy *(13)*.

All endoscopes require a light source, and these are generally universally available but require filters to avoid the hot infrared spectrum. Observation of the procedure requires a camera, monitor, and video system, which often incorporates recording systems. Monitors need to be positioned so that the surgeon, the assistant, and the operating room personnel can all view them. The cameras require gas sterilization and therefore can be either sterile or draped in a special plastic sheath so that their longevity is increased. Documentation of all endoscopic procedures is preferable and should be performed either on VHS tapes or digitally, as with the newer imaging technologies.

TECHNIQUES

All endoscopic procedures are performed under general anesthesia independent of patient age or disease. The anesthetic agents are chosen based on the presence or absence of increased intracranial pressure. Anticonvulsants are not routinely administered.

For procedures that require an anterior approach through a frontal burr hole, the patient is positioned supine and the head is immobilized in a rigid or semi-rigid fashion. For routine endoscopic third ventriculostomy (ETV), the patient's head is placed in a gel doughnut. The neck is slightly flexed to allow a direct trajectory into the third ventricle through the foramen of Monro and lateral ventricle. Modifications of this technique have been introduced so that one can also approach the posterior aspect of the third ventricle through an anterior burr hole.

For procedures requiring a posterior approach, the patient is positioned so that the head is lateral and the sagittal suture is parallel to the floor. This may require rigid fixation such as the Mayfield head holder or some other similar device or placement on a cerebellar head rest. This allows for ease of orientation and recognition of the normal anatomy, which is crucial in endoscopy. Approaches may be modified based on the patient's disease and medical condition.

All endoscopic procedures rely on the presence of fluid-filled spaces for adequate visualization, and therefore irrigation is essential to endoscopy. A number of authors have advocated continuous irrigation throughout any endoscopic procedure, but related complications have been described in the literature *(12,14,15)*, and therefore one has to be cautious and judicious in the use of continuous irrigation. The choice of fluid has also been a matter of discussion; generally Ringer's lactate has been recommended, although normal saline is equally safe as long as there is constant irrigation of the fluid through the CSF spaces.

Preoperative Assessment and Evaluation

Preoperative evaluation and planning for endoscopy requires magnetic resonance imaging (MRI) of the brain. This information provides adequate visualization of the intraventricular spaces, allows assessment of the size of the ventricles, and gives information as to the possible location of obstruction in the CSF spaces or the location of the cyst or tumor to be treated. On occasion, a contrast-enhanced dye study with injection of contrast into the ventricular system may provide more information regarding the communication between the ventricles, which can then lead to the appropriate choice of endoscopic procedure and endoscope. Computed tomography (CT) imaging of the brain alone is not sufficient prior to performing an endoscopic procedure unless there is a previous MRI of the brain and the CT scan is obtained only to document an increase in the ventricles, such as in a case of shunt malfunction in which an ETV is being considered.

If endoscopy is being performed in an attempt to remove a brain tumor, provisions need to be made for conversion of the procedure to an open craniotomy prior to the beginning of the operation (choice of incision, position, and immobilization of the head and appropriate consent).

Entry Sites for Endoscopy

The placement of the burr hole is dependent on the disease and the goals of surgery: is the fenestration (e.g., ETV) going to be accompanied by biopsy of an intraventricular tumor in a different location, will there be placement of an intraventricular device, will there be intraoperative microsurgery in addition to the endoscopy, and so on?

The approaches are generally via a frontal burr hole, which allows access to the frontal horns of the lateral ventricles, the foramen of Monro, and the third ventricle, or through a posterior occipital burr hole, which is usually utilized for lesions in the posterior aspect of the lateral ventricles and in the quadrigeminal cistern area. Burr holes placed in the forehead have also been recommended for approaches to the posterior part of the third ventricle and pineal area, as well as for aqueductoplasties. Laterally placed burr holes in the frontal area are utilized for septostomies and approaches to the midportion of the lateral ventricles. In some cases, more than one burr hole may be necessary, with a second endoscope or ventricular catheter placed for localization or additional illumination. Colloid cysts generally require two burr holes for adequate visualization and illumination, and the recent development of endoscopic resection of hypothalamic lesions also requires two burr holes.

Flexible Endoscopy

Flexible endoscopy is utilized for fenestration of multiloculated ventricles for which navigation in more than one ventricular space will be required. The choice of anterior or posterior approach depends on the patient's condition and ventricular anatomy. It is often helpful to have a second ventricular catheter placed as a guide, as the ventricular anatomy is frequently very abnormal and some of the normal landmarks may be distorted. This is especially true in patients who have had prior intraventricular hemorrhage or infection or have had long-standing shunts with previous revisions. Intraoperative imaging with ultrasound or frameless navigation to correlate the position of the endoscope with the ventricular anatomy is extremely helpful to ensure that the goals of surgery have been met. Flexible endoscopy can also be used to biopsy tumors or lesions in the posterior part of the third ventricle when the third ventricle is small or the placement of the burr hole does not allow the angulation of the rigid endoscope. Biopsy specimens with the flexible instruments are very small, and one requires experienced neuropathologists in such cases.

Rigid Endoscopy

Rigid endoscopy is the preferred method for most primary intracranial endoscopic procedures. The most common procedure is the ETV, which is performed via a frontal burr hole. As with all endoscopic procedures, the most important aspect is to identify normal anatomy and orient oneself. Once the normal anatomy is confirmed, the procedure is performed. Obscuration of the landmarks and lack of identification of the normal anatomy are contraindications to performing this procedure as the potential for serious neurovascular injury is great. Some authors have suggested utilization of additional imaging techniques to guide the endoscope accurately into the lateral ventricle or to predict the location of the basilar artery and the other vascular structures around the floor of the third ventricle *(16,17)*. One such system incorporates a sono probe at the tip of a catheter that is placed in the rigid endoscope sheath. It requires experience by the user and facility with interpretation of both endoscopic and ultrasound images but has potential in the treatment of multicystic hydrocephalus and may have more indications as future refinements to the technology are made. Contact ultrasonic probes have also been described as the method to make the perforation through the floor of the third ventricle *(18)*. Long-term safety data on this procedure are not available yet, and it is not known whether there are any injuries to the vessels from this probe.

Contact lasers have been used but are not recommended because of the potential of injury to the basilar artery and perforating vessels in the vicinity.

Rigid endoscopes are also the preferred endoscope for the fenestration of suprasellar arachnoid cysts and for the fenestration of intraventricular arachnoid cysts. The same principles of orientation and confirmation of anatomic landmarks apply here as with any endoscopic procedure.

Tumor biopsies can be performed with sufficiently large samples for tissue analysis. However, apart from colloid cyst removals, there are no documented cases of complete tumor resection performed entirely endoscopically, and it is primarily used as an assistive device. Because of the small size of the tumor samples with the endoscopic biopsy forceps, multiple samples usually need to be obtained. Large samples cannot be removed in one piece because of the small diameter of the working channel of the sheath, and another option is to remove the entire endoscope and sheath while holding on to the specimen itself. This has the disadvantage of removing and replacing the endoscope and sheath and the potential for additional injury to the brain.

Endoscopic imaging is becoming incorporated in aneurysm clipping and tumor resection when an open craniotomy with microsurgical resection is being performed *(19–22)*. A diagnostic endoscope with a sheath that has only one channel or no working channels is utilized, with different angles allowing for side views or a backward view. In these situations, it is very important that the endoscopist be familiar with the anatomy, orientation, and different images from the different angles of the endoscope since lack of familiarity will lead to misinterpretation of the images.

Endoscopes are investigated for use in the removal of intraparenchymal hemorrhage *(13,23)* and intraparenchymal tumors (Manwaring, 2002, personal communication). These applications are still in development, although with the integration of frameless neuronavigation into the endoscopy system, there appears to be some potential application of endoscopy in these cases. So far, the only tumors that have been biopsied and resected have been intraventricular tumors or tumors in the thalamus or walls of the ventricles so that the endoscope can have access to the tumor itself.

ENDOSCOPY FOR SPINAL AND OTHER PROCEDURES

Endoscopy has also been introduced in spinal surgery as a way to remove herniated spinal disks or fragments *(24,25)*. The endoscopes and techniques are different from those for intracranial procedures, although the same principles apply—knowledge of anatomy, size of scope with regard to size of area of interest, bleeding, and visualization. The limiting factors are the size of the endoscopes and entry sites as well as adequacy of visualization/bleeding.

Endoscopy is also used in peripheral nerve surgery *(26)*, although there are some controversies regarding its application for that condition.

FUTURE OF ENDOSCOPY

Endoscopy has clearly gained a place as an important tool in the armamentarium of neurosurgeons. The technical limitations seen in the beginning of the development of this field are being addressed, and a number of systems are available that will allow a neurosurgeon to perform the appropriate procedure. It is important to understand the limitations and advantages of all the systems so that one can make the correct choice of instruments and procedure. Knowledge of anatomy and orientation to the endoscopic images is crucial for the safe performance of these procedures. Appropriate preoperative evaluation of the anatomy with MRI is essential, and intraoperative assistance with frameless navigation systems and intraoperative visualization are very helpful and important adjuncts to the procedure. All these allow this procedure to fulfill its promise as a minimally invasive procedure with minimal morbidity to the patient and superior results.

Future developments will be technical and will incorporate imaging, the ability to perform endoscopy during microneurosurgical procedures with greater ease, and the ability to deliver drugs, clip aneurysms, remove brain tumors, and so on through a minimally invasive procedure.

REFERENCES

1. Lespinasse VL. Hydrocephalus and spina bifida, in *Lea & Febiger's Principles of Neurological Surgery*, (Davis L, ed.), Philadelphia, 1992, pp. 438–447.
2. Mixter WJ. Ventriculoscopy and puncture of the floor of the third ventricle. *Boston Med Surg J* 1923;188:227–278.
3. Ogata M, Ishikawa T, Horide R, et al. Encephaloscope: basic study. *J Neurosurg* 1965;22:288–291.
4. Fukushima T. Endoscopic biopsy of intraventricular tumors with the use of ventriculofiberscope. *Neurosurgery* 1978;2:110–113.
5. Moreau JJ, Ghorbel M, Moufid A, et al. Image-guided neuroendoscopy. *Neuro-Chirurgie* 2002;48:92–96.
6. Alberti O, Riegel T, Hellwig D, et al. Frameless navigation and endoscopy. *J Neurosurg* 2001;95:541–542.
7. Schroeder HW, Wagner W, Tschiltschke W, et al. Frameless neuronavigation in intracranial endoscopic Neurosurgery. *J Neurosurg* 2001;94:72–79.
8. Muacevic A, Muller A. Image-guided endoscopic ventriculostomy with a new frameless armless neuronavigation system. *Computer Aided Surgery* 1999;4:87–92.

9. Kehler U, Regelsberger J, Gliemroth J. Pros and cons of different designs of rigid endoscopes. *Minim Invasive Neurosurg* 2003;46:205–207.
10. Willems PW, Vandertop WP, Verdaasdonk RM, et al. Contact laser-assisted neuroendoscopy can be performed safely by using pretreated "black"fibre tips: experimental data. *Lasers Surg Med* 2001;28:324–329.
11. Vandertop WP, Verdaasdonk RM, van Swol CFP. Laser-assisted neuroendoscopy using a neodymium-yttrium aluminum garnet or diode contact laser with pretreated fiber tips. *J Neurosurg* 1998;88:82–92.
12. Handler MH, Abbott R, Lee M. A near-fatal complication of endoscopic third ventriculostomy: case report. *Neurosurgery* 1994;35:525–527.
13. Scholz M, Fricke B, Tombrock S, et al. Virtual image navigation: a new method to control intraoperative bleeding in neuroendoscopic surgery. Technical note. *J Neurosurg* 2000;93:342–350.
14. Fabregas N, Lopez A, Valero R, et al. Anesthetic management of surgical neuroendoscopies: usefulness of monitoring the pressure inside the neuroendoscope. *J Neurosurg* 2000;12:21–28.
15. Fabregas N, Valero R, Carrero E, et al. Episodic high irrigation pressure during surgical neuroendoscopy may cause intermittent intracranial circulatory insufficiency. *J Neurosurg Anesthesiol* 2001;13:152–157.
16. Resch KDM, Perneczky A, Schwarz M, et al. Endo-neuro-sonography: principles and 3-D technique. *Childs Nerv Syst* 1997;13:616–621.
17. Resch KDM. Endo-neuro-sonography: first clinical series (52 cases). *Childs Nerv Syst* 2003;19:137–144.
18. Paladino J, Rotim K, Stimac D, et al. Endoscopic third ventriculostomy with ultrasonic contact microprobe. *Minim Invasive Neurosurg* 2000;43:132–134.
19. Kato Y, Sano H, Behari S, et al. Surgical clipping of basilar aneurysms: relationship between the different approaches and the surgical corridors. *Minim Invasive Neurosurg* 2002;45:142–145.
20. Wang E, Yong NP, Ng I. Endoscopic assisted microneurosurgery for cerebral aneurysms. *J Clin Neurosci* 2003;10:174–176.
21. Barajas MA, Ramirez-Guzman G, Rodriguez-Vazquez C, et al. Multimodal management of craniopharyngiomas: neuroendoscopy, microsurgery, and radiosurgery. *J Neurosurg* 2002;97:607–609.
22. Abdeen K, Kato Y, Kiya N, et al. Neuroendoscopy in microvascular decompression for trigeminal neuralgia and hemifacial spasm: technical note. *Neurol Res* 2000;22:522–526.
23. Oka K, Go Y, Yamamoto M, et al. Experience with an ultrasonic aspirator in neuroendoscopy. *Minim Invasive Neurosurg* 1999;42:32–34.
24. Osman SG, Marsolais EB. Endoscopic transiliac approach to L5-S1 disc and foramen. A cadaver study. *Spine* 1997;22:1259–1263.
25. Tsou PM, Yeung AT. Transforaminal endoscopic decompression for radiculopathy secondary to intracanal noncontained lumbar disc herniations: outcome and technique. *Spine* 2002;2:41–48.
26. Okutsu I, Ninomiya S, Takatori Y, et al. Results of endoscopic management of carpal tunnel syndrome. *Orthop Rev* 1993;22:81–87.

2
MR Imaging of the Central Nervous System

Liangge Hsu, MD

INTRODUCTION

The development of magnetic resonance imaging (MRI) has vastly altered the field of radiology, particularly neuroradiology and by extension to a certain degree the practice of neurology and neurosurgery. Unlike the rapid implementation of X-rays after they were discovered by Wilhelm Roentgen in 1895, it took more than 40 yr before the clinical application of nuclear magnetic resonance (NMR) principles was realized. The fundamentals of NMR were first outlined by a Dutch physicist named G. J. Gorter in 1936 *(1,2)* and refined by Bloch and Purcell in 1946 *(3,4)* but it was not until 1973 when Lauterbur *(5)* suggested using magnetic field gradients and NMR to encode position information that the current clinical use of NMR medical imaging was established. Still, it required many years of contributions from the basic science fields of physics, chemistry, and engineering before the development and subsequent implementation of the clinical scanners that we use today.

Technical Setup of the Magnet

Every clinical imaging MR magnet requires a minimum of five coils for operation. The most important is the main gradient (in the *z* direction, along the length of the bore) with a field of B_0 that lines up all the hydrogen proton spins at Larmor frequency, which is defined as the product of field strength (*B*) and the gyromagnetic constant of the proton (γ). The Larmor frequency of the water proton (chosen because of its abundance in body tissue) is dependent on the magnetic field strength, calculated as 42.57 MHz at 1 T and 63.86 MHz at 1.5 T. Magnetic field strength is invariably described in Gauss (G, smaller field) and Tesla (T, larger field) where 1 T =10,000 G. To give a perspective on the scale, the earth's magnetic field is measured at approx 0.5 G. The goal of the magnet is for B_0 to give a spatial homogeneity of approx 10 ppm/40-cm sphere and temporal stability of 0.1 ppm/h.

The other four coils include a set of three orthogonal (*z* or slice-select, *y* or phase-encoding, *x* or frequency-encoding) gradients that can be turned on and off, which gives each proton spin a different time dependence that is essential for position encoding. The last coil is the radiofrequency (RF) coil, which

From: *Minimally Invasive Neurosurgery,* edited by: M.R. Proctor and P.M. Black © Humana Press Inc., Totowa, NJ

provides a uniform low-amplitude magnetic field near the Larmor frequency that can be switched on and off for excitation (short burst of RF at 0.1–10 kW for a few milliseconds) and for receiving or readout of signals (free induction decay 10–1000 ms) *(6–8)*.

Other varieties of more specialized RF coils include surface coils (placed close to the anatomical site), which are often smaller receive-only coils tailored to specific anatomical regions such as the orbit, temporal mandibular joint, extremities, and spine for increased signal-to-noise ratio (SNR) and at the same time using the larger body RF coil as transmitter. Phase-array coils are in essence multiple surface coils assembled to give an improved SNR but able to cover a larger area or field of view often used in the setting of total spine imaging *(9)*. The design of the orthogonal gradient coils is such that they are perpendicular to B_0 (except the z gradient), the most common being the quadrature configuration that yields an increase in SNR of the square root of 2.

During the early years, the permanent and resistive magnetic materials used were limited by their tremendous weight (tons) and inability to sustain a homogeneous magnetic field. Most, if not all, of the current mid- to high-field magnets (0.5–4 T) are made from superconducting alloys (niobium–titanium) that are wound into a coil configuration and whereby the magnetic field is generated by an electric current that passes through these coils. To maintain a temperature below the transition temperature of the superconducting alloy (10°K), liquid helium at 4°K is circulated around the coil while at the same time further buffering with the ambient temperature is accomplished by circulating liquid nitrogen at 77°K within the outer layer *(10)* (Fig. 1).

All magnetic fields are generated from electric currents and electric fields secondary to either changing electric current or charge accumulation. The magnetic field that a proton experiences depends on the cumulative sum of fields from all five coils. Coil design and configuration, the materials used in the manufacture of the magnet, electrical conductivity, and heat generated (by gradient coils) are a few of the variables that contribute to the imperfection of the field homogeneity and magnet inefficiency. In addition, eddy currents are often generated from the support material, RF coils, and at times even the mere presence of the patient within the magnet. These eddy currents in turn can be corrected by shimming or shielding via smaller coils that have opposite flowing electric current *(11,12)*.

Background of Magnetic Resonance Imaging

Unlike conventional X-rays, MRI is not a transmission technique but rather a technology whereby signal is generated from proton spins (primarily in cellular water and lipid and not DNA, protein, or bone) that have been perturbed from equilibrium. The voltage generated is secondary to the spin magnetization that is proportional to the static magnetic field strength and spin density. The tissue contrast thus generated results from small differences in tissue water concentration under nonequilibrium conditions. The term *spin relaxation* consists of both the time necessary for the spins to return to the equilibrium state and the transfer of energy among themselves and the surrounding environment.

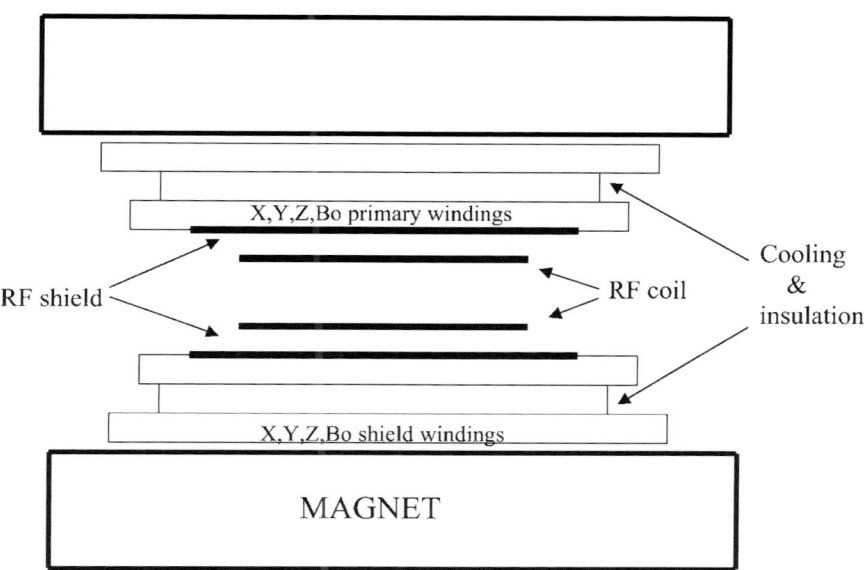

Fig. 1. Schematic diagram of a common setup of a shielded high-field superconducting magnet. RF, radiofrequency.

Two independent but simultaneous spin magnetization processes have been described: T1, or so-called longitudinal/spin-lattice, and T2, or transverse/spin-spin relaxations. After an RF pulse stimulation, the proton nuclei absorbs energy to move to an excited state which, in order to return to the ground state, energy needs to be transferred to neighboring nuclei or paramagnetic ions and molecules that are fluctuating or precessing at the *same* Larmor frequency. This energy transfer can occur between the nuclei of the same (intramolecular) or different molecules (intermolecular). A short T1 (300–500 ms) suggests an efficient energy transfer whereby there is approx 67% signal recovery in that period (Fig. 2). Lipid is a medium-sized molecule that tumbles at a rate closest to the Larmor frequency of bound water, thus possessing a short T1, and appears as bright signal on T1-weighted images. Free water tumbles too fast and large molecules too slow, both thereby exhibiting long T1 relaxation, leading to low signal on T1 images.

In contrast to spin-lattice relaxation, transverse magnetization describes the rate of loss of magnetic phase coherence secondary to magnetic field (local environment) imperfections in which not all nuclei are precessing at the same frequency. Larger molecules are more efficient at T2 relaxation (~67% signal loss in that period with faster signal loss, whereas free water (like cerebrospinal fluid [CSF]) has longer T2 (ms to s) and therefore exhibits bright signal on T2-weighted images (Fig. 3). Unlike T1 relaxation, transverse magnetization is independent of external field strength. The term *proton density* is merely a reflection of the number of proton spins in a particular region where the imaging parameters reflect neither T1 nor T2 weighting, i.e., long TR (repetition time)

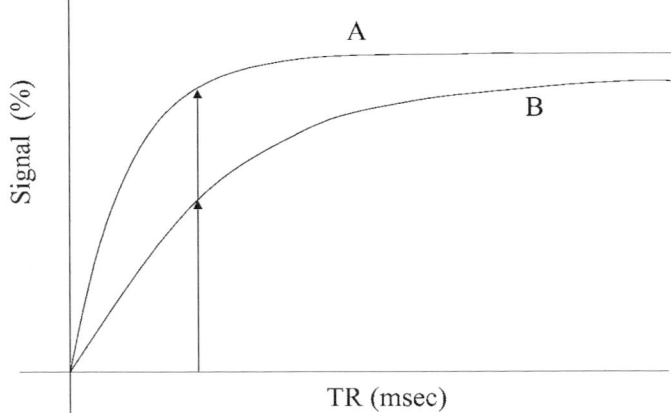

Fig. 2. Longitudinal magnetization returns to equilibrium with time constant T1. The T1 contrast between tissue A and B is greatest at short TR (600 ms) and TE.

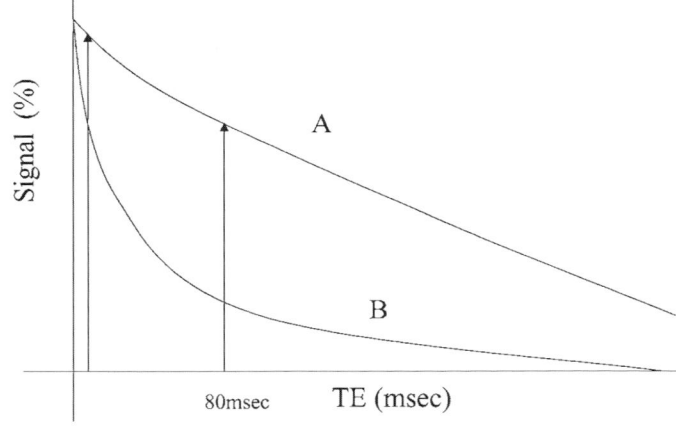

Fig. 3. The transverse magnetization decays to zero with time constant T2: a long TR and TE (80 ms) will maximize the tissue contrast.

but short TE (echo time), both of which will be discussed in more detail later in the chapter. *(13)*

IMAGE ACQUISITION

In understanding the concept behind T1 and T2 relaxation of the proton spins, it is perhaps time to discuss how the MR signal is formed and converted to an actual image. It is a complex process involving multiple parameters such as tissue T1 and T2 properties, strength of gradients, time and strength of the RF pulse, TR, and TE, all of which determine the final MR signal. The raw data acquired in k-space subsequently undergo a mathematical process called Fourier (2D or 3D) transformation to generate the final images.

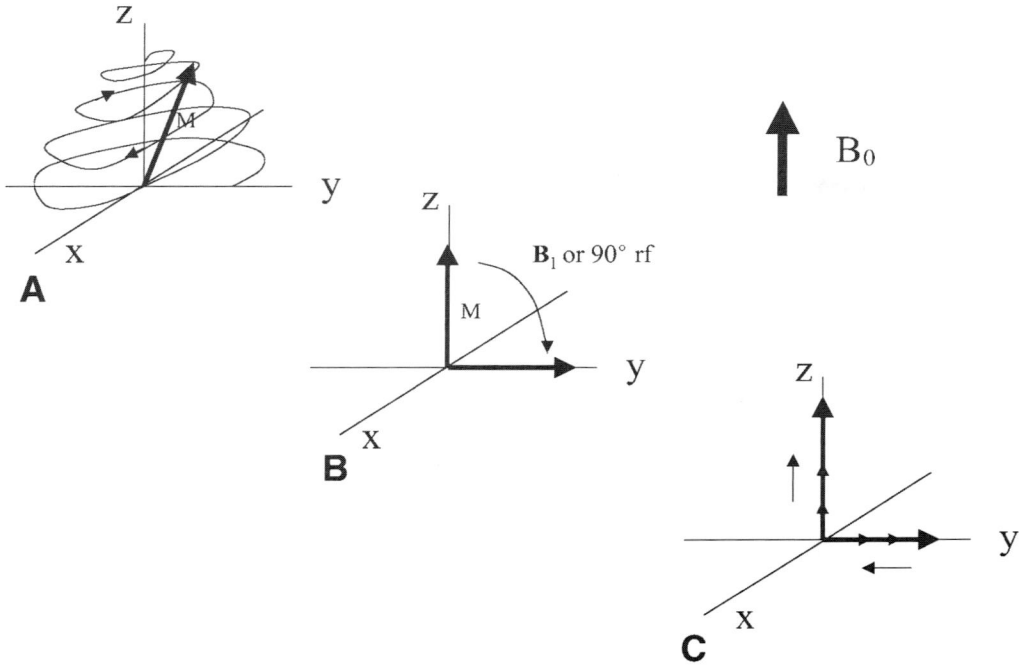

Fig. 4. (A) Magnetization vector **M** precesses toward the transverse (x–y) plane after RF pulse that generates a field of B_1 that is perpendicular to B_0. (B) View of the **M** vector after a 90° RF pulse with the observer within the rotating frame. (C) As the spin magnetization returns to equilibrium, the **M** vector can be split and viewed as two components whereby, if not for signal loss from phase coherence, the two components will return at the same rate.

Any atomic nucleus that consists of an odd number of protons or neutrons such as ^1H, ^{13}C, ^{23}Na, ^{19}F, and ^{31}P will have a net nuclear spin that acts like a small bar magnet aligned along the axis of the spinning nucleus. In the steady state the proton can only be in two equivalent energy states, either "up" or "down." As these protons randomly distribute themselves in the absence of an external magnetic field, these spins cancel each other out, leaving no net magnetism. If an external magnetic field (B_0) is present, a very small percentage of the protons will favor lining up with this external field, the sum of which generates a small net magnetization or vector **M**. It is this vector that is perturbed by a second RF field B_1 (applied perpendicular to B_0) that causes the spins to precess around this axis (Fig. 4A,B). The RF field is time varying in a sinusoidal pattern, and the frequency needs to be identical to the Larmor frequency of the spins in order to excite them. The Larmor frequency of the spins, as described before, is dependent on the gyromagnetic ratio and magnetic field strength. The rate and angle of precession of **M** is determined by the strength of B_1 and length of the pulse as B_1 is turned on and off. One often comes across an RF pulse represented by the precession angle that it causes, such as 90° and 180° in the classic spin-echo pulse sequence.

After the RF pulse or B_1 field has been turned off, the **M** vector or cumulative spins will again try to align back along B_0 axis, and it is this precession of magnetization to return to the equilibrium state that forms the MR signal. It is important to point out that it is best to view the **M** vector as having two components: the longitudinal (parallel to B_0 or z-axis) and the transverse (perpendicular to Bo or in the x–y plane), with the latter being the only component that contributes to the measured MR signal (Fig. 4C).

The T1 contrast in tissues is caused by the different local environment that the spins experience, whereas the transverse decay is slightly more complex: its decay is comprised of three components. The first is owing to T1 relaxation: the transverse portion decreases at the same time as the longitudinal vector returns to its original position. The other two causes of transverse magnetization decay are owing to both static and nonstatic magnetic field inhomogeneities; the former is caused by magnet design or materials used that cause different magnetic susceptibilities. This slight difference in local fields causes the nuclear spins to precess at a slightly different rate (though constant frequency as the inhomogeneity is constant) and thus lose phase coherence, (dephasing)/or fanning out to cancel each other. This form of signal loss also known as T2* decay; it can be reversed by applying a second refocusing RF pulse (180°) in the *transverse* plane to rephase such spins (Fig. 5). An analogy would be if different runners at constant but variable speeds set off say for 5 min; they then reverse direction and after another 5 min they will all end up back at the starting line at the same time. This is exactly what a spin-echo or spin-warp pulse sequence does consisting of a 90° RF pulse followed by 180° pulse just before the echo is recorded. Unlike those previously mentioned, the nonstatic inhomogeneities are microscopic and irreversible owing to the neighboring molecules that are in constant and variable motion, causing the spins to experience random frequency and changing fields over time. This and the reduction of transverse component owing to the T1 relaxation process are exponential and are described by T2, whereas the reversible loss as mentioned before is represented by T2* (Fig. 6).

The precessing vector **M** thus creates a time-varying magnetic field that will induce a voltage across a closed-looped wire according to Faraday's law. The intensity of the voltage (which is also the MR signal) is proportional to the magnitude of the net transverse magnetization vector and will be sinusoidal and also at Larmor frequency. It is appropriate here to illustrate again a classic pulse sequence called the spin echo or 90–180° or Carr-Purcell pulse. The terms TR and TE are also introduced: in a conventional spin-echo pulse sequence, TR is the repetition time or the time between two 90° pulses, whereas TE is the time during which the echo or data is collected after the 180° pulse. This acquisition of data is often represented by five lines, three for each of the x', y', and z-gradients, one for the RF pulse, and the last for readout of data (Fig. 7). The z-gradient (parallel to B_0) is also the slice-select gradient and is turned on at the same time as the 90° RF pulse. The z-gradient goes from the negative and then passes through zero and onto a positive slope where only the protons at a certain location along the z-axis with a local Lar-

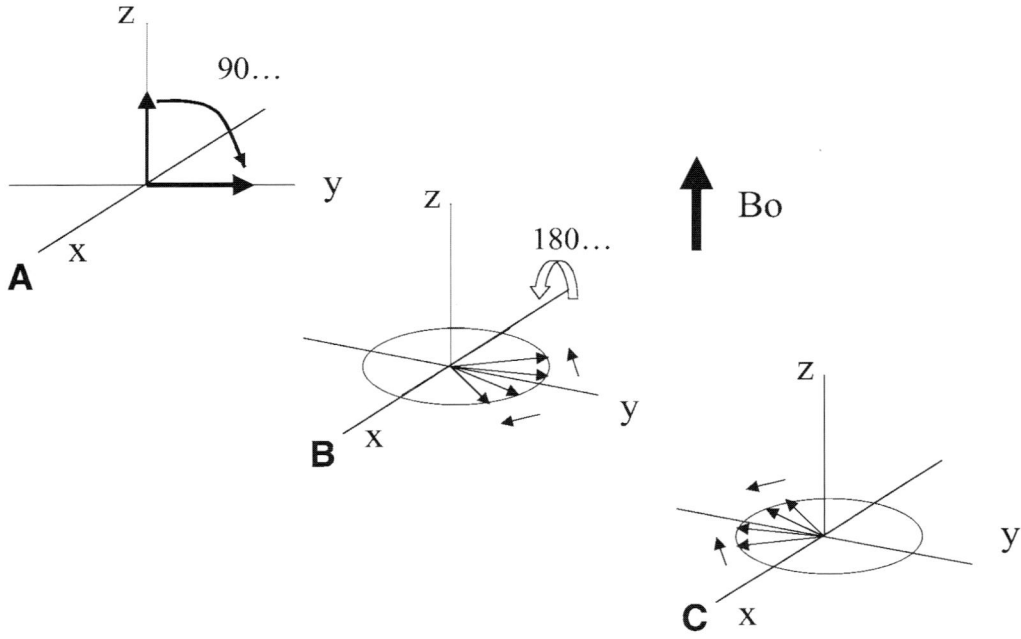

Fig. 5. (A) In the spin-echo sequence, a 90° RF pulse brings the **M** vector into the *x–y* plane. Different components of the transverse magnetization precess at slightly different rates owing to static/local field inhomogeneities. These will dephase **(B)** and cancel each other, resulting in a net zero vector if not for the 180° RF pulse that rephases them **(C)**.

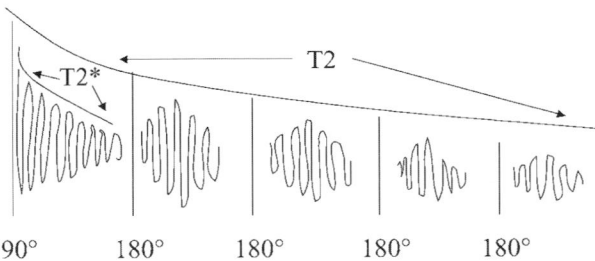

Fig. 6. T2* reflects the decay of echoes themselves with signal loss from both static and dynamic inhomogeneities. T2 decay represents the overall amplitude decay of the spin echo via dynamic inhomogeneities.

mor frequency matching the RF pulse will be excited (Fig. 8). The RF pulse is designed to consist of a defined range of frequencies that also corresponds to the slice thickness. By changing the RF frequency, different slices can be excited along the z-axis. The z-gradient is turned on at the same time as the 90° RF pulse, whereas the phase-encoding y-gradient is activated between the 90° and 180° RF pulse. The strength of the y-gradient is sequentially stepped up for each 90–180° encoding step, again usually from large negative to large positive values.

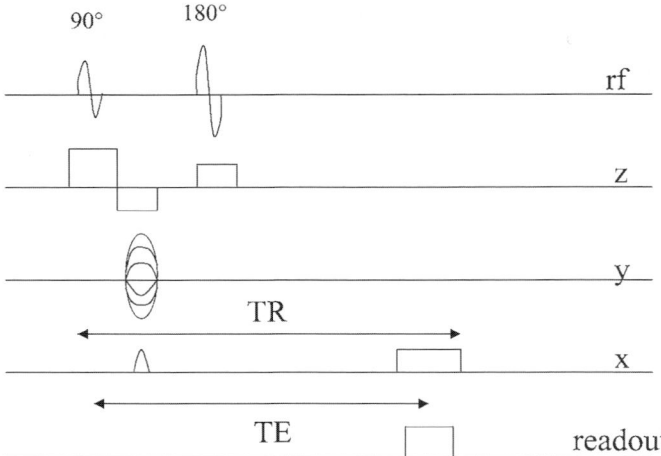

Fig. 7. A basic spin-warp or 90–180° pulse sequence. RF, radiofrequency pulse; z, the slice-select gradient; y, the phase encoding gradient; x, the frequency-encoding gradient.

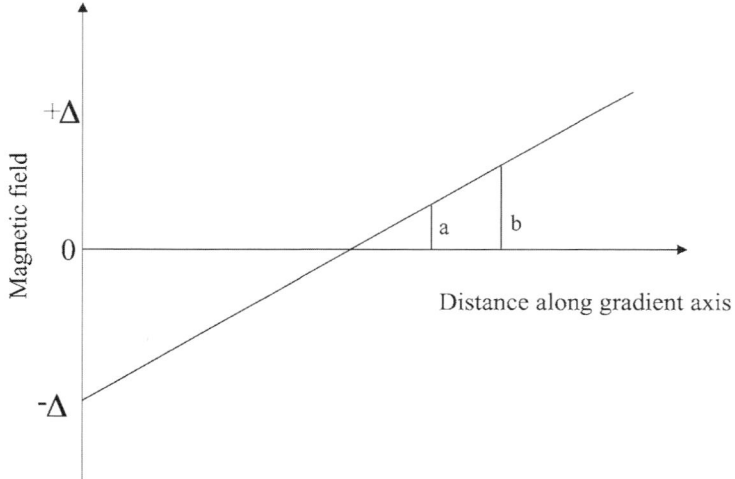

Fig. 8. Any one of the x, y, or z linear gradients causes the magnetic field to be a function of position along this axis. The different positions of a and b allow each to experience a slightly different local magnetic field, with b at slightly higher frequency.

After the 90° pulse as the spins precess and undergo relaxation, the signal generated needs to be encoded in such a way as to reflect their spatial position accurately within the imaged tissue. Two techniques called *frequency* and *phase encoding* are employed for this purpose, with the x-direction often assigned as the frequency or readout gradient and the y-axis as phase-encoding gradient. The understanding of the readout x-gradient is similar to that of the aforementioned z-gradient whereby the spins further to the right of the gradient will have a higher frequency than the more left-sided ones and will fall into position

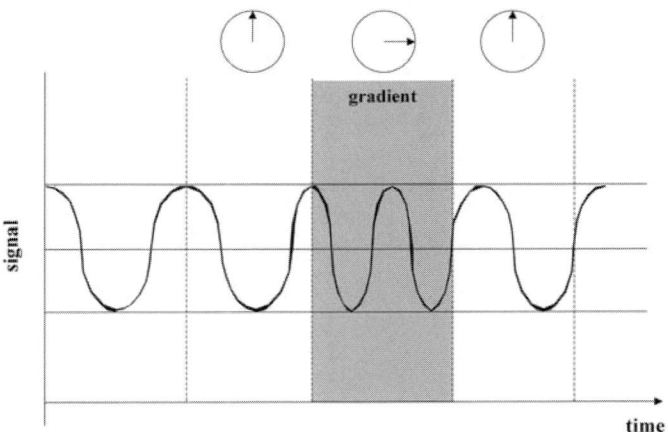

Fig. 9. Illustration of the effects of a transient gradient on the angle or phase of the vector magnetization. After the gradient is briefly turned on and off, there is a temporary increase in frequency; when the field returns to B_0, the frequency returns to the original value but with a 90° phase shift.

accordingly along this axis. Even though the x-position can be sorted out by different frequencies, that still leaves a whole column along the y-axis that all have the same frequency and are therefore unable to be differentiated into their individual positions. To circumvent this, the y-gradient is turned on very briefly and then shut off after the 90° RF pulse but before the 180° and readout step. This causes the spins to undergo an extra positive or negative rotation depending on their position and leading to a shift of phase or angle of the vector (Fig. 9). In order for Fourier transformation to resolve and localize each voxel in the y-axis, this step has to be repeated many times (corresponding to the number of y pixels or the matrix size in the final image, often in multiples of 128 such as 256 or 512, and so on), with a minimum of 128 times while using a different y-gradient strength each time *(14)*.

It is also necessary at this time to introduce the concept of *k*-space, a mathematical construct or the Fourier transformation data plane that illustrates the spatial frequency of a process spread out in space with a sinusoidal shape and consisting of signal pattern at different spatial frequencies. Spatial frequency is therefore measured in cycles per unit length and is what a phase-encoding gradient pulse imposes on the spin vectors. In other words the *k*-space is a 2D array of raw data with the data placed one line at a time during each readout pulse for each different y-gradient. A very important point to note is that there is *not* a one-to-one correlation between a point in *k*-space and the final image. Every point in *k*-space contributes to every pixel of the image and vice versa. It also turns out that the points at the edges of *k*-space determine resolution or sharpness of the image whereas the points near the center of *k*-space are responsible for the brightness or contrast of the final image (Fig. 10). The number of phase-encoding steps (y-gradient) determines the number of lines in *k*-space, the value of the steps contributes to the closeness of the lines, and the maximum (positive

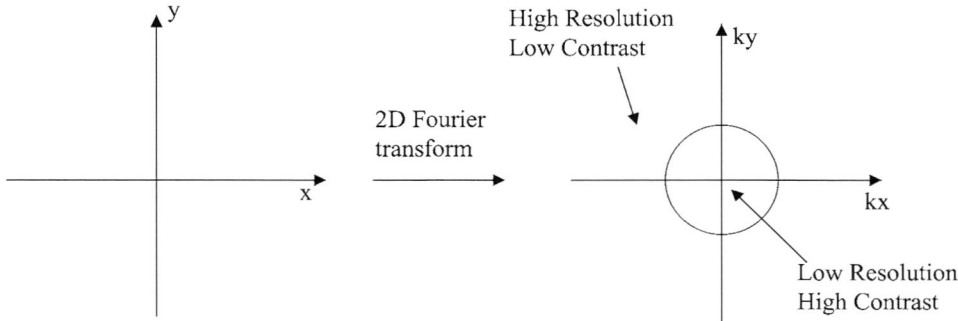

Fig. 10. In k-space k_x and k_y define the spatial frequency; the center of k-space contributes to contrast, whereas the periphery contributes to the resolution of the final image.

or negative) value defines the size of k-space. The length or duration of the line in k-space is proportional to the product of duration and strength of the readout or x-gradient.

The way that the data points are filled in k-space and the order in which they are filled can also be manipulated by the way the pulse sequence is designed and thus allows one to control the resolution and contrast of the image acquired. There is also a direct one-to-one relationship between data points in k-space and gradient strength. A larger negative or positive gradient fills the lower left and upper right edges of k-space, respectively, contributing to higher resolution of the image. A large k-space also gives the image a higher resolution, but if only the central part of k-space is filled the resolution will decrease. After the filling of k-space, 2D or sometimes 3D Fourier transformation can be performed to give the final MR image (15).

From the above discussion, one notes that the time to fill k-space will equal $N \times TR \times NEX$ where N is the number of phase-encoding steps, TR the repetition time, and NEX the number of times the slice is sampled. The essence of MRI and pulse sequence design is the balancing and optimizing of the amount of imaging time and final image quality. A shorter acquisition time will minimize the potential for patient motion, increase throughput, and decreases strain on the gradient coils. All the different pulse sequences that are discussed in the following sections such as fluid-attenuated inversion recovery (FLAIR), fat suppression, diffusion, perfusion, fast scan, MR angiogram (MRA), and MR venogram (MRV) are designed to optimize certain data acquisitions but often also come with the penalty of time.

IMAGING SEQUENCES

Besides the basic conventional spin-echo T1 (TR: 400–600 ms; TE: 15–30 ms) and T2 (TR: 2500–8000 ms; TE: 90–120 ms) weighted imaging, a whole variety of specially designed pulse sequences are also available and tailored toward answering specific questions or gathering clinically relevant information. At our institution, every brain MRI includes T1, T2, FLAIR, and diffusion pulse

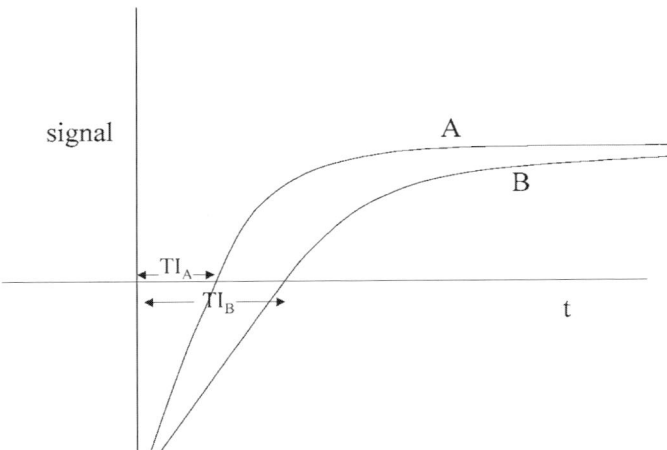

Fig. 11. Following a 180° inversion pulse, tissues A and B have different rates of T1 recovery and cross the zero signal (inflection point) at different times (TI).

sequences. Other additional sequences include postcontrast T1 (for infectious and inflammatory causes or tumor), gradient echo (GRE)/susceptibility (for hemorrhage and in the case of the cervical spine for its myelographic effect), fat suppression, MRA, or MRV (for stroke and sinus thrombosis) and in selected cases such as multiple sclerosis the use of magnetization transfer (MT) imaging. Fast scan techniques such as fast spin-echo (FSE) and echoplanar imaging (EPI) are also employed under appropriate situations that require very short TR and TE times such as in dynamic/perfusion and functional MRI. MR spectroscopy and functional MR are discussed in detail in Chapters 3 and 4, respectively.

Inversion Recovery (FLAIR)/Fat Suppression (STIR)

Inversion recovery is a technique making use of the difference in T1 recovery of tissue protons, especially water and fat, thus also representing one of the ways to suppress fat. Very simply, the sequence design consists of a nonselective 180° RF pulse followed by the regular slice-selective 90–180° spin-echo pulses. This initial 180° pulse cause the main vector to flip 180° from the original vertical position that then starts to recover/relax. As different tissue protons recover and cross the zero line at different times, the timing of when to record the echo or read out determines whether water or fat will give a signal. The time it takes for the relaxing proton to traverse the zero line or inflection point is designated as TI or inversion time (Fig. 11). In other words, the FLAIR sequence is in effect a water suppression technique as the echo is acquired at TI of CSF (~2000 ms). Only "normal" water will show loss of signal, as in CSF or nonproteinaceous cyst. Pathological increases in water content such as cytotoxic or vasogenic edema and demyelinating processes will appear as high signal areas on FLAIR. One can therefore recognize the advantage of such a sequence to facilitate the ease of identifying small lesions, especially those that are in proximity to CSF, as in the case of multiple sclerosis and white matter disease *(16,17)* (Figs. 12 and 13).

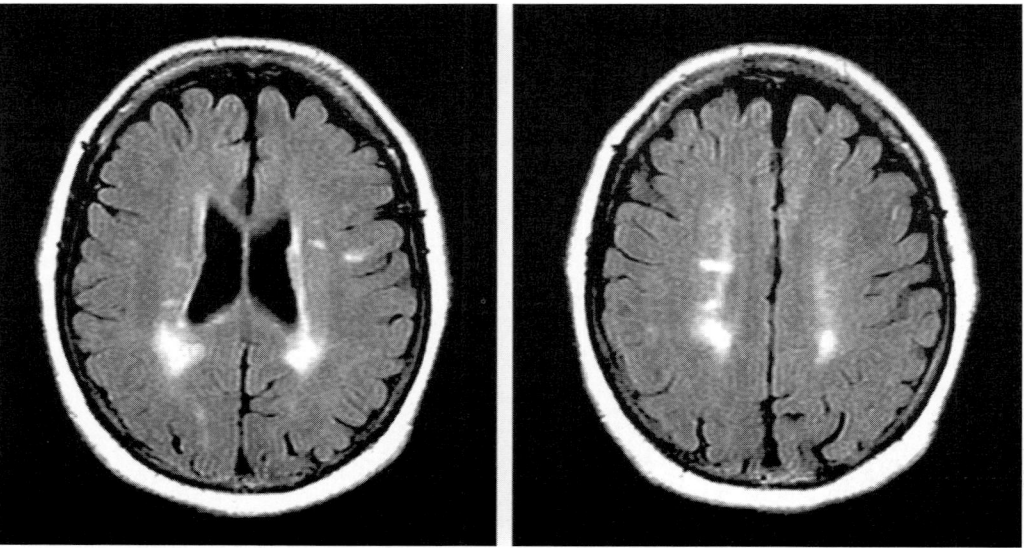

Fig. 12. FLAIR image of the brain shows distinctive plaques in the periventricular white matter in a patient with multiple sclerosis.

If the data is acquired after a period of approx 160 ms (TI of fat), a fat-suppressed image will ensue, a sequence also known as short tau inversion recovery (STIR). As in the case of most MR sequences, it is almost always a tradeoff in which the inversion technique costs time and is particularly sensitive to CSF and other motion artifacts. This, therefore, necessitates a more cautious interpretation of abnormal signal on FLAIR imaging; at the same time, different techniques have also been proposed to correct such artifacts *(18)*. Other methods of fat suppression are also available including opposite phased imaging and frequency-selective saturation. The former applies to a gradient-echo pulse sequence whereby the relative phases of water and fat protons change from successive echo times owing to their different resonant frequencies. When they are in phase, their signals are additive; when they are out of phase, the signal from the pixel reflects their difference, and the contribution from fat is essentially cancelled. This method is more useful for small fatty containing lesions. *(19)* (Fig. 14). In contrast, frequency-selective saturation is a method used for large areas of fat whereby a slice-selective RF pulse with a value the same as the resonance frequency of lipid is applied followed immediately by a spoiling gradient pulse to dephase all the selected lipid signal. Fat suppression is especially useful in orbit imaging and in the differentiation of fat-containing lesions (Figs. 15 and 16). Another important clinical use of fat suppression is in the setting of arterial dissection: T1 with a fat suppression technique facilitates the visualization of bright signal blood within the vessel wall that is surrounded by high-signal fatty tissue (Fig. 17).

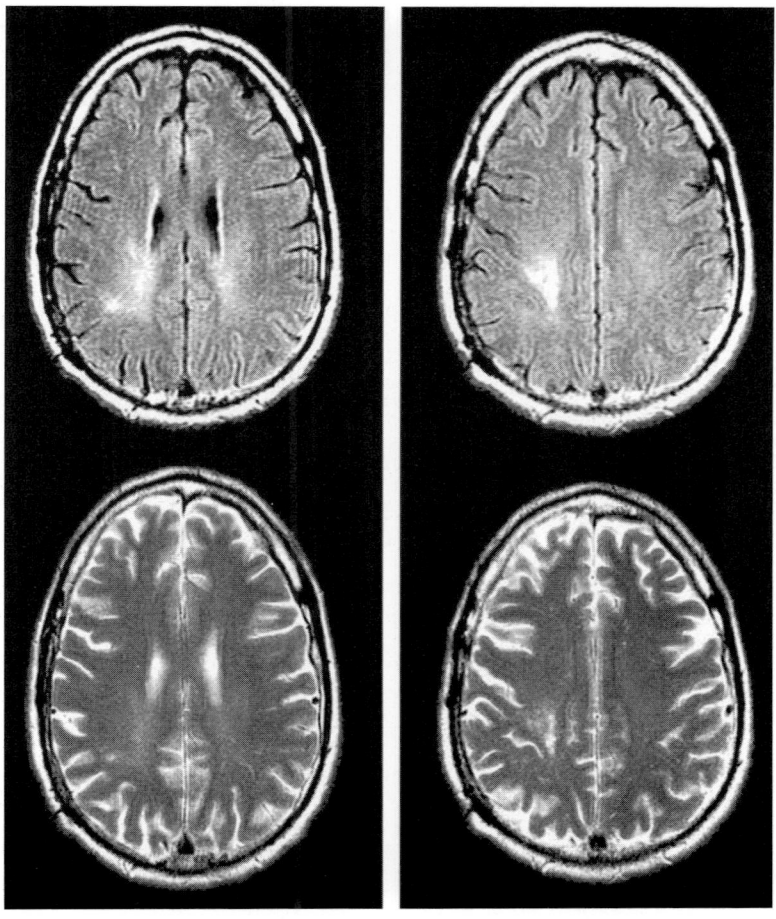

Fig. 13. T2 weighted (bottom) compared to FLAIR (top) images illustrate the better ease of localization of white matter disease against a grayer background of the latter.

Diffusion

The diffusion-sensitive sequence exploits the normal microscopic brownian motion (random thermal molecular movement) of free water in living tissues. The rate of diffusion of a molecule over a short distance is determined by the diffusion coefficient D measured in square centimeters per second. Owing to the difficulty in distinguishing non-energy-dependent vs energy-dependent transport mechanisms in living tissue, the term *apparent* diffusion coefficient (ADC) is used. Diffusion-weighted images are acquired using a pair of sequential equal strength but opposite polarity gradient pulses employed before and after the 180° degree of a standard spin-echo pulse sequence (first described by Stejskal and Tanner in 1968). After the first gradient pulse, motion causes spins to acquire a phase shift that the second gradient pulse (a spacing of 40–60 ms) cannot fully correct or rephase to the original position, thus causing significant signal loss. In other words, for a stationary molecule, the second gradient pulse

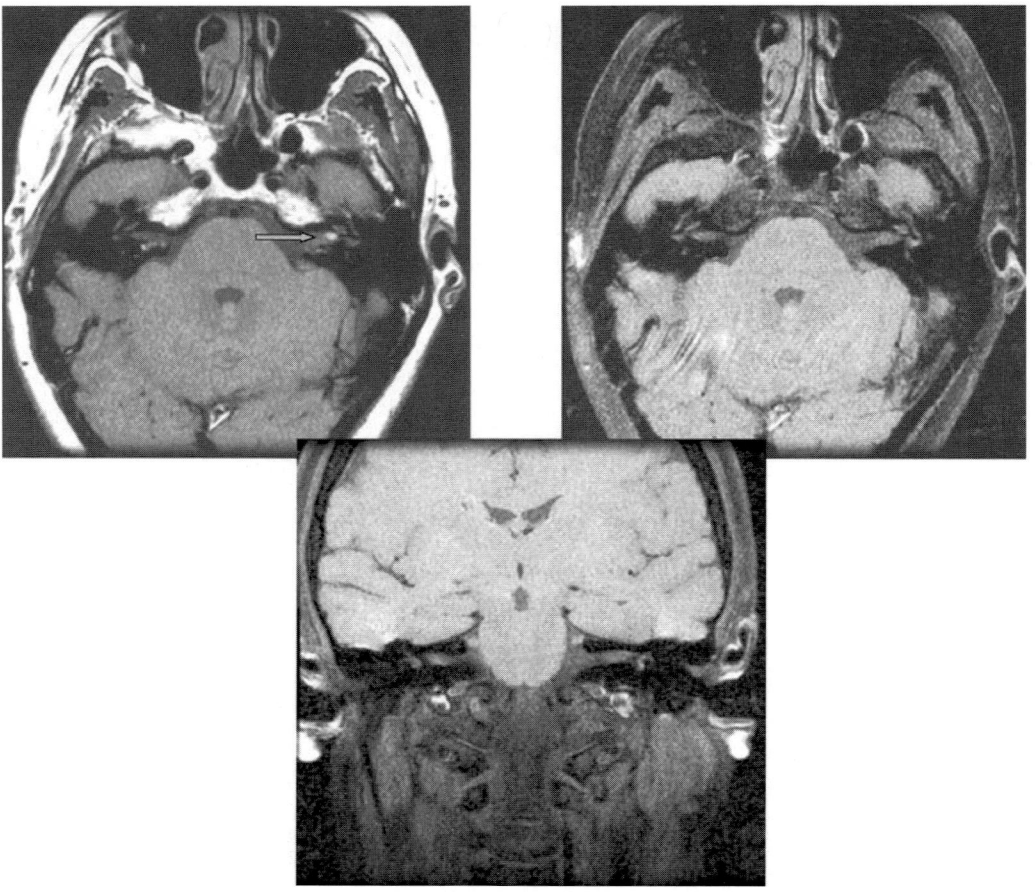

Fig. 14. Fat suppression (top right and bottom) of a small, high-signal left IAC lesion on noncontrast T1 images consistent with a lipoma.

will completely put it back to the original state as if no extra pulse gradients were ever applied.

The timing and strength of these gradient pulses determine the b value factor (amount of diffusion weighting): the signal loss is proportional to the exponent of $-bD$ according to the Stejskal and Tanner equation *(20)*. The ADC at each voxel can then be calculated by measuring signal intensity using two different b values (often with $b = 0$, i.e., without diffusion weighting, and $b = 1000$). Clinically, three sets of images are available, an ADC map (restricted diffusion or low ADC as in acute stroke shows signal loss), a $b = 0$ map serving as a baseline signal because the diffusion pulse sequence is slightly T2 weighted, and diffusion-weighted images (DWIs; $b = 1000$) in which truly restricted areas appear bright against a gray background). The most mobile water molecules such as in CSF and cysts will have the most signal loss and will appear bright on ADC (high diffusion coefficient) and $b = 0$ maps but as low signal on the $b = 1000$ images. Both ADC and $b = 0$ maps are useful to rule out the T2 "shine-through"

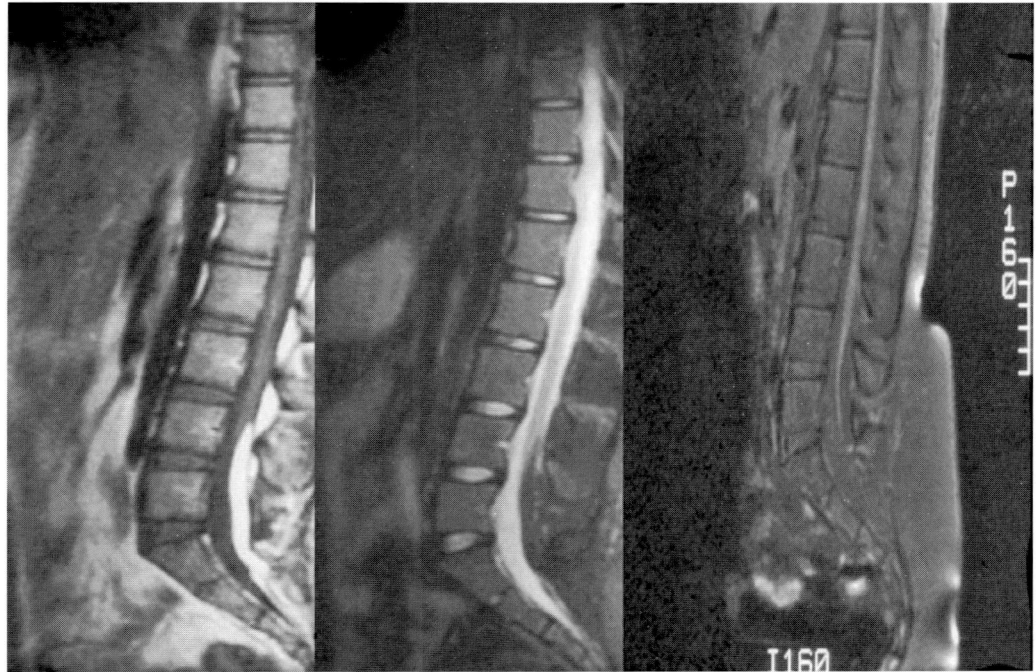

Fig. 15. T1, T2, and fat suppression images (left to right) of a lumbar sacral intradural lipoma (L4–S1).

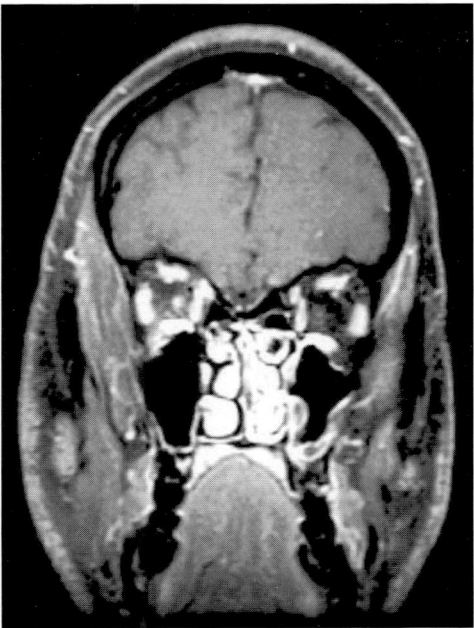

Fig. 16. Coronal T1 postcontrast fat saturation image of the orbit shows enhancement of the right optic nerve secondary to optic neuritis.

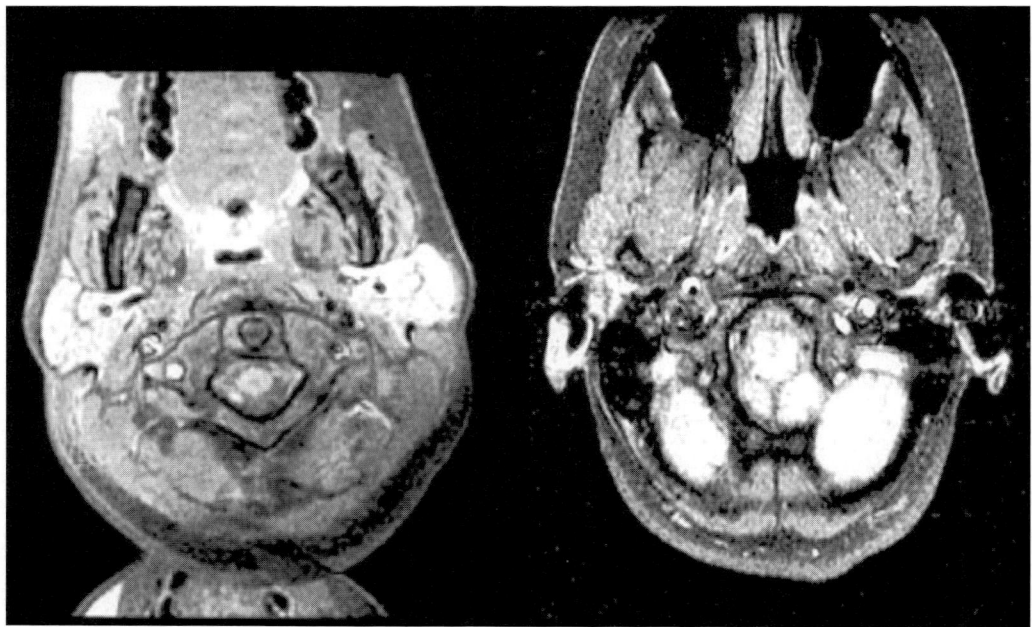

Fig. 17. Increased signal within the right vertebral artery (left) and the wall (bright cresentic area) of the right internal carotid artery (right) on T1 fat saturation images consistent with dissection.

phenomenon, whereby an area with increased T2 signal may appear bright on diffusion images. If the area is truly restricted, the ADC map will show a corresponding dark signal and the $b = 0$ map should show a less bright area than the $b = 1000$ image. As a reference the ADCs of CSF, gray matter, and white matter are 2.7, 0.8, and 0.6×10^{-5} cm^2/sec respectively *(21)* (Fig. 18).

In acute infarct, restricted diffusion can be seen as early as 30 min after onset of symptoms and remains bright on DWI for 10–11 d from the event. The cause of low ADC in acute ischemia is not well understood although the two most prevalent theories include the loss of critical perfusion causing failure of the sodium ATP pump with subsequent shifting of extracellular water to the intracellular compartment thereby reflecting a relative loss of free water in the tissue and therefore relative restriction. Alternatively, a loss of function of intracellular organelles may lead to the loss of normal orderly "streamlined" intracellular transport and thus cause a relative increased restriction. As infarction evolves, the ADC in the affected area becomes elevated over time and in fact goes above the normal level. This so-called pseudo-normalization presents as an area of subacute to chronic infarct that appears as a normal signal on DWI *(22)*. In other words, infarcted areas remain as high signal on $b = 1000$ images for about 10–12 d from the precipitating event. Old infarct appears as CSF or low signal on diffusion images (Fig. 19). Although diffusion imaging is most useful in diagnosing acute infarction, many other diseases can also show some degree of restricted diffusion. Any process that causes cytotoxic edema such as herpes

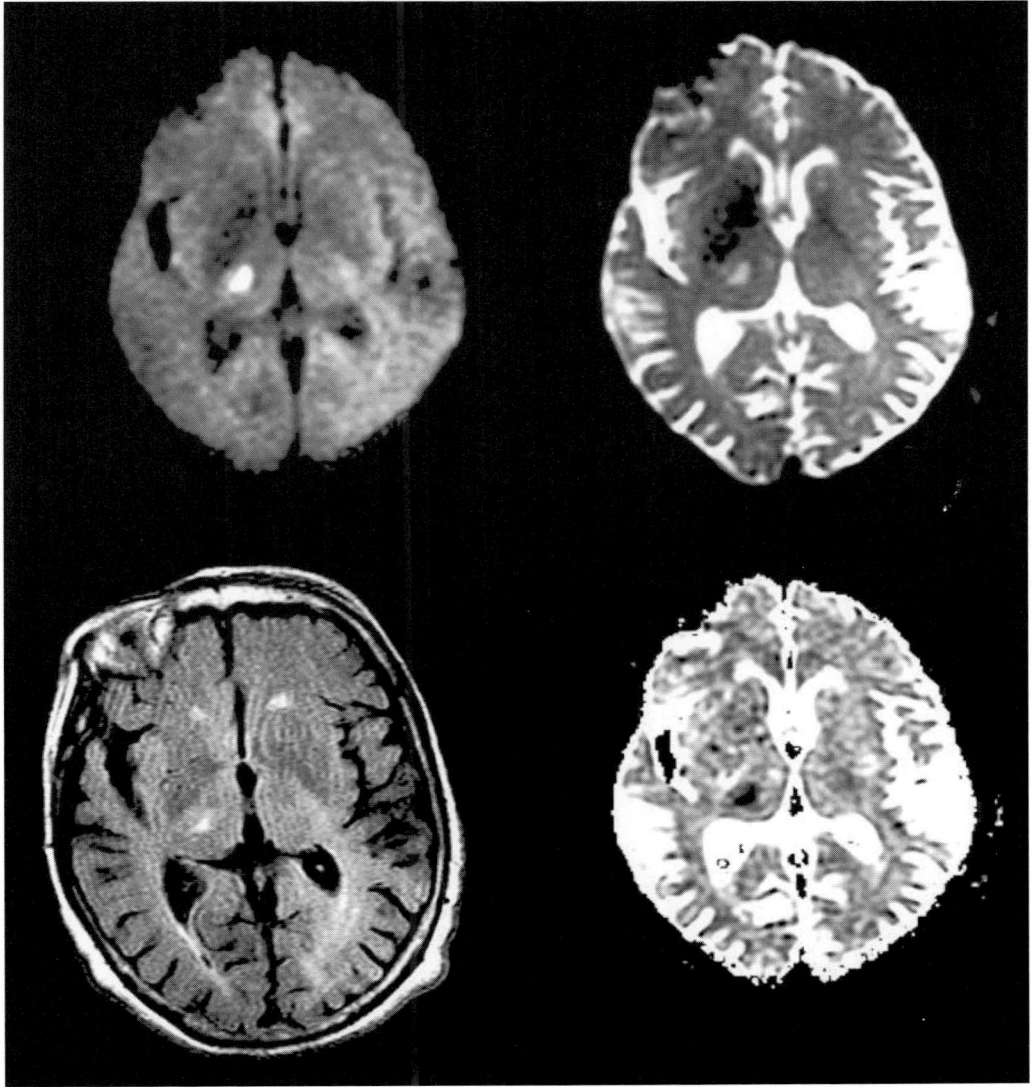

Fig. 18. Diffusion-weighted ($b = 1000$), $b = 0$, ADC, and FLAIR images (clockwise from upper left) of an acute right thalamic infarct.

encephalitis, Creutzfeld–Jakob disease *(23)*, diffuse axonal injury (Figs. 20–22), or increased viscosity and cellular matrix such as in abcess and epidermoid cyst will all demonstrate increased signal on DWI *(24,25)* (Figs. 23 and 24).

The diffusivity of water at a given point can also be described by a 3×3 matrix of numbers or "tensor" (D), as water mobility is independent in three dimensions (Fig. 25). Water diffusion in free liquid is the same in all directions and is therefore termed isotropic. In tissue, especially the brain, water mobility may be preferential in one direction such as along the axon in white matter tracts, which is known as anisotropic diffusion. The white matter tracts them-

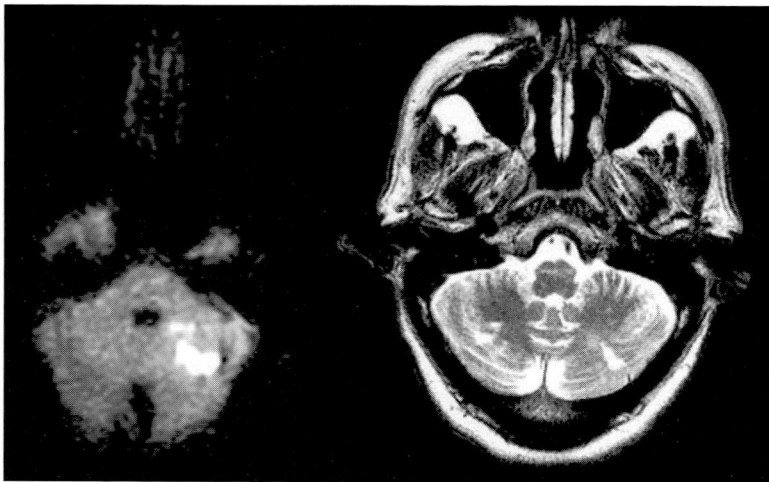

Fig. 19. Subacute to chronic right and acute left cerebellar infarct on diffusion-weighted (b = 1000; left image) and T2 images (right image).

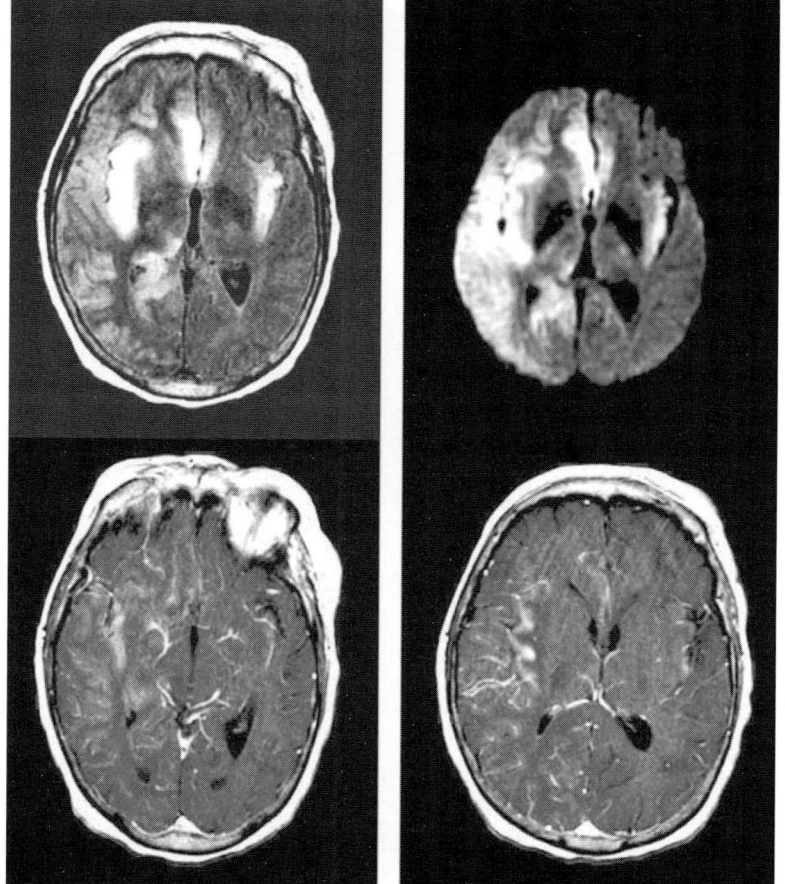

Fig. 20. FLAIR, diffusion-weighted (b = 1000), and postcontrast T1 images (clockwise from top left) of bilateral cingular and insular involvement of herpes encephalitis.

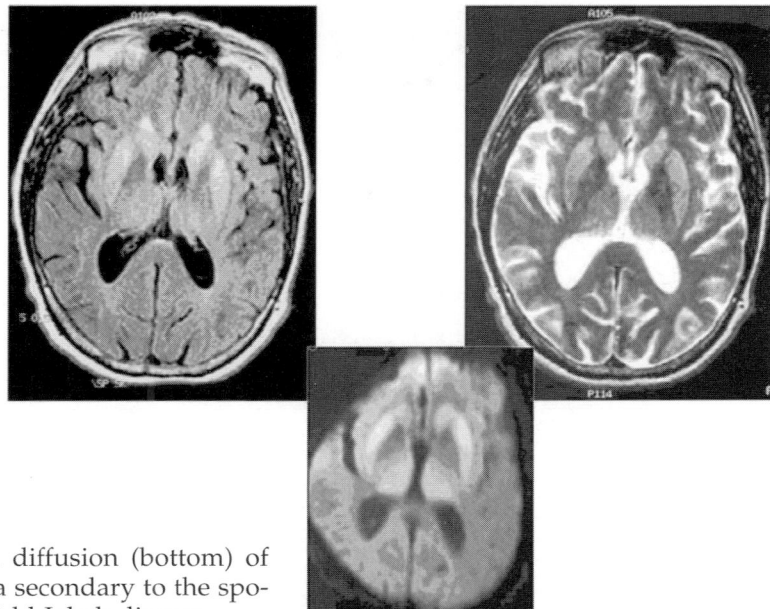

Fig. 21. Restricted diffusion (bottom) of bilateral basal ganglia secondary to the sporadic form of Creutzfeld-Jakob disease.

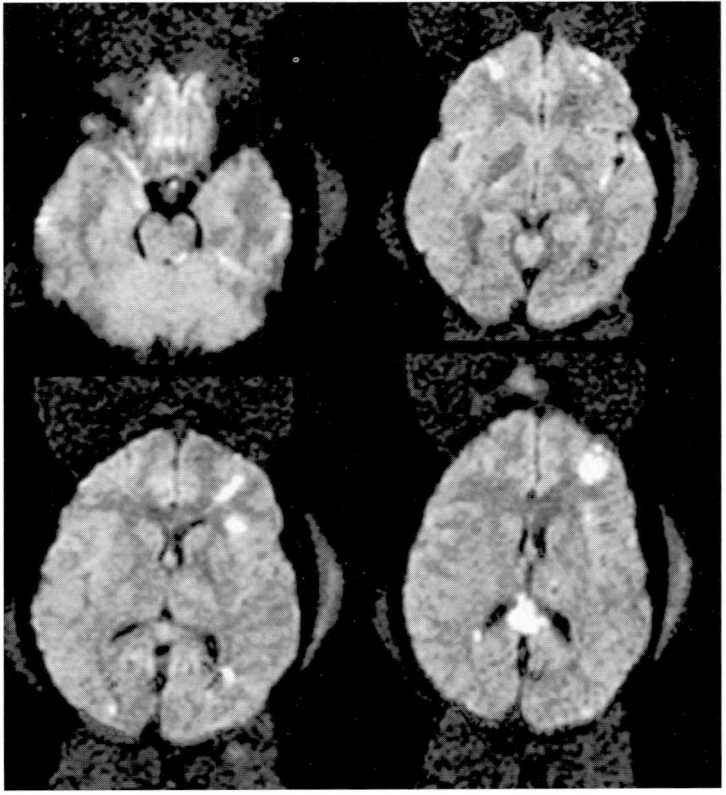

Fig. 22. Restricted diffusion in left midbrain, bifrontal, splenial, and parietal areas in diffuse axonal injury (clockwise from top left).

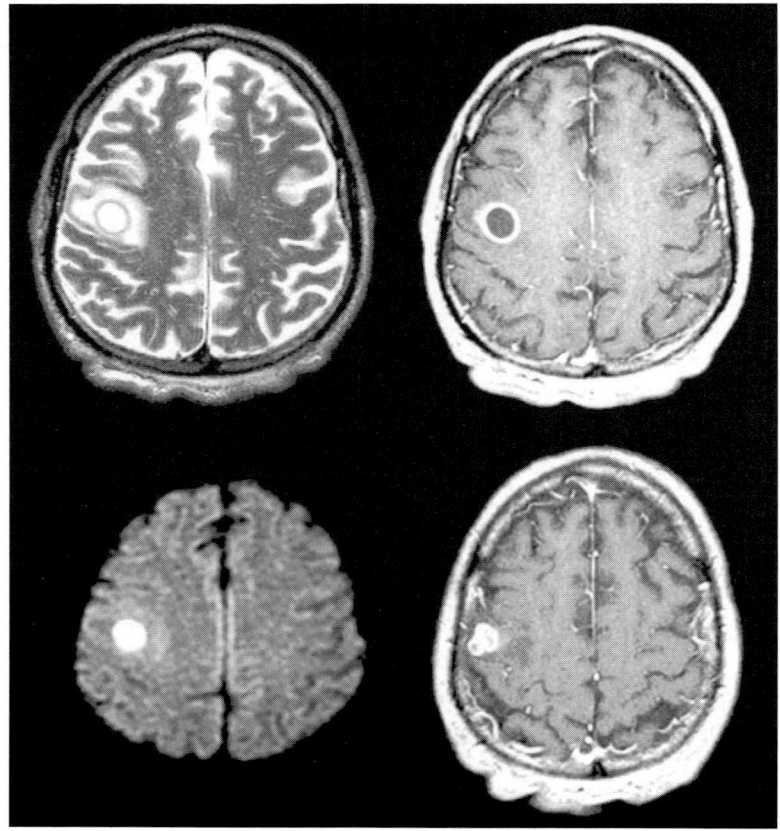

Fig. 23. Axial T2, postcontrast T1, and diffusion-weighted images (clockwise from top left) of a typical brain abcess of the right frontal lobe.

selves can also be oriented in various directions in space. Accordingly, a minimal of six different non-coplanar direction measurements is necessary to determine the tensor elements owing to the existence of six independent variables. In clinical practice, most scanners are equipped to perform the "trace" of diffusion tensor by acquiring DWIs in three directions and averaging these to give trace-weighted diffusion images. In other words, the diffusion tensor information can be applied in two ways; along the scalar aspect, the values can be combined to give indices reflecting the degree of anisotropy, whereas in the directional aspect, orientations of the principal diffusion axis allow the inference of the orderly microstructure of tissues such as myocardial fibers and white matter tracts in the brain. The latter has the potential of mapping white matter tracts in diseased CNS conditions or even more so in the setting for pre- and intraoperative evaluation of the proximity of essential white matter tracts to brain tumors *(26)* (Fig. 26).

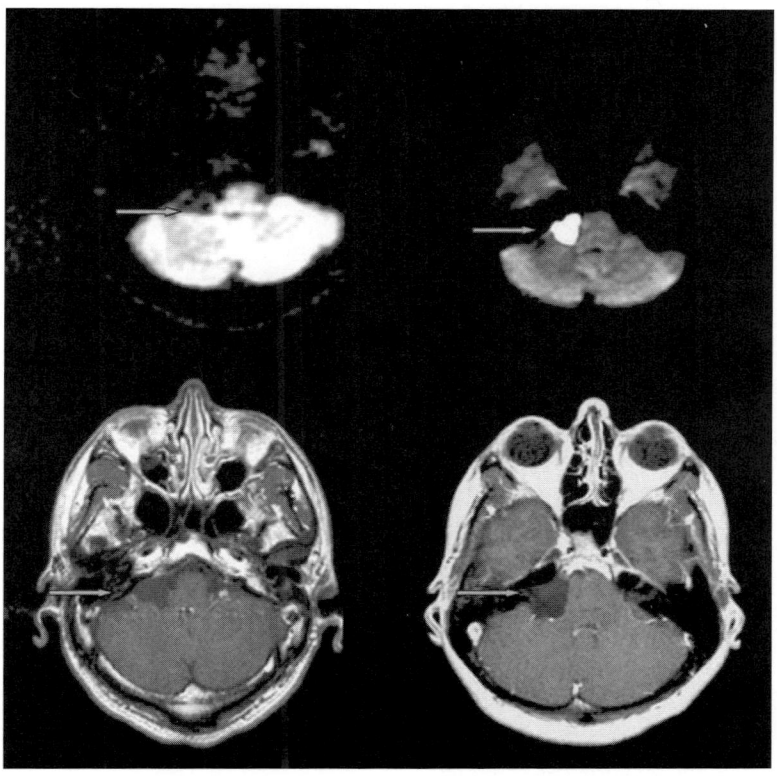

Fig. 24. Low signal on diffusion of right cerebellar pontine (CP) angle arachnoid cyst (left, top) compared with high signal right epidermoid (right, top) with their respective postcontrast images (bottom).

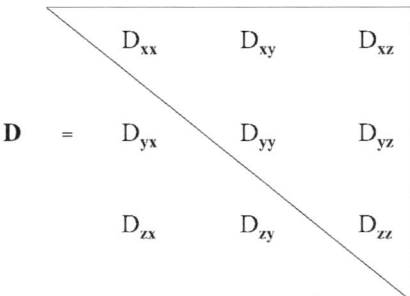

Fig. 25. The tensor matrix consists of nine components; practically, only six are used because D_{zx} D_{yx} and D_{zy} are the same as D_{xz} D_{xy} and D_{yz}. The "trace" of the tensor can be represented by D_{xx} D_{yy} and D_{zz}.

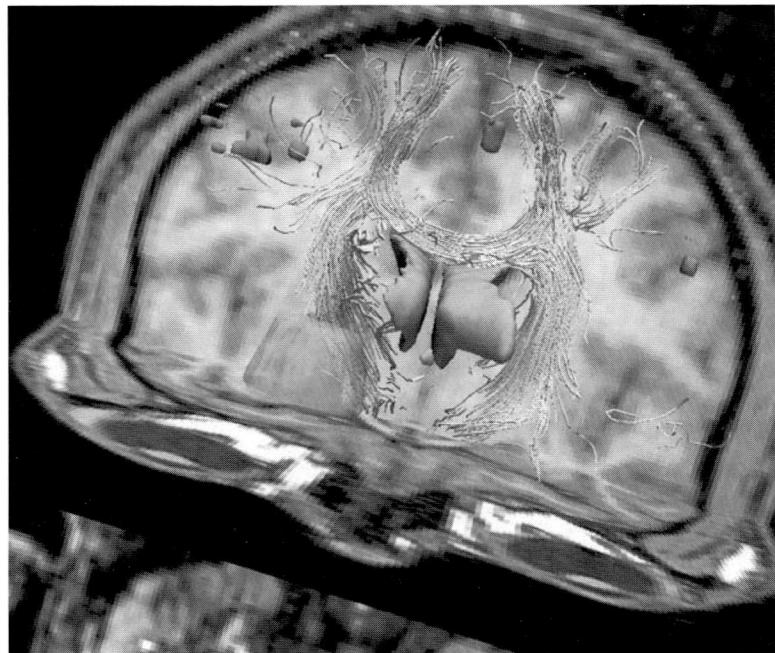

Fig. 26. Tensor diffusion representation of white matter fiber tracts along the corpus callosum and cortical spinal tract as they are deviated by a deep right frontal tumor.

Flow (MRA and MRV)

One of the main advantages of MR over other imaging modalities is the ability to evaluate flow (blood or CSF) in a noninvasive manner with or without the need for contrast agents. Moving spins exhibit two properties that are fundamental to the understanding of flow effects in MRI. *Time of flight* describes the position change of spins as they move in and out of the imaging volume (slice or pixel) during the pulse sequence, i.e., the effect of time elapsed between RF labeling and sampling of moving spin magnetization (Fig. 27). Time-of-flight effects can result in either signal increase or decrease depending on the pulse sequence's repetition time, the T1 of flowing fluid and stationary tissue, the velocity of the fluid, and slice thickness. The aim is to maximize the signal of the flowing spins and minimize the stationary background tissue signal.

When spins within the voxel are repeatedly excited and the TR (time between two 90° pulse) is shorter than the T1 of stationary tissue, there will be very little contribution of tissue signal, as there is not sufficient time for longitudinal relaxation and recovery of magnetization vector for the next RF pulse. In contrast, for the fully relaxed or unsaturated inflowing spins that have not been excited and are moving into the volume between 180° and the next 90° RF pulse, much signal will be generated. The proportion of unsaturated vs satu-

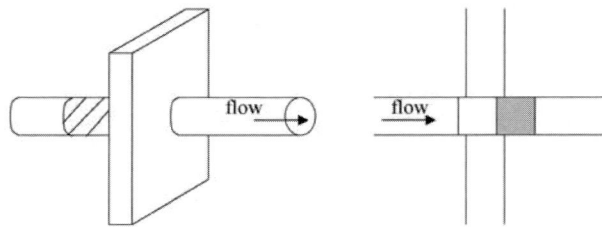

Fig. 27. In the time-of-flight (TOF) technique, the maximum signal results from an inflowing velocity that completely replaces the imaging slice with fresh or unsaturated spins.

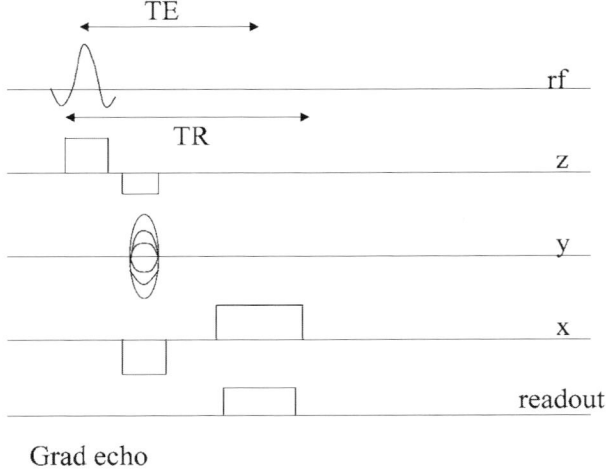

Fig. 28. A basic gradient-echo pulse sequence design.

rated spins will then ultimately determine the final average signal within the pixel volume. The relationship among the slice thickness, TR, and velocity is described by the formula V_{max} = slice thickness/TR where V_{max} represents the maximum inflowing velocity that completely replaces the slice with fresh spins at TR and therefore generates the most signal. A velocity too low or a slice too thick will result in a higher proportion of saturated spins and therefore decreased overall signal. For a velocity greater than V_{max}, there will be a loss of signals, as more unsaturated spins are exiting than entering the slice between the 90° and 180° RF pulse. This is particularly important in spin-echo sequences: both 90° and 180° RF pulse are slice selective, and a 90° "pulsed" spin that exits the slice before the 180° RF pulse will therefore not give a signal. In addition, a longer TE will also favor signal loss as the spins are more likely to have left the imaging volume (27,28).

In contrast to spin echo, gradient-echo sequences (Fig. 28) operate within the T2* envelope where the signal is generated by gradient reversal that is non-slice selective. Any spin that has been excited during the initial slice or slab excitation will give a signal even after it has traveled out of the imaging volume. In

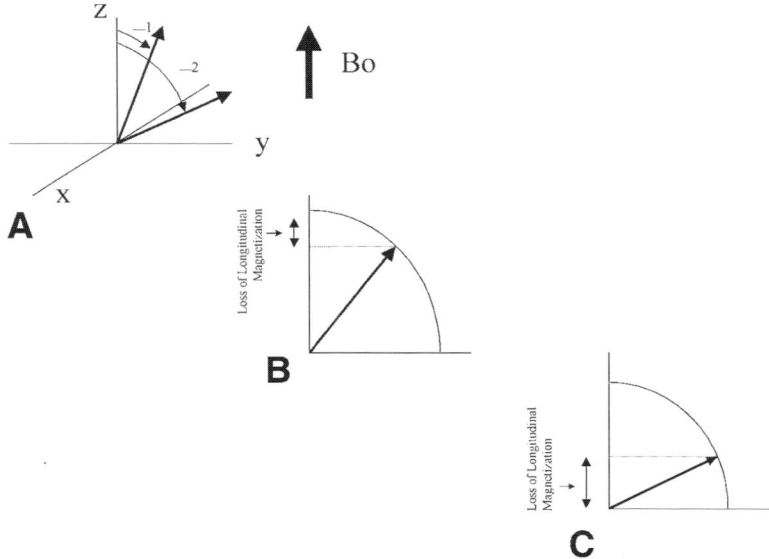

Fig. 29. (A–C) In gradient echo, the size of the flip angle affects the degree of longitudinal magnetization, loss being greater with larger angles. The resulting partially recovered magnetization vector then becomes the "starting" vector for the next pulse. This is particularly applicable in the steady-state gradient-echo sequence.

other words, gradient-echo imaging maximizes the high signal of incoming spins while minimizing the outflow signal loss. The flip angle (α) is important in gradient-echo imaging, in which a larger angle contributes to more effective saturation of stationary spins, especially those with longer T1 magnetization (Fig. 29). One should also note that when flow velocity is not constant or cyclic, there would be loss (and less often gain) in signal owing to turbulence in both CSF (Fig. 30) and vascular flow.

Besides TOF, the other property that is important in understanding flow in MRI is phase shift effects owing to the phase changes that the spin experiences as it moves through magnetic gradients. There can be signal loss caused by cancellation of signal from phase dispersion from different spin velocities, signal increase at even-numbered echoes, and artifacts such as ghosting caused by misregistration of phase shifts from velocity changes. Normally, in stationary tissue the net phase shift caused by the gradients (except the phase-encoding direction) is zero, as the gradients are symmetrical in strength and duration and spins are refocused by the 180° RF pulse in spin-echo sequences. When flowing spins have the same velocity, the phase shift is uniform within the voxel, and signals actually add together constructively. Variable velocities owing to acceleration or direction change produce a net signal loss caused by phase spread or dispersion. There can also be a temporal variation such as in the respiratory and cardiac cycle, in which more rapid flow in systole causes more intravoxel dephasing and therefore more signal loss. One can almost assume that in turbulent or complex flow there will be

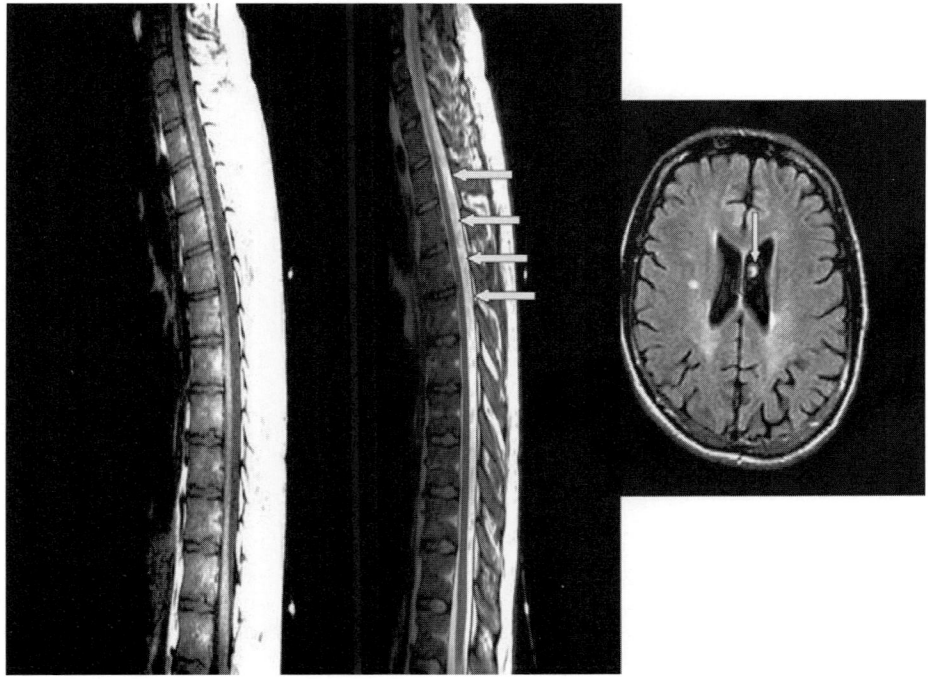

Fig. 30. CSF flow artifact along the posterior aspect of the T-spine on T2 images manifested as multiple amorphous areas of decreased signal within the CSF that is not substantiated on T1 images (left). Unilateral and often bilateral increased or decreased oval area of signal abnormality within the lateral ventricles caused by flow artifact from CSF traversing the foramen of Monro (right).

lack of signal from phase dispersion, often occurring at sites such as the carotid bulb, the siphon, or sites of vessel tortuosity (Fig. 31). Various methods have been employed to counteract such higher order motion including gradient moment nulling, creating different gradient waveforms and timing, and employing respiratory and cardiac gating; these techniques are beyond the scope of this chapter (27,29).

MRA and MRV are made possible by means of exploitation of the TOF and phase shift properties mentioned above. The TOF method is based on longitudinal magnetization and in and out flow effects; the other method is the *phase-encoding technique*. In TOF, we have already discussed that the TR is kept short to minimize the background signal although tissues with very short T1 such as fat or methemoglobin in subacute hemorrhage will cause "shine-through" (Fig. 32). This is often noted on TOF MRA source images, in which the orbital and subcutaneous fat appears bright and is "cut out" on postprocessing images to give the illusion that only the vessels of interest were imaged (Fig. 33). It is thus imperative to note that the TOF technique is really a measure of signal from spins with short T1 or unsaturated spins and is therefore an *indirect* measurement of flow. This is in contrast to the phase-encoding technique, which

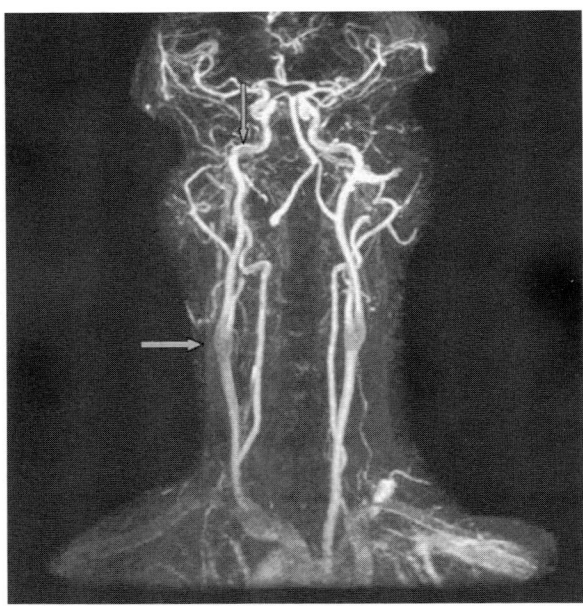

Fig. 31. Bilateral subtle loss of flow signal at the carotid bulb and petrous carotid on TOF MRA owing to flow turbulence.

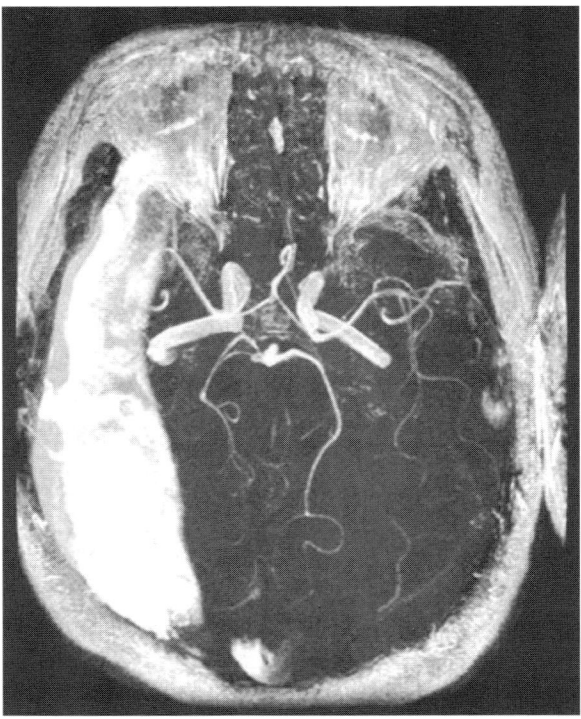

Fig. 32. 3D TOF image of the circle of Willis shows "shine-through" of subcutaneous and intraorbital fat as well as a large right subdural hematoma owing to the short T1 effects of fat and subacute blood.

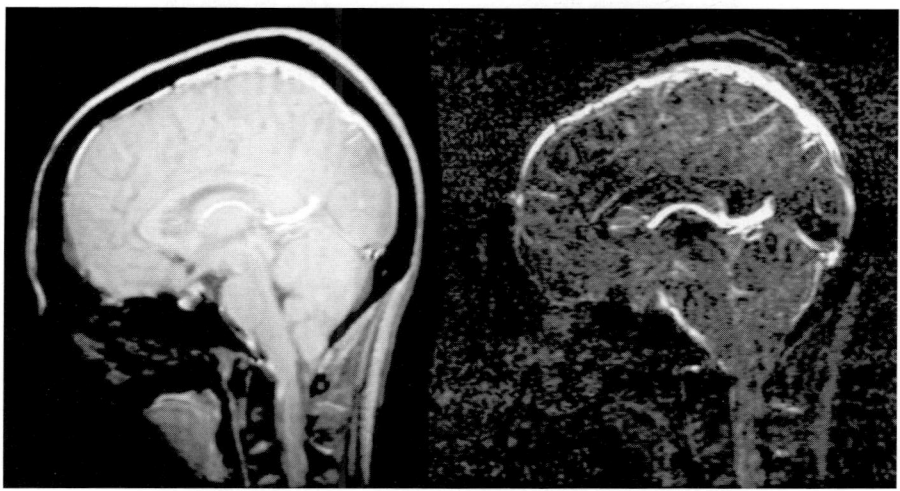

Fig. 33. Normal 3D TOF MRA of the circle of Willis before and after postprocessing.

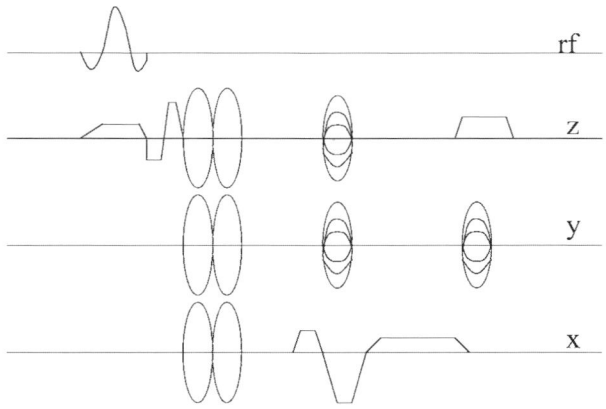

3D phase contrast MRA

Fig. 34. A simplified version of a 3D phase-contrast MRA pulse sequence. rf, radiofrequency.

shares the same basis as the previously mentioned technique of phase encoding along the *y*-axis. The only difference is that instead of position data acquired along the *y*-direction, velocity is encoded. This is achieved by applying two equal and opposite sign gradient pulses (bipolar pulses) whereby the phase shift in stationary tissue is effectively cancelled out and only moving spins will show a phase shift proportional to the distance traveled (Fig. 34). In other words, a single gradient pulse measures the spin position at the center of the pulse, and a bipolar gradient measures the distance traveled between the centers over time. The major drawback of this technique, which actually measures

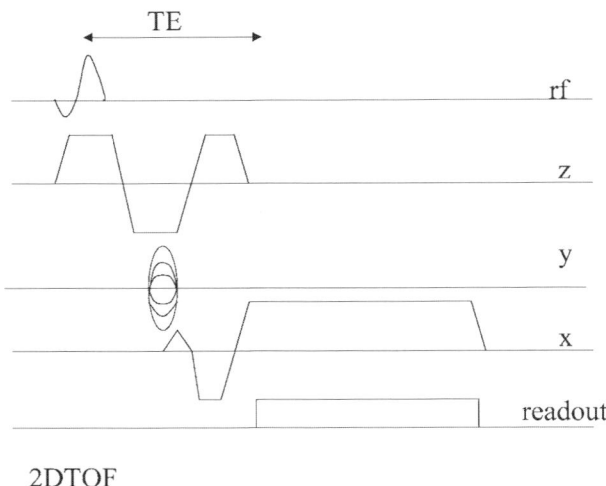

2DTOF

Fig. 35. Example of a CSF flow study using the phase contrast technique to determine whether there is increased flow through the aqueduct. rf, radiofrequency.

velocity and is therefore a direct measurement of flow, compared with TOF, is that three dataset acquisitions are necessary in three orthogonal directions, therefore tripling the imaging time *(30)*. The advantage of this technique is that it is a true measure of velocity and is invaluable in distinguishing slow flow from thrombus (in which short T1 thrombus and slow flow will appear as high signal on TOF) and that it is also the method used for CSF flow study primarily for determining shunt placement for patients suspected of normal pressure hydrocephalus *(31)* (Fig. 35).

Even with the various advantages of the phase-contrast technique, TOF remains the method of choice for most MR vascular flow studies (not CSF flow) primarily because of the time-saving factor. As one can expect, this method does not distinguish the direction of flow and therefore both arterial and venous flow will be depicted on the images. To obtain only arterial (MRA) or venous (MRV) flow, a saturation band is used that is essentially a thin slab of gradient that is turned on and placed proximal to the direction of the flow that one wants to suppress. The flowing spins are therefore saturated before entering the imaging volume and will not contribute to any signal formation. For MRV, the saturation band will be placed proximal to the common carotid arteries; for MRA, it is deployed at the cranial end of the head to suppress venous spins that flow in the caudal direction.

Both 2D and 3D TOF techniques can be employed for MRA; each has its strength and weaknesses. Two-dimensional TOF (Fig. 36) is essentially made up of sequential thin slices oriented perpendicular to the flow of the vessel. Because of the thickness of the slices, 2D TOF is sensitive to slow flow (applicable for evaluation of carotid stenosis) but requires maximum gradient strength and thus pays the price of longer TE and greater susceptibility to spin dephasing. In comparison, 3D TOF consists of a relatively thick slab that allows

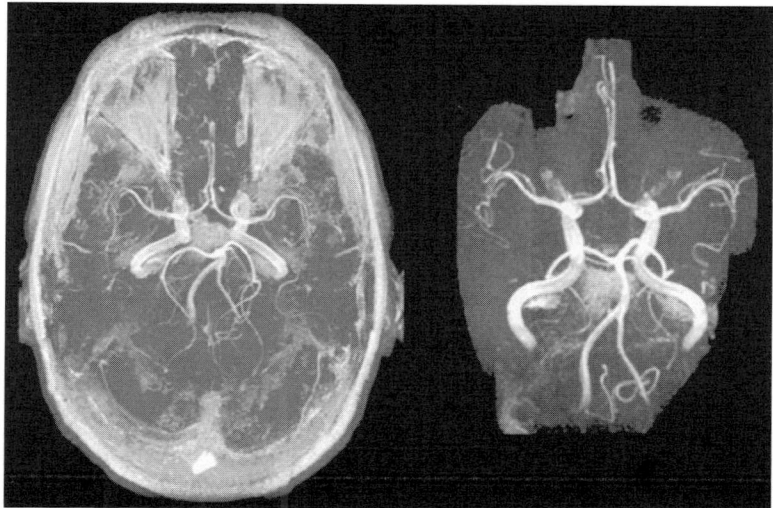

Fig. 36. A typical 2D TOF pulse sequence.

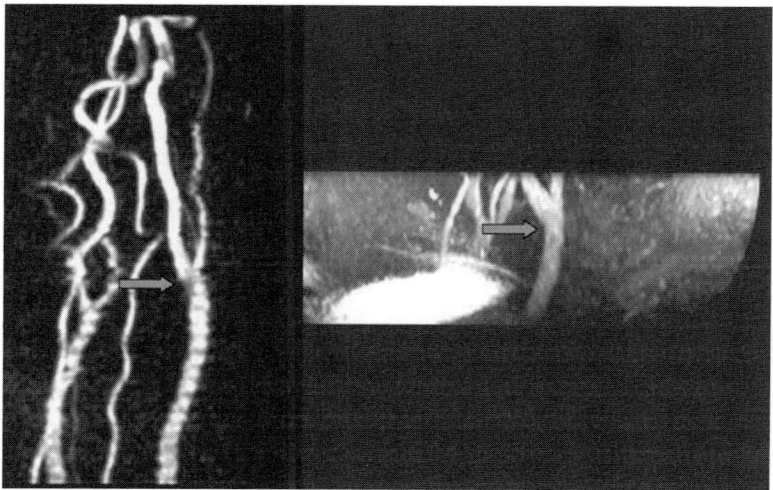

Fig. 37. 2D (left) and 3D (right) TOF MRA of the neck showing less intravoxel dephasing or signal loss at the carotid bulb in the latter, avoiding potential erroneous diagnosis of carotid artery stenosis.

for better SNR, a shorter TE, and less intravoxel dephasing (Fig. 37). On the other hand, the drawback is the risk of insensitivity to slow flow conditions: by the time the spin has traveled from one end of the slab to the other it has already become saturated. Clinically, 3D TOF of the circle of Willis is used mostly for the diagnosis and screening of aneurysms and vascular malformations; 2D TOF MRA or MRV is employed for evaluation of carotid bifurcation stenosis and suspected cases of venous sinus thrombosis, respectively (Figs. 38–40).

Both TOF methods are also inherently insensitive to the problem of in-plane flow, i.e., flow that is parallel to the imaging plane. To counteract this, the

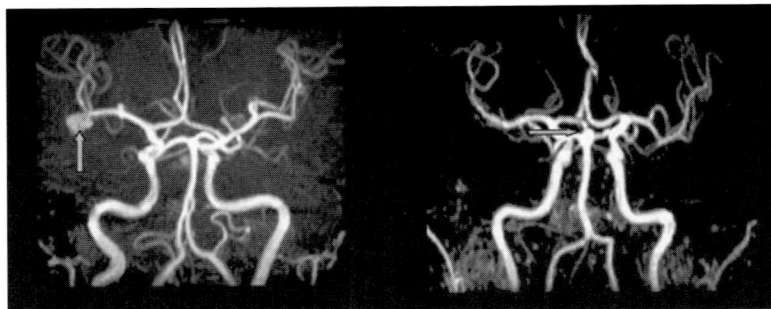

Fig. 38. 3D TOF MRA of the circle of Willis depicting right middle cerebral artery bifurcation and basilar tip aneurysms in two different patients (left and right).

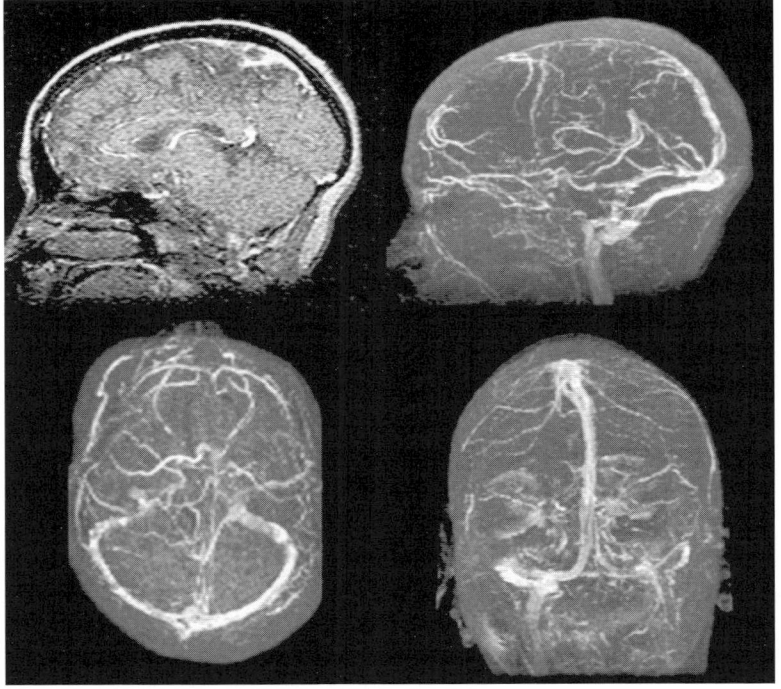

Fig. 39. Source and reconstructed 2D TOF images of a normal MR venogram in three orthogonal planes (clockwise from top left).

administration of gadolinium DTPA a contrast agent that shortens T1, is used to strengthen the signal from the longitudinal relaxation of blood as it remains within the circulation. This also permits the acquisition of data in the coronal or sagittal or other oblique planes, allowing for more coverage with fewer slices and less time (for example, from the aortic arch all the way to the intracranial vessels with the source images acquired in the coronal plane) and eliminating the issue of in-plane flow (Fig. 41). One of the occasional disadvantages of contrast MRA is that the indiscriminant T1 shortening results in a technique that

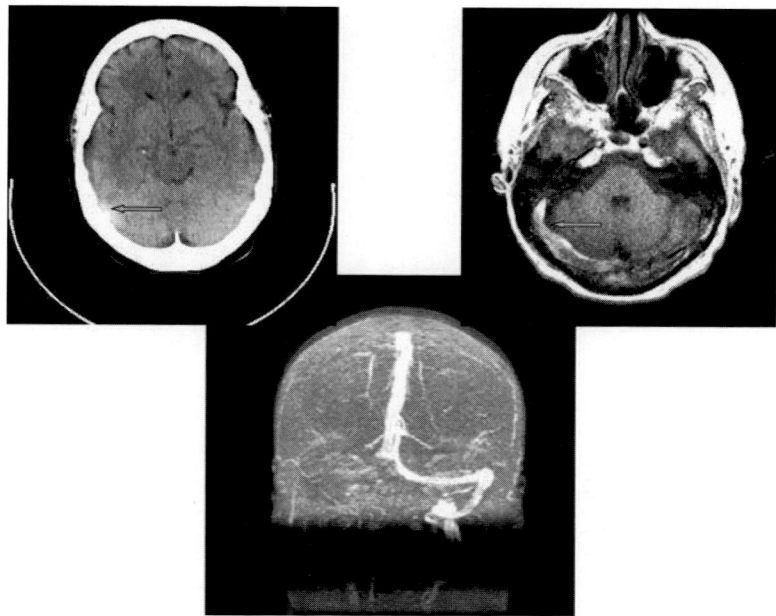

Fig. 40. Axial CT (high attenuation), T1 noncontrast MR (high signal), and 2D TOF MRV images of a right lateral sinus thrombosis (clockwise from top left).

emphasizes the opacification of the vessel and in essence (like computed tomography angiogram) may decrease the functional aspect of MRA. In other words, if there is high-grade stenosis at the carotid bifurcation, there is often decreased flow signal distally, especially for the intracranial vessels in the noncontrast setting. With the T1 shortening effect of gadolinium, these intracranial vessels may show signal, thereby underestimating the severity of disease. In addition, as contrast flows into the venous system, the timing of the bolus administration and data acquisition becomes crucial in the success or failure of the study (Fig. 42). Various methods such as contrast test bolus, varying gradient shapes, and *k*-space sampling have been developed to counteract these problems. Ultimately one needs to be cautious in the interpretation of these different methods of flow data acquisition, as in addition to the aforementioned factors, artifacts or signal loss from the pulsatile, tortuous, and calcified or diseased nature of the vessels can further confound the overall picture *(32,33)*.

Fast MR Imaging

The advantages of fast MRI in the clinical setting are evident to any clinician or radiologist who has dealt with a patient who cannot keep still within the scanner. Various techniques have been developed the most commonly encountered being GRE or fast GRE (Fig. 43), FSE, and EPI. In GRE, the lack of a 180° refocusing pulse is the main difference from a conventional spin echo sequence. Instead of an RF refocusing pulse, the signal is formed by gradient pulse with the MR signal decaying as a function of T2*. In other words, rather than T2

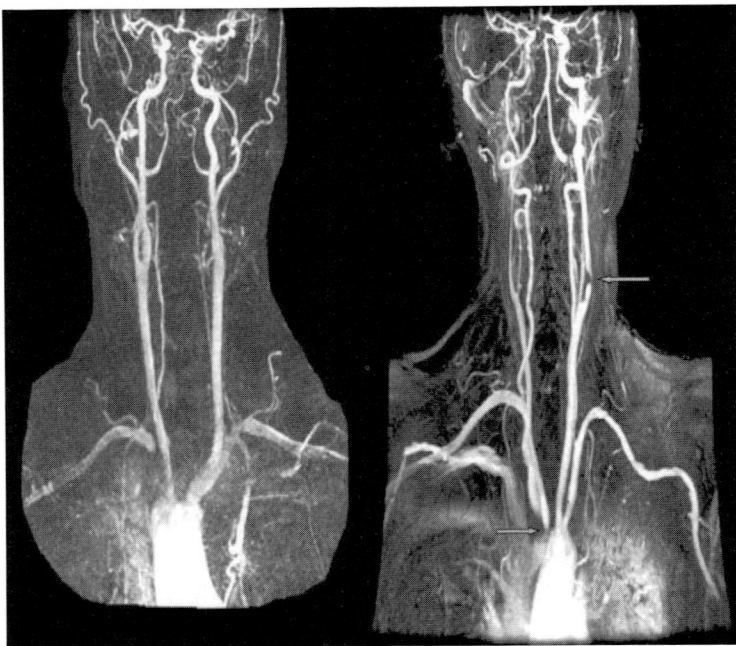

Fig. 41. Normal 3D TOF coronally acquired reconstructed contrast MRA of the arch and neck and most of circle of the Willis (left). High-grade stenosis of the left proximal internal carotid artery and proximal right common carotid artery at the takeoff from the arch, resulting in functionally decreased flow signal of the distal right internal carotid artery in a different patient (right).

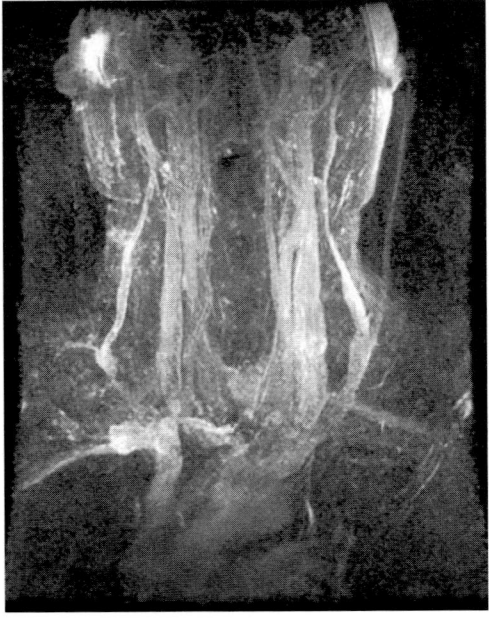

Fig. 42. Coronal postcontrast 3D TOF MRA of the neck demonstrating the consequence of missed timing of contrast bolus resulting in an uninterpretable image owing to overlapping of the arterial and venous phases.

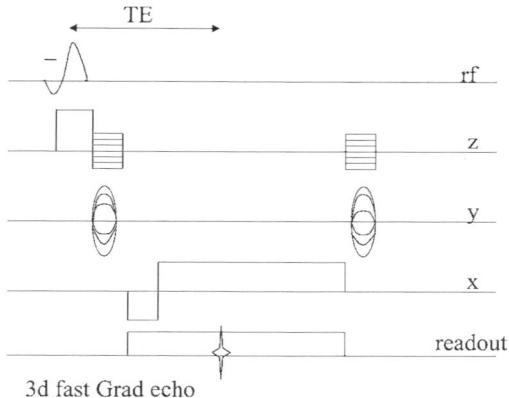

Fig. 43. Diagram of a 3D fast gradient echo sequence. rf, radiofrequency.

decay GRE works within a much smaller envelope (Fig. 6): for a T2-weighted GRE image the TE will be 35 ms instead of 80 ms. As illustrated in Fig. 28, a frequency-encoding gradient lobe (with half the area) first dephases the transverse magnetization followed by a second gradient lobe with opposite polarity, thus rewinding the spins phases. In GRE, the RF pulse used is often less than 90° in order to conserve the longitudinal magnetization for subsequent excitation, as the TR is short. This flip angle thus serves as another parameter to optimize the image contrast; having a small angle has essentially the same effect on tissue contrast as decreasing TR. For a T1-weighted GRE, a larger flip angle (60°) is used, whereas a smaller one is used for T2 weighted imaging (15°). The TE and flip angle therefore also determine tissue contrast, with the exception that when TR is extremely short (30 ms) a steady-state phenomenon comes into play owing to the presence of residual transverse magnetization that is recycled into the subsequent excitation.

To make the scanning even faster, one can further decreases TR (8–10 ms with 5–15° flip angles) or acquire more than one set of data per excitation. As one can predict, with the shorter time comes the penalty of poor SNR, image contrast, and saturation. The shorter time also means that more signal is acquired from pulses early in the echo train than later. This in turn allows for the influence of k-space sampling on image contrast whereby if the central k-space is sampled during the stronger signal from the earlier echo train, the resulting image will have better contrast but poorer resolution.

Both FSE and EPI accomplish imaging in a short period by acquiring more datasets per excitation. A basic EPI obtains all the data for an image in a single excitation about 35–50 ms and is essentially a gradient-echo sequence. An RF pulse is turned on at the same time as the slice-select gradient to generate magnetization in a single slice. The frequency gradient is then turned on, alternating in polarity as the echo train is generated (Fig. 44). For the filling of k-space for each of these echoes, the phase-encoding gradient is turned on very briefly (blipped) starting from the maximum negative value and again with alternat-

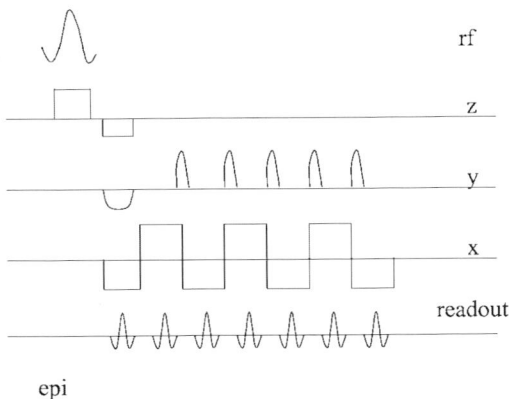

Fig. 44. Basic echo planar (EPI) pulse design. rf, radiofrequency.

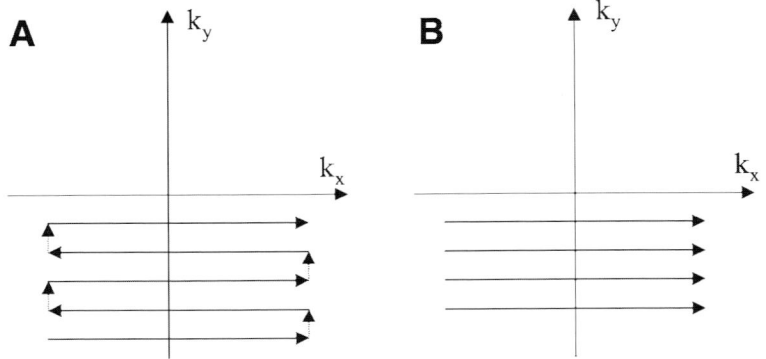

Fig. 45. (A,B) Diagram of filling of lines in k-space in EPI and FSE sequence consisting of four echo train lengths respectively.

ing polarity for each blip (Fig. 45A). In other words, the whole k-space is filled after a single shot of this echo train; 128 phase-encoding steps will require an echo train of 128 echoes. In order for the echo train to be shorter than T2* decay, the hardware demands stronger and faster gradients than the standard MR fare, resulting in expensive upgrades. Various different modifications of a basic EPI sequence have been developed including variations of k-space filling to save more time but minimizing image degradation.

FSE is in essence the spin-echo version of EPI. Again, it starts with a 90° pulse, but the pulse sequence in FSE is followed by a train of 180° pulses, unlike conventional spin echo (CSE) with its subsequent 90–180° pulses consisting of one phase encoding each. This in turn generates a train of spin echoes each with an independent phase encoding (Fig. 46). For example, in a CSE sequence with four echoes, each echo is phase-encoded in the same way and is stored in separate memory locations with four images generated after reconstruction. In FSE with a four-echo train length (ETL), each echo is phase-encoded differently with all the data placed into the same memory location, thus generating a single

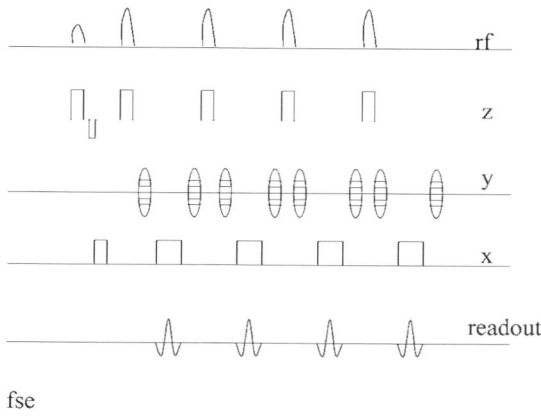

Fig. 46. Basic FSE sequence. rf, radiofrequency.

image (Fig. 45B). The scan time for FSE, however, will only be a fourth that of CSE. To perform independent phase-encoding for each echo, before each readout gradient, a phase encoding gradient imparts phase prep, if you will, to the transverse magnetization. Then immediately after readout, a second gradient of equal and opposite amplitude rewinds it back to zero for the next prep gradient. (Fig. 46). As there are contributions from various TEs, the final contrast of the image is determined by the TE of the echo that fills the center part of k-space (Fig. 10). The scanner tries to match the echo that is closest to the desired TE (selected by the operator) and maps it to the center of k-space. On the images, the difference between CSE and FSE includes less susceptibility to metal and blood products in an FSE sequence as well as fat remaining relatively bright on FSE T2 images *(34–36)*.

MR Perfusion

As mentioned above, functional MR is primarily discussed in Chapter 4, although MR perfusion will be touched on briefly here. Unlike MRA or MRV, which essentially deal with bulk flow, MR perfusion focuses more on the tissue level or microscopic blood flow. A contrast agent such as gadolinium DTPA is used in MR perfusion for its T2 (T2*) effects, which causes signal loss in the area of perfusion owing to dephasing of spins from the susceptibility effect of the contrast bolus as it rapidly traverses the capillary beds *(37)*. Relative rather than true cerebral blood volume (CBV) maps are constructed using the tracer kinetic principle, as the arterial input function is not usually measured. Integration of a signal time curve is performed for each voxel: the signal loss is dependent on the contrast concentration and density of vessels per volume of tissue. An actual quantification of CBV can be accomplished by applying arterial input function at a region of interest over a major blood vessel such as the middle cerebral artery. Semiquantitative cerebral blood flow can also be computed by applying deconvolution methods to simultaneous tissue and vessel concentration time curves, with the latter acquired by the indicator dilution theory.

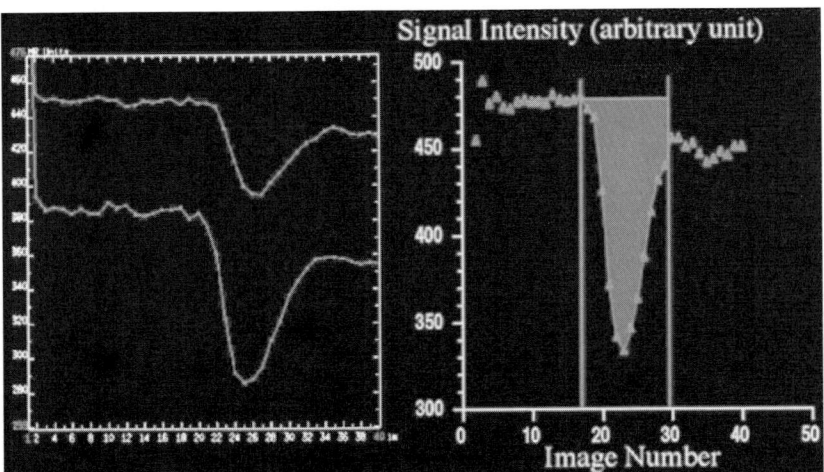

Fig. 47. Perfusion imaging demonstrating a plot of signal loss curve against time. On the left, the bottom curve shows normally perfused tissue and the top curve represents ischemic tissue with decreased and delayed signal loss owing to decreased delivery of contrast agent. The right diagram illustrates the area "under" the signal curve, which is integrated to calculate the relative cerebral blood volume (rCBV).

For MR perfusion fast MRI techniques are used including gradient echo, EPI, and FSE sequences. The latter has the advantage in tumor perfusion imaging as it is more sensitive to microvasculature, unlike GRE imaging, which often incorporates artifact from surrounding larger vessels. The change in T2 relaxation rate, or dR_2 is defined as $-\ln(S/S_0)/\text{TE}$, where S is the signal intensity and S_0 the baseline signal. This dR_2 vs time curve for every pixel is then mathematically integrated to generate the relative (r)CBV map (Fig. 47). The main clinical application of perfusion is in the setting of stroke, in which the dR_2 vs time curve can be used to calculate time to peak (TTP), mean transit time (MTT), relative cerebral blood volume (rCBV) and relative cerebral blood flow (rCBF). From these parameters one hopes to derive information or perhaps a threshold whereby viable ischemic tissue can be salvaged (the penumbra region where there is mismatch of diffusion and perfusion). In an area of infarct, one would expect a slower rise or shallower slope of the curve, slower TTP and MTT, and decreased rCBF *(38)*.

One of the major limitations of this MR perfusion technique occurs in areas that are leaky or necrotic or that have extensive breakdown of the blood–brain barrier. The more direct contact of contrast with tissue vs that within capillaries accentuates the T1 effects of gadolinium, thus counteracting T2 effects and resulting in erroneous lower rCBV. This is especially problematic in the tumor setting when one is attempting to derive information on the more vascular or aggressive portion of the tumor or to differentiate tumor growth from treatment changes. Even though numerous methods have been used to correct this problem (such as a corrective algorithm, a presaturation of leaky areas with a small amount of preinjected dose of contrast, use of stronger T2 effect contrast agents,

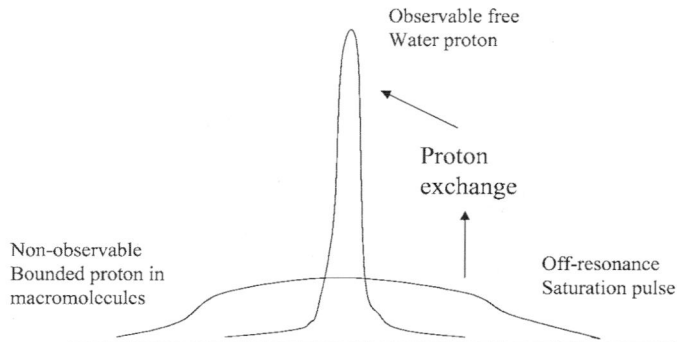

Fig. 48. Theory behind magnetization transfer showing exchange of off-resonant proton with free water proton as a means to suppress background.

and lessening the T1 effect by increasing TR and decreasing flip angle), the leakage problem has still not been successfully eliminated. Other remedies include noncontrast spin-labeled pulse sequences that tag the incoming spins using RF pulse that are subsequently imaged downstream. These spin-labeled inversion recovery EPI sequences carry their own set of drawbacks. Because of limitations from both hardware and software and because of cost–benefit issues, MR perfusion has not been as clinically successful as MR diffusion and is not a routine clinical tool at this time. Further investigation is necessary before MR perfusion can become an accurate means of determining high metabolic areas within tumor or the differentiation of active tumor from treatment changes (39).

Magnetization Transfer

The MT technique is often used to increase the contrast between the background and regions of interest. Very simply, a pulsed or continuous off-resonance low-power RF pulse is applied to saturate the bounded hydrogen protons in proteins and/or macromolecules. Because of the chemical exchange of these bounded protons with free water protons, some of this saturation will be transferred and exchanged by bulk water, thus causing a decrease in MR signal of the water/background (Figs. 48 and 49). The rate of this proton MT can be quantified pixel by pixel (40). In other words, the MT contrast is a reflection of the efficiency of such proton exchange that can be altered in pathological states such as multiple sclerosis in which all imaging sequences may appear normal to the eye but will have abnormal measured MT ratios (41).

ARTIFACTS

As with other imaging modalities and especially with MR, the many variables that contribute to the complexity of image acquisition also make the imaging susceptible to artifacts. These can be caused by field or frequency shifts, aliasing or sampling error, instrument irregularities, and motion from the patient. Chemical shift is the most recognized example of artifact owing to frequency shift. As was discussed in earlier sections, the proton resonates at a spe-

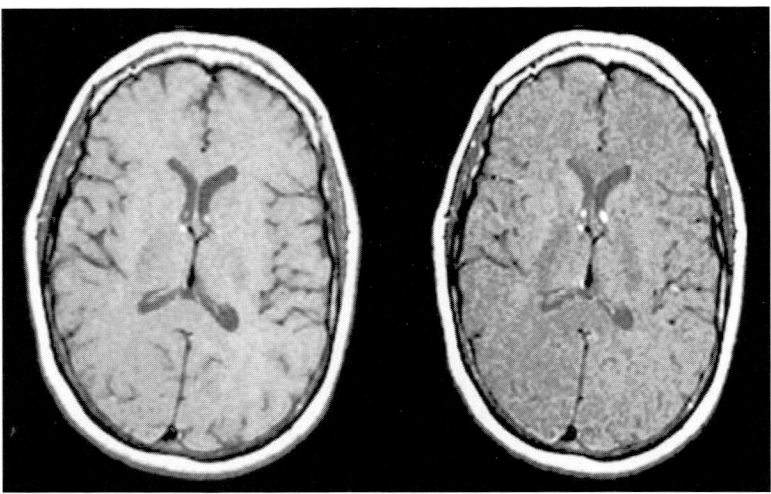

Fig. 49. Axial T1 noncontrast MR of the brain (left) with corresponding magnetization transfer image (right) at the same level showing suppression of the background with slightly better distinction of gray and white matter. Note also the CSF flow artifact of high signal at the foramen of Monro.

cific frequency that is dependent on the strength of the external field and its local environment. It is the interactions with the surrounding local molecules that causes chemical shift, most noticeably between that of water and fat. The hydrogen proton of the water molecule has a slightly different electron or magnetic shielding than those of the methylene group in fatty acids; therefore a small precessional frequency shift results. In a 1.5-T magnet this chemical shift of 3.5 ppm translates approximately into a separation of 224 Hz that is detected in the frequency-encoding or readout direction (42).

This chemical shift between water and fat manifests on imaging as spatial misregistration whereby as the imager is centered at water frequency, fat will be mapped at a slightly different site than its true spatial location, being most obvious at a water–fat interface such as the orbit and kidney. When the chemical shift misregistration is equal to or more than the size of a pixel, a dark or bright band will appear at the interface. The dark band on the lower frequency side of the interface is caused by shifting of fat proton to a lower frequency and away from the fat–water interface. On the higher frequency side of the interface, a bright band appears owing to the resulting overlapping water and lipid signals (Figs. 50 and 51). There are several ways to minimize this effect including changing the frequency-encoding direction, the field of view, or the bandwidth or employing fat suppression techniques. On the other hand, the chemical shift artifact itself can be exploited to clinical advantage to identify fat containing central nervous system lesions such as teratomas and dermoids (Fig. 52) and in differentiating fat from other high-signal T1 substances.

Aliasing or sampling error is best exemplified by truncation artifact/edge ringing and image foldover. The truncation phenomenon occurs when there is

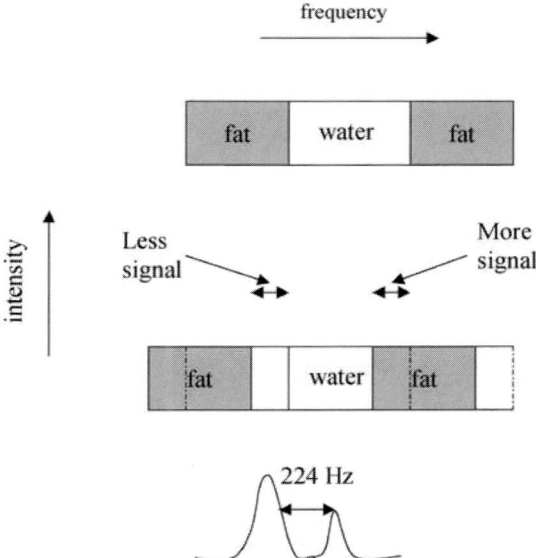

Fig. 50. Chemical shift artifact depicted by the difference of 224 Hz between water and fat in a 1.5-T magnet. The shifting of fat to a lower frequency causes a thin band of signal loss at the fat–water interface and a similar band of high signal at the higher frequency water–fat interface.

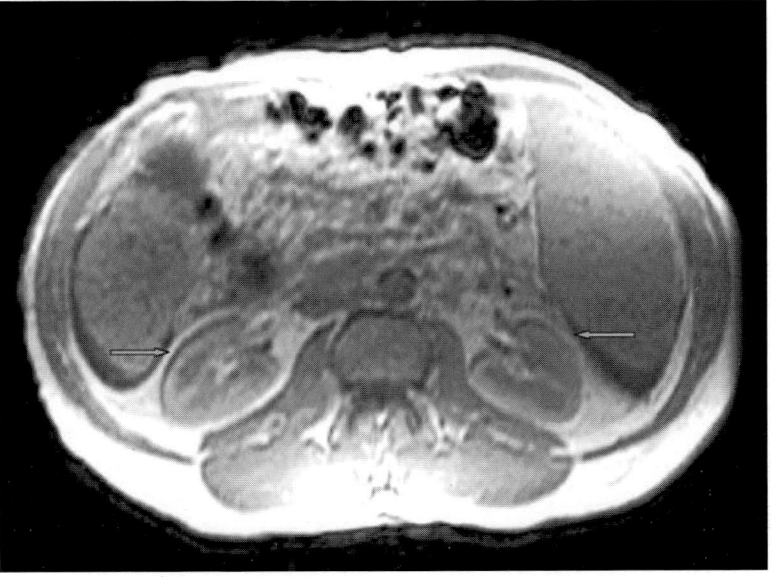

Fig. 51. Typical appearance of a thin band of signal loss at the rightward fat–kidney and corresponding brighter band at the leftward kidney–fat interface secondary to fat–water chemical shift artifact. Frequency encoding is in the left to right direction.

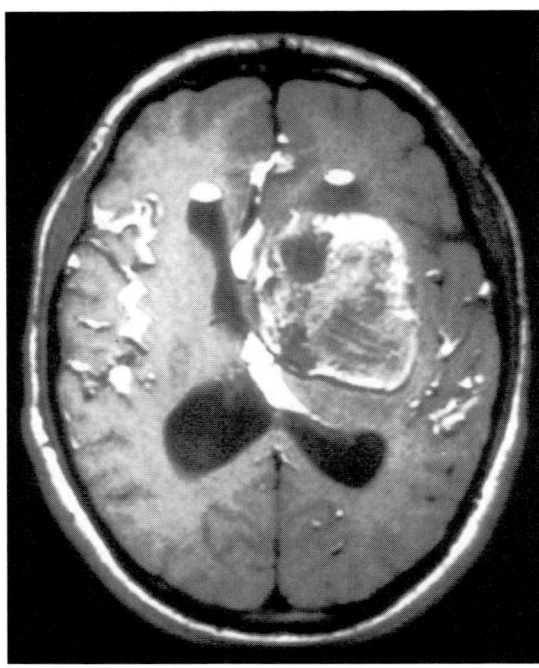

Fig. 52. Axial noncontrast T1 image of a dermoid ruptured into the CSF space, again showing a thin band of signal loss at the bottom of the lesion as the frequency direction is in the anterior–posterior direction as opposed to left to right as in Fig. 51.

a discontinuity in a function as it jumps abruptly from one value to another. This applies to a step function in a Fourier series: the function has a constant value until it reaches the point at which it jumps suddenly to another constant value. When the Fourier series consists of such a function represented by a finite number of terms, broad oscillations will occur about the point of abrupt change or truncation. The oscillations are squeezed closer as the number of terms increases. In other words, the step-like changes in signal intensities cannot be accurately portrayed by the limited bandwidth of the Fourier series. On imaging, this is most evident during spine imaging by alternating parallel light and dark lines or ripples conforming to the anatomical contour owing to the abrupt signal variations from sharp edges such as fluid/soft tissue/bony interface *(43)* (Fig. 53).

Image foldover or wraparound is caused by too small a field of view (FOV). To facilitate data reconstruction, the space outside the FOV is filled by identical copies of data from within. In other words, when the object is larger than the FOV, there will be spillover, appearing as wraparound (Fig. 54). To counteract this problem, one has to make sure either that the object to be imaged is completely included within the FOV or that the frequency- or phase-encoding data are oversampled, to create an image that is twice the size, with the portions of the image outside the selected FOV discarded. On gradient images, a "zebra"

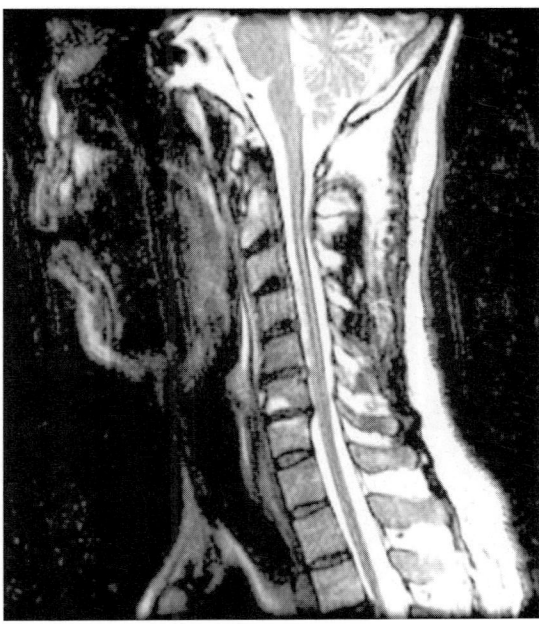

Fig. 53. Sagittal T2 image of the cervical spine illustrating the multiple parallel lines of a Gibbs artifact that mimic a linear intramedullary increased signal abnormality.

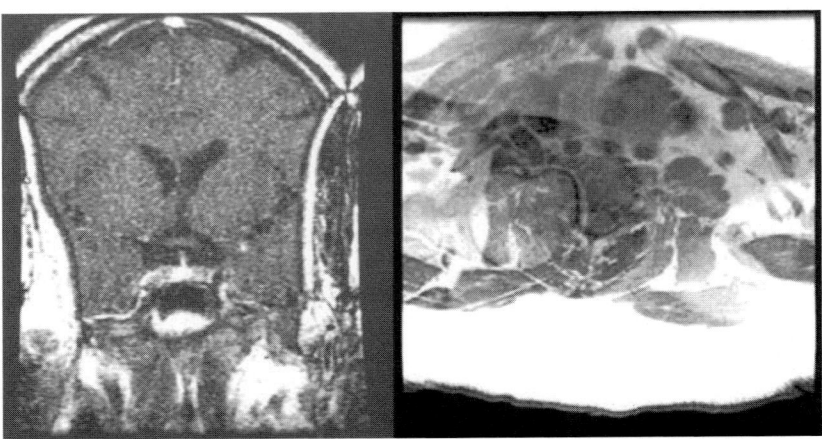

Fig. 54. Foldover or wraparound artifact that obscures the normal anatomy in the brain (left) and cervical spine (right).

pattern is created owing to interference between the aliased parts and the main image.

Artifacts caused by instrument or hardware malfunction include magnetic inhomogeneity with signal dropoff (from faulty shielding or foreign material on or within the patient), data clipping and spikes, broadband noise, and ghosting owing to temporal instability, just to mention a few. Inhomogeneity leads to

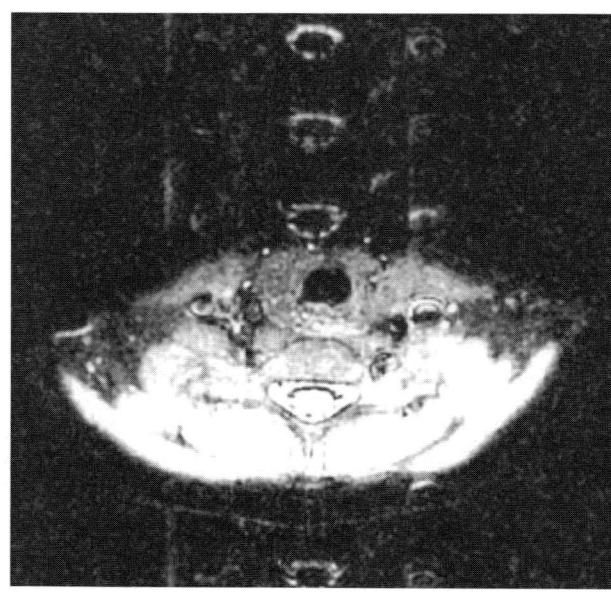

Fig. 55. Ghosting artifact in the neck represented by parallel "ghosts" of pulsating structures such as the internal carotid arteries and CSF-filled thecal sac in the spinal canal.

distortion of the image geometry that is particularly relevant in fat suppression imaging as this method depends on the frequency offset of fat and water within a homogeneous field. The inhomogeneous field broadens both the fat and water peaks, causing overlap and blurring.

Ghosting can be caused by any motion or suboptimal pulse sequence design of gradient profile owing to flow-related phase shifts. Periodic motion from the respiratory or cardiac cycle or arterial pulsatile flow can cause displacement and mismapping of spins along the phase encoding gradient. On imaging they appear as a series of "ghosts" conforming to the shape of the structure of motion along the phase-encoding axis (Fig. 55). On the other hand, this artifact can be exploited in the clinical setting to identify aneurysms: their periodic pulsations will give rise to ghosting, thus differentiating them from calcification or bony structures (Fig. 56). Various solutions to this issue have been proposed, including respiratory and cardiac gating, patient sedation, switching phase- and frequency-encoding direction, and fast scanning techniques. Flow artifact from CSF pulsation has previously been discussed.

Foreign material either inside or outside the patient can also contribute to signal and image distortion owing to the susceptibility phenomenon, whereby a material is partially magnetized when placed within a magnetic field. These include metallic objects, dental ware, cosmetics that contain ferromagnetic material, tattoos, bullets, or medical devices (Figs. 57–59). MR-compatible materials may torque or heat up during scanning, rendering them unsafe even if they do not cause significant distortion of the image. It is therefore imperative

MR Imaging of the CNS

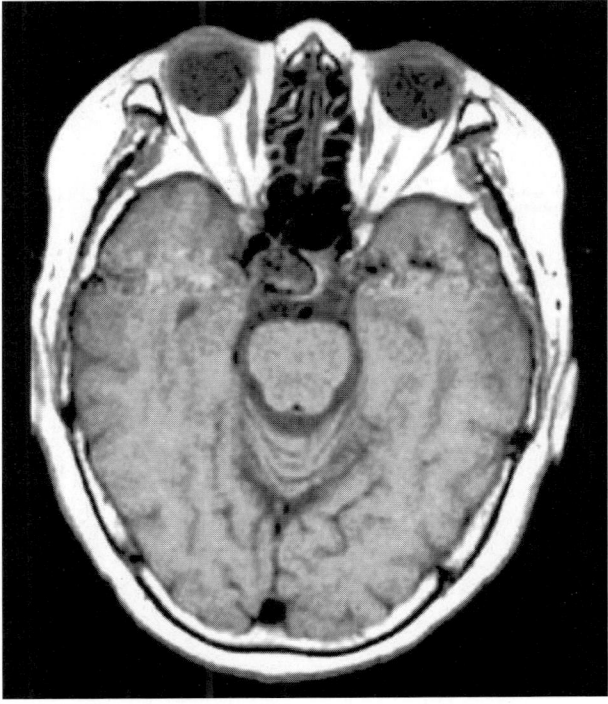

Fig. 56. Pulsation artifact aiding in the diagnosis of a right cavernous carotid aneurysm on noncontrast T1 MR image.

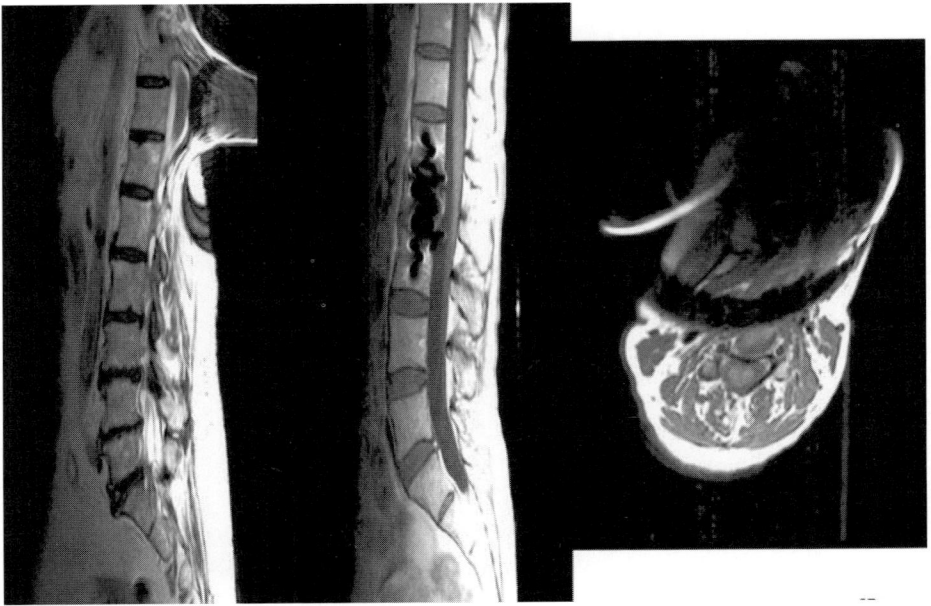

Fig. 57. Artifacts from metallic hooks (left), surgical spine instrumentation (middle), and a denture (right) that distort normal anatomy on MR images.

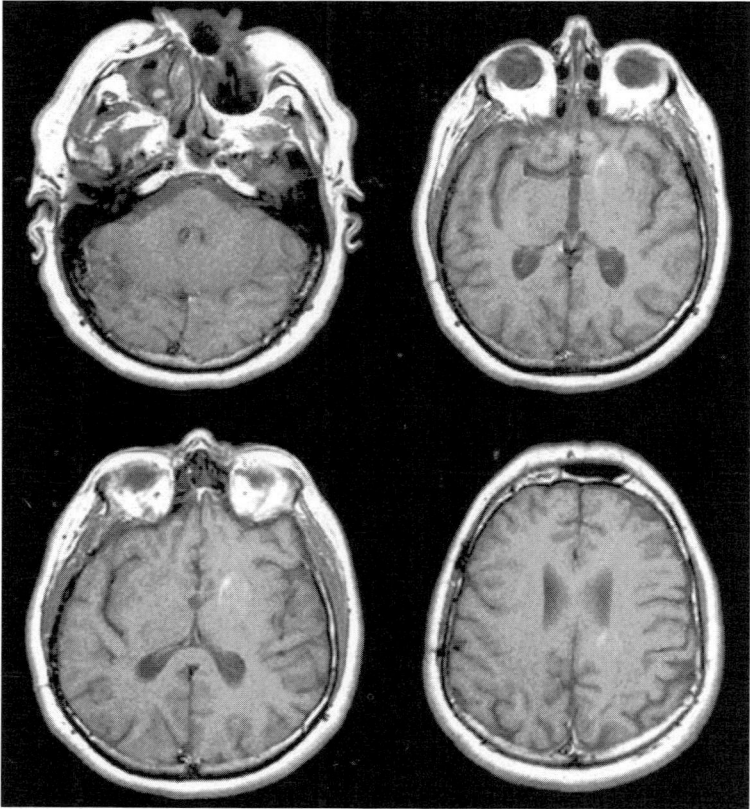

Fig. 58. Sequential depiction of an inverted U-shaped bright signal in dental artifact that goes anteriorly to posteriorly as the images progress from the skull base to the convexity (left to right, top to bottom).

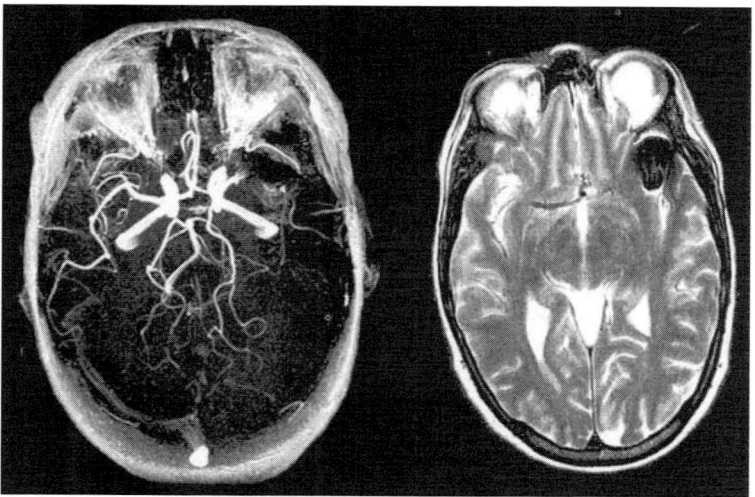

Fig. 59. An apparent loss of flow signal of the left middle cerebral artery owing to an aneurysm clip artifact rather than occlusion of the vessel seen here on MRA (left) and T2 MR images (right).

MR Imaging of the CNS

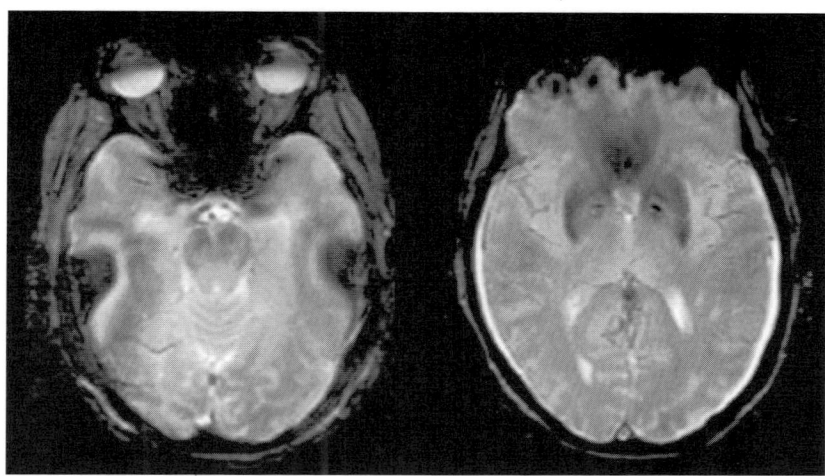

Fig. 60. Gradient-echo pulse sequence showing loss of signal from susceptibility at the air bone interface as well as bringing out the mineralization signal loss of the basal ganglia bilaterally.

that all patients be prescreened for potential foreign material within or on them before they are placed into the scanner. Gradient sequences are more sensitive to such artifacts than spin-echo sequences because of the lack of a 180° refocusing RF pulse. Again the susceptibility phenomenon can be exploited: a gradient sequence increases sensitivity to small foci of mineralization, cavernomas, and hemorrhage, because of their paramagnetic properties, which allows them to "bloom," appearing as an area of signal void with the extent of the area being exaggerated compared with the actual size of the abnormality *(44)* (Figs. 60–62).

HEMORRHAGE

The appearance of hematoma on MRI depends on the oxidized state of the hemoglobin and iron and whether it is within or outside the erythrocyte, which in turn translates into factors such as age, location, and source of the hematoma. The term magnetic susceptibility describes the magnetic response or induced magnetic field that a substance generates when placed in a constant magnetic field. A diamagnetic material generates a weak field that is opposite to the applied field, whereas a paramagnetic substance produces an augmented induced field in the same direction as the applied one. Oxyhemoglobin like most body tissue, is diamagnetic with iron in the ferrous state (Fe^{2+}); deoxy (Fe^{2+})/methemoglobin (ferric/Fe^{3+}) and hemosiderin (Fe^{3+}) are all paramagnetic *(45)*.

The varying signals of hemorrhage on T1 and T2 imaging are explained by the relaxivity (proximity of water proton and availability of unpaired electrons of iron) and susceptibility of the various stages and compartments of hemoglobin within an evolving hematoma. The relaxivity effects of the dipole–dipole interactions with a paramagnetic substance are better detected on short TR and TE, i.e., T1-weighted images, with more efficient relaxation generating a higher signal. In contrast, the selective T2 susceptibility signal loss

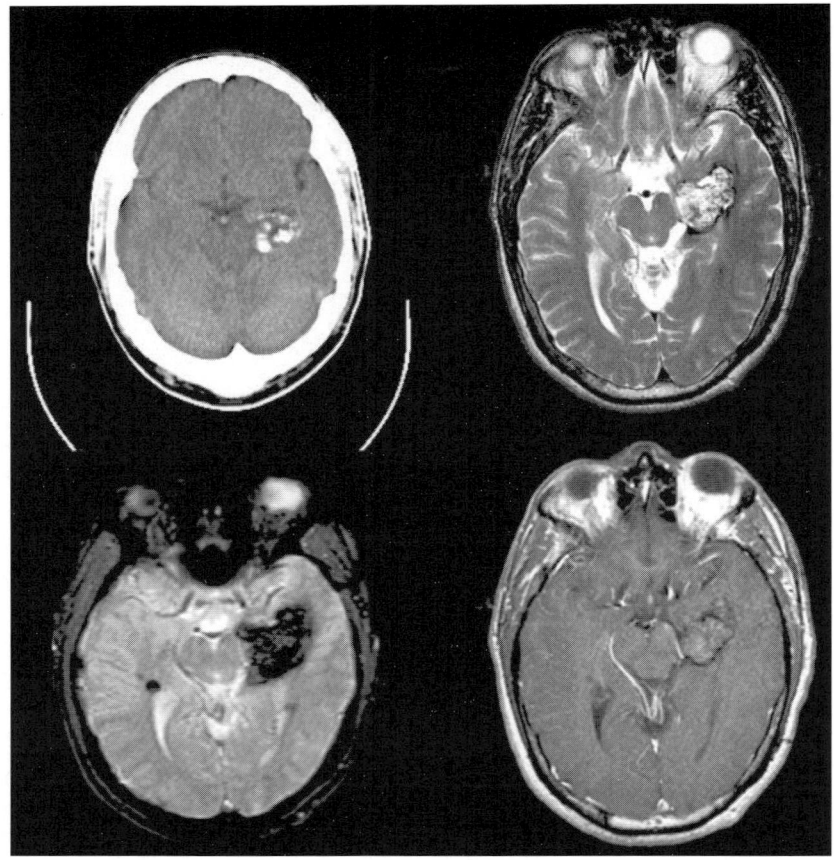

Fig. 61. Axial noncontrast computed tomography (top left), T2-weighted (top right), gradient-echo (bottom left), and postcontrast T1 (bottom right) MR images showing a calcified large left medial temporal lobe cavernoma. Note that other, smaller lesions including the right periatrial area are only apparent on gradient-echo or susceptibility sequence.

that was earlier termed irreversible nonstatic inhomogeneity does not affect T1 and cannot be corrected with the 180° RF pulse of the spin-echo sequence. In the context of hematoma, this T2 loss is owing to frequency variations produced by diffusing water molecules into and out of erythrocytes, resulting in phase incoherence and dispersing of spin signals. In terms of the selection of pulse sequence for imaging of hematoma, gradient echo is the most sensitive, with "blooming" caused by paramagnetic properties; one should be aware that the area of signal loss is in fact larger than the actual size of the hemorrhage. Fast EPI in either the spin-echo or the gradient mode is also sensitive to the susceptibility effects of hemorrhage, followed by CSE; FSE is the least sensitive among the various sequences.

In hyperacute hematoma (within the first few hours), the iron within the red blood cell (RBC) is in the ferrous state, with six paired electrons, thus rendering oxyhemoglobin diamagnetic without either relaxativity or susceptibility. On T1

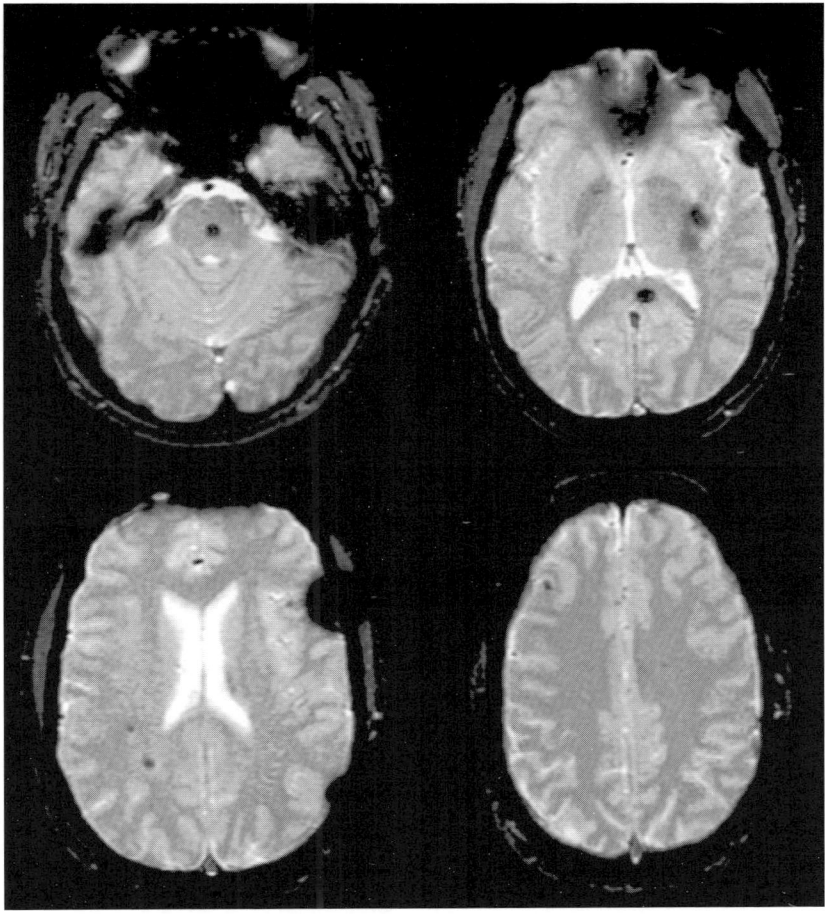

Fig. 62. Numerous small hemorrhagic foci in the brainstem, splenium of corpus callosum, and gray–white junctions on gradient-echo images in a patient with diffuse axonal injury.

it appears as iso- or slightly hypointense to the brain probably because of the protein content and high signal on T2 owing to a lack of signal loss from susceptibility. In the clinical setting, it is rare to encounter hematoma at this stage; it is much more common to detect hemorrhage in the acute (deoxyhemogloblin–hours to days) and subacute (methemoglobin–days to months) stages. A hematoma causes compression of surrounding tissue, decreasing perfusion and oxygen delivery and leading to deoxygenation, thus converting the heme ferrous ion from a six-ligand system to a five-ligand system consisting of four unpaired electrons and rendering it paramagnetic. As this ferrous ion in a quaternary structure is still screened from water molecules by the globin protein, dipole–dipole relaxation cannot occur and therefore the hematoma remains iso/hypointense on T1 images. On the other hand, the packaging of deoxyhemoglobin within RBC causes susceptibility variations within the RBC compared

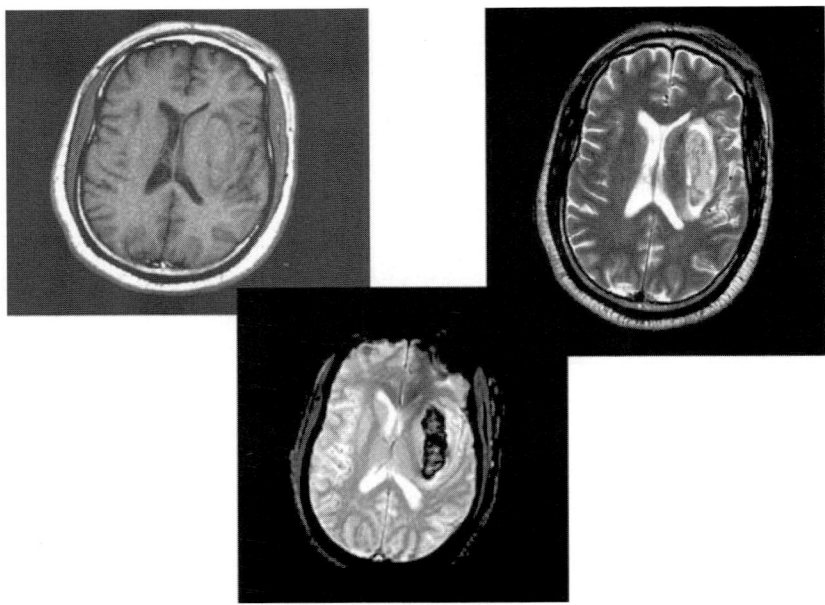

Fig. 63. Axial noncontrast T1 (top left), T2 (top right), and gradient-echo (bottom) images of acute hemorrhage at the oxy–deoxyhemogloblin stage being isointense to brain on T1 and iso- to hypointense on T2.

with the extracellular plasma thus resulting in signal loss on T2 images. In fact, the hypointensity on T1 is actually owing to T2 shortening. With retraction of the clot, protein is also known to promote both T1 and T2 relaxation. In other words deoxyhemoglobin exhibits susceptibility but not relaxativity properties *(46–48)* (Fig. 63).

As the metabolic status of the hematoma further declines to the subacute stage, deoxyhemoglobin is converted to methemoglobin: the iron is in the ferric state with one unpaired electron. This paramagnetic center is now also accessible to water protons, therefore promoting both T1 and T2 relaxation. Methemoglobin will appear as bright signal on T1 images; the T2 appearance depends on whether there has been lysis of the RBC. In the early subacute stage (first several days to a week), intracellular methemoglobin is still experiencing the same packaging susceptibility effects mentioned for deoxyhemoglobin and will therefore manifest as low signal (like air) on T2 images (Fig. 64). After cell lysis one would then expect the extracellular methemoglobin to allow dipolar relaxation to occur, thereby shortening both T1 and T2 relaxation times. On T1 it remains high signal; in fact, the T1 effect dominates at this stage, and with the lack of packaging susceptibility effect extracellular methemoglobin actually appears as high signal on T2 (Fig. 65). As more RBCs are lysed within the hematoma, it also becomes a very high-proton-density area with the released iron chelated by proteins such as lactoferrin and transferrin, all of which remain paramagnetic *(49)*.

MR Imaging of the CNS

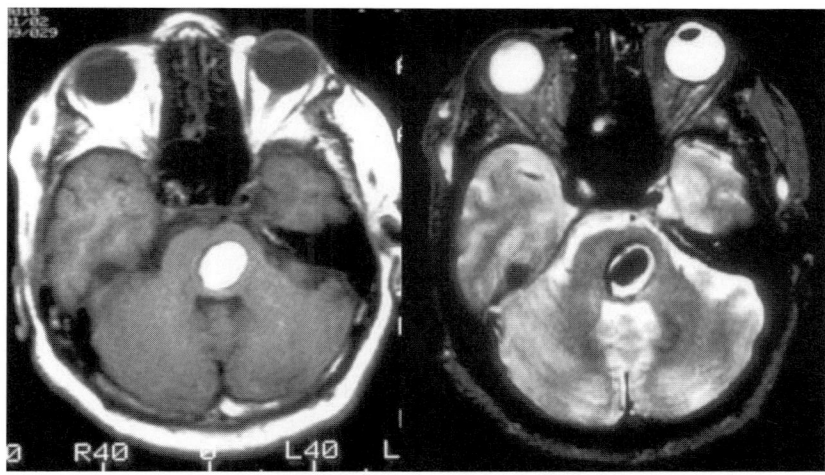

Fig. 64. Increased T1 (left) and decreased T2 (right) signal representing intracellular methemoglobin from a patient with subacute pontine hemorrhage.

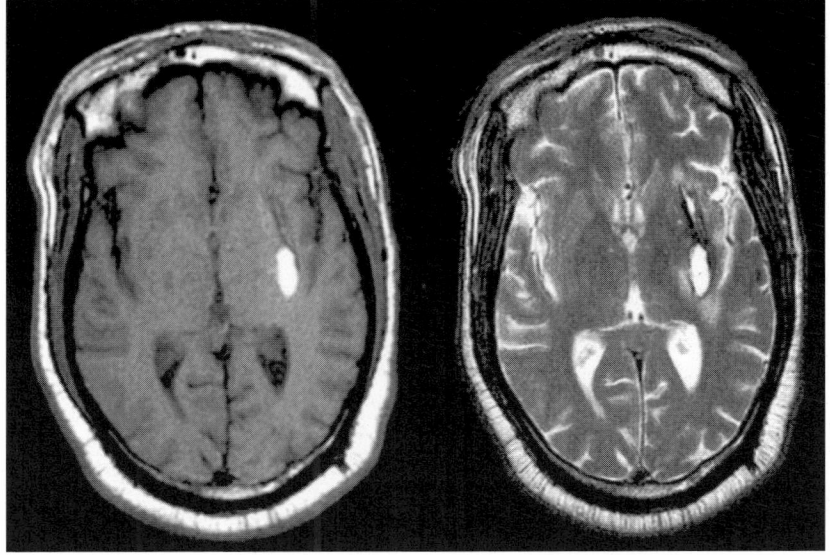

Fig. 65. Axial T1 (left) and T2 (right) images both of which show increased signal at the left posterior basal ganglia from hypertensive bleed secondary to extracellular methemoglobin.

Eventually the iron is stored in ferritin with excess iron in the form of hemosiderin, forming aggregates that are paramagnetic and inaccessible to water molecules, whereby they do not have relaxivity but retain susceptibility effects. Hemosiderin will thus appear hypointense on both T1 and T2 images. This is also what one often observes at the outer margins of hematoma where the iron from breakdown products of methemoglobin accumulates as hemosiderin in

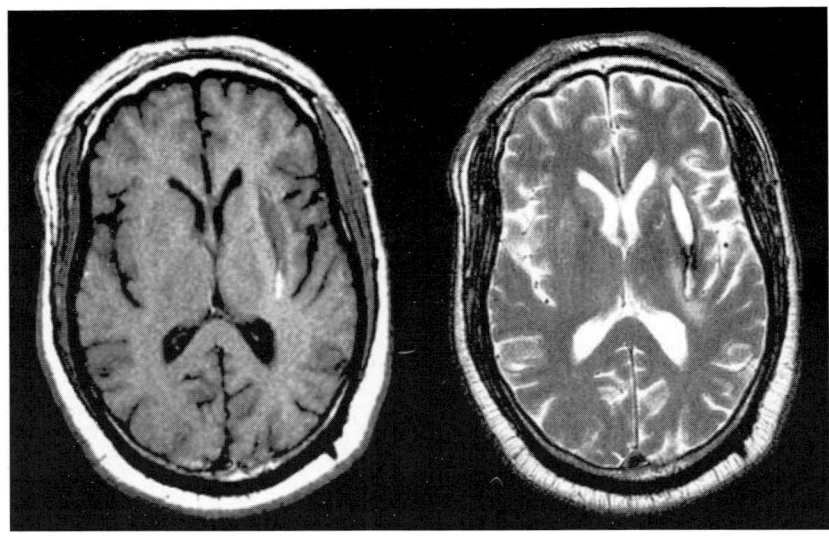

Fig. 66. Same patient as in Fig. 65 with older left anterior basal ganglia bleed showing CSF-like signal on T1 (left) and T2 (right) with a peripheral rim of dark hemosiderin.

macrophages or glial cells (Fig. 66). From this discussion, one would expect the different stages to evolve from the center of the hematoma to the periphery, from oxyhemoglobin to deoxyhemoglobin to methemoglobin (intra- to extracellular), and finally to the chronic stage of hemosiderin. It is important to point out that these stages of hematoma apply to parenchymal bleed; hemorrhage in other compartments of central nervous system such as the subarachnoid space and extraaxial locations will follow a different temporal evolution. This is partly owing to the different oxygen tensions in these nonparenchymal locations, which are suboptimal for the conversion of oxyhemoglobin to deoxyhemoglobin to methemoglobin *(46,47)* (Fig. 67).

Subpial deposition of hemosiderin can arise from recurrent or chronic subarachnoid hemorrhage from tumor or vascular lesions that can appear as a thin dark line of "etching" along the surface of the brain and spinal cord *(50)*. (Fig. 68) Another clinically important situation is the differentiation of a simple hematoma from one with an underlying cause such as a tumor or vascular lesion. A markedly heterogenous collection of signals owing to different stages of bleed that are not in the expected orderly concentric distribution, delayed evolution of blood products, a disrupted, absent, or irregular hypointense outer rim, and persistent surrounding edema all suggest an underlying lesion especially applicable to tumor *(51)* (Fig. 69). For some tumor and vascular lesions such as cavernoma, it is sometimes necessary to wait until the hematoma has resolved before the underlying lesion can be observed. Overall, a T2* susceptibility pulse sequence is used to detect small foci of hemorrhage whatever the cause that otherwise may be missed on all the other available MR pulse sequences (Figs. 61, 62, and 70).

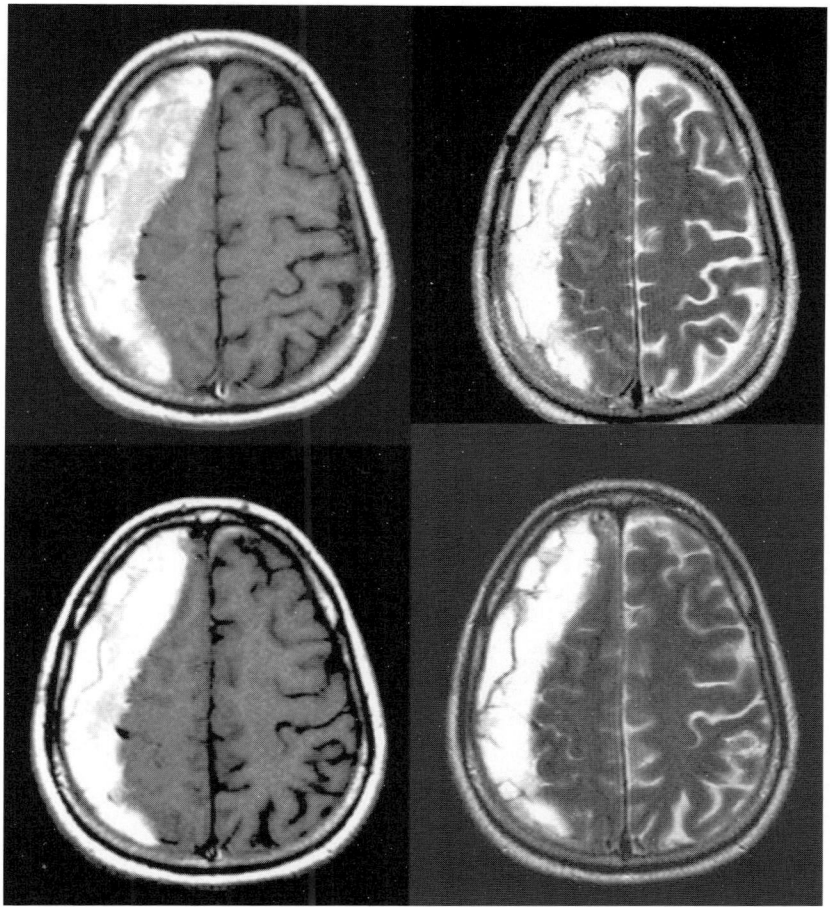

Fig. 67. A large right subdural hematoma with a more inhomogeneous mixture of signal owing to different stages of hemorrhage and differences of oxygenation. (T1, left; T2, right)

CLINICAL APPLICATIONS

Finally, besides the basic commonly used MR sequences for brain imaging already discussed, under certain clinical situations other different parameters are employed that are tailored to the site of anatomical interest or intrinsic properties of the area imaged. Examples include imaging of the internal auditory canal, cranial nerves, leptomeninges, and pituitary gland: thin sections (3 mm) in various orthogonal planes and various contrast agents are used (Figs. 71–74). Occasionally when one is attempting to locate a small pituitary microadenoma or for bringing out early enhancing areas within a tumor to facilitate a better biopsy or resection, dynamic imaging can be applied with fast imaging to monitor contrast delivery to these areas of interest. For seizures, 3D volume coronal spoiled GRASS (SPGR) and FLAIR sequences are added to the basic protocol for better detection of small temporal tumors or mesial temporal sclerosis (Fig. 75).

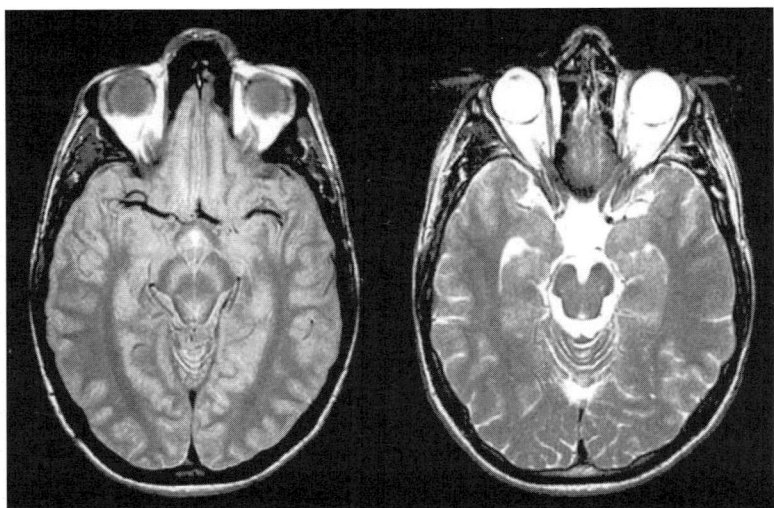

Fig. 68. Hemosiderosis with a thin line of dark "etching" along the brainstem owing to chronic hemorrhage from a distal spinal ependymoma that bled.

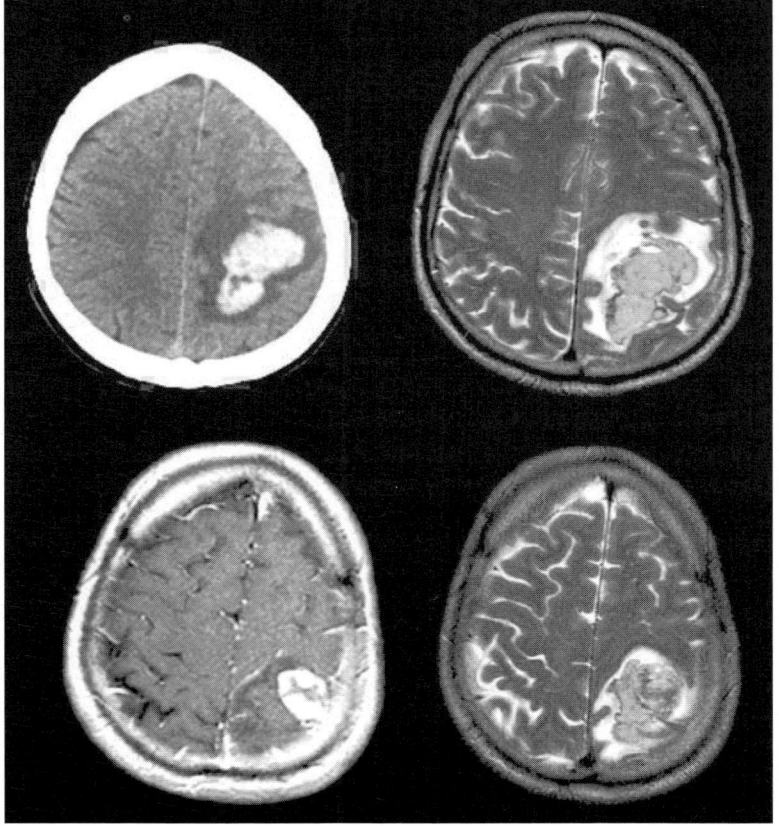

Fig. 69. Axial noncontrast computed tomography (top left), T2 (right), and postcontrast (bottom left) T1 MR images demonstrate a hemorrhagic renal metastasis with inhomogeneous signal (with blood fluid level top right) that does not follow the concentric temporal evolution pattern of simple hematoma.

MR Imaging of the CNS

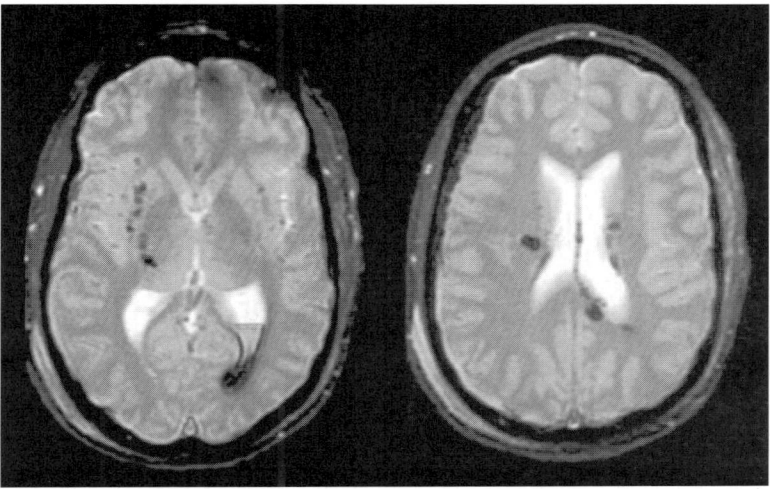

Fig. 70. Axial gradient-echo/susceptibility images of subarachnoid and intraventricular bleed.

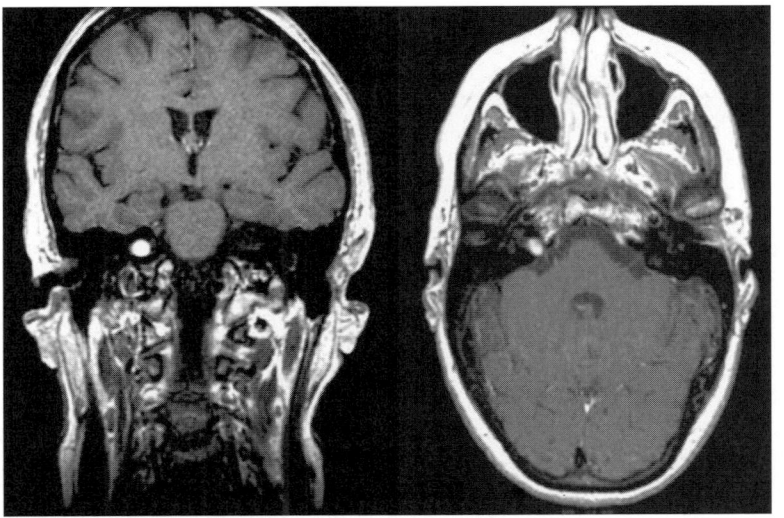

Fig. 71. Coronal (left) and axial (right) thin-section (3-mm) postcontrast images showing an enhancing right intracanalicular acoustic schwannoma.

For spinal imaging, STIR sequences are currently often used in the setting of trauma for detecting subtle fractures and ligamentous injuries (Figs. 76 and 77). Phase-array capability also allows imaging of the entire spine in a short period to access abnormalities in all (epi- and intradural and intramedullary) spinal compartments (Figs. 78–80). In addition, both MRA and diffusion techniques can be utilized for the diagnosis of spinal arterial venous malformations and spinal cord infarcts, although within certain limitations (Figs. 81 and 82).

In summary, this has been a brief discussion of some of the fundamentals of MRI and its clinical applications. The emphasis and the future of MRI will be

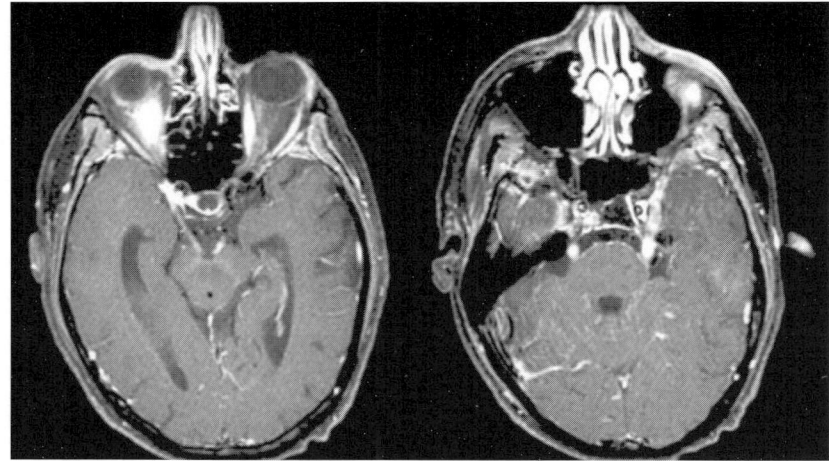

Fig. 72. Axial postcontrast T1 images illustrating bilateral enhancement of cranial nerves III (left) and V (right) in a patient with lymphoma.

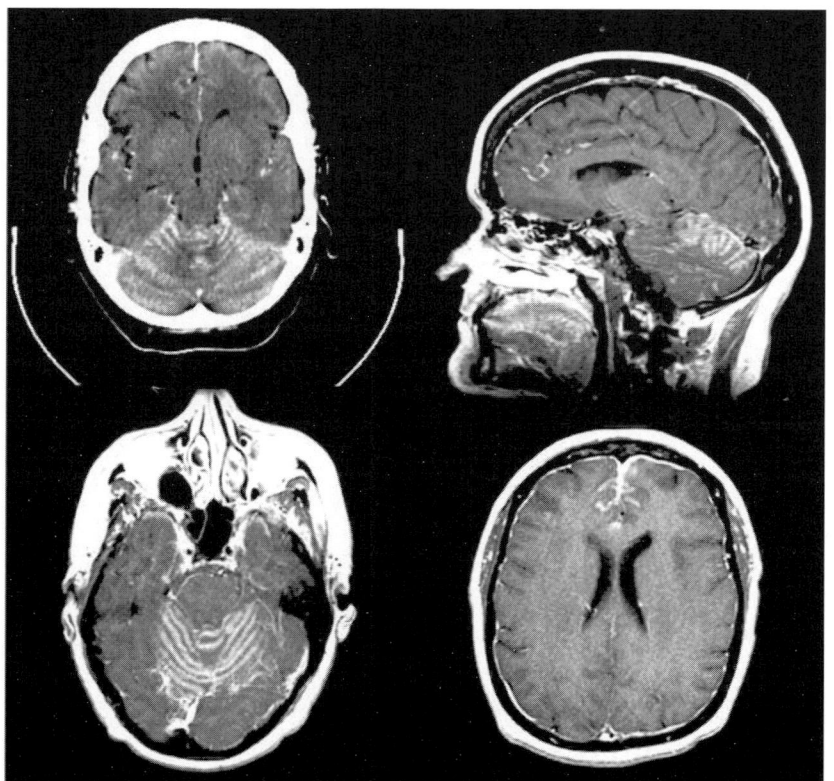

Fig. 73. Diffuse leptomeningeal enhancement on computed tomography (top left), sagittal (top right), and axial (bottom) T1 MR images in a breast cancer patient.

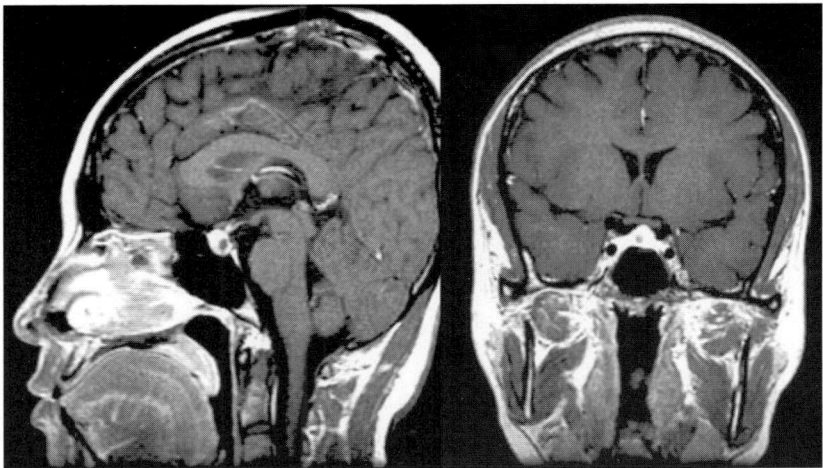

Fig. 74. Sagittal (left) and coronal (right) thin-section (3-mm) images through the pituitary gland illustrating delayed enhancement of a right microadenoma.

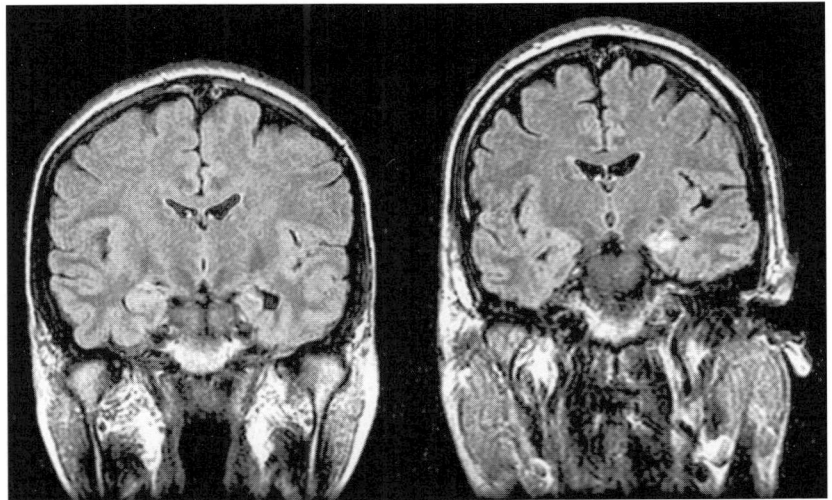

Fig. 75. Coronal FLAIR MR images of mesial temporal sclerosis with an enlarged left temporal horn (left) and increased signal of the left hippocampus (right).

geared toward even more powerful magnets for faster scanning, higher image resolution, and perhaps combination with newer MR contrast agents (MIONs, which are small, iron oxide-based nanomolecules), with the ultimate goal of molecular imaging for diagnostic, monitoring, and therapeutic purposes. Currently, high-field (3–9 T) imaging is still in the early stages, especially the very high fields that are mostly used in the experimental setting. They do have the potential of providing much better resolution for tensor diffusion imaging of white matter tracts, in MRA imaging of smaller distal vasculatures, and also

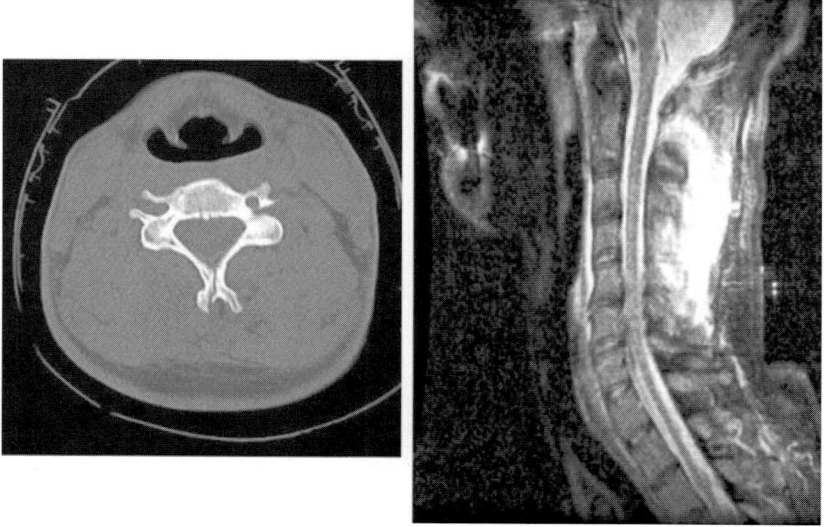

Fig. 76. Computed tomography (left) and sagittal STIR (right) images of the cervical spine showing a subtle C6 vertebral body and spinous process fractures with marked increased signal of the paraspinal soft tissue and interspinous ligaments (C2–C6).

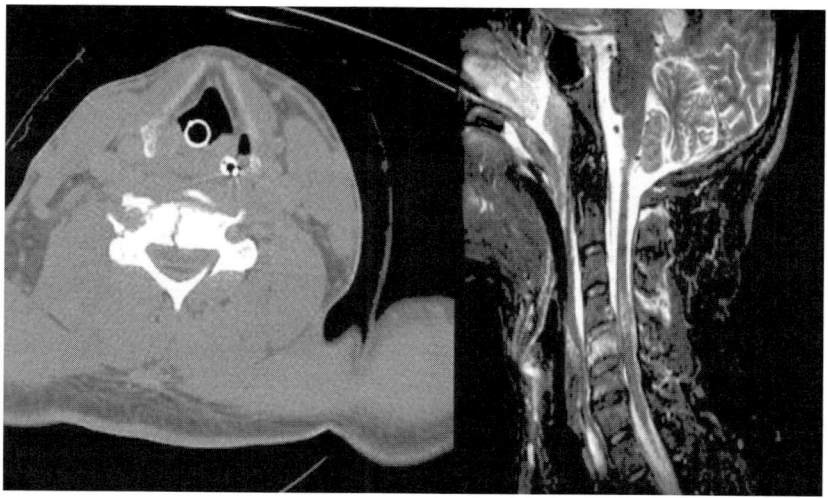

Fig. 77. Axial computed tomography (left) and sagittal STIR (right) MR images revealing fractures of C5 and C6 vertebral bodies with increased marrow signal consistent with edema and loss of normal dark linear integrity of the posterior longitudinal ligament and abnormal cord signal all consistent with traumatic injury.

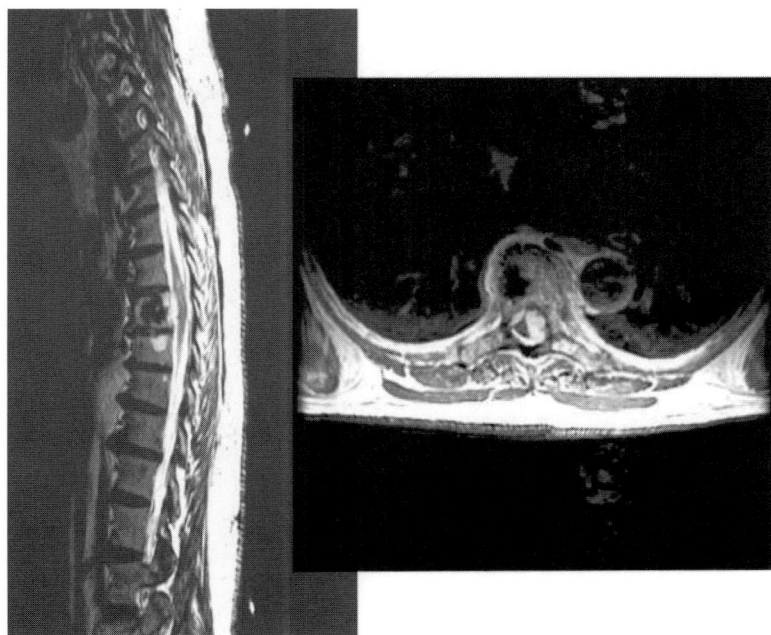

Fig. 78. Sagittal T2 (left) and axial postcontrast (right) MR images show bony metastasis to mid thoracic spine with enhancing epidural component causing cord compression.

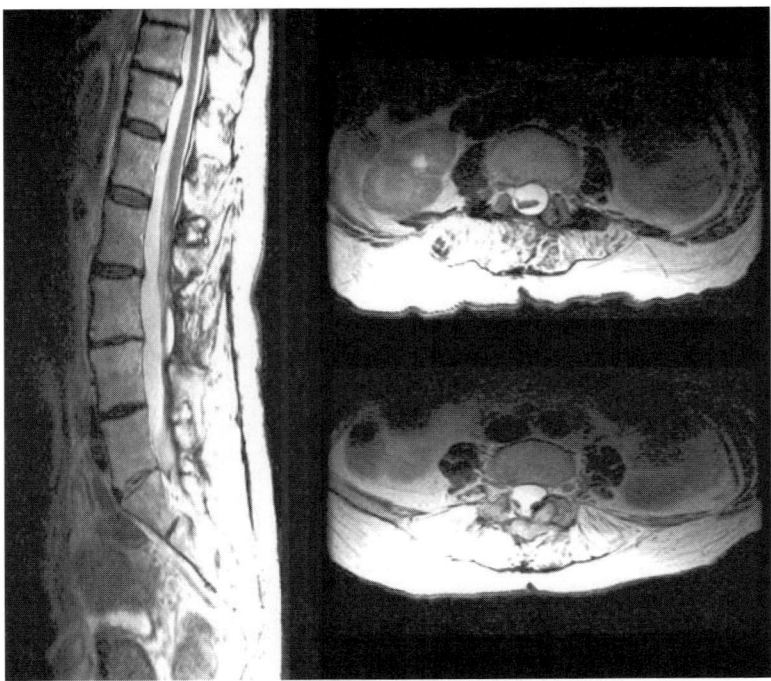

Fig. 79. Sagittal (left) and axial T2 (right) MR images in a patient with arachnoiditis seen here with clumping of the nerve roots and an almost "empty sac" appearance (bottom right).

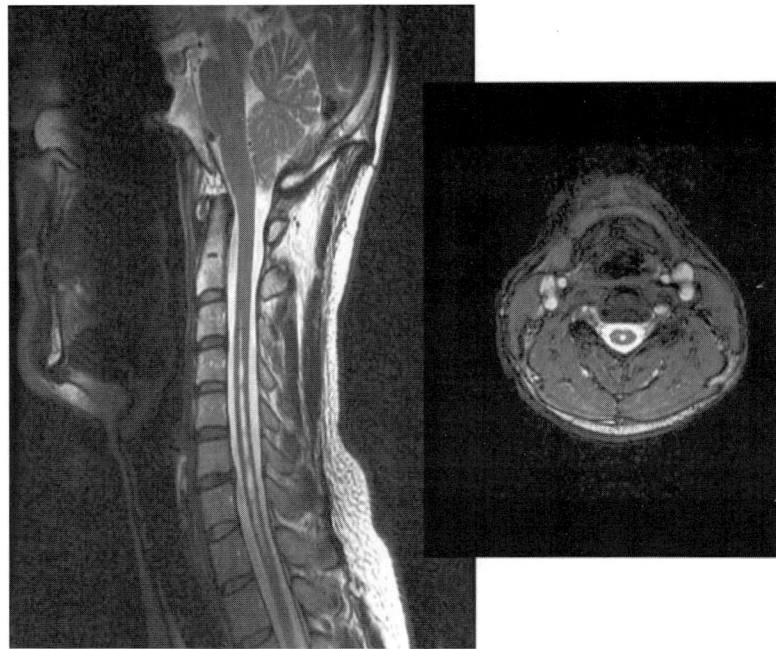

Fig. 80. Sagittal (left) and axial T2 (right) images show an elongated increased intramedullary signal lesion that follows the CSF on all pulse sequences, consistent with cervical thoracic syringohydromyelia.

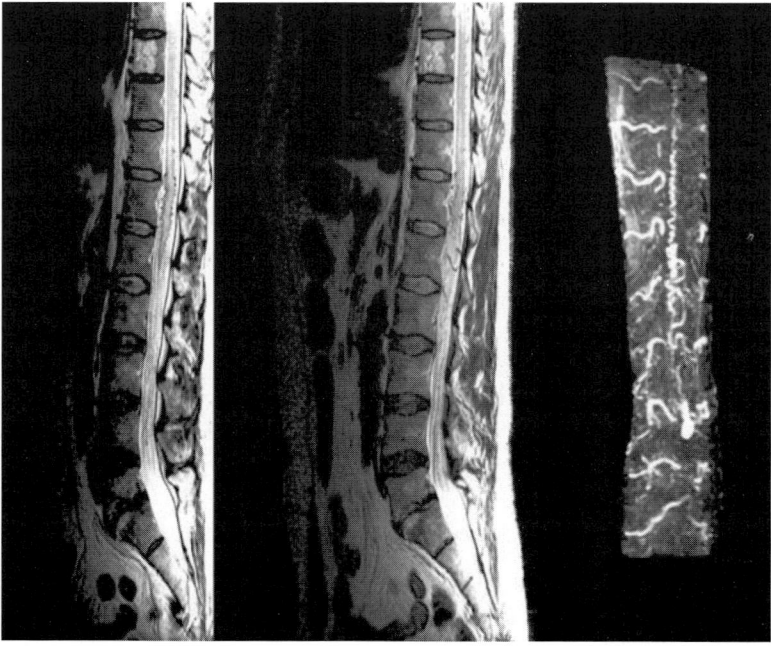

Fig. 81. Sagittal T2 (left, middle) and TOF (right) MRA of the spine depicting abnormal intramedullary T2 signal of the distal cord with multiple serpiginous flow voids and corresponding flow signal on MRA consistent with a spinal arteriovenous malformation.

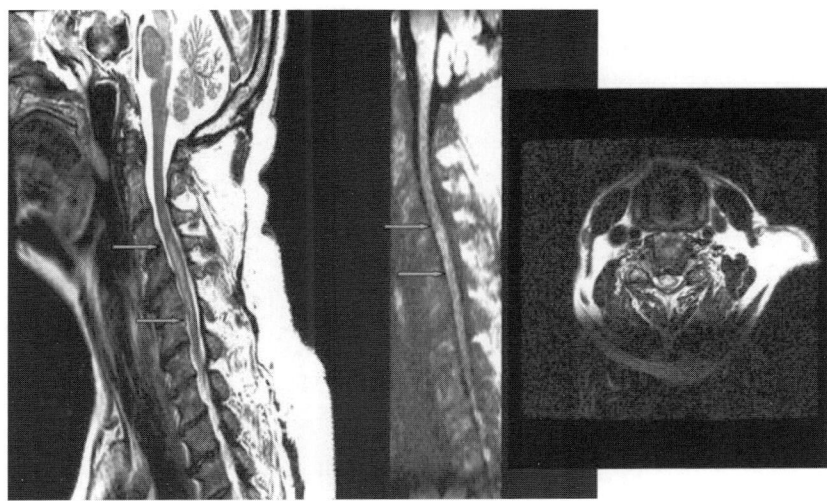

Fig. 82. Sagittal T2 (left), diffusion (middle), and axial (right) T2 images of the cervical spine show abnormal increased signal at C4 and C5 representing cord infarction.

especially in functional MR, spectroscopy, and perfusion applications. The latter is reflected in the ability of high-field MR scanners to image a slice of tissue in 3–4 ms; in other words, the entire brain can be imaged in 1 s compared with approx 10 slices/s in a 1.5-T magnet. Other advantages of high-field imaging include an increase in SNR and the fact that it allows the use of a lower dose of contrast agent to achieve the same effect. On the other hand, the main drawbacks of high-field magnets are the increased sensitivity to susceptibility effects, especially at the bone/air/soft tissue interface and the higher energy deposition to body tissues.

REFERENCES

1. Gorter CJ. Negative result of an attempt to detect nuclear magnetic spins. *Physica* 1936;3:995–998.
2. Gorter CJ, Broer LJF. Negative result of an attempt to observe nuclear magnetic resonance in solids. *Physica* 1942;9:591–596.
3. Purcell EM, Torrey HL, Pound RV. Resonance absorption by nuclear magnetic moments in a solid. *Phys Rev* 1946;69:37–38.
4. Bloch F, Hansen WW, Packard M. The nuclear induction experiment. *Phys Rev* 1946;70:474–485.
5. Lauterbur PC. Image formation by induced local interaction: examples employing nuclear magnetic resonance. *Nature* 1973;242:190–191.
6. Schenck JF, Leue WM. Instrumentation: magnets, coils and hardware, in *Magnetic Resonance Imaging of the Brain and Spine*, 2nd ed. (Atlas SW, ed.), Lippincott-Raven, Philadelphia, 1996, pp. 1–26.
7. Turner R. Gradient coil design: a review of methods. *Magn Reson Imaging* 1993;11: 903–920.

8. Schenck JF. Radiofrequency coils: types and characteristics, in *The Physics of MRI*, Medical Physics, vol. 21 (Bronskill MJ, Sprawls P, eds.), American Institute of Physics, Woodbury, NY, 1993, pp. 98–134.
9. Schenck JF, Hart HR Jr, Foster TH, et al. High resolution magnetic resonance imaging using surface coils, in *Magnetic Resonance Annual* (Kressel HY, ed.), Raven Press, New York, 1986, pp. 123–160.
10. Wilson MN. *Superconducting Magnets*. Clarendon Press, Oxford, 1983.
11. Roemer PB, Hickey JS. Self shielded gradient coils for nuclear magnetic resonance imaging. US patent 4,737,716:1988.
12. Mansfield P, Chapman B. Active magnetic screening of gradient coils in MR imaging. *J Magn Reson* 1986;66:573–576.
13. Wehrli FW, McGowan JC. The basis of MR contrast, in *Magnetic Resonance Imaging of the Brain and Spine*, 2nd ed. (Atlas SW, ed.), Lippincott-Raven, Philadelphia, 1996, pp. 29–48.
14. Joseph PM. Principles of image formation, in *Magnetic Resonance Imaging of the Brain and Spine*, 2nd ed. (Atlas SW, ed.), Lippincott-Raven, Philadelphia, 1996, pp. 49–63.
15. Mezrich R. A perspective on K-space. *Radiology* 1995;195:297–315.
16. Kwong KK, McKinstry RC, Chien D, et al. CSF-suppressed quantitative single shot diffusion image. *Magn Reson Med* 1991;21:157–163.
17. De Coene B, Hajnal JV, Gatehouse P, et al. MR of the brain using fluid attenuated inversion recovery (FLAIR) pulse sequences. *AJNR* 1992;13:1555–1564.
18. Herlihy AH, Hajnal JV, Curati WL, et al. Reduction of CSF and blood flow artifacts on FLAIR images of the brain with *k*-space reordered by inversion time at each slice position. *AJNR* 2001;22;896–904.
19. Delfaut EM, Beltran J, Johnson G, et al. Fat suppression in MR imaging: techniques and pitfalls. *Radiographics* 1999;19:373–382.
20. Stejskal E, Tanner J. Spin diffusion measurements: spin echoes in the presence of a time-dependent field gradient. *J Chem Physics* 1965;42:288–292.
21. Rowley HA, Grant PE, Roberts TPL. Diffusion MR imaging: theory and applications. *Neuroimaging Clin North Am* 1999;2:343–361.
22. Beauchamp N, Ulug AM, Passe TJ, et al. MR diffusion imaging in stroke: review and controversies. *Radiographics* 1998;18:1269–1283.
23. Damaerel P, Heiner L, Robberecht W, et al. Diffusion weighted MRI in sporadic Creutzfeld Jakob disease. *Neurology* 1999;52:205–208.
24. Kim Y, Chang K, Kim H, et al. Brain abcess and necrotic or cystic brain tumor: discrimination with signal intensity on diffusion-weighted imaging. *AJR* 1998;171: 1487–1490.
25. Tsuruda J. Chew WM, Moseley ME, et al. Diffusion-weighted MR imaging of the brain: value of differentiating between extra-axial cysts and epidermoid tumors. *AJNR* 1990;11:925–931.
26. Makris N, Worth AJ, Sorensen AG, et al. Morphometry of in vivo human white matter association pathways with diffusion-weighted magnetic resonance imaging. *Ann Neurol* 1997;42:951–962.
27. Bradley WG, Waluch V. Blood flow: magnetic resonance imaging. *Radiology* 1985; 154:443–450.
28. Keller PJ. Time-of-flight magnetic resonance angiography. *Neuroimaging Clin North Am* 1992;2:639–656.
29. Heiserman JE. MR angiography: toward faster and more accurate methods. *Neuroimaging Clin North Am* 1999;2:253–261.
30. Dumoulin CL Phase-contrast magnetic resonance angiography. *Neuroimaging Clin North Am* 1992;2;657–676.

31. Bradley WG Jr, Whittemore AR, Kortman KE, et al. Marked cerebrospinal fluid void: indicator of successful shunt in patients with suspected normal hydrocephalus. *Radiology* 1991:178:459–466.
32. Tsuruda J, Saloner D, Norman D. Artifacts associated with MR neuroangiography. *AJNR* 1992;13:1411–1422.
33. Foo TKF, Ho V, Choyke PL. Contrast-enhanced carotid MR angiography: imaging principles and physics. *Neuroimaging Clin North Am* 1999;2:263–284.
34. Keller PJ. Fast(er) MR imaging. *Neuroimaging Clin North Am* 1999;2:243–252.
35. Hennig J, Nauwth A, Friedburg H. RARE imaging: a fast imaging method for clinical MR. *Magn Reson Med* 1986;3:823–833.
36. Cohen MS, Weisskoff RM. Ultra-fast imaging. *Magn Reson Imaging* 1991;9:1–37.
37. Rosen BR, Belliveau JW, Aronen HJ, et al. Susceptibility contrast imaging of cerebral blood volume. Human experience. *Mag Reson Med* 1991;22:293–299.
38. Sorensen AG, Buonanno FS, Gonzalez RG, et al. Hyperacute stroke: evaluation with combined multi-section diffusion weighted and hemodynamically weighted echo-planar MR imaging. *Radiology* 1996;199:391–401.
39. Aronen HJ, Gazit IE, Louis DN, et al. Cerebral blood volume maps of gliomas: comparison with tumor grade and histologic findings. *Radiology* 1994;191:41–51.
40. Mcgowan JC, Schnall MD, Leigh J. Magnetization transfer imaging with pulsed off-resonance saturation: contrast variation with saturation duty cycle. *J Magn Reson Imaging* 1994;4:79–82.
41. Filippi M, Campi A, Dousset V, et al. A magnetization transfer imaging study of normal-appearing white matter in multiple sclerosis. *Neurology* 1995;45:478–482.
42. Hood M, Ho V, Smirniotopoulos JG, et al. Chemical shift: the artifact and clinical tool revisited. *Radiographics* 1999;19:357–371.
43. Whittemore AR. The Gibbs phenomenon. *AJR* 1990;154:204.
44. Sobol WT. Artifacts in magnetic resonance imaging. *Appl Radiol* 1994;Aug:11–17.
45. Cohen MD, McGuire W, Corey DA, et al. MR appearance of blood and blood products: an in vitro study. *AJR* 1986;146:1293–1297.
46. Barkovich AJ, Atlas SW. Magnetic resonance imaging of intracranial hemorrhage. *Radiol Clin North Am* 1988;26:801–820.
47. Bryant RG, Marill K, Blackmore C, et al. Magnetic relaxation in blood and blood clots. *Magn Reson Med* 1990;13:133–144.
48. Gomori JM, Grossman RI, Yu-Ip C, et al. NMR relaxation times of blood: dependence on field strength, oxidation state and cell integrity. *J Comput Assist Tomogr* 1987;11:684–690.
49. Gomori JM, Grossman RI, Hackney DB et al Variable appearances of subacute intracranial hematomas on high-field spin-echo MR. *AJNR* 1987;8:1019–1026.
50. Gomori JM, Grossman RI, Bilaniuk LT, et al. High-field MR imaging of superficial siderosis of the central nervous system. *J Comput Assist Tomogr* 1985;9:972–975.
51. Atlas SW, Grossman RI, Gomori JM, et al. Hemorrhagic intracranial malignant neoplasms: spin echo MR imaging. *Radiology* 1987;164:71–77.

3
Proton MR Spectroscopy

Amir A. Zamani, MD

INTRODUCTION

Nuclear magnetic resonance spectroscopy (MRS) has been in use in biochemistry labs for more than 50 yr. In its earlier years, it was used primarily for in vitro chemical analysis of small samples. Magnetic resonance imaging (MRI) is a powerful imaging technique that combines exquisite sensitivity to soft tissue contrast with the ability to demonstrate anatomy in many different planes and projections. MRS as a technique for in vivo sampling of biological tissue provides another piece of information, revealing the biochemical changes occurring in the pathological region. The advantages of MRS in comparison with other techniques that provide metabolic information (such as positron emission tomography [PET] or single-photon emission computed tomography [SPECT]) lies in the fact that MRS can be obtained during the same session as MRI. With newer MRS techniques it is possible to sample the entire lesion and its surroundings and cross-reference them to MR images; this enables us to obtain spectra belonging to many small region of the lesion (generally about 1 cm^3). The spectra obtained with this whole brain technique can be compared with spectra obtained from the same exact location after therapeutic intervention, thus allowing us to see the effect of certain therapeutic interventions.

MRS can be used in differentiation of similar-appearing pathology (infarct from tumor, tumor from abscess). In certain pathological conditions the MR spectrum is virtually diagnostic. Moller-Hartmann et al. *(1)* report that added information provided by spectroscopy led to approx 15% more correct diagnoses and 6% fewer incorrect diagnoses.

In our current discussion, we consider only proton MRS. Sodium, carbon, and phosphorus MRS have yet to find wide clinical application.

PHYSICS OF SPECTROSCOPY

Spectroscopy is based on chemical shifts. A proton (hydrogen nucleus) in a magnetic field (for example, 1.5 T) has a precession frequency governed by Larmor's equation (64 MHz at 1.5 T). In fact, the local magnetic field experienced by the proton is not exactly the same as the external magnetic field. This is because the adjacent orbiting charged particles (for example, electrons)

From: *Minimally Invasive Neurosurgery,* edited by: M.R. Proctor and P.M. Black © Humana Press Inc., Totowa, NJ

produce their own magnetic field, which add to, or subtract from, the external magnetic field. Thus the resonance frequency of a proton is different (shifted) from what is expected in the given external field. The degree of shift, expressed in parts per million (ppm), depends on the chemical structure of the material. For example, the chemical shift of a proton in the radical $-CH_3$ is different from that of a proton in the radical $-CH_2^-$.

Like conventional MRI, imaging in MRS begins with the MR signal. Radio waves at an exact frequency will cause the protons in the magnetic field to go to higher energy levels. These higher energy levels are unstable, and protons give up the extra energy in the form of a signal, the amplitude of which diminishes with time (free induction decay). In order to produce spectra on which the differences in chemical shifts are recorded, the received MR signal is subjected to Fourier transform to change it from a plot of intensity vs time to a plot of intensity vs frequency (change from time domain to frequency domain). To ensure that the shifts in frequency reflect different chemical structures only, one has to ensure the homogeneity of the external magnetic field over the imaging region. Indeed, ensuring that the magnetic field is homogenous is key to obtaining good spectra (2).

To obtain spectra from important metabolites in the brain, it is essential to suppress signal generated by water. In biological specimens the concentration of water is 1000–10,000 times greater than that of these metabolites; thus its signal, if not suppressed, will overwhelm the spectrum. A variety of water suppression techniques are available.

From what has been said so far, it is clear that successful spectroscopy depends on good suppression of water as well as achieving external field homogeneity (2). The process of doing both has been simplified in most modern scanners by performing a *prescan*. At the end of this, the imager measures the degree of water suppression as well the homogeneity of the field. If these are satisfactory, the actual acquisition of spectra is allowed to begin.

Contrast enhancement is an essential part of MR evaluation of many lesions. Spectroscopy usually begins after this enhancement. Does this process change the spectra in a way detrimental to identification of the peaks? The effects of enhancement on spectra are subject to much debate, but overall it is believed that in most instances, these effects are negligible.

The important metabolites detected by MRS include *N*-acetyl aspartate (NAA), creatine, choline, lactate, myoinositol, and mobile lipids (3,4).

NAA is a marker of neuronal population and function, and this metabolite in adult brain is confined to neurons. Whenever neurons die (for example, in ischemic infarction) or are displaced by other elements (for example, in tumors), the NAA peak is diminished.

Creatine is in constant equilibrium with phosphocreatine and is a marker of oxidative metabolism of the cells. The concentration of creatine is tightly regulated and is not easily affected by disease processes. For this reason, it acts as a yardstick against which other peaks are measured. Brain does not produce its creatine; it is transported to the brain from liver and kidney.

A choline peak at 3.2 ppm is a combination of multiple metabolites (free choline, phosphocholine, phosphatidyl choline, and glycerophosphocholine). Some of these metabolites are degradation products of cell membranes; some others are metabolites used in the synthesis of membranes. Because of increases in cell membrane turnover, the choline peak is elevated in all brain tumors. Many investigators point to a high choline/creatine ratio as nonspecific spectroscopic evidence of neoplasia.

Lactate is normally produced in small amounts. These small amounts are usually undetected by MRS. Whenever the glucose metabolism becomes essentially anaerobic, lactate in detectable amounts is produced. Lactate at 1.3 ppm is a doublet peak at TE of 140 ms. With a TE of 40 ms, the lactate peak is all entirely above the baseline. This change with different TEs is essential in positive identification of the lactate peak.

Plasma membrane lipids are seen in conditions associated with necrosis. The peak owing to these may extend over a large segment of the spectrum and overlaps the lactate peak. They do not have the characteristic doublet appearance of lactate and become far less noticeable with a longer TE (for example, 270 ms).

Glutamate is an abundant amino acid and a metabolite related to detoxification of ammonia. It is also an excitatory neurotransmitter.

Myoinositol at 3.6 ppm is a cerebral osmolyte. It may be a degradation product of myelin and possibly a marker for glial cells.

NORMAL SPECTRUM

The postprocessing of data produces spectra with a typical appearance, although there are some variations related to the age of the patient and the site of sampling (Fig. 1). The NAA peak at 2.00 ppm is the dominant peak; the choline peak at 3.2 ppm and the creatine peak at 3.0 ppm are almost half as tall as the NAA peak. There is no lactate peak. Myoinositol at 3.6 ppm and glutamate peaks may be discernible.

PATHOLOGICAL CONDITIONS

Infarction

One of the common questions encountered is differentiation of an infarct from a tumor. Some tumors such as low-grade astrocytomas and anaplastic astrocytomas may have an appearance similar to an infarct and can be erroneously diagnosed as infarcts under these conditions. Correct diagnosis can be aided by obtaining spectroscopy. Another scenario is development of an infarct around the time of resection of a tumor. Apparently, this is not uncommon; some authorities believe the incidence of this event to be as high as 10%. In these situations, positive identification of an infarct can usually be accomplished with diffusion-weighted imaging. Spectroscopy can also be helpful.

Neurons are very sensitive to ischemia. As soon as delivery of oxygen and nutrients ceases, anaerobic glycolysis takes over. As a result, lactate is produced and is easily detectable by spectroscopy by its characteristic doublet appearance at 1.3 ppm.

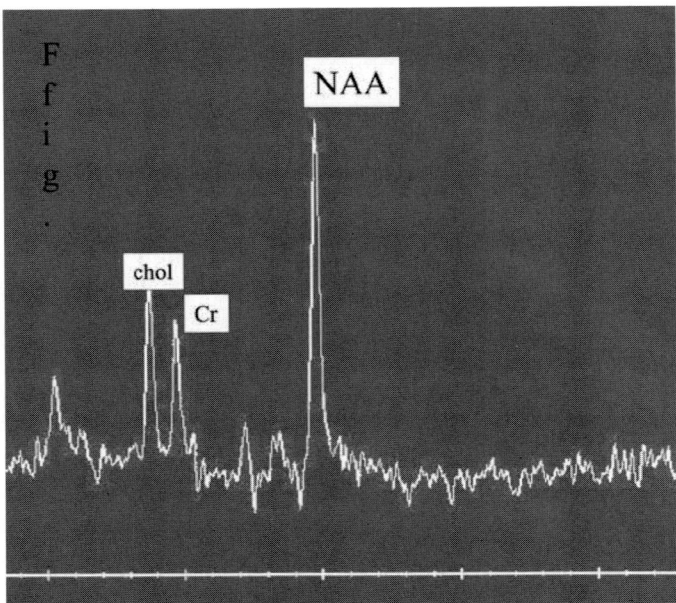

Fig. 1. Normal spectrum. chol, choline; Cr, creatine; NAA, N-acetyl aspartate.

Soon after this (in about 30–60 min), the NAA peak begins to diminish (6). Loss of neurons is irreversible, and as a result, the NAA peak remains low while the lactate peak gradually diminishes only to increase again in the subacute and chronic stages because of migration of macrophages that are naturally rich in lactate. Figure 2 demonstrates an acute infarct. Figure 3 demonstrates a tumor that was erroneously diagnosed as an infarct initially. MRS revealed the true nature of the lesion.

Brain Tumors

According to some authors, spectroscopy is abnormal in every case of brain tumor. This is probably too optimistic, as every practitioner of MRS will testify. It is safe to state that spectroscopy is abnormal in the great majority of brain tumors.

Tumors of the brain are either extraaxial or intraaxial and in each case, they replace the normal neuronal population. As expected, there is a reduction in NAA. Some tumors show spectra in which there is a peak at 2.0 ppm. This is probably because they contain material structurally akin to NAA. NAA is strictly confined to adult neurons.

Tumors also cause a large peak of choline, apparently caused by rapid turnover of cell membranes with accumulation of material used in the synthesis of membranes, or material generated by degradation of cell membranes. A high peak of choline is seen in both intraaxial and extraaxial tumors. In the intraaxial tumors, it can be seen in both tumors of glial origin and others, for example, metastases and lymphomas. A high choline peak, however, is not confined to neoplastic conditions and can be seen in other diseases, for example in

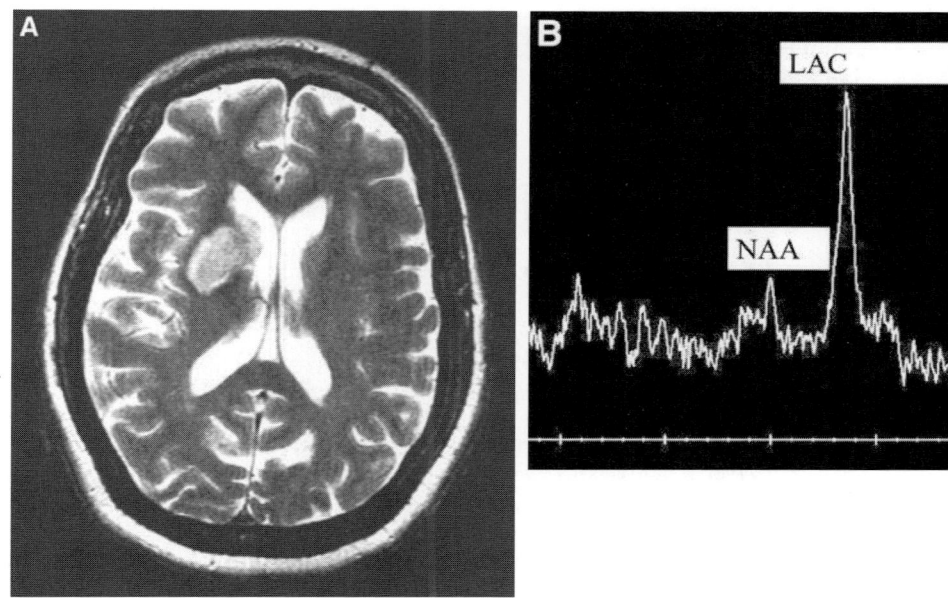

Fig. 2. (A) Right basal ganglionic acute infarct. (B) The corresponding single-voxel spectroscopy shows decreased N-acetyl aspartate (NAA) and a prominent lactate (LAC) peak. A TE of 40 ms was used.

demyelinating plaques of tumefactive multiple sclerosis (see Demyelinating Disease following). Among gliomas, the choline peak may be higher in anaplastic astrocytomas than glioblastomas. One important observation made by many investigators is that in tumors, the site with the highest choline peak does not necessarily correspond to the site of enhancement; this site may reside outside the enhancing portion of the lesion. This fact is potentially significant in choosing an appropriate site for biopsy.

Lactate peak and mobile lipid peaks are seen in more malignant tumors and in those with necrosis. The cystic spaces within a tumor are high in lactate. One note of caution is that even in more benign lesions, after a therapeutic intervention (radiation and/or surgery) a lactate peak may appear (7–10).

Different portions of tumor may have different spectroscopic signatures. Tumors tend to be inhomogeneous, and a complete spectroscopic picture cannot be obtained with single-voxel spectroscopy, hence the need to develop 2D and 3D spectroscopy methods that are more complicated. In many centers, these are fairly routine now, and with 3D volume spectroscopy, the entire brain can be sampled in less than 20 min.

Figures 4 and 5 demonstrate spectroscopy of a glioma and a meningioma, respectively.

The spectra produced by metastases, lymphomas, and malignant gliomas may be quite similar. It is noteworthy that spectra obtained in peritumoral regions in glioma show increased choline. This increased choline is not seen in peritumoral regions of metastases (11). Castillo et al. (12) report that myoinositol

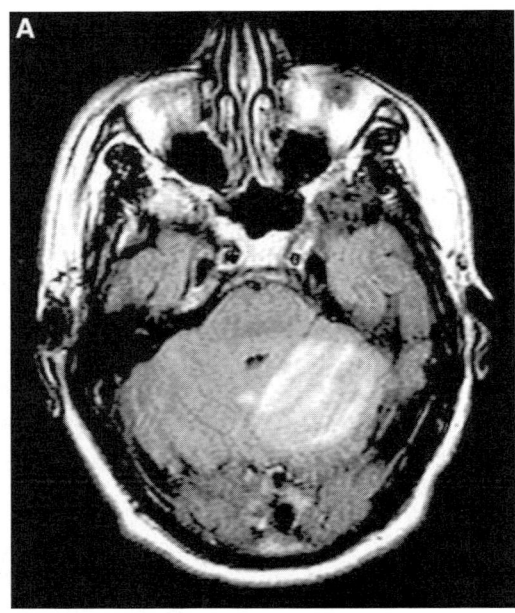

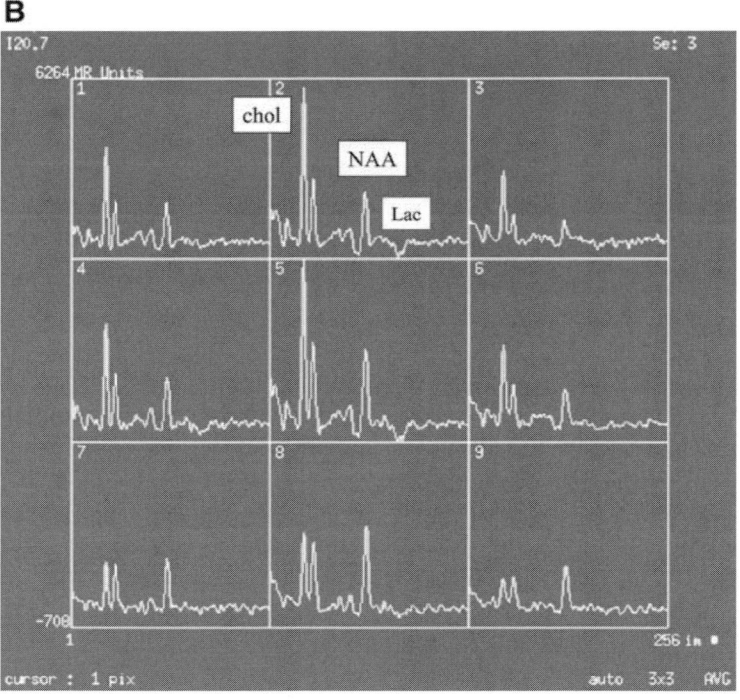

Fig. 3. Medulloblastoma of left cerebellum. **(A)** A left cerebellar lesion with sharply defined margins and a quadrilateral shape, suggesting an infarct. Note mild mass effect in the fourth ventricle. **(B)** Corresponding spectra from a multivoxel study with a TE of 140 ms shows increased choline (chol), a depressed N-acetyl aspartate (NAA) peak, and a small lactate (LAC) peak. The spectra are strongly in favor of a neoplastic process. Compare with surrounding normal voxels, for example, voxel #9 in the bottom right.

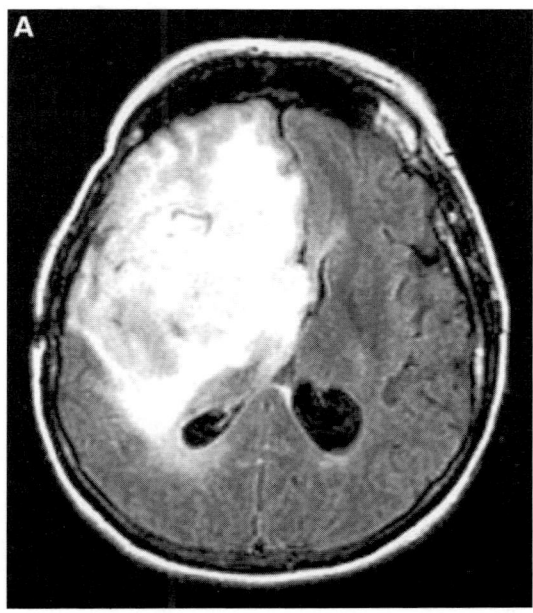

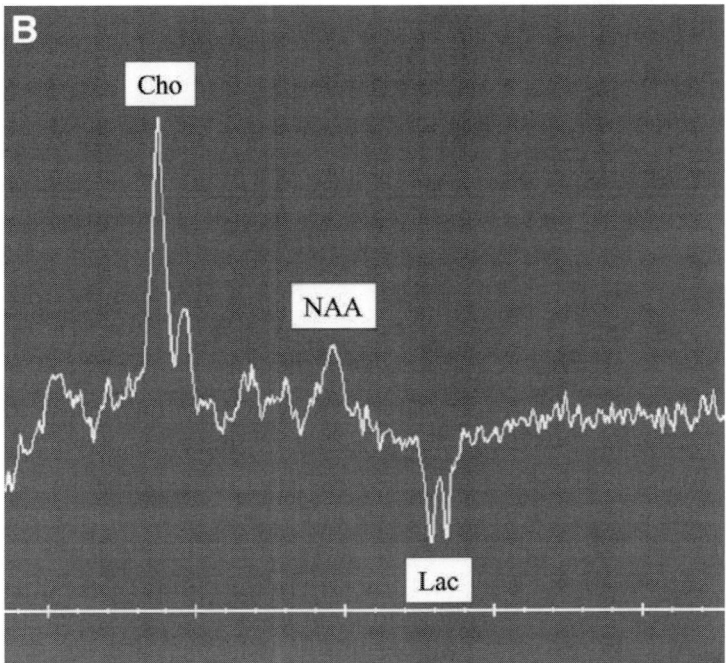

Fig. 4. (A) A large hemispheric tumor with mass effect. **(B)** MR spectroscopy shows elevated choline, decreased NAA, and a lactate peak.

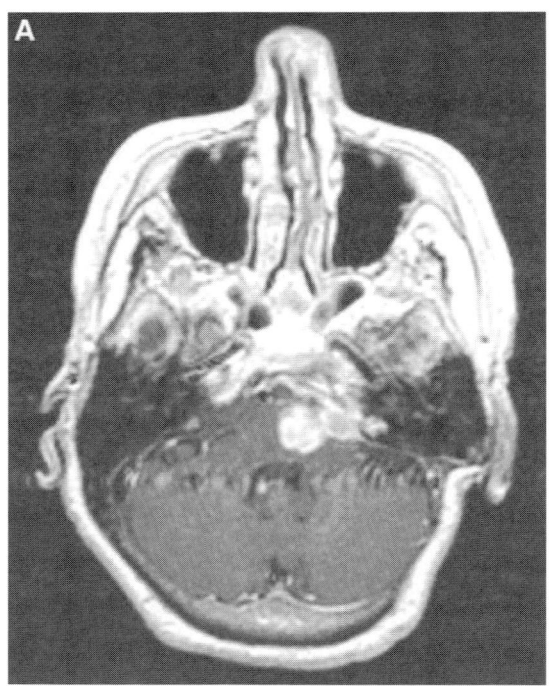
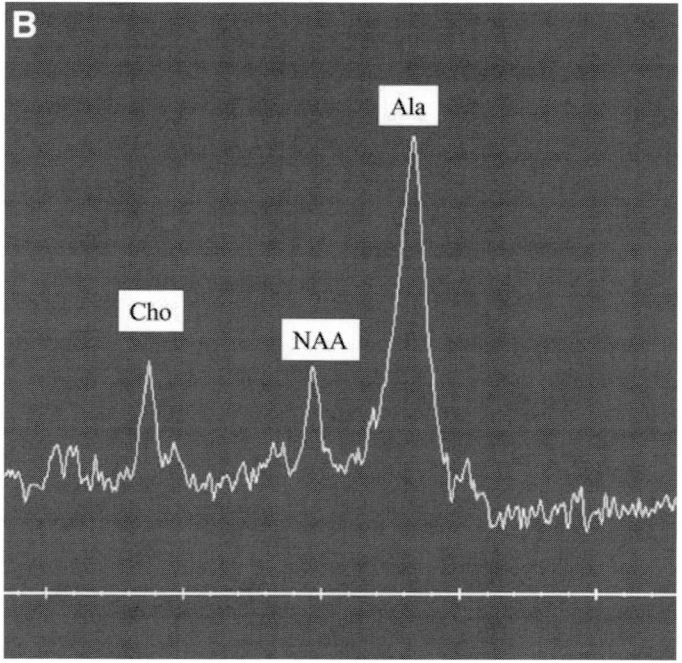

Fig. 5. Spectroscopy of a meningioma. **(A)** A posterior fossa meningioma. **(B)** Spectroscopy demonstrates increased choline (Cho), and decreased N-acetyl aspartate (NAA). An alanine (Ala) peak is an inconsistent finding in meningiomas.

is present in all tumors arising from the central nervous system and is absent in metastases. With anaplastic astrocytomas and glioblastomas, there is a trend toward lower myoinositol levels compared with those of low-grade astrocytomas *(12)*. In addition, within the glial family of tumors, it is not currently possible to differentiate between different cell lines, for example, between oligodendrogliomas and astrocytomas.

Radiation Necrosis

Perhaps the purest form of brain radiation necrosis can be seen in patients with head and neck cancer whose brain is injured because of its proximity to the primary site of tumor. Such brain lesions may be seen in temporal and frontal lobes. Radiation necrosis produces a rather flat spectrum because of reduction in the amount of NAA and choline. Lactate may be seen, however. Several investigators have shown that in *severe* radiation necrosis there may be an elevated choline peak. This choline peak makes differentiation of recurrent tumor from radiation necrosis difficult *(13)*.

Abscesses and Other Infections

Necrotic tissue seen in some tumors has a different spectroscopic signature compared with that seen in pyogenic infections. Several investigators have shown this, both in vitro and in vivo. Bacteria producing pyogenic infections possess enzymes that are capable of breaking proteins into amino acids. Identification of cytosolic amino acids (leucine, isoleucine, and valine) by spectroscopy is essential in appreciating the pyogenic nature of a lesion. These amino acids produce a peak at 0.9 ppm *(14)*. This peak, upright when spectroscopy is obtained with a TE of about 40 ms, becomes inverted with a TE of 140 ms. Several authors have shown a similar appearance with cysticercosis. Besides these amino acids, lactate and acetate may be seen. Figure 6 shows spectroscopy of a pyogenic abscess.

Tuberculous infections lack such amino acids. Lipids and lactate may be seen. Herpes simplex encephalitis causes significant reduction of NAA and a lactate peak. With AIDS encephalitis, there is an irreversible loss of NAA *(15)*.

Demyelinating Disease

In active lesions (those with enhancement), there is a mild elevation of choline, and a lactate/lipid peak may be seen *(16,17)*. A highly elevated, towering choline peak may be seen in some case of fulminant demyelination *(5)*. Because of similarities with brain tumors, MRS may not be able to differentiate the two. Decreased NAA is a bad sign that (along with T1 black holes, and low magnetization transfer ratio) may signal loss of neurons and poor prognosis.

Epilepsy

The role of spectroscopy in evaluation of patients with medically refractory seizure is controversial. Currently, scalp electroencephalography and tailored MR can be used effectively to localize lesions and help with lateralization. In a certain percentage of patients, these strategies may fail or may provide discordant

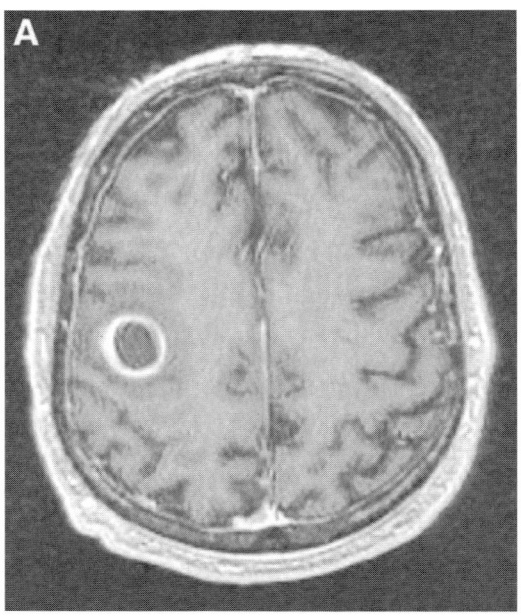
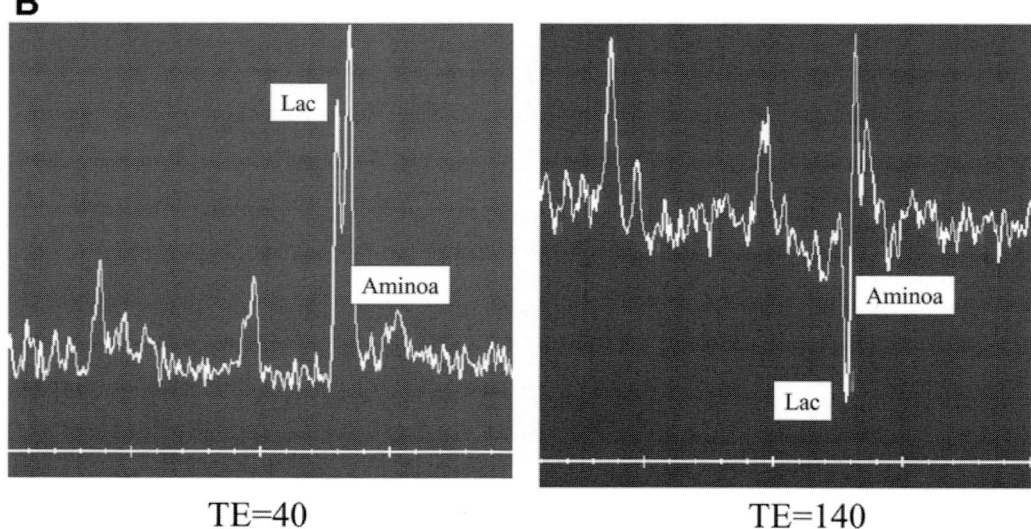

Fig. 6. (A) MRS of a well-defined lesion with a thin rim of contrast enhancement and surrounding edema. Spectroscopy was accomplished with TEs of 40 and 140 ms. (B) Note reversal of the peak belonging to cytosolic amino acids (Aminoa) at 0.9 ppm when TE is switched from 40 to 140 ms. This lesion was a nocardia brain abscess. Lac, lactate.

results. In these patients PET imaging, SPECT imaging, and MRS can be used *(18)*. Several studies have demonstrated a reduction in the choline-to-NAA ratio in the temporal lobes responsible for seizure. Achten et al. *(19)* have found the NAA/chol+Cr ratio to be even more helpful than PET in lateralization. Capizzano et al. *(20)* report that in patients with mesial temporal lobe epilepsy, in the ipsilateral hippocampus the absolute NAA was 18.5% lower compared with that in the contralateral side. Asserting that metabolic changes can be found in other parts of the temporal lobe and brain, these authors found that lateralization could improve if whole temporal lobe data, rather than hippocampal data, were employed *(20)*. Also, a lactate peak may be seen in the immediate postictal period in the responsible temporal lobe and in lesser amounts in the contralateral temporal lobe. Whether these observations will lead to universal employment of MRS in the evaluation of patients with refractory seizures remains to be seen.

REFERENCES

1. Moller-Hartman W, Heminghaus S, Krings T, et al. Clinical application of proton magnetic resonance spectroscopy in the diagnosis of intracranial mass lesions. *Neuroradiology* 2002;44:371–381.
2. Mukherji SK. *Clinical Applications of MR Spectroscopy*. Wiley-Liss, New York, 1998.
3. Castillo M, Kwok L. Mukherji SK. Clinical applications of proton MR spectroscopy. *AJNR* 1996;17:1–15
4. Miller BL. A review of chemical issues in 1-H NMR spectroscopy: N-acetyl-L-aspartate, creatine, and choline. *Nucl Magn Reson Biomed* 1991;4:47–52
5. Rand SD, Prost R, Li SJ. Proton MR spectroscopy of the brain. *Neuroimaging Clin North Am* 1999;9(2):379–395.
6. Baker PB, Gillard JH, VanZijji PCM, et al. Acute stroke: evaluation with serial proton MR spectroscopic imaging. *Radiology* 1994;192:723–732.
7. Castillo M, Kwock L. Proton MR spectroscopy of common brain tumors. *Neuroimaging Clin North Am* 1998;8:733–752.
8. Burtscher IM, Holtas S. Proton magnetic resonance spectroscopy in brain tumors: clinical applications. *Neuroradiology* 2001;43:345–352.
9. Nelson SJ, Vigneron DB, Dillon WP. Serial evaluation of patients with brain tumors using volume MRI and 3D 1-H MRSI. *NMR Biomed* 1999;12:123–128.
10. Bulakbasi N, Kocaoglu M, Ors F, et al. Combination of single-voxel proton MR spectroscopy and apparent diffusion coefficient calculation in the evaluation of common brain tumors. *AJNR* 2003;24:225–233
11. Law M, Cha S, Knopp EA, et al. High-grade gliomas and solitary metastases: differentiation by using perfusion and proton MRI. *Radiology* 2002;222:715–721.
12. Castillo M, Smith K and Kwock L: Correlation of Myo-inositol levels and grading of cerebral astrocytomas. *AJNR* 2000;21:1645–1649.
13. Chan Yl, Yeung DKW, Leung SF, et al. Proton magnetic resonance spectroscopy of late delayed radiation-induced injury of the brain. *J Magn Reson Imaging* 1999;10:130–137.
14. Grand S, Passaro G. Ziegler A, et al. *Necrotic tumor versus brain* abscess: importance of amino acids detected at 1-H MR spectroscopy. Initial results. *Radiology* 1999;213:785–793.
15. Chong WK, Sweeney B, Wilkinson ID, et al. Proton MR spectroscopy of the brain in HIV infections: correlation with clinical, immunologic, and MRI findings. *Radiology* 1993;188:119–124.
16. Ross B, Michaelis T. Clinical application of magnetic resonance spectroscopy. *Magn Reson Q* 1994;10:191–247.

17. Arnold DL, Matthews PM, Francis GS, et al. Proton magnetic resonance spectroscopic imaging for metabolic characterization of demyelinating plaques. *Ann Neurol* 1992;31:235–241.
18. Castillo, M. Imaging intractable epilepsy: How many tests are enough? Editorial. *AJNR* 1999;20:534–535.
19. Achten E, Santens P, Boon P, et al. Single-voxel proton MR spectroscopy and positron emission tomography for lateralization of refractory temporal lobe epilepsy. *AJNR* 1998;19:1–8.
20. Capizzano AA, Vermathen P, Laxer KD, et al. Multisection proton MR spectroscopy for mesial temporal lobe epilepsy. *AJNR* 2002;23:1359–1368.

4
Functional Brain Mapping Options for Minimally Invasive Neurosurgery

Alexandra J. Golby, MD and Kathleen A. McConnell, MD

INTRODUCTION

Minimally invasive intracranial neurosurgery depends on the ability to localize accurately the operative target and its relationship to any neighboring eloquent areas. There are several methods of mapping cortical function, including the intracarotid amytal injection test (IAT or Wada test), positron emission tomography (PET), magnetoencephalography (MEG), direct electro-cortical stimulation (ECS), transcranial magnetic stimulation (TMS), and functional magnetic resonance imaging (fMRI). Some of these tests (PET, FMRI, and MEG) are *activation* techniques, meaning they demonstrate brain activation, which occurs when the subject performs a particular behavioral task. In contrast, the tests traditionally used for the determination of eloquent cortex (ECS, IAT) are essentially *deactivation* techniques, meaning that a temporary brain lesion is created pharmacologically or electrically and behavioral effects are measured. Deactivation studies are well suited to the pre-resection evaluation of cortical function because they mimic the effects of resection of the tissue; however, their use is limited by their invasiveness. Transcranial magnetic stimulation is a promising and relatively less invasive deactivation technique that can be performed through an intact skull.

Each brain mapping modality offers different strengths and weaknesses in terms of spatial and temporal resolution, repeatability, and invasiveness. Many of these techniques are relatively new and unexplored; however, they promise to offer far more options in terms of functional mapping to neurosurgeons and their patients. It is likely that the most accurate and useful information will eventually be gained by combining techniques that are complementary. For example, the excellent spatial resolution of fMRI can be integrated with the fine temporal resolution obtained with MEG to get more information than with either technique alone. Combining these techniques with frameless stereotactic neuronavigation and coregistration of datasets will allow the integration of data from different modalities. Not only will this provide useful complementary information but this effort will also allow the cross-validation of methods that depend on different physiologic signals.

From: *Minimally Invasive Neurosurgery*, edited by: M.R. Proctor and P.M. Black © Humana Press Inc., Totowa, NJ

INACTIVATION METHODS

Intracarotid Amytal Testing

The IAT was originally developed to determine language dominance in preoperative epilepsy patients who were candidates for temporal lobectomy (1). The IAT remains the current gold standard technique for presurgical determination of language dominance, especially in patients who are suspected of mixed or unusual language dominance. The IAT involves catheterization of the internal carotid artery and injection of sodium amobarbital, which anesthetizes those regions of the cerebral hemisphere supplied by the carotid artery while the patient undergoes a battery of neuropsychological tests. After the appearance of contralateral hemiparesis indicating hemispheric anesthetization, several tests of language and memory function are rapidly administered. Failure in a cognitive domain indicates that it is supported by the hemisphere that was injected.

Although the IAT was developed as a test of language dominance, its use has been extended to testing for memory competence of the medial temporal structures and in the preoperative determination of language dominance in patients with pathological processes other than epilepsy. Patients who have an anomalous circle of Willis, which may result in contralateral injection and anesthesia of the opposite hemisphere, may have inaccurate results from the test. The IAT is also limited in its ability to make fine distinctions in neurocognitive abilities. Both the time constraints imposed by the temporary nature of the induced cerebral anesthesia and the practical constraints imposed by having to test the patient in an angiography suite limit the scope and sensitivity of neuropsychiatric testing that can reasonably be accomplished. The IAT is able to predict lateralization of memory and language functions but cannot *localize* these functions within the hemisphere. Its use is restricted to determining language dominance patterns and predicting and avoiding global amnesia in patients who cannot support memory with the contralateral mesial temporal lobe (MTL) (2). However, the validity of the Wada test in predicting postoperative memory deficits has been questioned based both on anatomic grounds (in most people the MTL is perfused by the posterior cerebral artery and not by the internal carotid artery) and on clinical outcomes (3,4). This invasive procedure carries a 0.6–1% risk of stroke related to the catheterization (5) as well as puncture site complications in 0.5–10% (6). In addition, the test is quite stressful to patients owing to the temporary hemiparesis and cognitive testing procedures required during the procedure.

Electrocortical Stimulation

Direct ECS testing remains the gold standard method for mapping brain function in preparation for surgical resection. For simple motor mapping, intraoperative cortical stimulation may be performed with the patient under general anesthesia but without muscular paralysis. In this case, low-frequency stimulation causes muscular contractions when they are delivered to the motor cortex. The motor strip may also be localized using somatosensory evoked potentials (SSEPs) and determining the region of phase reversal, although this method is not suited to detailed evaluation of motor function and somatotopy. To test language functions, however, it is necessary that the patient remain awake and able to perform certain tasks such as counting or naming. Meanwhile the surgeon stimulates the cortical surface, inducing a transient disruption in function that mimics the effects of actual resection. This technique requires a wide craniotomy, which exposes the tumor and adjacent eloquent cortical regions suspected of being jeopardized by the resection.

There are special anesthetic, surgical, and neuropsychological considerations when one is performing intraoperative cortical mapping. Awake craniotomy for language mapping is typically performed using a combination of local anesthetic field block and short-acting general agents to induce a rapidly reversible hypnotic state. Once the scalp, skull, and dura are opened and the cortical surface exposed, the surgeon localizes the tumor either grossly or with the aid of neuronavigation or ultrasound and marks the boundaries using sterile surface markers. During the cortical stimulation testing, the patient is awake and asked to perform simple tests such as counting or moving fingers to command while the surgeon stimulates the cortical surface using bipolar stimulating electrodes with a 5-mm tip separation. Stimulation parameters are typically set at 60-Hz biphasic square wave pulses (1 ms/phase) with variable peak-to-peak current amplitudes between 2 and 10 mA. The surgeon first maps the relevant somatosensory cortical regions by eliciting sensory or motor responses in the face and hand. To map language areas, the surgeon asks the patient to count or name objects and records those areas in which cortical stimulation induces speech arrest or other error. In their study of 40 patients undergoing removal of gliomas in the dominant temporal lobe, Haglund et al. *(7)* reported that for patients without language deficits preoperatively, 87% had no deficits postoperatively using the above methods. Most surgeons feel that a reasonably safe limit of resection is to allow a 1-cm margin around cortical areas that appear to be functionally eloquent.

In spite of the excellent spatial and temporal resolution of this technique for cortical mapping, the most obvious drawback is that it requires a craniotomy. This technique, therefore, does not allow for *pre*surgical planning, but is reserved for intraoperative assessment and confirmation of results obtained from preoperative studies. ECS mapping also requires that the patient be able to cooperate in performing these tasks during an awake craniotomy. Most children and some adults are unable to tolerate being awake for such a procedure. Even cooperative patients may have trouble maintaining task performance over the course of the investigation. Awake craniotomy generally requires dedicated and specially trained neuroanesthesia support and a sufficient caseload to provide training and expertise and hence may not be available in many centers. Cortical stimulation testing is also limited by the difficulty of examining the sulcal depths, which comprise as much as two-thirds of the cortical surface *(8)*, the deep structures of the mesial temporal lobe, or the underlying white matter. For example, it is not uncommon for patients who have undergone cortical mapping and resection respecting the boundaries of the eloquent cortex to be left nevertheless with neurological deficits secondary to damage to associated white matter tracts.

ECS can also be performed extraoperatively. This option is used primarily for epilepsy surgery for the mapping of the seizure focus through the chronic (~1 wk) implantation of intracranial electrodes. During this period, cortical stimulation for the determination of eloquent cortex is usually also performed. In order to pursue intracranial electrode placement, there must be sufficient evidence to limit the possible sites of epileptogenesis. On the basis of the scalp electroencephalogram (EEG) and other data, sites are selected for implantation with either depth or subdural electrodes. Depth electrodes are implanted using stereotactic guidance and are most commonly used to monitor the medial temporal lobe structures. Subdural electrodes, arranged in grids and strips, may be used to record from large areas of cortex including intrahemispheric or subtemporal locations.

Each technique has its strengths and limitations in terms of risk, accessible brain areas, and ease of placement, making individualized determination of the appropriate method important *(9)*. In both cases, the electrodes can be used to stimulate as well as record, thereby allowing extraoperative functional mapping *(10)*. When indicated, this technique has the advantage of allowing significant time and a sufficiently relaxed and cooperative patient to allow detailed cognitive testing. However, this technique, like intraoperative ECS, can only sample from limited regions and is therefore not suitable for certain investigations. Because of the necessity of an additional operative session and risks of hemorrhage, infection, or cerebral edema in 1–2 % of patients, this technique has limited indications. In addition, the need for intracranial recording has declined as other less invasive preoperative studies have been developed and validated that allow patients to proceed directly to resective surgery without this step.

Transcranial Magnetic Stimulation

TMS uses electromagnetic energy to stimulate cortical neurons through the intact skull. Combined with a frameless stereotactic system, it has the potential to map brain function in a manner similar to ECS but without the risk of craniotomy. The TMS apparatus consists of a power supply that charges a large bank of capacitors, which are then rapidly discharged through a circular or figure-eight coil; the charged coil produces a powerful and focal magnetic field pulse on the order of 1–2 T. The TMS pulses are typically 200 μs in duration, and the power is concentrated in a band around 5 kHz, well below the frequencies at which body-related field attenuation occurs *(11)*. Therefore, the electromagnetic energy of the TMS pulse is able to pass unimpeded through the scalp and skull to the cortical surface or to deeper structures. On the cellular level, magnetic stimulation by TMS functions very much like electrical stimulation with ECS. The resting membrane potential of excitable cellular membranes is maintained at about –70 mV by the relative intra- and extracellular concentrations of Na^+, K^+ and Cl^- ions maintained by the Na–K pump and passive diffusion. Moving a charge across this membrane, either directly with electrical stimulation or indirectly by magnetic stimulation, creates a transmembrane potential. If this potential reaches about –40 mV, it triggers an action potential in the target neurons and causes motor or sensory responses if the TMS is targeted to sensorimotor regions or speech arrest if the TMS is directed to language regions.

The use of TMS for brain mapping is still in the very early stages of development. In 1998, Krings et al. *(12)* examined the motor cortical representation of 12 muscles of the trunk and upper and lower extremities of 18 healthy controls using TMS combined with a frameless stereotactic system (FSS), allowing the investigators to orient their stimulation sites to the central sulcus rather than to less precise bony landmarks. They observed distinct but overlapping areas of muscle representation for each of these 12 muscles. The also found that the cortical maps changed with increasing stimulus intensity: more muscles became excitable, motor-evoked potential (MEP) amplitude increased, size of the responsive area increased, and latency of the MEP decreased. In 1999, Boroojerdi et al. *(13)*, again using the combination of TMS with FSS, investigated whether the accepted anatomical landmarks on cross-sectional imaging for the location of the intrinsic hand muscles (hand knob shaped like an omega) correlated with the functional areas for hand as mapped by TMS. In all four healthy controls, they observed that the centers of gravity for each MEP elicited by transcranial electric stimuli fell within the anatomical area predicted by the hand-knob gyral configuration and also fell within the area of fMRI activation produced by voluntary hand clenching.

TMS has also been shown to be useful for mapping in the preoperative setting. Krings et al. *(14)* observed good correlation between the stereotactic TMS motor maps of two patients with tumors near the central sulcus and the corresponding intraoperative motor maps produced using ECS. More recently, the same group has examined the efficacy of using TMS–FSS to map motor function in patients with mass lesions near the central sulcus as compared with motor maps produced using fMRI *(15)*. In their cohort of 10 patients they observed that the peak parenchymal fMRI activation and the cortical area where TMS elicited the maximum MEPs averaged within 0.6 cm of each other, thus demonstrating that even in cases of diseased brain, TMS and fMRI, despite having entirely different physiologic bases, yield concordant (although not identical) results.

TMS may also become a useful method for the preoperative assessment of cortical language organization, however, significant obstacles and outstanding questions remain. Michelucci et al. *(16)* performed an early study using TMS to determine language dominance in 14 patients with epilepsy. They obtained results that were concordant with hand preference in only half of the patients, concluding that TMS lacked sensitivity. At that time, it was also not uncommon for TMS to cause significant undesirable side effects such as seizures or transient neurologic deficits. Epstein et al. *(17)* in a review of TMS studies for language mapping, reported that TMS appeared to lead to speech arrest when performed over the facial motor cortex rather than over Broca's area. This suggests that the mechanism behind TMS-induced speech arrest is not a true aphasia but rather a disruption of motor function. In a later study, they also found that language lateralization by TMS did not replicate Wada test results and that right hemisphere or bilateral lateralization were unexpectedly prevalent in the TMS results (18). In addition, there is currently an incomplete understanding of the effects of TMS on cognitive cortical areas, as some stimulation paradigms cause inhibition of function, whereas others appear to facilitate function (19). Based on these findings, a clinical role for TMS language mapping is not yet fully established. There is, however, ongoing interest in refining this technique. For example, Knecht et al. (20) have demonstrated that language function disruption by unilateral TMS is less severe in individuals with more bilateral language representation by functional imaging. These results suggest that a more distributed cortical language representation may be protective in cases of brain damage.

TMS is a promising modality for surgical planning because, like ECS, it mimics the effect of resection but can be performed noninvasively and repeatedly. The use of TMS as a tool for mapping brain function is still very much in its infancy. Although the electromagnetic pulse generated by TMS is very focal, it is still difficult to determine exactly where on the cortex the pulse is targeted, although the continued development of the combination of TMS with frameless stereotactic neuronavigation devices promises to ameliorate this difficulty somewhat. As with fMRI, it also remains to be seen what effects medications, aging, tumor infiltration, or other patient variables will have on an individual's response to TMS Finally, as is the case with many other brain mapping techniques, TMS requires costly special equipment and dedicated personnel.

ACTIVATION METHODS

Magnetoencephalography

MEG is a noninvasive method of measuring brain activity by measuring the magnetic fields that accompany neuronal activity. Neural activity can be described as the generation and propagation of ion currents. The longitudinal current flow generated by several thousands of neurons firing synchronously can be detected at the scalp surface using a biomagnetometer. Unlike fMRI, which measures brain function indirectly by imaging cerebral vascular response to neuronal activity, MEG is based on electrical activity akin to EEG. Like EEG, MEG has excellent temporal resolution on the order of 1 ms. Unlike surface EEG, however, the MEG signal is not attenuated by the skull and scalp and has an excellent spatial resolution of approx 2 mm (21). MEG data are gathered using a biomagnetometer made up of wire induction coils arranged in an array covering the entire head. The magnetic fields produced by neural activity induce electric currents in these coils and can be used to reconstruct an image of the distribution of evoked neural electrical activity of brain function in real time. Magnetic source imaging is the coregistration of MEG data to a structural image to facilitate the anatomic–functional correlations and to incorporate this information into stereotactic neuronavigation systems (22).

MEG scanners require dedicated personnel as well as magnetic and radiofrequency-shielded rooms similar to those for conventional MRI. MEG is extremely vulnerable to environmental magnetic noise including the earth's magnetic field and the magnetically noisy environment in hospitals. Currently, MEG scanners are very expensive (>$2 million capital equipment costs) and have limited availability. Their use at this time is mainly restricted to centers pursuing research programs.

In neurosurgical practice MEG is used primarily in the presurgical evaluation of epilepsy patients to localize epileptogenic foci as well as functional areas that must be preserved during resection. For practical reasons, MEG scans are limited to interictal observations, but several studies have reported good correspondence between MEG recorded interictal spikes and seizure foci. Minassian et al. *(23)* reported, in a series of 11 children with neocortical epilepsy, a strong regional correspondence between the location of MEG-identified interictal spikes and ictal activity confirmed by subdural grid electrode recordings. Wheless et al. *(24)* compared the accuracy of MEG for locating seizure activity with MRI, scalp video EEG, and interictal and ictal subdural grid electrode recording as determined by each method's ability to predict the clinical success of surgical resection. They found that MEG was second only to ictal grids and strips in predicting a positive surgical outcome but made no direct comparison between the anatomic location of seizure foci determined by each method *(24)*. Mamelak et al. *(25)* compared MEG interictal data to intracranial electrode monitoring in 23 epilepsy patients. They found that MEG accurately localized seizure foci to the correct lobe and was therefore useful in guiding the placement of subdural electrodes, particularly in neocortical epilepsy *(25)*.

MEG is also routinely used not only for identification of epileptogenic foci but also for functional mapping of sensorimotor cortex *(26)*. MEG functional mapping of the auditory and visual cortex has also been performed. MEG task design is similar to the blocked design of fMRI experiments in that a stimulus is presented multiple times in alternating patterns of task and rest. The resulting evoked neuromagnetic signals are then averaged over several epochs to separate the signal produced by a focal population of active neurons from background activity. Identification of the central sulcus is most frequently achieved using passive sensory tasks such as electrical stimulation of the median nerve or tactile or vibratory stimulation of the hand and lower lip or tongue. Motor mapping is less common because MEG data acquisition requires smooth, well-controlled hand movements such as flexion and extension of one or more digits of the hand, which can be difficult for patients to perform.

The neurosurgical use of MEG has more recently expanded to stereotactic and image-guided surgery to aid in the safe resection of lesions threatening eloquent cortex *(27,28)*. Several studies report good correlation between properative MEG functional data and intraoperative maps of sensory- and motor-evoked potentials and electrocortical mapping *(29–33)*. Several groups have merged functional MEG data with anatomic data in order to locate functional cortex near and within cortical lesions including arteriovenous malformations, gliomas, and brain metastases. Rezai et al. reported a technique of integrating MEG functional mapping data for both motor and sensory tasks into a stereotactic database for use intraoperatively as well as for preoperative planning. Their system combined MEG data with computed tomography (CT) scans,

MRIs, and digital angiography in an interactive stereotactic system and was used in 10 patients undergoing surgical resection of lesions involving the sensorimotor cortex. Similarly, McDonald et al. *(34)* report the successful combination of both fMRI and MEG data into a frameless stereotactic system that also incorporates digital registration of cortical stimulation sites. These techniques allow the simultaneous viewing of both structural and functional brain anatomy and their spatial relationship to brain lesions, which may allow the surgeon to resect more aggressively without violating functional cortical areas.

Positron Emission Tomography

PET was the primary functional imaging modality used in neuroscience research prior to fMRI and was the basis for the development of in vivo mapping studies of human functional cognitive anatomy. Positron emission tomography for functional mapping involves injecting a radioactive tracer, usually ^{15O}water, during the performance of both a behavioral task of interest and a control task. When brain areas are activated by a given task, there is a consequent increase in local cerebral blood flow. By comparing tracer uptake during the two conditions on a voxel-by-voxel basis, it is possible to make inferences about which regions are activated by performance of the task. PET may also be used to quantify resting or ictal metabolic activity; for these purposes a radioisotope with a longer half-life such as 18-fluorodeoxy glucose (FDG) is used.

The physiologic basis and methodology of PET are analogous to those of fMRI. In comparison with fMRI, however, PET has a relatively poor signal-to-noise ratio (SNR). That is, the signal of interest is only minimally distinguishable from background activity, or noise, generally requiring averaging of scans across multiple subjects or sessions in order to make a statistically significant observation about task-driven increases in metabolic activity for a given brain region. This low SNR makes PET a poor method for the presurgical mapping of an individual patient. Additionally, the spatial and temporal resolution of PET is only moderate. PET also requires the injection of radioactive tracers, making it an invasive procedure. This restricts the number and duration of PET scans on the same subject in order to avoid excessive radiation exposure and makes PET unsuitable in children and certain other populations.

Certain limitations intrinsic to PET constrain its use as a method to map complex task-related brain function. Since PET depends on the systemic distribution, half-life, and metabolic binding of its radioligand to its target pathway, PET is limited to examining those functions that can be sustained for several minutes, giving it very poor temporal resolution. The spatial resolution of PET is also quite limited owing to camera limitations and SNR-imposed limits on voxel size. Despite these limitations, PET has been used, and continues to be used, in many studies of brain function in both healthy subjects and patients. The extensive experience with PET as an activation test of brain function has also aided in the rapid development of fMRI as a technique owing to similarities in study design, analysis, statistical methodology, and interpretation (*see* fMRI section next).

PET has been used successfully in many brain mapping studies including investigation of somatosensory and motor function, vision, language *(35)*, and memory and learning *(36–38)*. Patient studies have investigated the effects of various pathological conditions (e.g., Alzheimer's disease *[39–41]*) as well as changes that accompany recovery of function *(42–44)*. PET has been used to perform preoperative mapping of primary somatosensory motor cortex, language areas, and visual cortex *(45)*. However, because of the aforementioned limitations, PET has generally been supplanted by fMRI in preoperative evaluation of eloquent cortex.

PET may also be used to examine metabolic abnormalities for the preoperative determination of seizure onset localization using FDG PET to quantify glucose metabolism *(46,47)*. Interictally, regions of relative hypometabolism correlate highly with areas of epileptogenic tissue. The high sensitivity of PET is able to detect areas of hypometabolism that appear structurally normal on MRI and that may even demonstrate no histopathological abnormalities after resection. Ictal studies involve injecting the radioligand during a seizure, which may demonstrate hypermetabolism (although single-photon emission tomography [SPECT] is more commonly used in this setting owing to its relative simplicity). In the presurgical evaluation of candidates for epilepsy surgery, FDG PET data are combined with clinical information, scalp EEG, and structural MRI (1) to detect the appropriate side for anterior temporal lobectomy, (2) to select intracranial areas for microelectrode recording or grid placement if extracranial EEG provides insufficient localizing evidence, and (3) to establish the prognosis for seizure control following anterior temporal lobectomy *(48,49)*.

Functional Magnetic Resonance Imaging

fMRI is an emerging noninvasive brain mapping technique. It has been used extensively in cognitive science to study the brain basis of neurologic processes and is becoming more integrated into clinical practice as methodological issues are resolved and experience is accumulated across multiple centers. A major difference between fMRI (or PET) studies and IAT, intraoperative ECS, and TMS is that the former are tests of activation with certain tasks, whereas the latter are based on performance failure during brain inactivation. Inactivation tests are the standard for presurgical planning because they mimic the effects of surgical resection. Unfortunately, except for TMS, these techniques are highly invasive. Also, inactivation tests are not as amenable to the study of normal physiology or to task specificity as activation tests. Moreover, they do not allow detailed information to be available prior to surgery. Other issues include the inability to investigate the sulcal depths as well as underlying white matter tracts. fMRI has the potential to provide useful information on all these fronts non-invasively and preoperatively. Validation of the utility and accuracy of fMRI activation tasks in surgical planning is a major goal of fMRI research efforts.

Technique

Functional MRI localizes neural activity by measuring its correlate, regional cerebral blood flow. The most commonly used technique is blood oxygen level-dependent (BOLD) contrast imaging. When brain regions are activated during the performance of any activity, a neurally mediated vasodilation of capillaries and postcapillary venules occurs. This results in a relative increase in the ratio of oxygenated to deoxygenated hemoglobin owing to blood flow oversupply relative to increased neuronal utilization of oxygen *(50)*. Because of the different magnetic properties of deoxyhemoglobin (paramagnetic) and oxyhemoglobin (diamagnetic), it is possible to measure these changes as alterations in the BOLD signal intensity on T2*-weighted images *(51,52)*. Pixels whose signal intensity varies with the timing of stimulus presentation (with appropriate hemodynamic delay) represent activation by the task *(53,54)*. Statistical inferences are made using correlation coefficients, statistical parametric mapping (SPM), or other methods to find those areas whose activity varies with the task paradigm. This information may then be overlaid on anatomic images forming functional maps. fMRI has spatial and temporal resolution far in excess of Wada or PET studies, particularly when using high field strengths *(55)*. Moreover, fMRI is noninvasive and readily repeatable, as opposed to cortical stimulation testing. Patients can be studied sequentially, allowing the impact of surgery or other intervention to be assessed.

An alternative fMRI technique, known as perfusion imaging, detects changes in blood flow via a contrast *(56)* or spin-tagged bolus *(57)*. Contrast-based techniques are relatively quick to perform, but require the injection of contrast material and are therefore not completely noninvasive. Spin-labeling techniques have the advantage of providing absolute blood flow values, which are being used for certain specific applications but are quite time consuming. Perfusion-based techniques have the advantages of being both highly specific and less sensitive to motion artifact than BOLD. However, because of decreased sensitivity compared with BOLD, their use is limited to mapping areas with very strong intrinsic signal such as the motor cortex. Postprocessing for motion correction and statistics are similar to those of BOLD imaging. Perfusion imaging is affected by tumor vascularity and enhancement caused by blood–brain barrier breakdown. These effects are the basis for using these techniques to assess tumor histology, but the use of perfusion techniques for functional mapping in tumor patients may be confounded by these unknown effects *(58)*.

Although many centers have all the necessary equipment to perform, analyze, and present fMRI studies, there are sufficiently complex issues of methodology to warrant caution, perspective, and rigorous quality control when implementing a new clinical fMRI program. fMRI can be performed on standard 1.5-T (or less) clinical MRI scanners. Higher field strengths such as the 3-T scanners currently being installed in some research and clinical facilities yield higher SNRs, allowing shorter scan times, more investigations, or better spatial resolution. The addition of faster gradients can allow faster acquisition times, thereby increasing signal or providing finer temporal resolution. As mentioned above, fMRI maps cortical function by measuring blood flow changes induced by neuronal activation in response to specific tasks. Thus the design and presentation of these task paradigms are vital to the success of the fMRI localization for a given function.

Currently, fMRI analysis is highly labor intensive, requiring personnel specially trained to administer the functional test paradigms, acquire the fMRI data, and perform data transfer and analysis. Functional MRI datasets are also very large, typically occupying up to a gigabyte or more of memory per study, so fMRI analysis also requires significant dedication of computer hardware and memory space. Turnkey software is being developed, but currently most data analysis is performed with a combination of freely available software (e.g., SPM *[59]*), commercial packages, and programs developed in-house. Finally, the interpretation of fMRI results requires an understanding of the fairly sophisticated statistical analyses required to process the data in addition to an understanding of the fMRI acquisition protocol, behavioral paradigms, and the patient's clinical status.

ADVANTAGES

Functional MRI holds great promise for noninvasive mapping of the human brain in vivo. Unlike PET, fMRI is both noninvasive and readily repeatable. This can allow multiple investigations to map several brain functions fully, to investigate changes in brain activity under different conditions (e.g., medications) or to study the recovery process. Compared with PET, fMRI has a significantly higher SNR, allowing statistically powerful mapping of a single subject as required of a presurgical evaluation *(60)*. fMRI data can also be combined with diffusion tensor imaging (DTI) of white matter tracts in and around lesions, allowing the visualization not only of the areas of cortical activation but also of the white matter tracts functionally connecting them to other areas (*see* the Diffusion Tensor Imaging section following for more information on DTI). In the future, fMRI may allow nonoperative and minimally invasive approaches to a variety of neurological problems by refining targeting of destructive lesions (e.g., radiosurgery, focused ultrasound, or radiofrequency ablation) and stimulation or neuromodulating procedures.

CHALLENGES

fMRI has its own limitations. As fMRI localizes neural activity by measuring its correlate, regional cerebral blood flow, findings may be affected by the many physiologic variables that influence cerebral perfusion or neurovascular coupling. Many of these variables remain to be studied, such as the effects of medications, changes occurring with normal aging, metabolic abnormalities, and the effect of mass lesions. Such limitations have so far limited the acceptance of fMRI in the clinical realm. Applying fMRI to neurosurgical problems also presents an opportunity to test directly the correlations between brain activity and the fMRI signal. Therefore, efforts to validate fMRI against the gold standard of intraoperative ECS are extremely important.

Surprisingly complex issues arise when one is performing, interpreting, and applying fMRI studies in a clinical setting *(61)*. The complexity and resultant questions increase as one progresses from mapping relatively straightforward motor areas to less well understood cognitive areas. Outstanding questions and challenges include the following:

1. *Interpretation of activations.* There may be multiple areas outside the conventionally designated eloquent cortex that respond to a particular behavioral paradigm. It is unclear how to differentiate areas that *participate* in a task from areas that are *required* for the performance of this task. For example, whereas the cingulate gyrus has shown activation in a wide variety of cognitive paradigms including language production *(62)*, resection of this structure does not result in a corresponding deficit. How to interpret this type of activation from a surgical planning standpoint may be unclear.
2. *Validity.* The precision of the spatial localization obtained by fMRI is still being studied and is probably affected by many patient variables. There are growing numbers of reports comparing fMRI and cortical mapping. However, these studies frequently define activations as much as 10 mm apart as "overlapping," even though this is a significant distance when one is trying to determine the limits of surgical resection. Krings et al. *(63)* sought to validate fMRI by comparing motor hand maps produced using four functional mapping techniques: PET, TMS, ECS, and fMRI. The fMRI maps strongly correlated with the maps produced by these other techniques; ECS-derived and fMRI maps fell within 1 cm of each other in 31 of 49 subjects and were neighboring (<2 cm) in 14 of 49. In the remaining patients, fMRI maps were uninterpretable because of low SNR or motion artifact *(63)*. Several studies have examined the potential alterations in the somatotopic arrangement of the motor homunculus patients with tumors impinging on this area. fMRI reliably predicted cortical areas for hand and foot activation determined at the time of surgery by ECS from 82 to 92% of the time *(64,65)*.
3. *Reliability.* Whether results obtained from fMRI studies are reproducible and reliable has significant implications for both its scientific and clinical applications. Whereas there is good evidence that on a group level activations associated with a given cognitive task are stable across institutions *(66)* and sessions *(67)*, significant questions remain regarding the intrasubject reliability of given activations *(68,69)*. A study of intersession differences concluded that a single fMRI study session provides only a snapshot in time of brain activation *(68)*. As more data are acquired across several sessions, the certainty of activation of particular voxels increases. Another study indicated it may require approximately five sessions to achieve good statistical certainty *(70)*.
4. *Statistical thresholding.* Functional maps derived from fMRI studies represent statistical probabilities that voxels are activated by a given task. This means, among other interpretation caveats, that the extent of activation will vary according to the statistical threshold is used. The significance threshold that corresponds in extent to the functional cortex found at operation by cortical mapping is dependent on the individual and cannot be predicted *(71)*. When one is planning surgical resections immediately adjacent to eloquent cortex, the issue of how far to carry the resection depends critically on the extent of active cortex (Fig. 1; *see* Color Plate 1 following p. 112).
5. *Influence of lesion type.* Another important issue that merits further investigation is the effect of different types of lesions on the function maps generated by fMRI. It is reasonable to suppose that the functionality of adjacent brain will be different in infiltrative vs displacing lesions. Schreiber et al. *(72)* examined the alterations in fMRI maps for hand function in glial and nonglial space-occupying lesions. Motor cortex activation ipsilateral to nonglial lesions increased by 14%, in contrast to a 36% decrease with infiltrating gliomas. Their observations support the conclusion that gliomatous infiltration significantly alters cerebral hemodynamics and/or cor-

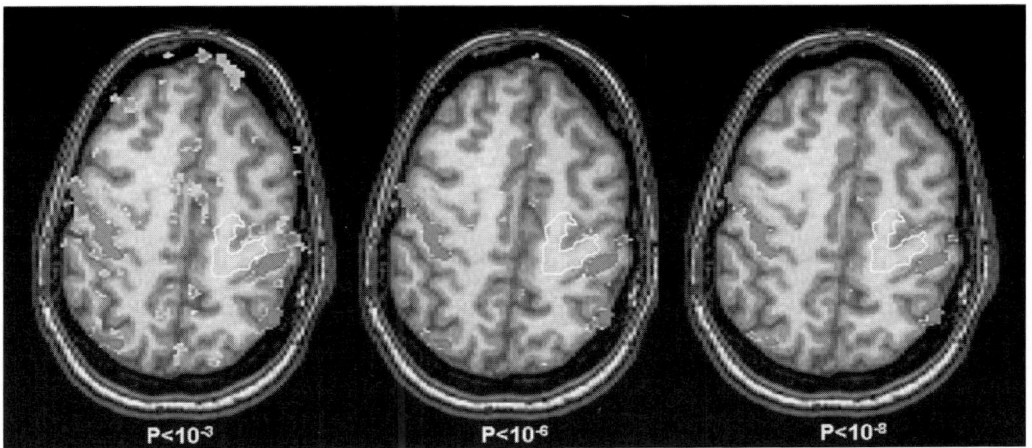

Fig. 1. Statistical maps of fMRI activation during a motor task in a patient with a low-grade lesion (yellow outline) involving the precentral area demonstrate the effect of varying the statistical threshold. As the threshold is made more stringent, the number of pixels exceeding the threshold diminishes, and the activation shown appears to shrink away from the tumor margin. (Courtesy of Drs. Lawrence Panych and Seung-Schik Yoo, Brigham and Women's Hospital Department of Radiology. See Color Plate 1 following p. 112.)

tical function, whereas nonglial lesions tend to displace but not destroy cortical neurons (72). Krings et al. (73) compared alterations in fMRI activation among tumor patients with varying degrees of hand weakness. They observed significant decreases in activation proportional to the severity of hand paresis but increases in the secondary motor areas remote from the tumor. They concluded that tumor tissue can interfere with cerebral hemodynamics and/or neural activity (73).

6. *Selection of task paradigm.* The choice and execution of a task paradigm as well as its associated "rest" condition will greatly affect the resultant activations. For simple motor mapping, true rest is probably an appropriate baseline task, but when exploring cognitive processes the choice of an appropriate baseline task becomes much more complex. In an auditory listening task to map language, for example, a resting baseline would result in more activation in areas such as the auditory cortex, which are outside of primary language areas. In comparison, the use of a high-level baseline listening task such as listening to nonlinguistic stimuli would result in less activations in areas participating in nonlanguage auditory processing. Another critically important determinant of success in any fMRI study of patients is that they be asked to perform tasks that they are *capable* of performing (74). E.g., if a patient has a hemiparesis that interferes with his or her ability to perform a finger-tapping task, then any results from the study may be invalid.

Behavioral Protocols

The BOLD signal change associated with task activation averages 2% increase from background activation or noise. Therefore, to produce statistically significant observations, one must typically acquire and compare several sets of images ranging from 100 to more than 300 scans of the region of interest. For preoperative mapping and patient studies, the most common task paradigms use a block design in which activation tasks alternate with rest periods. This series is repeated through several cycles for an acquisition time of 3–10 min. A functional run may be repeated to increase SNR, or other functions may be investigated during typical fMRI scanning protocols, which last up to an hour. Block designs are generally used because they have excellent SNR, are easy for patients who may have cognitive or motor abnormalities to understand and to perform, and are fairly unaffected by changes in the hemodynamic response to neural activation *(75)*. In addition, these types of studies are fairly straightforward to analyze, in contrast to some of the complex single-trial techniques gaining acceptance in cognitive science research.

These parameters limit the types of tasks that can be used for fMRI analysis to simple tasks that are discrete and repeatable. Most subjects are unable to tolerate sustaining the task/rest paradigm for extended periods, so fMRI scanning sessions tend to be limited to studying only one or two discrete functions. Because fMRI is highly sensitive to motion artifact that can irreparably corrupt data acquisition, tasks must be limited to activity that does not produce significant head movement. Most simple motor tasks below the shoulders do not interfere with BOLD acquisition (but see ref. 76, which suggests that there is measurable head movement with motor tasks and that it may be worse in patient populations). Any tasks associated with movements of the face and tongue can produce corrupting movement and artifact. This restriction on movement limits the usefulness of fMRI for speech testing to subvocal language generation, which does not allow for monitoring of patient performance and also may not engage all the cortical areas involved in overt speech production. It also complicates the comparison of fMRI studies with ECS for the purposes of validating fMRI in language studies, as ECS mapping necessarily uses speech performance and speech arrest as end points. However, several groups are developing techniques that overcome the difficulties associated with the use of overt speech generation *(77,78)*.

Current Applications

Motor and Somatosensory: A few studies in small numbers of patients have demonstrated good concordance between fMRI localization of primary motor and somatosensory cortices and cortical stimulation *(63,79–85)*. Krings et al. *(63)* compared motor activation maps produced by various functional imaging techniques (fMRI, PET, TMS, and ECS) in an effort to describe the relative accuracy of each method. They found that out of 50 patients, only 1 had fMRI-localized areas of activation, which contradicted the areas of activation demonstrated using these other techniques. In a separate study, the same group described difficulties with fMRI functional mapping encountered during this group's extensive experience (194 patients over 3 yr) with patient mapping *(86)*. They report that fMRI mapping identified the motor regions in 85% of all investigated paradigms and only 11% failed to show fMRI activation. They further report that motion artifact was the most common reason for fMRI failure and that motor tasks involving the proximal limbs were more likely to produce such artifact than were tasks involving distal muscles. Interestingly, they also found that motion artifact correlated with the degree of paresis, implying that those patients who are most severely affected neurologically might be more difficult to map successfully.

Pujol et al. *(87)* report similar observations: they found selective and reproducible fMRI patterns of activation in 82% of 42 patients with space-occupying lesions. Of the 22 patients who proceeded to surgery, a 100% correspondence was found between the fMRI areas of activation and those identified by ECS. They failed to identify the central sulcus in 18% of these cases owing to damage to the primary sensorimotor region caused by the patients' lesions; this was correlated with the severity of hand paresis.

Atlas et al. *(82)* examined areas of activation surrounding gliomatous lesions compared with the contralateral side in such a way as to be able to demonstrate alterations in fMRI patterns of activation produced by tumor infiltration. They found displacement and decreased volumes of activation compared with the unaffected hemisphere. In an attempt to develop and validate improved methods of fMRI mapping in patients whose activation maps might be altered by brain pathology, Hirsch et al. *(84)* developed and tested an integrated battery of fMRI tasks in 63 healthy control subjects and 125 tumor patients. Sensitivity, as defined by the ability of specific tasks to activate the target regions, was 100% for motor cortex in control subjects. However, for patients harboring tumors, these figures were somewhat lower. As would be expected, both patients and controls demonstrated higher sensitivity in those cortical areas that are highly localized such as sensorimotor areas. Further work is needed to validate fMRI against the gold standard of cortical mapping in the more complex area of the supplementary motor cortex and to determine whether fMRI may provide additional information not available from cortical stimulation.

VISION

Functional MRI has been used extensively in neuroscience studies to map primary and secondary visual areas. Primary visual areas can be robustly activated by photic stimulation *(88)*, flashing checkerboard patterns, or other simple or complex visual stimuli. Preoperative mapping, although not commonly employed in this area, can provide a clear map of the retinotopic architecture of the striate cortex. Perhaps even more useful will be the development of DTI localization of the optic radiations in the temporal and parietal lobes.

LANGUAGE

The ability to define language areas accurately preoperatively is an important determinant of surgery for various pathological processes in both the frontal and temporal lobes. fMRI has been used both to lateralize *(89–96)* and to localize *(82,84,97–101)* eloquent language areas in the brain, to compare these techniques with the IAT, and to awake intraoperative cortical mapping.

Lateralization studies thus far have found excellent, although not constant, agreement between the two modalities (Fig. 2; *see* Color Plate 2 following p. 112). The most complex and difficult to interpret cases are those in which there is incomplete dominance with bilateral representation. To date, there is no consensus on which types of language paradigms (e.g., silent word generation, semantic tasks, reading, auditory comprehension) and analysis methods (e.g., lateralization

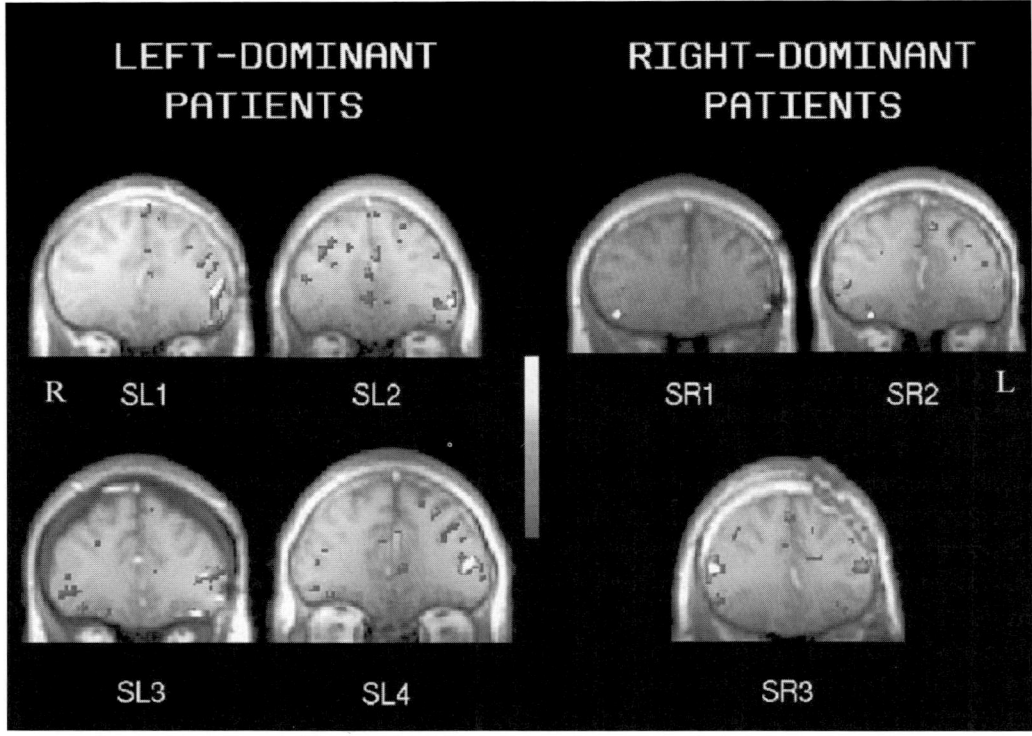

Fig. 2. Validation of fMRI as a clinical tool for assessing language lateralization and localization. Seven patients, previously Wada tested to assess hemispheric language dominance, were scanned in an fMRI experiment while they performed alternating semantic and nonsemantic tasks. fMRI lateralization was consistent with the Wada test results in all patients. The figure illustrates one coronal section for each patient, with the left side of the brain depicted on the right side of the section. Voxels depicted in the red–yellow color scale represent regions of the brain in which the semantic task produced statistically significantly greater activation than did the nonsemantic task. (From Desmond et al. [1995], ref. 91, by permission of Oxford University Press. *See* Color Plate 2 following p. 112.)

indices for the whole hemisphere vs for just Broca's area, maximum correlation values vs number of active voxels or extent) are most valid, reliable, and practical.

The few existing studies of language *localization* demonstrate that these paradigms are less robust than motor mapping *(84)* and also that the most valid results will probably be obtained with methods that combine several complementary behavioral paradigms *(101)*. These studies include only small numbers of patients who have undergone both fMRI and intraoperative language mapping and, like the lateralization studies, demonstrate very good, but not exact, agreement with intraoperative findings. Before fMRI can replace awake craniotomy, larger patient series will have to be performed, standardized techniques developed, and systematic study of the effect of patient variables undertaken. Nevertheless, presently, fMRI of language areas can serve as an adjunct to intraoperative mapping, allowing informed surgical decisions and directed cortical mapping.

MEMORY

The study of memory processes with fMRI has proved quite challenging, even in healthy subjects. One reason for this difficulty is that memory-encoding systems are believed to be almost continually engaged in encoding new events into memory, thereby making the isolation of these processes with comparison to an appropriate baseline task difficult. In addition, memory is not a unified process but rather a series of processes including encoding, storage, and retrieval, each of which are necessary for normal memory performance. Failure in any one of these domains will result in a clinical deficit on memory testing.

Despite these obstacles, the determination of memory lateralization and localization is an important clinical goal. Indeed, because of the relative difficulty of testing memory processes from both a behavioral and anatomic standpoint, the development of preoperative and noninvasive methods is particularly important. Moreover, memory changes, particularly of verbal memory, in patients undergoing dominant temporal lobectomy, remain one of the most perplexing and difficult to avoid postoperative neuropsychiatric complications (102).

To date, there have only been a few studies comparing fMRI with the IAT in the assessment of memory lateralization in patients with MTL epilepsy. Using a scene-encoding task, Detre et al. (103) found that activation asymmetries in the MTL concurred with IAT-determined memory competence in all cases, including two cases in which memory was paradoxically located ipsilateral to the seizure focus. In another study, Bellgowan et al. (104) reported that MTL activation during a verbal encoding task can differentiate between patients with left (L) MTLE and right (R) MTLE. They found that RMTLE patients had LMTL activation during verbal encoding but that LMTLE patients did not. However, these findings were on the group level only and do not allow inferences to be made on an individual subject basis. Moreover, interpretation of a lack of activation, rather than an altered pattern of activation, can be problematic as there can be many technical reasons for not finding activations.

Golby et al. (105) studied the lateralization of encoding of different types of stimuli by fMRI compared with the IAT. Using a novelty encoding paradigm that investigated memory for stimuli varying in their capacity to be verbalized (faces, scenes, designs, and words), fMRI and IAT lateralization were concordant in eight of nine MTLE patients. They also demonstrated the reorganization on a group level of material-specific memory to the contralateral temporal lobe: patients with LMTLE activated the *right* MTL during verbal encoding (Fig. 3; *see* Color Plate 3 following p. 112), whereas healthy control subjects and patients with RMTLE normally activated the *left* MTL during verbal encoding. In the future, these types of studies may allow the quantification of surgical risk to memory and the potential tailoring of medial temporal resection. fMRI may also be useful in predicting postoperative seizure outcome. Killgore et al. (106) have found that when combined, fMRI and IAT provided complementary data that resulted in improved prediction of postoperative seizure control compared with either procedure alone.

Further studies using this and other paradigms will be necessary to determine whether the amount of functional reorganization can be quantified and whether

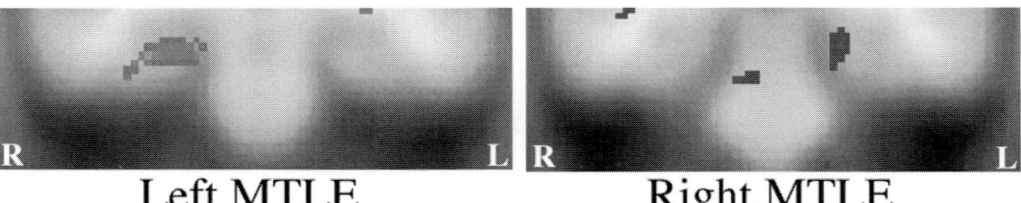

Fig. 3. Patients with left and right mesial temporal lobe epilepsy (MTLE) were studied with fMRI during encoding of various stimuli. The figure presents statistical maps of group-level activation during word encoding for the two groups. Patients with right MTLE activate the left hippocampal region during language encoding, similar to healthy control subjects (not shown). Patients with left-sided MTLE, however, have activation in the right hippocampal region during word encoding consistent with reorganization of material-specific verbal encoding processes to the contralateral MTL. (*See* Color Plate 3 following p. 112.)

this is predictive of postoperative outcome. Moreover, these studies appear to be particularly challenging to administer, analyze, and interpret and will require significant modification before they can become part of a routine preoperative evaluation. For example, as part of a protocol attempting to use fMRI comprehensively to test several neurologic functions, Deblaere et al. *(78)* were able to demonstrate anterior hippocampal activation in only four of nine subjects.

Diffusion Tensor Imaging

Injury to the white matter tracts connecting the motor, somatosensory, visual, and language cortices causes significant neurological deficits similar to injuries involving the corresponding cortex. To achieve the goal of maximal safe resection while preserving neurologic function, knowledge of white matter tract location and the relationship to a lesion is as important as defining the lesion's relationship with eloquent cortical areas. However, conventional structural MRI does not provide information on the location of white matter tracts and their relationship to the lesion.

The trajectory and location of white matter tracts can be detected by means of anisotropic DTI. This imaging method is based on measuring the diffusion of water protons in the cerebral white matter. The cerebral white matter consists of a network of tightly packed fiber tracts with different orientations. Owing to the cell membranes and myelin sheaths, water proton diffusion is facilitated parallel to the fibers and restricted perpendicular to them. It follows that by imaging water proton diffusion, one can obtain an image of these structures depicting both their orientation and possible alteration by pathologic processes *(107)*. Theoretically, three types of lesion/fiber tract interactions may occur: fiber tract displacement, fiber tract infiltration, and fiber tract destruction. In our experience with DTI, all three scenarios have been encountered, isolated or in combination (Fig. 4; *see* Color Plate 4 following p. 112). Each of these is likely to be associated

Functional Brain Mapping Options

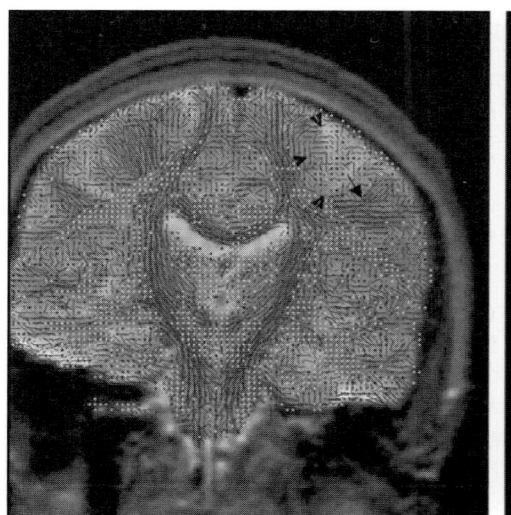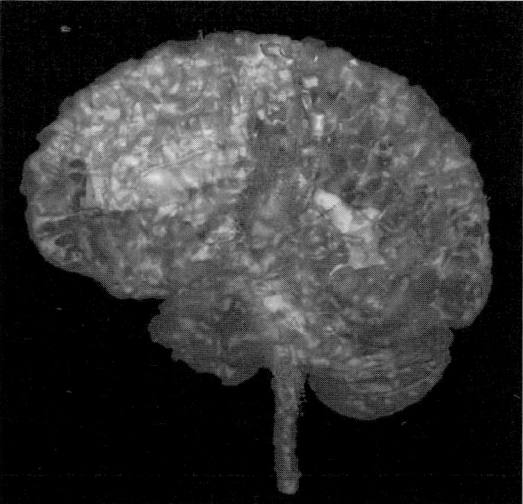

Fig. 4. Diffusion tensor imaging of white matter tracts in a patient with a low-grade glioma demonstrates disruption of white matter tracts in the supplementary motor area by the tumor (arrowheads). Left panel shows a 2D representation displaying tensors. Right panel presents a 3D rendering showing tumor in green, functional activation in yellow and tractography of the corticospinal tract in red. (Courtesy of Dr. Ian-Florin Talos, Brigham and Women's Hospital, Department of Radiology. *See* Color Plate 4 following p. 112.)

with different consequences if fiber tracts are disrupted during surgery. Recent work has demonstrated the ability to trace the corticospinal tract and its relation to the brain tumor *(108)*. By combining DTI with fMRI it is possible to demonstrate both a particular functional area and its connections to other areas.

FUTURE DIRECTIONS

Techniques such as fMRI and TMS, which do not require craniotomy, will be essential for the further development of less invasive techniques for treating neurosurgical disease. For instance, in order to perform endovascular, radiosurgical, or focused ultrasound procedures safely in the vicinity of eloquent cortex, an accurate preprocedure map is necessary. Therefore, the development of diagnostic brain mapping techniques should proceed in parallel to the development of new therapeutic techniques. Certainly, we can anticipate that the combination of more refined understanding of individual functional anatomy and less invasive techniques will open up entirely new avenues of neurosurgical treatment. One intriguing possibility is the use of imaging techniques to target the site of functional neurosurgical procedures. For example, the ongoing investigations into the neural basis of chronic pain may allow the further refinement of neurosurgical procedures for the treatment of pain. Already, fMRI has been used noninvasively to refine the target for epidural primor motor stimulation in the treatment of pain *(109)*.

CONCLUSIONS

There has been a tremendous recent increase in the options and techniques available for functional brain mapping. It is important that any clinicians who rely on the results of functional imaging studies be aware of the strengths and weakness of the various modalities. An important consideration is the fundamental differences between studies based on the disruption of neural activity (inactivation studies) and those that demonstrate brain activation related to a particular behavior (activation studies). Further considerations include the resolution (both spatial and temporal), reliability, validity, invasiveness, and repeatability of each method. There are now an unprecedented variety of choices in functional mapping modalities that can be used to augment, and in some cases replace, more conventional invasive procedures. Combining complementary modalities will minimize each method's weaknesses while maximizing the amount and quality of useful information available to the neurosurgeon. The continued development and refinement of functional brain mapping will provide the road map to allow the application of new minimally invasive therapeutic techniques.

REFERENCES

1. Wada J, Rasmussen T. Intracarotid injection of sodium amytal for the lateralization of cerebral speech dominance: experimental and clinical observations. *J Neurosurg* 1960;17:226–282.
2. Jones-Gotman M. Commentary: psychological evaluation-testing hippocampal function, in *Surgical Treatment of the Epilepsies* (Engel J Jr, ed.), Raven, New York, 1987, pp. 203–211.
3. Dodrill CB, Ojemann GA. An exploratory comparison of three methods of memory assessment with the intracarotid amobarbital procedure. *Brain Cogn* 1997;33: 210–223.
4. Loring D, Lee G, Meador K, Flanigin H, Smith J. The intracarotid amobarbital procedure as a predictor of memory failure following unilateral temporal lobectomy. *Neurology* 1990;40:605–610.
5. Hankey GJ, Warlow CP, Sellar RJ. Cerebral angiographic risk in mild cerebrovascular disease. *Stroke* 1990;21:209–222.
6. Hessel SJ, Adams DF, Abrams HL. Complications of angiography. *Radiology* 1981; 138:273–281.
7. Haglund MM, Berger MS, Shamseldin M, Lettich E, Ojemann GA. Cortical localization of temporal lobe language sites in patients with gliomas. *Neurosurgery* 1994;34:567–576; discussion 576.
8. Cosgrove GR, Buchbinder BR, Jiang H. Functional magnetic resonance imaging for intracranial navigation. *Neurosurg Clin N Am* 1996;7:313–322.
9. Hamer H and Morris H. Indications for invasive video-electroencephalographic monitoring, in *Epilepsy Surgery* (Luders HO, Comair YG, eds.), Lippincott Williams & Wilkins, Philadelphia, 2001, pp. 559–566.
10. Mueller WM and Morris GL, 3rd. Intraoperative and extraoperative identification of eloquent brain using stimulation mapping. *Neurosurg Clin N Am* 1993;4: 217–222.
11. Bohning D. Introduction and overview of TMS physics, in *Transcranial Magnetic Stimulation in Neuropsychiatry* (George M, Belmaker R, eds.), American Psychiatric Press, Washington, DC., 2000, pp. 13–44.

12. Krings T, Naujokat C, von Keyserlingk DG. Representation of cortical motor function as revealed by stereotactic transcranial magnetic stimulation. *Electroencephalogr Clin Neurophysiol* 1998;109:85–93.
13. Boroojerdi B, Foltys H, Krings T, Spetzger U, Thron A, Topper R. Localization of the motor hand area using transcranial magnetic stimulation and functional magnetic resonance imaging. *Clin Neurophysiol* 1999;110:699–704.
14. Krings T, Buchbinder BR, Butler WE, et al. Stereotactic transcranial magnetic stimulation: correlation with direct electrical cortical stimulation. *Neurosurgery* 1997;41:1319–1325; discussion 1325–1326.
15. Krings T, Foltys H, Reinges MH, et al. Navigated transcranial magnetic stimulation for presurgical planning—correlation with functional MRI. *Minim Invasive Neurosurg* 2001;44:234–239.
16. Michelucci R, Valzania F, Passarelli D, et al. Rapid-rate transcranial magnetic stimulation and hemispheric language dominance: usefulness and safety in epilepsy. *Neurology* 1994;44:1697–700.
17. Epstein CM. Transcranial magnetic stimulation: language function. *J Clin Neurophysiol* 1998;15:325–332.
18. Epstein CM, Woodard JL, Stringer AY, et al. Repetitive transcranial magnetic stimulation does not replicate the Wada test. *Neurology* 2000;55:1025–1027.
19. Sparing R, Mottaghy FM, Hungs M, et al. Repetitive transcranial magnetic stimulation effects on language function depend on the stimulation parameters. *J Clin Neurophysiol* 2001;18:326–330.
20. Knecht S, Floel A, Drager B, et al. Degree of language lateralization determines susceptibility to unilateral brain lesions. *Nat Neurosci* 2002;5:695–699.
21. Pizzella V and Romani G. Principles of Magnetoencephalography, in *Advances in Neurology: Magnetoencephalography* (Sato S, ed.), Raven, New York, 1990, pp. 1–9.
22. Fagaly R. Neuromagnetic instrumentation, in *Advances in Neurology: Magnetoencephalography* (Sato S, ed.), Raven, New York, 1990, pp. 11–32.
23. Minassian BA, Otsubo H, Weiss S, Elliott I, Rutka JT, Snead OC 3rd. Magnetoencephalographic localization in pediatric epilepsy surgery: comparison with invasive intracranial electroencephalography. *Ann Neurol* 1999;46:627–633.
24. Wheless JW, Willmore LJ, Breier JI, et al. A comparison of magnetoencephalography, MRI, and V-EEG in patients evaluated for epilepsy surgery. *Epilepsia* 1999;40:931–941.
25. Mamelak A, Lopez N, Akhtari M, Sutherling W. Magnetoencephalography-directed surgery in patients with neocortical epilepsy. *J Neurosurgery* 2002;97:865–873.
26. Lewine J, Orrison W, Halliday A, et al. Magnetoencephalography: functional imaging in epilepsy, in *Neuroimaging in Epilepsy: Principles and Practice* (Cascino G, and J. CR Jack JCR, eds.), Butterworth-Heinemann, Boston, 1996, pp. 193–207.
27. Rezai AR, Hund M, Kronberg E, et al. The interactive use of magnetoencephalography in stereotactic image-guided neurosurgery. *Neurosurgery* 1996;39:92–102.
28. Orrison WW Jr. Magnetic source imaging in stereotactic and functional neurosurgery. *Stereotact Funct Neurosurg* 1999;72:89–94.
29. Gallen CC, Bucholz R, Sobel DF. Intracranial neurosurgery guided by functional imaging. *Surg Neurol* 1994;42:523–530.
30. Gallen CC, Schwartz BJ, Bucholz RD, et al. Presurgical localization of functional cortex using magnetic source imaging. *J Neurosurg* 1995;82:988–994.
31. Kamada K, Takeuchi F, Kuriki S, Oshiro O, Houkin K, Abe H. Functional neurosurgical simulation with brain surface magnetic resonance images and magnetoencephalography. *Neurosurgery* 1993;33:269–272; discussion 272–273.

32. Rezai AR, Hund M, Kronberg E, et al. Introduction of magnetoencephalography to stereotactic techniques. *Stereotact Funct Neurosurg* 1995;65:37–41.
33. Sutherling WW, Crandall PH, Darcey TM, Becker DP, Levesque MF. Barth DS, The magnetic and electric fields agree with intracranial localizations of somatosensory cortex. *Neurology* 1988;38:1705–1714.
34. McDonald J, Chong B, Lewine J, et al. Integration of preoperative and intraoperative functional brain mapping in a frameless stereotactic environment for lesions near eloquent cortex. *J Neurosurg* 1999;90:591–598.
35. Leblanc R, Meyer E, Bub D, Zatorre RJ, Evans AC. Language localization with activation positron emission tomography scanning. *Neurosurgery* 1992;31:369–373.
36. Dolan RJ and Fletcher PC, Dissociating prefrontal and hippocampal function in episodic memory encoding. *Nature* 1997;388:582–585.
37. Tulving E, Markowitsch HJ, Craik FE, Habib R, Houle S. Novelty and familiarity activations in PET studies of memory encoding and retrieval. *Cereb Cortex* 1996;6:717–719.
38. Haxby JV. Medial temporal lobe imaging [news; comment]. *Nature* 1996;380:669–670.
39. Backman L, Andersson JL, Nyberg L, Winblad B, Nordberg A, Almkvist O. Brain regions associated with episodic retrieval in normal aging and Alzheimer's disease. *Neurology* 1999;52:1861–1870.
40. Mielke R and Heiss WD. Positron emission tomography for diagnosis of Alzheimer's disease and vascular dementia. *J Neural Transm Suppl* 1998;53:237–250.
41. Tohgi H, Yonezawa H, Takahashi S, et al. Cerebral blood flow and oxygen metabolism in senile dementia of Alzheimer's type and vascular dementia with deep white matter changes. *Neuroradiology* 1998;40:131–137.
42. Imahori Y, Fujii R, Kondo M, Ohmori Y, Nakajima K. Neural features of recovery from CNS injury revealed by PET in human brain. *Neuroreport* 1999;10:117–121.
43. Heiss WD, Kessler J, Thiel A, Ghaemi M, Karbe H. Differential capacity of left and right hemispheric areas for compensation of poststroke aphasia. *Ann Neurol* 1999;45:430–438.
44. Calautti C, Leroy F, Guincestre JY, Marie RM, Baron JC. Sequential activation brain mapping after subcortical stroke: changes in hemispheric balance and recovery. *Neuroreport* 2001;12:3883–886.
45. Viñas FC, Zamorano L, Mueller RA, et al. [^{15}O]-water PET and intraoperative brain mapping: a comparison in the localization of eloquent cortex. *Neurol Res* 1997;19:601–608.
46. Duncan JS. Imaging and epilepsy. *Brain* 1997;120:339–377.
47. Hajek M, Antonini A, Leenders KL, Wieser HG. Mesiobasal versus lateral temporal lobe epilepsy: metabolic differences in the temporal lobe shown by interictal 18F-FDG positron emission tomography. *Neurology* 1993;43:79–86.
48. Manno EM, Sperling MR, Ding X, et al. Predictors of outcome after anterior temporal lobectomy: positron emission tomography. *Neurology* 1994;44:2331–2336.
49. Radtke RA, Hanson MW, Hoffman JM, et al. Temporal lobe hypometabolism on PET: predictor of seizure control after temporal lobectomy. *Neurology* 1993;43:1088–1092.
50. Fox PT and Raichle ME. Focal physiological uncoupling of cerebral blood flow and oxidative metabolism during somatosensory stimulation in human subjects. *Proc Natl Acad Sci USA* 1986;83:1140–1144.
51. Kwong KK, Belliveau JW, Chesler DA, et al. Dynamic magnetic resonance imaging of human brain activity during primary sensory stimulation. *Proc Natl Acad Sci USA* 1992;89:5675–5679.

52. Ogawa S, Lee TM, Nayak AS, Glynn P. Oxygenation-sensitive contrast in magnetic resonance imaging of rodent brain at high magnetic fields. *Magn Reson Med* 1990;14:68–78.
53. Detre JA, Leigh JS, Williams DS, Koretsky AP. Perfusion imaging. *Magn Reson Med* 1992;23:37–45.
54. Bandettini PA, Wong EC, Hinks RS, Tikofsky RS, Hyde JS. Time course EPI of human brain function during task activation. *Magn Reson Med* 1992;25:390–397.
55. Gati J, Menon R, Ugurbil K, Rutt B. Experimental determination of the BOLD field strength dependence in vessels and tissue. *Magn Reson Med* 1997;38:296–302.
56. Rosen BR, Belliveau JW, Vevea JM, Brady TJ. Perfusion imaging with NMR contrast agents. *Magn Reson Med* 1990;14:249–265.
57. Barbier EL, Silva AC, Kim SG, Koretsky AP. Perfusion imaging using dynamic arterial spin labeling (DASL). *Magn Reson Med* 2001;45:1021–1029.
58. Essig M, Wenz F, Scholdei R, et al. Dynamic susceptibility contrast-enhanced echo-planar imaging of cerebral gliomas. Effect of contrast medium extravasation. *Acta Radiol* 2002;43:354–359.
59. Neurology WDoC, *SPM99*, London, 1990.
60. Toga A, Ojemann G, Ojemann J, Cannestra A. Intraoperative brain mapping, in *Brain Mapping: The Methods* (Toga A, Mazziotta J, Frackowiak R, eds.), Academic, New York, 1996, pp. 75–105.
61. Desmond J and Chen S. Ethical issues in the clinical application of fMRI: factors affecting the validity and interpretation of activations. *Brain Cogn* 2002;50:482–497.
62. Cabeza R and Nyberg L. Imaging cognition: an empirical review of PET studies with normal subjects. *J. Cogn. Neurosci.* 1997;9:1–265.
63. Krings T, Schreckenberger M, Rohde V, et al. Metabolic and electrophysiological validation of functional MRI. *J Neurol Neurosurg Psychiatry* 2001;71:762–771.
64. Fandino J, Kollias SS, Wieser HG, Valavanis A, Yonekawa Y. Intraoperative validation of functional magnetic resonance imaging and cortical reorganization patterns in patients with brain tumors involving the primary motor cortex. *J Neurosurg* 1999;91:238–250.
65. Lehericy S, Duffau H, Cornu P, et al. Correspondence between functional magnetic resonance imaging somatotopy and individual brain anatomy of the central region: comparison with intraoperative stimulation in patients with brain tumors. *J Neurosurg* 2000;92:589–298.
66. Casey BJ, Cohen JD, O'Craven K, et al. Reproducibility of fMRI results across four institutions using a spatial working memory task. *Neuroimage* 1998;8:249–261.
67. Noll DC, Genovese CR, Nystrom LE, et al. Estimating test-retest reliability in functional MR imaging. II: Application to motor and cognitive activation studies. *Magn Reson Med* 1997;38:508–517.
68. McGonigle DJ, Howseman AM, Athwal BS, Friston KJ, Frackowiak RS, Holmes AP. Variability in fMRI: an examination of intersession differences. *Neuroimage* 2000;11:708–734.
69. Yoo S, Wei X, Dickey C, et al. Evaluation of reproducibility in sensorimotor activation: long-term fMRI study, in *ISMRM, 10th Scientific Meeting and Exhibition*, Honolulu, 2002.
70. Maitra R, Roys SR, Gullapalli RP. Test-retest reliability estimation of functional MRI data. *Magn Reson Med* 2002;48:62–70.
71. Roux FE, Ibarrola D, Tremoulet M, et al. Methodological and technical issues for integrating functional magnetic resonance imaging data in a neuronavigational system. *Neurosurgery* 2001;49:1145–1156; discussion 1156–1157.

72. Schreiber A, Hubbe U, Ziyeh S, Hennig J. The influence of gliomas and nonglial space-occupying lesions on blood- oxygen-level-dependent contrast enhancement. *AJNR Am J Neuroradiol* 2000;21:1055–1063.
73. Krings T, Topper R, Willmes K, Reinges MH, Gilsbach JM, Thron A. Activation in primary and secondary motor areas in patients with CNS neoplasms and weakness. *Neurology* 2002;58:381–390.
74. Price CJ and Friston KJ. Scanning patients with tasks they can perform. *Hum Brain Mapp* 1999;8:102–108.
75. Carusone LM, Srinivasan J, Gitelman DR, Mesulam MM, Parrish TB. Hemodynamic response changes in cerebrovascular disease: implications for functional MR imaging. *AJNR Am J Neuroradiol* 2002;23:1222–1228.
76. Seto E, Sela G, McIlroy WE, et al. Quantifying head motion associated with motor tasks used in fMRI. *Neuroimage* 2001;14:284–297.
77. Huang J, Carr TH, Cao Y. Comparing cortical activations for silent and overt speech using event-related fMRI. *Hum Brain Mapp* 2002;15:39–53.
78. Deblaere K, Backes WH, Hofman P, et al. Developing a comprehensive presurgical functional MRI protocol for patients with intractable temporal lobe epilepsy: a pilot study. *Neuroradiology* 2002;44:667–673.
79. Krings T, Buchbinder BR, Butler WE, et al. Functional magnetic resonance imaging and transcranial magnetic stimulation: complementary approaches in the evaluation of cortical motor function. *Neurology* 1997;48:1406–1416.
80. Mueller WM, Yetkin FZ, Hammeke TA, et al. Functional magnetic resonance imaging mapping of the motor cortex in patients with cerebral tumors. *Neurosurgery* 1996;39:515–520; discussion 520–521.
81. Puce A, Comparative assessment of sensorimotor function using functional magnetic resonance imaging and electrophysiological methods. *J Clin Neurophysiol* 1995;12:450–459.
82. Atlas SW, Howard RSd, Maldjian J, et al. Functional magnetic resonance imaging of regional brain activity in patients with intracerebral gliomas: findings and implications for clinical management. *Neurosurgery* 1996;38:329–338.
83. Roux FE, Ranjeva JP, Boulanouar K, et al. Motor functional MRI for presurgical evaluation of cerebral tumors. *Stereotact Funct Neurosurg* 1997;68:106–111.
84. Hirsch J, Ruge MI, Kim KH, et al. An integrated functional magnetic resonance imaging procedure for preoperative mapping of cortical areas associated with tactile, motor, language, and visual functions. *Neurosurgery* 2000;47:711–21; discussion 721–722.
85. Kober H, Nimsky C, Moller M, Hastreiter P, Fahlbusch R, Ganslandt O, Correlation of sensorimotor activation with functional magnetic resonance imaging and magnetoencephalography in presurgical functional imaging: a spatial analysis. *Neuroimage* 2001;14:1214–1228.
86. Krings T, Reinges MH, Erberich S, et al. Functional MRI for presurgical planning: problems, artefacts, and solution strategies. *J Neurol Neurosurg Psychiatry* 2001; 70:749–760.
87. Pujol J, Conesa G, Deus J, Lopez-Obarrio L, Isamat F, Capdevila A, Clinical application of functional magnetic resonance imaging in presurgical identification of the central sulcus. *J Neurosurg* 1998;88:863–869.
88. Fried I, Nenov VI, Ojemann SG, Woods RP. Functional MR and PET imaging of rolandic and visual cortices for neurosurgical planning. *J Neurosurg* 1995;83: 854–861.
89. Gerschlager W, Lalouschek W, Lehrner J, Baumgartner C, Lindinger G, Lang W. Language-related hemispheric asymmetry in healthy subjects and patients with

temporal lobe epilepsy as studied by event-related brain potentials and intracarotid amobarbital test. *Electroencephalogr Clin Neurophysiol* 1998;108:274–282.

90. Binder JR, Swanson SJ, Hammeke TA, et al. Determination of language dominance using functional MRI: a comparison with the Wada test. *Neurology* 1996; 46:978–984.
91. Desmond JE, Sum JM, Wagner AD, et al. Functional MRI measurement of language lateralization in Wada-tested patients. *Brain* 1995;118:1411–149.
92. Benson RR, FitzGerald DB, LeSueur LL, et al. Language dominance determined by whole brain functional MRI in patients with brain lesions. *Neurology* 1999; 52:798–809.
93. Ramsey NF, Sommer IE, Rutten GJ, Kahn RS. Combined analysis of language tasks in fMRI improves assessment of hemispheric dominance for language functions in individual subjects. *Neuroimage* 2001;13:719–733.
94. Lehericy S, Cohen L, Bazin B, et al. Functional MR evaluation of temporal and frontal language dominance compared with the Wada test. *Neurology* 2000;54: 1625–1633.
95. Hertz-Pannier L, Gaillard WD, Mott SH, et al. Noninvasive assessment of language dominance in children and adolescents with functional MRI: a preliminary study. *Neurology* 1997;48:1003–1012.
96. Hund-Georgiadis M, Lex U, von Cramon DY. Language dominance assessment by means of fMRI: contributions from task design, performance, and stimulus modality. *J Magn Reson Imaging* 2001;13:668–675.
97. Benson RR, Logan WJ, Cosgrove GR, et al. Functional MRI localization of language in a 9-year-old child. *Can J Neurol Sci* 1996;23:213–219.
98. Stapleton SR, Kiriakopoulos E, Mikulis D, et al. Combined utility of functional MRI, cortical mapping, and frameless stereotaxy in the resection of lesions in eloquent areas of brain in children. *Pediatr Neurosurg* 1997;26:68–82.
99. Tomczak RJ, Wunderlich AP, Wang Y, et al. fMRI for preoperative neurosurgical mapping of motor cortex and language in a clinical setting. *J Comput Assist Tomogr* 2000;24:927–934.
100. Fernandez G, de Greiff A, von Oertzen J, et al. Language mapping in less than 15 minutes: real-time functional MRI during routine clinical investigation. *Neuroimage* 2001;14:585–594.
101. Rutten GJ, Ramsey NF, van Rijen PC, Noordmans HJ, van Veelen CW. Development of a functional magnetic resonance imaging protocol for intraoperative localization of critical temporoparietal language areas. *Ann Neurol* 2002;51:350–360.
102. Rausch R. Epilepsy surgery within the temporal lobe and its short-term and long-term effects on memory. *Curr Opin Neurol* 2002;15:185–189.
103. Detre JA, Maccotta L, King D, et al. Functional MRI lateralization of memory in temporal lobe epilepsy. *Neurology* 1998;50:926–932.
104. Bellgowan PS, Binder JR, Swanson SJ, et al. Side of seizure focus predicts left medial temporal lobe activation during verbal encoding. *Neurology* 1998;51: 479–484.
105. Golby AJ, Poldrack RA, Illes J, Chen D, Desmond JE, Gabrieli JD. Memory lateralization in medial temporal lobe epilepsy assessed by functional MRI. *Epilepsia* 2002;43:855–863.
106. Killgore WD, Glosser G, Casasanto DJ, French JA, Alsop DC, Detre JA. Functional MRI and the Wada test provide complementary information for predicting postoperative seizure control. *Seizure* 1999;8:450–455.
107. Mamata H, Mamata Y, Westin CF, et al. High-resolution line scan diffusion tensor MR imaging of white matter fiber tract anatomy. *AJNR Am J Neuroradiol* 2002;23: 67–75.

108. Holodny AI, Ollenschleger MD, Liu WC, Schulder M, Kalnin AJ. Identification of the corticospinal tracts achieved using blood-oxygen-level-dependent and diffusion functional MR imaging in patients with brain tumors. *AJNR Am J Neuroradiol* 2001;22:83–88.
109. Sol J, Casaux J, Roux F, et al. Chronic motor cortex stimulation for phantom limb pain: correlations between pain relief and functional imaging studies. *Stereotact Funct Neurosurg* 2001;77:172–176.

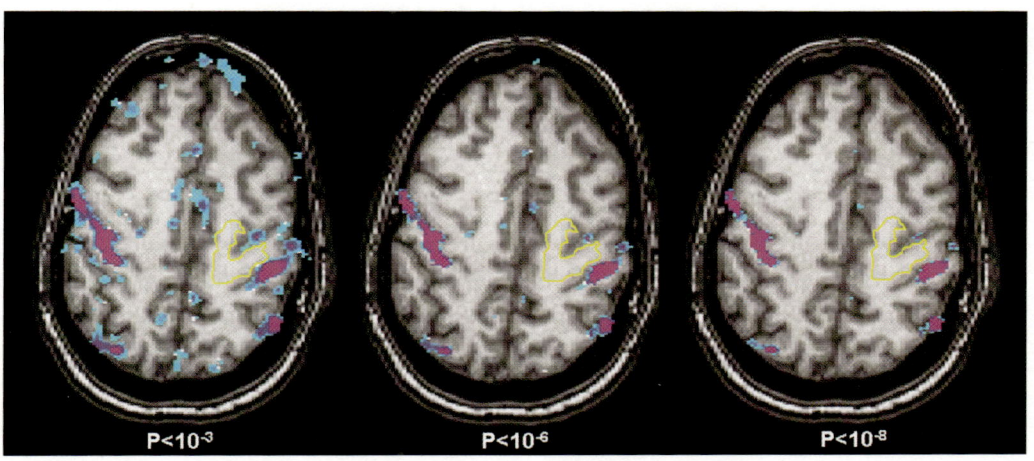

Color Plate 1, Fig. 1, Chapter 4. Statistical maps of fMRI activation demonstrate effect of varying the threshold. (*See* full caption on p. 99 and discussion on p. 98.)

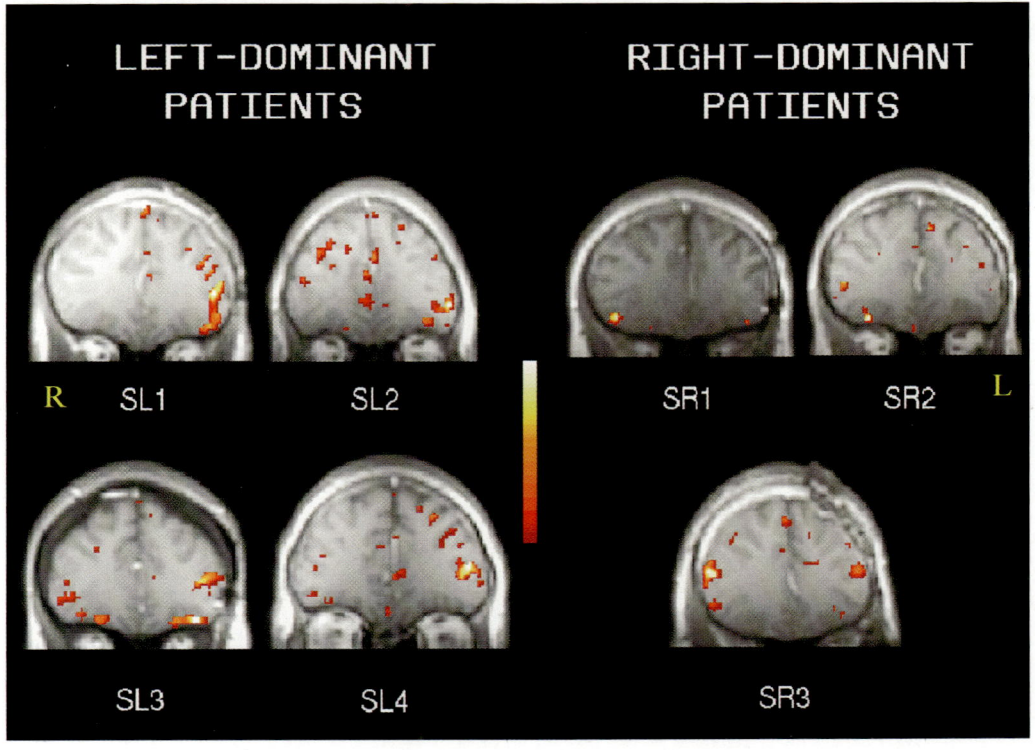

Color Plate 2, Fig. 2, Chapter 4. Validation of fMRI as a clinical tool for assessing language lateralization and localization. (*See* full caption on p. 102 and discussion on pp. 101–102. By permission of Oxford University Press.)

Word encoding activation

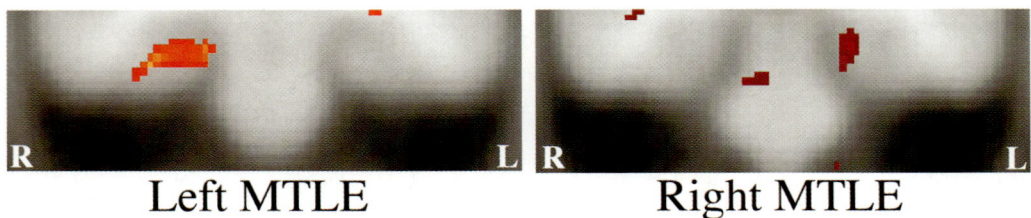

Left MTLE   Right MTLE

Color Plate 3, Fig. 3, Chapter 4. fMRI studies of patients with left and right MTLE encoding various stimuli. (*See* full caption on p. 104 and discussion on p. 103.)

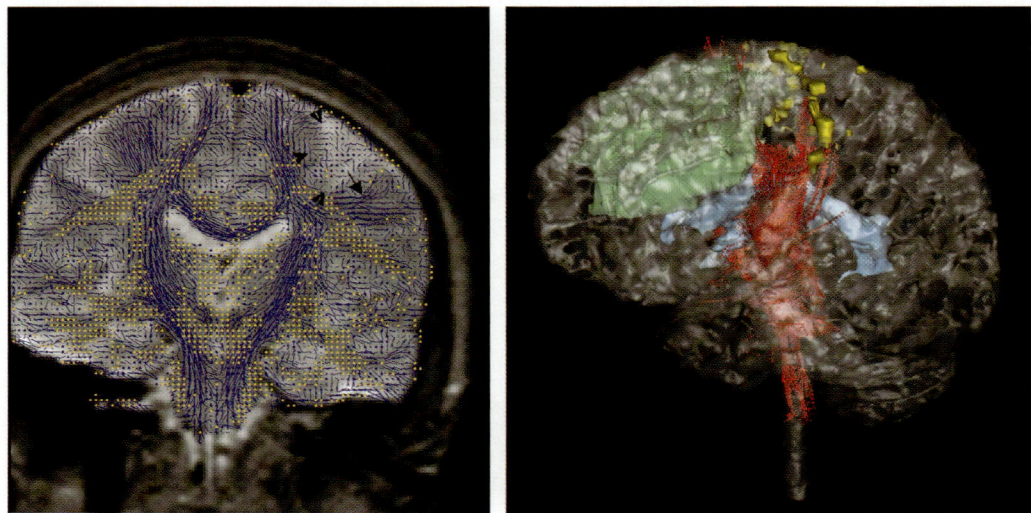

Color Plate 4, Fig. 4, Chapter 4. Diffusion tensor imaging of white matter tracts in low-grade glioma. (*See* full caption on p. 105 and discussion on p. 104. Courtesy of Dr. Ian-Florin Talos.)

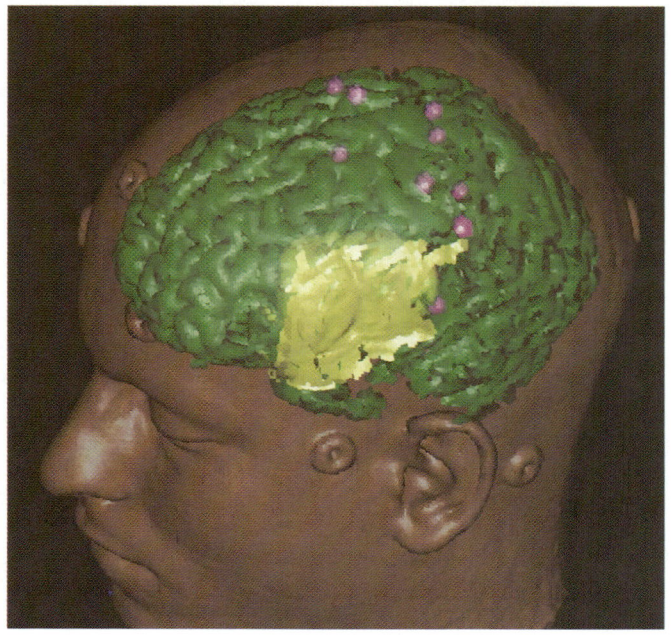

Color Plate 5, Fig. 5, Chapter 5. Computer model showing magnetoencephalography. (*See* full caption on p. 124 and discussion on p. 123.)

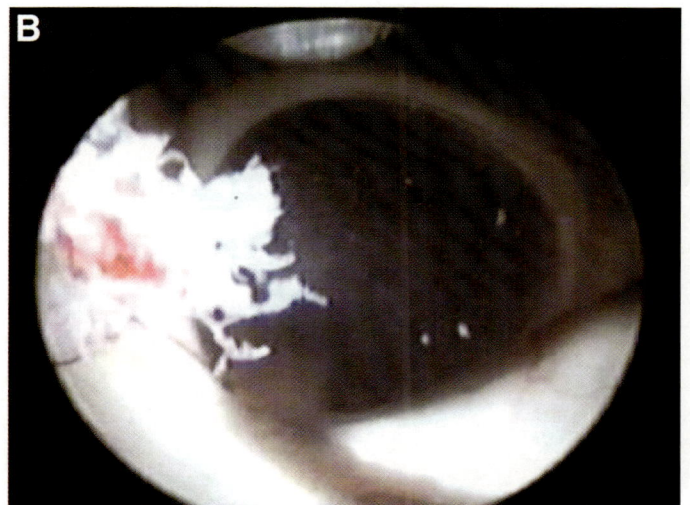

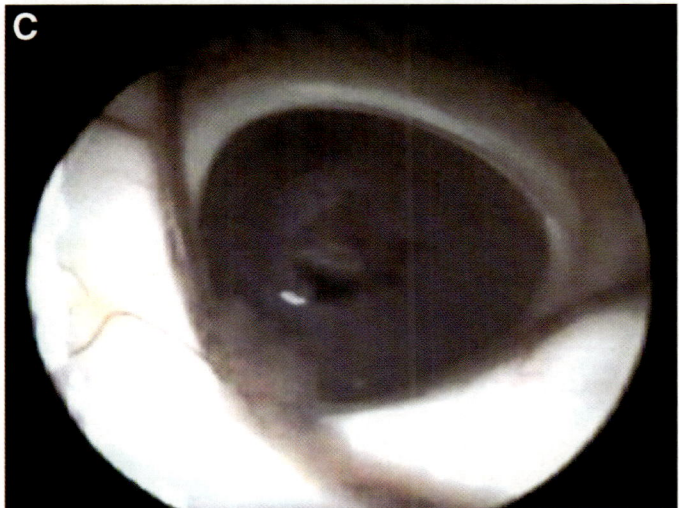

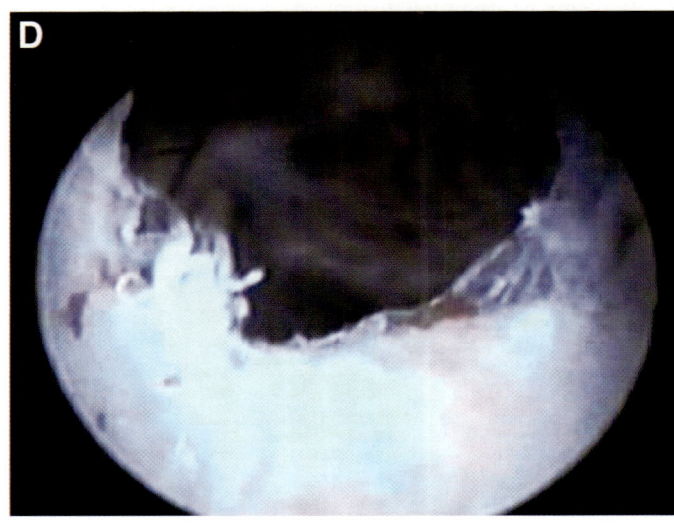

Color Plate 6, Fig. 1, Chapter 15. MRI series of fenestration of large suprasellar cyst. (*See* full caption on p. 324 and discussion on p. 323. Courtesy of Dr. Liliana Goumnerova.)

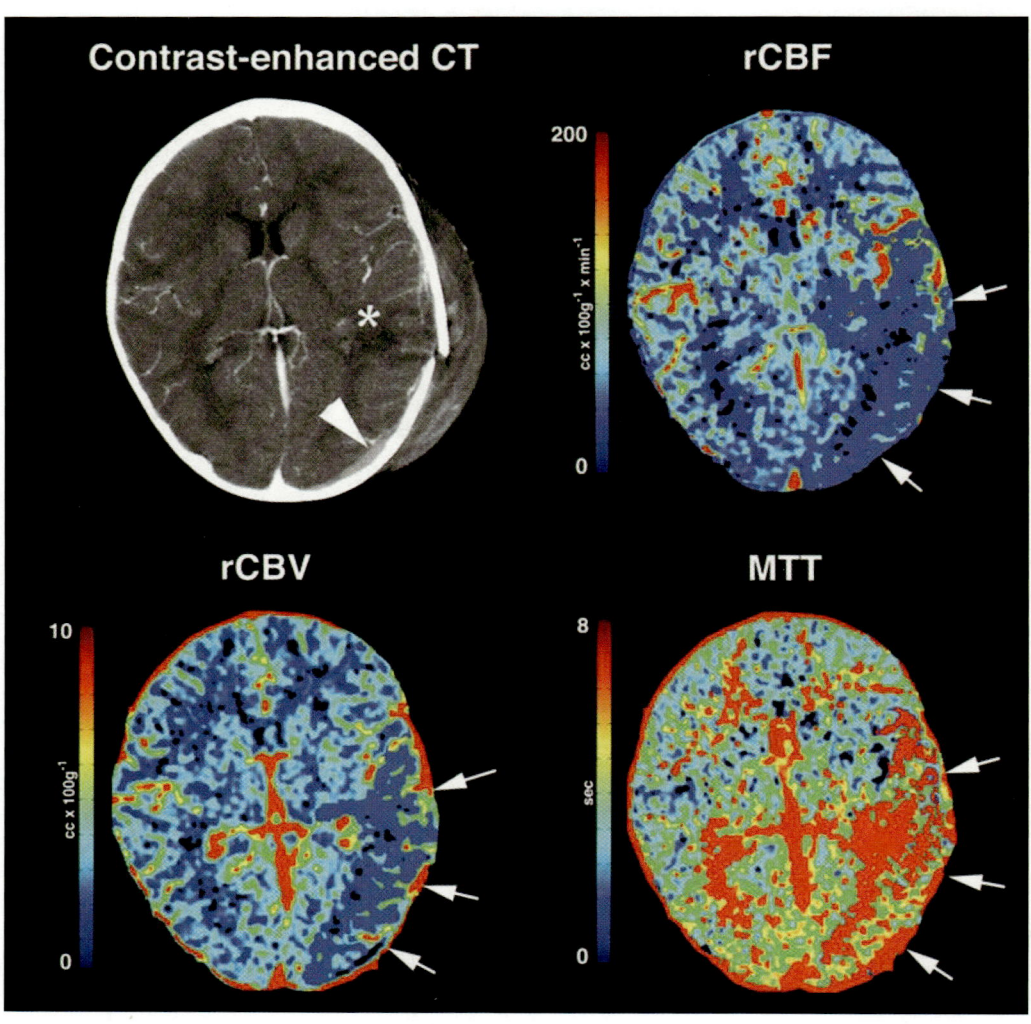

Color Plate 7, Fig. 5, Chapter 20. Comparison of perfusion-CT and conventional studies of patient with Glasgow Coma Scale score of 9. (*See* complete caption and discussion on pp. 409,410.)

5
Image Guidance in Minimally Invasive Neurosurgery

Richard D. Bucholz, MD, FACS and Lee McDurmont, BS

INTRODUCTION

Surgeons deal with an unavoidable conflict on a daily basis. As physicians, they are bound by the Hippocratic oath to first avoid doing any harm to their patients. However, the very act of surgery implies an exposure of the internal anatomy of the patient and cannot be performed without inflicting harm to tissues superficial to the surgical target. To justify inflicting such harm, a surgeon must balance damage done by the possible good done for the patient and proceed only if the benefit exceeds the damage done. In effect, a surgeon can remain true to the oath if the patient experiences no net harm after the procedure has been performed. Viewed in this fashion, the external tissues are not only a barrier to exposure but also present the rate-limiting step for many interventions, as the harm done to these tissues during exposure may rule out the marginal benefit of many procedures.

In order to increase the number of conditions justifiably treated by surgery, it is to be expected that surgeons actively pursue methods to minimize harm. The development of anesthesia, for example, was a pivotal development, in that the pain and suffering of an awake procedure limited surgery to only the most dire and life-threatening situations; even in those extreme situations, surgery had to be of the most basic sort, as finesse and refinement would only come at an unacceptable cost of prolonging the agony for the patient. The advent of anesthesia was therefore a powerful enabling technology that vastly increased the utilization of surgery in the treatment of disease throughout the body. More recently, the technology of endoscopy has greatly increased the number of procedures performed by diverse surgical specialists, as the diminished invasiveness of endoscopic procedures justifies surgery in medically fragile patients, or in patients in which the benefit may be questionable, and therefore the prolonged recuperation of a traditional, open procedure is not justified. Many knee arthroscopies are performed, for example, in patients who would never consider undergoing the risk of open knee surgery.

To further the cause of noninvasiveness, one must understand why surgery, by nature, requires invasiveness. Surgery differs from medical interventions in

From: *Minimally Invasive Neurosurgery,* edited by: M.R. Proctor and P.M. Black © Humana Press Inc., Totowa, NJ

that the pathology is exposed to allow direct intervention or alteration, as opposed to indirect intervention through the use of medication. In order to reach the pathology, the surgeon must recognize, and become oriented to, the patient's anatomy en route to the target structure, so as not to veer off course and cause collateral damage to surrounding tissue. Once at the target pathology, to allow definitive treatment, a specific amount of exposure is needed to treat the lesion. Surgical invasiveness is therefore the result of two needs: orientation with respect to normal anatomy and sufficient exposure of abnormal anatomy so as to ensure definitive treatment. For the purposes of this chapter, the first need will be called visualization and the second therapeutic access.

It is easy to see how image-guided surgery, which employs high-resolution images of a patient's anatomy to navigate the course of a procedure, would prove helpful in decreasing the invasiveness required to obtain visualization during the course of a procedure. Less obvious, but perhaps even more powerful, is the ability of image guidance to permit a therapeutic intervention with minimal invasiveness using a technology that requires less access. To examine how image-guided surgery enhances the cause of minimal invasiveness, it is useful to review the history of the field and reach an understanding of the forces that helped develop instrumentation to its current state.

Somewhat surprisingly, image guidance has its beginnings in the field of stereotaxis, which actually initially *increased* the invasiveness of surgery through the use of stereotactic frames. These devices, bolted to the head prior to imaging, allowed the use of preoperative images for navigation by registering the images to the surgical field, a process discussed in more detail in the Registration section next. Frames developed specifically for cranial applications with current imaging modalities include the Brown-Roberts-Wells (BRW) system, for use with computed tomography (CT) *(1)* (Fig. 1), and the Leksell frame as adapted for use with magnetic resonance imaging (MRI) *(2)*. Such frames were painful when applied to the patient, prolonged the interventional procedure by coupling surgery to the act of imaging, and could hardly be considered as anything but invasive. Widespread use of image guidance did not occur until alternative means for registering images to surgery became easily available. These techniques, which can be gathered together under the concept of registration, are a major source of error in image guidance and are key issues when one is considering the overall desirability of image guidance for a particular patient.

This chapter reviews how image guidance can allow minimally invasive techniques to proliferate and also addresses modern methods that reduce the invasiveness of image guidance itself. As the role of image guidance is still evolving, the organization of this chapter reflects current developments that employ this technique in the three surgical necessities that require invasiveness: registration, visualization, and therapeutic access.

REGISTRATION

The process of registration consists of the establishment of a rigid relationship between two coordinate systems: that by which the images were obtained

Imaging Guidance

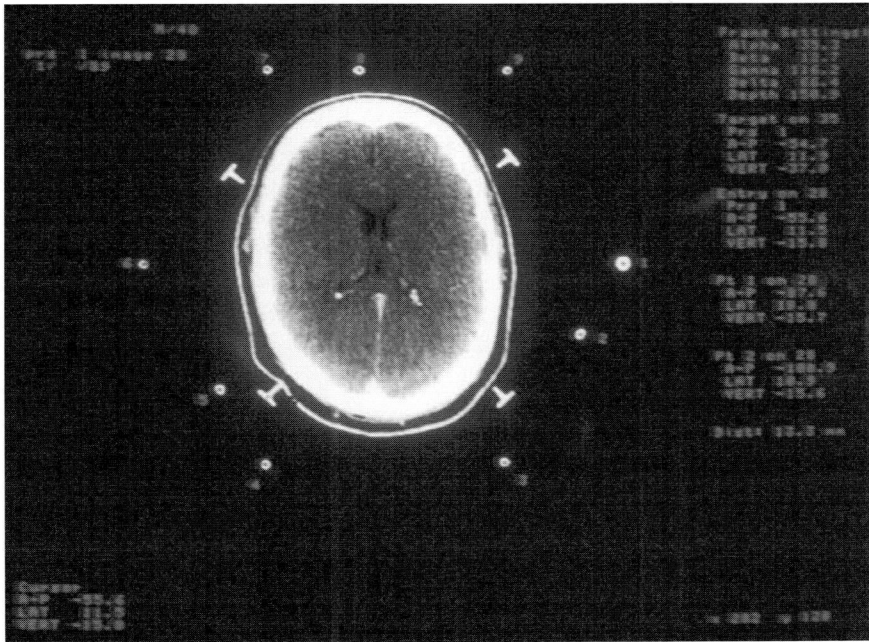

Fig. 1. Computer registration of the rods of a BRW frame visualized in CT imaging.

and that superimposed on the surgical field. Once images have become registered to the patient, the surgeon can translate from any point on the patient to the same point on the images, and vice versa, using a transformation matrix dictated by the registration process. This process, easily allowed by computers, permits the surgeon to plan a procedure on the preoperative images and superimpose the plan onto the patient's anatomy. In this fashion, registration can be viewed as a Rosetta Stone that allows translation between the 3D space of the images (a virtual space) and the anatomical structure of the patient (a real space).

By its very nature, image guidance requires registration in order to render the images of the patient's anatomy useful to the surgeon. Registration can be performed by a number of different methods, and, as with all factors relating to surgery, there is a tradeoff between accuracy and ease of use. Easier methods are, as a rule, less accurate; highly accurate methods are more difficult to employ and are generally more invasive for the patient. Furthermore, registration methods can require significant computational ability and therefore were not feasible prior to the introduction of computers into the operating room. As even the most computationally complex registration algorithms are easily performed by standard computers available today, computational demands will not be taken into consideration in the following discussion. This requirement for computer power for registration did, however, limit image guidance in its early history to devices that required little in the way of computer power. These simpler and more traditional methods are familiar to many neurosurgeons, who often regard them as being inherently more accurate. However, it is important to realize that traditional methods are not necessarily more accurate because they are less complex. Computationally demanding registration techniques, even those not immediately comprehensible by the surgeon, may actually afford greater accuracy compared with traditional techniques. The intense use of computation power does not imply that a process is inherently less accurate, and accuracy can only be determined by a rigorous study of accuracy in side-by-side comparisons of two registration techniques.

The most direct registration method involves the use of intraoperative imaging. By taking an image in the operating room, with a surgical instrument or implant in place, one can immediately check suitability of position without resorting to any computational method or registration technique; the image literally speaks for itself. Employed in this way, intraoperative imaging has been used to reduce the invasiveness of many procedures, including the use of fluoroscopy during transsphenoidal pituitary surgery *(3)*, placement of intracranial electrodes *(4)*, breast needle biopsies *(5)*, and minimally invasive spine surgery *(6)*. The vast majority of experience with intraoperative imaging involves fluoroscopy, given its ready availability and ease of use. A major limitation of intraoperative fluoroscopy is its inherently 2D nature (the same limitation also being applicable to ultrasound) and the tissue contrast of the images obtained. Even though a rough appreciation of location in three dimensions can be obtained by taking a matching pair of images obtained approximately orthogonal to one other, precise 3D localization is not possible with standard fluoroscopy. Furthermore, fluoroscopy is in general useless for determining location relative to soft tissue targets, as the soft tissue contrast of this imaging modality is very limited. As a result, there has been considerable interest in using inherently 3D imaging techniques intraoperatively.

A few centers have used intraoperative CT but have found this technique to be useful only for localization of radiologically detectable structures such as bone or implants, as the ability of CT to detect soft tissue is almost as impaired as that associated with fluoroscopy *(7)*. This has motivated a significant research effort into the use of intraoperative MRI, using modified scanners that allow access to the patient, scanners that allow the patient to be moved into the scanner, or miniature scanners that can be placed about the head of the patient. This considerable variation in approach, with some centers using high-field magnets *(8)* and other centers using magnets with far weaker field strengths, specifically designed for use in the operative situation *(9)*, indicates that no consensus has been reached as to the most useful intraoperative MRI device (*see* Chapter 6).

Regardless of the technology used, it should be noted that imaging does not occur simultaneously with surgery. Instead, a preliminary set of scans is obtained for guidance, and then surgery is performed, followed by a second course of imaging, which is analyzed to decide what further surgery should be performed. The serial nature of this process interrupts the normal flow of surgery to accommodate imaging, which increases the overall duration of surgery and thus has the unintended effect of increasing the invasiveness (in terms of anesthesia time) of the procedure. In addition, as the position of the instrumentation needs to be related to the images taken in the operating room, some form of tracking mechanism is mandatory. The technique of tracking is usually identical to the means employed by image guidance systems used for navigation with preoperative images. As long as the use of these navigational systems is required, there is no reason that preoperative images could not be employed as well, especially if they convey information not easily obtained in the operating room, such as functional localization. Furthermore, the quality of intraoperative imaging, particularly with the lower strength magnets, is almost invariably inferior to images obtained with purely diagnostic machines. Therefore, most systems provide some means of relating the intraoperative images to the preoperative diagnostic studies to allow enhanced interpretation. As has been experienced with fluoroscopy, the quality of imaging used for therapy does not have to match the quality of images used for diagnosis.

Alternatively, if only preoperative images are to be used, some form of registration is needed. When stereotactic surgery was first employed, computational capabilities were limited, and registration was obtained by making the coordinate systems of the images and the operating room identical *(10)*. This was accomplished by attaching a frame to the patient's anatomy, which established the plane of origin of the preoperative images. A localizer was attached to this frame that produced marks in the images obtained and established the coordinate system of the frame within the images. The technique became more extensively employed when 3D imaging techniques, such as CT, became available. As early tomographic devices had inaccuracies in their stepping procedures between subsequent scans, the localizers employed were modified with the addition of redundant image markers, called fiducials, that allowed the precise orientation of each scan in relation to each of the other images and the frame itself *(11)*. The redundancy of this marking system, added to the rigid nature of the attachment of the frame to the head, led to a reasonably accurate registration technique that had the additional benefit of holding the patient stable during both imaging and surgery. This rigidity makes these systems preferable even today when one is dealing with uncooperative or confused patients. However, the need to have the frame and localizer in position during imaging made the routine use of stereotaxis very difficult, and few surgeons availed themselves of the accuracy of these systems.

In the late 1980s two developments allowed the use of less invasive registration methods for image guidance. First, CT scanners were improved in their ability to step accurately in the z-dimension between scans. Second, computational capabilities sufficiently inexpensive to be used routinely in the operating room became available to translate instantaneously between two coordinate systems arranged at random angles and displacements with respect to each other. By introducing at least three points in the images, which have to be clearly seen on the imaging modality employed, point fiducials can be employed to replace the redundant fiducials of framed systems. If these points are then touched in the operating room with a device that could precisely determine position in 3D space (a device called a 3D digitizer), the second set of coordinates can be paired with the position of the same fiducials on the images to produce a translational matrix. Increasing the number and spacing of point fiducials generally results in improved accuracy. Important assumptions inherent in such a process are that the fiducials would approximate as close as possible a point in 3D space and that the relative position of the fiducials with respect to the underlying anatomy does not vary between the process of imaging and the end of the surgical procedure.

This technique allows the easy dissemination of stereotactic technique to almost all intracranial procedures. A major concern remains the technique of attaching the fiducials to the patient. As many procedures do not require high accuracy, a common technique is to use self-adhesive fiducials applied to the scalp. Given the mobility of the scalp, the need for a rigid relationship between the fiducials to each other and the underlying anatomy during imaging and registration is only partially satisfied. This error can be reduced by using a multiplicity of fiducials and a process that selects those fiducials that seem to have maintained a rigid relationship between one another. However, for maximal accuracy of registration, the need for a fixed relationship between registration and imaging can only be achieved with fiducials attached to the skull. It has been demonstrated that use of such fiducials matches, if not exceeds, the accuracy of frame-based registration *(12)*. Given this demonstrated accuracy, it is surprising that frames are still used for applications, such as functional neurosurgery, that are perceived as requiring the utmost in accuracy. It is to be anticipated that all applications will eventually use point-based registration methods, given the ease with which these techniques can be used and the decrease in discomfort experienced by the patient. Clearly, the act of incising the scalp and screwing a fiducial into the skull simply to achieve registration cannot be perceived as adding to the concept of minimal invasiveness; when using point-based fiducial registration, an important tradeoff between accuracy and minimal invasiveness must be considered by the surgeon.

A final method exists that is highly accurate and completely noninvasive. If two X-ray sources, oriented at approximately right angles to each other, are employed to take an image of an anatomical structure at the junction of their beams using either radiographic film or radiosensitive digital devices, the two resultant 2D images can be employed to determine the exact position and orientation of the anatomical structure in space. To perform registration, a high-resolution CT scan of the anatomical part is required. By using a projection algorithm, multiple "virtual radiographs" of the CT dataset can be produced, emulating various angles of source and detector location around the anatomic part. By comparing this library of "virtual radiographs" with the actual radiographs taken in the procedure suite, the exact location of the head relative to the source and detectors can be determined. This registration technique is used for the CyberKnife, discussed in the Therapeutic Intrevention section; as it is totally noninvasive, it can be repeated as necessary with no risk to the patient. This capability allows for fractionated stereotactic radiosurgery and is highly accurate *(13)*, but has not as yet been employed in the operating room.

Registration has therefore gone through a cyclical process. It was initially avoided entirely by using intraoperative 2D imaging and then enhanced using 3D preoperative images that were employed through the use of an invasive, but accurate, stereotactic frame. Use of scalp-based markers eliminated the use of the frame in all procedures except those needing the highest accuracy; skull-based markers will eventually eliminate the use of the frame in all procedures owing to their high accuracy, but at the expense of some invasiveness in terms of pain in placing these markers. Finally, a method now exists to use 2D intra-operative radiographs to register high-resolution 3D preoperative images in a completely noninvasive technique. Technology has therefore addressed the issue of maximizing registration accuracy while essentially eliminating registration invasiveness.

VISUALIZATION

Just as surgery balances harm and good to achieve a therapeutic response, a procedure must balance the exposure of normal and abnormal tissue. Exposure of normal tissue is, for the most part, needed only to orient the surgeon and avoid damage to critical structures near the surgical target. In traditional craniotomy, for example, exposure of specific cortical structures is routinely employed to allow the surgeon to estimate where the target lesion is located underneath the cortical surface. Other examples are seen in gallbladder surgery, in which it is needed to visualize the hepatic artery and to avoid damage to these critical structures, as well as during intracranial aneurysm surgery, in which visualization of perforators is required to avoid incorporating them into the clip that occludes the aneurysm.

Employed in an ideal fashion, image guidance should completely obviate the need to expose tissue to orient the surgeon, as orientation would occur entirely through imaging. In reality, even with the best imaging technologies available, exposure of structures smaller than the resolution of the imaging employed is still required to avoid inadvertent collateral damage to tissue surrounding the pathology being targeted by the procedure. For example, it is impossible to visualize the striate arteries with a diameter of 0.5 mm using CT scans of 1 mm thickness. Therefore, visualization of small (<1 mm) structures is still required. It must be appreciated that exposure of normal tissue for visualization comes at a cost in terms of risk, and therefore, invasiveness, to the patient. The simple exposure of normal brain tissue, for example, may allow the tissue to desiccate, with subsequent damage. Also, exposure of normal tissue for orientation usually requires larger incisions, which are associated with more postoperative pain. Finally, exposure of normal tissue can allow inadvertent damage as instrumentation is moved in and out of the surgical field.

Image guidance is ideal for minimization of exposure of normal tissue, owing to its ability to project the location of deep-seated structures to the surface of the patient, allowing determination of the best path to the target with minimal exposure of normal tissue. An example of such use is given in Fig. 2. This MRI of a patient with a convexity meningioma was obtained with scalp-based fiducials and contrast enhancement. Although resection of such a tumor is straightforward, the addition of image guidance allows the use of a linear incision directly over the lesion, creating a scalp flap of precisely the size and shape necessary to resect the lesion. Furthermore, given the proximity of the

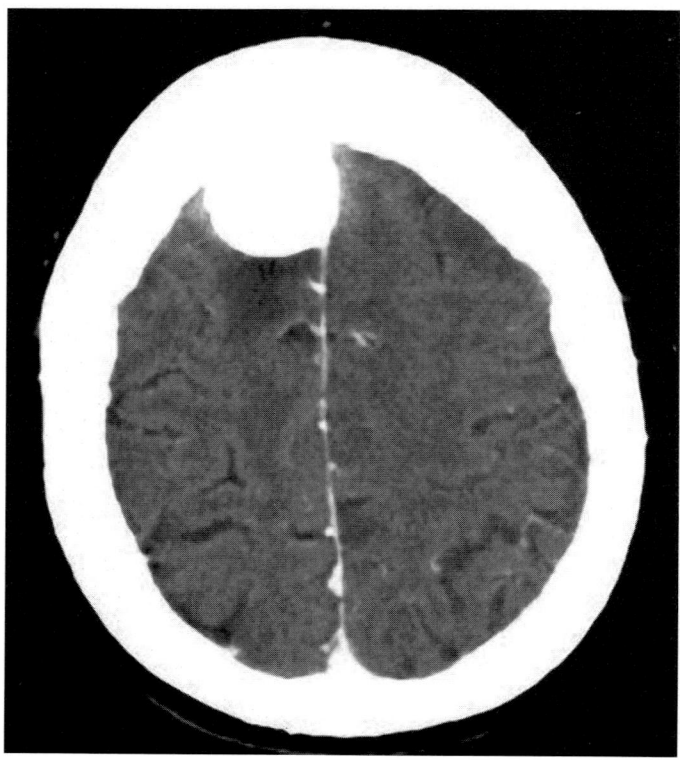

Fig. 2. Contrast-enhanced CT scan of a frontal parafalcian meningioma.

tumor to the sagittal sinus, the surgeon can either choose not to expose the sinus and position the skull flap as close as possible to the edge of this structure, or choose to make the bone flap extend over the sinus and avoid placing burr holes over the sinus, which could lead to significant blood loss. The dura can then be opened precisely to expose only the junction of the tumor and the underlying brain. In this way, essentially no normal cortex is exposed except that directly beneath the tumor, which is exposed following resection. This approach also minimizes the amount of dura resected with the tumor and limits the need for a tissue graft to cover the postresection dura defect.

When dealing with intrinsic tumors of the brain, not only does minimum exposure of normal tissue play a role, but minimization of risk to functional brain tissue is also key. Image guidance can orient the path of surgery so that the initial exposure is directly over the most superficial portion of the tumor. Alternatively, when the shortest path to the tumor is through cortical tissue with specific functional significance (previously termed "eloquent cortex"), damage to which will result in an irreversible neurologic deficit, image guidance can orient the course of surgery so that it is carried out along a path designed to minimize, if not completely eliminate, exposure and retraction of such critical tissue. Figure 3 shows an MRI of a large mesial temporal lobe lesion in the dominant left temporal lobe. The approach to this lesion was

Imaging Guidance

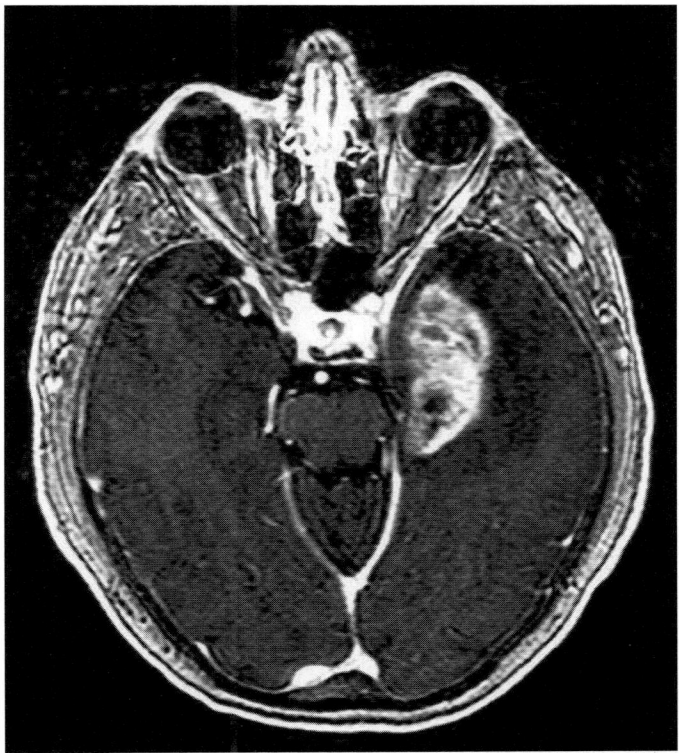

Fig. 3. Gadolinium-enhanced MRI of a medial temporal lobe tumor.

through the anterior temporal lobe, sparing the dominant speech cortex on the posterolateral aspect of the temporal lobe, and allowing for a complete resection with no postoperative neurological deficit (Fig. 4).

When one is using image guidance to avoid eloquent cortex (such as the calcarine cortex or the precentral motor cortex), it is important to realize that the position of eloquent cortex in a specific patient may be significantly different from its location in the normal population. By studying individuals with strokes, as well as stimulation studies of patients undergoing craniotomy while awake, a standardized map of the location of key functions within the brain has been produced, which can be presented in the form of an atlas with these functions superimposed on an "averaged" brain. Neurosurgeons rely on these atlases to avoid such structures when planning surgical interventions. Sometimes when a surgical target is believed to be located within tissue located at a key functional area, removal of the target may be felt to entail such a high risk of postoperative deficit that intervention is considered to be ill advised. This concept has become embodied by the lay public as the so-called inoperable brain tumor, although it should be apparent that any brain tumor is removable and thus technically operable; the true determinant of operability is the attendant risk to the patient, and a more appropriate term would be "unacceptable risk." Therefore, a key factor in deciding the operability of a particular lesion is the relative location of eloquent cortex.

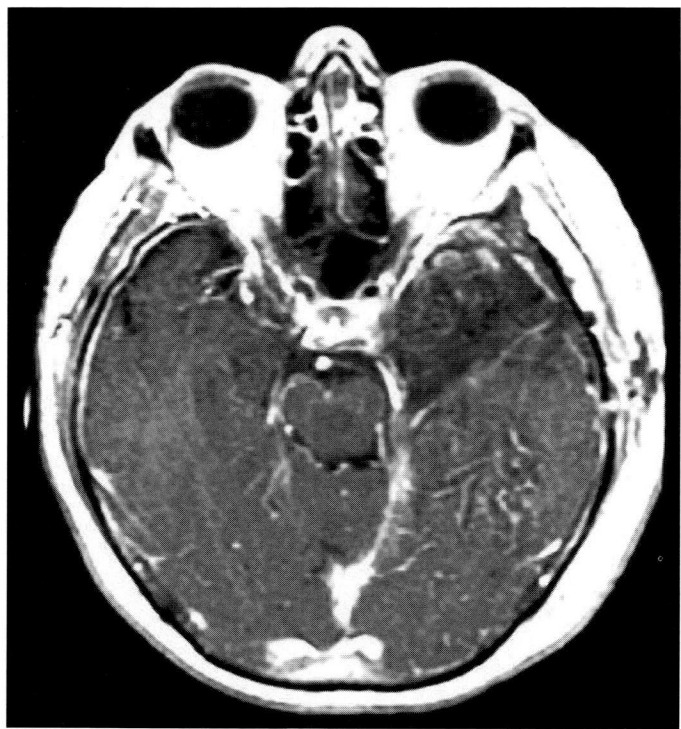

Fig. 4. Gadolinium-enhanced MRI of the patient in Fig. 3 taken postoperatively.

Although brain atlases are appropriate when contemplating surgery on individuals with anatomically normal brains, surgery is usually performed on patients experiencing mass effect and anatomical distortion, owing to either structural or congenital lesions. Given the distortion of brain anatomy in the presence of mass lesions, by using functional imaging, a lesion that was previously considered to present too high a risk can become the target for a procedure if eloquent cortex has been shifted out of harm's way. Conversely, without functional imaging, a surgeon may decide to intervene in an apparently straightforward case and cause a massive neurological deficit because eloquent cortex is moved directly into the path of the surgical intervention. Therefore, when dealing with lesions in and around eloquent cortex, it is essential to employ imaging that allows the depiction of the function at risk, as opposed to basing surgery on structural imaging only. The use of functional imaging to guide an operation that was previously felt to be impossible using traditional techniques is an example of surgery completely enabled by the use of appropriately selected image guidance. (*See* Chapter 4 for functional imaging.)

There are several choices for imaging function as opposed to structure. One of the most commonly used techniques is positron emission tomography (PET). This technique detects metabolic activation of specific areas while the patient being imaged performs a specific task. It has been used extensively as a research tool to delineate normal functional anatomy for elaboration of an atlas of normal human brain *(14)*. Disadvantages of PET scanning are that is requires radioactive tracers, which are costly to produce and short lived, and that the detectors employed have a relatively low resolution, on the order of 2.5–3 mm. Many centers have now established the use of functional magnetic resonance imaging (fMRI), which employs a baseline study subtracted from an activated signal while the patient performs specific tasks *(15)*. Metabolic activation of cortex causes a change in the MRI characteristics of tissue, and the subtracted images demonstrate the location of these activated areas. fMRI is now being employed by image-guided systems in many centers to depict eloquent cortex in an attempt to modify surgical interventions around these areas. The resolution of fMRI is considerably better than that of PET, on the order of 2–2.5 mm.

A major limitation of both fMRI and PET is that both require metabolic changes in the brain in order to detect functional localization. Thus these imaging techniques actually depict epiphenomena of functional activity but do not depict the signal generated by the function itself. Attempts to use electroencephalography (EEG) to localize function have been frustrated by the high resistance of the human skull, which makes it difficult to localize the origin of specific electrical impulses caused by functional activity *(16)*. This limitation is not seen in magentoencephalography (MEG). Rather than using electrical waves associated with specific functions, MEG uses a series of highly sensitive magnetometers to determine the origin of magnetic activity that arises during a functional event. MEG, therefore, offers the promise of precisely depicting the location of functional cortex so that it can be avoided during the course of an image-guided procedure. An example of such an intervention is given in Fig. 5 (*see* Color Plate 5 following p. 112). In this example, a 28-yr-old patient presented with a lesion felt by many to be inoperable, in that it was located in the left posterior frontal lobe. Evaluation was performed with MEG, which demonstrated that the motor and speech cortex were not involved with this lesion. This was confirmed by placing a grid over the cortex and stimulating the cortex postoperatively. When the MEG data were confirmed, the complete resection of a grade III oligodendroglioma was carried out using image guidance. The patient is now 6 yr postop, with no evidence of recurrence.

Another important aspect of MEG is that it can be used to depict the location of abnormally functioning tissue, resection of which may benefit the patient. A typical example of this capability is the localization of an epileptogenic focus responsible for the generation of seizures intractable to medication. By accurately depicting an abnormal focus, resection of the focus may lead to cure of the seizure activity. As this tissue is usually structurally normal, but functionally abnormal, only by coupling MEG to an image guidance system can the surgeon be led to this focus accurately.

In conclusion, image guidance can be used not only to visualize the target of a surgical intervention, be it a structural or functional abnormality, but also to avoid critical tissue that must be preserved in order to avoid neurological deficit. When used in this way, image guidance may actually allow surgery to be performed safely on lesions that were hitherto felt to be inoperable owing to perceived surgical risks based on assumptions as to the location of critical func-

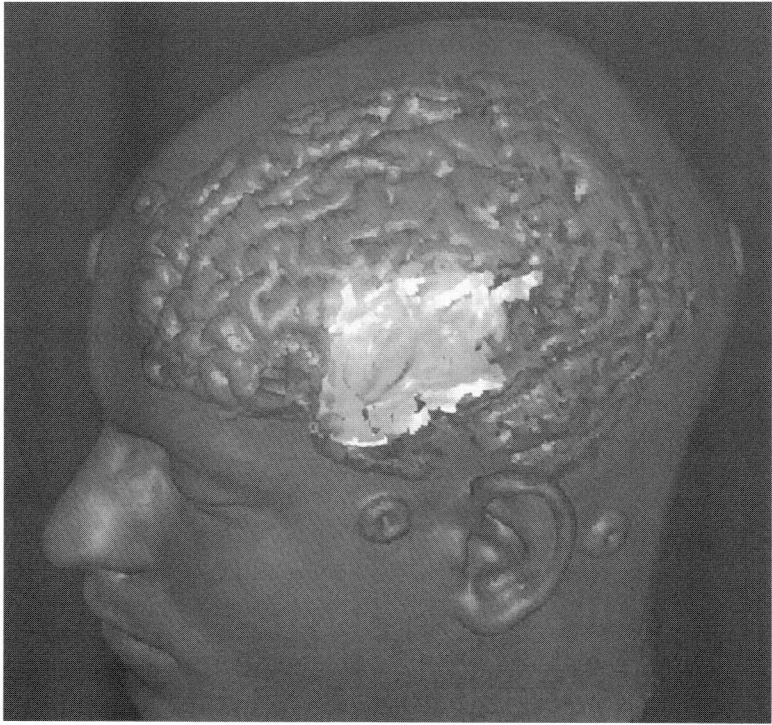

Fig. 5. Computer model showing a lesion in yellow and MEG dipole locations in purple. (*See* Color Plate 5 following p. 112.)

tional tissue. In any case, the use of image guidance, with appropriate choice of guiding imaging, enables the use of minimally invasive concepts to be employed. In this way, image guidance can be seen as analogous to an endoscope or microscope as a powerful enabler of minimal invasiveness.

THERAPEUTIC INTERVENTION

As defined above, the concept of therapeutic intervention is the "elbow room" needed to achieve therapy. In the treatment of abdominal aortic aneurysm, for example, conventional technique requires a large abdominal opening to resect the lesion and placement of a graft. Using the image guidance technique of angiography, coupled with the use of a novel technology consisting of the intravascular stent, this conventional maximally invasive procedure can be replaced by one performed through a small incision in the groin. Therefore, the reduction in "elbow room" needed to effect a cure often involves image guidance plus a new technology that requires accurate placement to be effective. Image guidance has been used to alter conventional procedures and to allow minimally invasive procedures that, in the absence of image guidance, may not be possible, owing to the medical status of the patient, or the very nature of the lesion. Such procedures, which are not possible with conventional techniques, fall into two general categories: those that have as their target tissue that cannot be visualized with conventional technique, such as deep brain stimulation, and procedures using as an effector an agent that cannot be employed within the usual confines of the operating room. A classic example of this latter category is stereotactic radiosurgery (also discussed in Chapter 11).

Conventional neurosurgery in many instances was designed to address a structural target that, in many cases, had to be removed. A classic example is resection of an intracranial tumor. As these lesions can be seen by the naked eye once exposed, conventional surgery was performed with direct visualization and removal of the target. In the previous sections, examples of how this process can be made less invasive have been given. However, neurosurgery has now evolved to the point at which restoration of function, as opposed to removal of a lesion, is the target of many procedures. An example of this effort is deep brain stimulation for movement disorder. This technique, which has been found to ameliorate the symptomatology associated with the central tremor of Parkinson's disease, is now performed at many academic medical centers *(17)*.

The technique falls under the concept of minimal invasiveness in that an electrode is inserted into the brain and, through stimulation of tissue, functional restoration can occur, as opposed to the sectioning of brain performed conventionally. Guidance for such a procedure usually involves a high-resolution preoperative MRI dataset coregistered to a CT scan, which can be registered using either framed or frameless techniques. The electrode is guided first by these images and then by cellular recordings obtained in the operating room. On obtaining a recording from the electrode consistent with the target tissue characteristics, a final position of the electrode is determined. Such intraoperative recordings do not usually fall within the general concept of imaging, and a more appropriate term for the field would therefore be *information-guided therapy*. Deep brain stimulation is, therefore, an example of a minimally invasive technique that is entirely enabled through the appropriate use of information-guided techniques.

An example of the use of an agent not currently employed in the operating room is stereotactic radiosurgery. As first proposed by Leksell *(18)*, this technology employs a stereotactic frame to register 3D images to a device consisting of multiple cobalt sources, which are collimated and focused on a specific point in 3D space. The patient's head is held by the stereotactic frame and positioned so that the focused irradiation directly overlays the target selected within the patient's brain. By moving the patient through a prescribed set of points, a highly convoluted and tightly focused dose of radiation can be delivered to the patient through a planning process called dosimetry. The result is that a lethal dose of radiation can be given to the target with an extremely sharp roll-off, thereby allowing destruction of tissue deep within the head that is not particularly radiosensitive. Stereotactic radiosurgery therefore uses anatomy and image guidance to achieve a therapeutic effect, as opposed to any innate radiosensitivity of the target tissue itself.

Stereotactic radiosurgery has revolutionized neurosurgical practice for the treatment of many benign lesions, which are completely resistant to conventional radiation therapy. As these lesions have a sensitivity to radiation similar to that of surrounding brain tissue, conventional radiation therapy, which irradiates the entire organ, cannot achieve a cure without incurring significant collateral damage. These lesions can now be effectively treated with a completely minimally invasive technique. Classic examples of such a lesion are eighth cranial nerve schwannomas *(19)*. These lesions were formerly approachable only through a rather involved surgical intervention, which often required retraction and visualization of delicate neural structures. This has now been largely replaced by a minimally invasive technique in which a stereotactic frame is applied, the patient is imaged, a dose plan is calculated, and a lethal dose of radiation given to the tumor. The results of stereotactic radiosurgery, especially for the elderly population, are seemingly identical to those of surgical intervention, and the complication rate is far less. Therefore, stereotactic radiosurgery is a prime example of a minimally invasive technique made completely possible through image guidance.

Just as framed stereotactic radiosurgery has revolutionized the performance of neurosurgery, frameless stereotactic radiosurgery promises to bring the benefits of highly focused radiation therapy to sites throughout the entire body. The CyberKnife is a robotically mounted linear accelerator that can be positioned and oriented with a high degree of accuracy *(13,20)*. By the use of multiple positions of the linear accelerator, a highly conformal, tightly focused dose of radiation can be delivered that is identical in nature to that produced by Leksell's Gamma Knife device. As the current registration process requires only that the lesion be in proximity to a skeletal element so that it can be imaged with the radiographic devices located within the CyberKnife suite, the CyberKnife overcomes the limitation of the Gamma Knife unit in that it can be applied to any bony structure throughout the entire body. An extremely exciting prospect for the CyberKnife is the ability of the device to accommodate movement of tissue during the delivery of radiation. New registration techniques are being developed that should allow the CyberKnife to treat soft tissue lesions that actively deform and to translate between pretreatment imaging and the therapeutic intervention. It can be foreseen that the CyberKnife will allow completely minimally invasive techniques to be applied anywhere in the body, accommodating the movement of tissue while subjecting the patient to minimal risk.

CONCLUSIONS

This chapter has shown the importance of image guidance in furthering the application of minimally invasive techniques throughout the body. Registration for image guidance has become significantly simplified and should no longer present an obstacle, as with the use of stereotactic frames in the past. Visualization of target tissues, as well as normal tissues to be avoided during the course of surgery, has been made possible through advances in imaging technologies, which are coupled to the operation. With the advent of functional imaging technologies, such as MEG, the promise that these technologies may be scaled to the molecular level suggests potentially fascinating interventions based on molecular abnormalities delivered by image-guided techniques on a microscopic scale. Finally, image guidance allows the use of novel therapeutic interventions, such as deep brain stimulation and radiation therapy, permitting the completely noninvasive amelioration of symptomatology or destruction of tissue, which would be impossible in the absence of image guidance.

In a very real way, the future of therapeutic intervention can only be achieved with the infrastructure provided by information-guided therapy. It can be anticipated that demands for minimization of risks and maximization of benefit will be realized only through the innovative use of information-guided technology.

REFERENCES

1. Brown RA, Roberts TS, Osborn AG. Stereotaxic frame and computer software for CT-directed neurosurgical localization. *Invest Radiol* 1980;15:308–312.
2. Leksell L, Leksell D, Schwebel L. Stereotaxis and nuclear magnetic resonance. *J Neurol Neurosurg Psychiatry* 1985;48:14–18.
3. Pergolizzi RS Jr, Nabavi A, Schwartz RB, et al. Intra-operative image guidance during trans-sphenoidal pituitary resection: preliminary results. *J Magn Reson Imaging* 2001;13:136–141.
4. Hogan RE, Lowe VJ, Bucholz RD. Triple-technique (MR imaging, single-photon emission CT, and CT) coregistration for image-guided surgical evaluation of patients with intractable epilepsy. *Am J Neuroradiol* 1999;20:1054–1058.
5. Liberman L. Percutaneous image-guided core breast biopsy. *Radiol Clin North Am* 2002;40:483–500.
6. Cleary K, Clifford M, Stoianovici D, Freedman MT, Mun SK, Watson V. Technology improvements for image-guided and minimally invasive spine procedures. *IEEE Trans Inform Tech Biomed* 2002;6:249–261.
7. Lee JYK, Lunsford LD, Subach BR, Jho HD, Bissonette DJ, Kondziolka D. Brain surgery with image guidance: current recommendations based on a 20-year assessment. *Stereotact Funct Neurosurg* 2000;75:35–48.
8. Hall WA, Liu H, Martin AJ, Pozza CH, Maxwell RE, Truwit CL. Safety, efficacy and functionality of high-field strength interventional magnetic resonance imaging for neurosurgery. *Neurosurgery* 2000;46:632–641.
9. Lenz GW. Interventional magnet and system design at low field, in *Interventional MRI* (Lufkin RB, ed.), Mosby, St. Louis, 1999, pp. 8–14.
10. Gildenberg PL. Whatever happened to stereotactic surgery? *Neurosurgery* 1987;20: 983–987.
11. Maciunas RJ, Fitzpatrick JM, Galloway RL, et al. Beyond stereotaxy: extreme levels of application accuracy are provided by implantable fiducial markers for interactive image-guided neurosurgery, in *Interactive Image-Guided Neurosurgery* (Maciunas RJ, ed.), American Association of Neurological Surgeons, Park Ridge, IL, 1993, pp. 259–270.
12. Maurer CR, Fitzpatrick JM, Wang MY, Galloway RL, Maciunas RJ, Allen GS. Registration of head volume images using implantable fiducial markers. *IEEE Trans Med Imaging* 1997;16:447462.
13. Chang SD, Main W, Martin DP, Gibbs IC, Heilbrun PM. An analysis of the accuracy of the CyberKnife: a robotic frameless stereotactic radiosurgical system. *Neurosurgery* 2003;52:140–146; discussion 146–147.
14. Corbetta M, Miezin FM, Dobmeyer S, Shulman GL, Petersen SE. Selective and divided attention during visual discriminations of shape, color, and speed: functional anatomy by positron emission tomography. *J Neurosci* 1991;11:2383–2402.

15. Cordesa D, Haughton VM, Arfanakis K, et al. Mapping functionally related regions of brain with functional connectivity MR imaging. *Am J Neuroradiol* 2000; 21:1636–1644.
16. Krenkel W. The EEG in tumors of the brain, in *Handbook of Clinical Neurology*, vol. 16 (Vinken PJ, Bruyn GW, eds.), Elsevier, Amsterdam, 1974, pp. 418–454.
17. The Deep-Brain Stimulation for Parkinson's Disease Study Group. Deep-brain stimulation of the subthalamic nucleus or the pars interna of the globus pallidus in Parkinson's disease. *N Engl J Med* 2001;345:956–963.
18. Leksell L. The stereotaxic method and radiosurgery of the brain. *Acta Chir Scand* 1951;102:316–319.
19. Leksell L. A note on the treatment of acoustic tumors. *Acta Chir Scand* 1969;137: 763–765.
20. Adler JR Jr, Chang SD, Murphy MJ, et al. The Cyberknife: a frameless robotic system for radiosurgery. *Stereotact Funct Neurosurg* 1997;69:124–128.

6
Intraoperative Imaging Using the Siemens 0.2- and 1.5-Tesla MR Systems

Christopher Nimsky, MD and Rudolf Fahlbusch, MD

INTRODUCTION

Intraoperative imaging is an important tool in modern minimally invasive neurosurgery. Intraoperative imaging, especially in combination with some kind of neuronavigational device, correlating the virtual image data to the real patient world in the operating room, serves as intraoperative quality control, supporting the goal of maximum tumor resection with least morbidity.

Magnetic resonance imaging (MRI), in comparison with computed tomography (CT) and ultrasound, provides multiplanar imaging with a high soft tissue resolution. It is generally accepted that MRI is the method of choice for the preoperative diagnostic evaluation of intracranial tumors and patients with epilepsy. However, when the MR technology was introduced into clinical diagnostics, the closed-bore superconducting cylindrical design of MR scanners, with relatively long imaging times and difficult patient access, prevented their intraoperative application.

Therefore, intraoperative imaging evaluating the extent of a tumor resection was introduced into neurosurgery by ultrasound imaging *(1–3)* and CT *(4–9)*. Their efficacy was investigated in the early 1980s *(7,8)*. However, imaging quality and lesional resolution, especially in CT for soft tissue, were not quite satisfactory.

In the mid 1990s, widespread interest arose in intraoperative imaging in the neurosurgical community, since the development of open configured MRI systems made it possible to adapt these systems to the operating room. Intraoperative MRI in neurosurgery was first introduced by Black and Jolesz in 1995 at the Brigham and Women's Hospital in Boston with a dedicated MRI system for intraoperative use (Signa SP, 0.5 T), which was developed in a collaboration with the General Electric Corporation *(10)*. Removing the central segment of a cylindrical MR system has solved the problem of patient access. This so-called "double doughnut" design allows patient access through the vertical gap of the scanner. As an alternative approach, we adapted a diagnostic low-field MR scanner (Magnetom Open, 0.2 T) for intraoperative use: it was originally designed for diagnostic purposes only. This implementation was a cooperative

From: *Minimally Invasive Neurosurgery,* edited by: M.R. Proctor and P.M. Black © Humana Press Inc., Totowa, NJ

effort of the Siemens Corporation with the Departments of Neurosurgery at the Universities of Erlangen and Heidelberg *(11,12)* at the end of 1995. The scanner has a biplanar magnet design using a resistive magnet. The C-shape design with a horizontal gap allows a wide patient access.

Our primary concept was based on the installation of the MR scanner in a twin operating room, in combination with pointer- and microscope-based neuronavigation systems (Stealth, Medtronic and MKM, Zeiss). This setup allows frameless stereotaxy based on anatomical data. Furthermore, it is also possible to integrate functional data from magnetoencephalography (MEG) and functional MRI (fMRI) for intraoperative identification of eloquent brain areas, which is now known as "functional neuronavigation" *(13–15)*.

Intraoperative image quality and sequence spectra of the various low-field MR scanners cannot compete with the routine pre- or postoperative imaging quality standards set by high-Tesla machines. This led to the development of a new concept to adapt a standard high-field MR scanner to our operating environment, while preserving the benefits of standard microsurgical equipment and microscope-based neuronavigational guidance with integrated functional data. The active magnetic shielding of modern high-field MR systems results in a steep decrease in the magnetic field, so that the 5-G line is close to the scanner, facilitating the intraoperative application of these high-field devices.

This chapter summarizes our concept and different setups for intraoperative low- and high-field MRI and gives an overview of our clinical experience in low-field intraoperative MRI, which is compared with our preliminary data using the new high-field system.

LOW-FIELD INTRAOPERATIVE MRI

As demonstrated by other groups *(10,11,16–20)* the use of MR scanners in the operating environment seems to be safe and reliable, as well as applicable to neurosurgical procedures, even if these procedures have to be adapted to the MR environment to a certain extent. Even intraoperative patient transport, which was necessary in our first conceptual design combining intraoperative imaging with microscope-based neuronavigation, did not cause any problems. The development of new navigation microscopes, which can be used in the fringe field of the MR scanner *(21)*, allowed us to abandon the cumbersome and time-consuming intraoperative patient transport. It is now possible to integrate full microscope-based neuronavigational support with the concept of surgery in the fringe field, which was first applied in transsphenoidal surgery *(12,22)* and afterwards proposed for open cranial surgery *(23)*.

There are two main designs for intraoperative MRI. In the first, the patient is placed directly inside the scanner, using a system specially designed for intraoperative use, like the Signa SP "double-doughnut" scanner *(10,24)*, which offers almost real-time imaging with the drawback of restricted patient access. The 0.12-T PoleStar N-10 (Odin Technologies, Yokneam, Israel) has a similar design: the disk-shaped magnets are placed below the operating table and moved upward for scanning *(25,26)*. In the second type, the standard diagnostic scanners adapted to the operating environment require some kind of patient transport. The patient is operated on either in the fringe field of the scanner, lying on the movable MR tray *(21)*, or on a rotating operating table *(27)*, or else surgery is performed in a separate operating room, as in the twin operating room setup, necessitating a longer intraoperative patient transport *(11,12)*. Both of these designs are implemented with the 0.3-T AIRIS II scanner (Hitachi Medical Corporation, Tokyo, Japan) *(28)*.

Presently we consider that intraoperative MRI is indicated for the surgical treatment of gliomas (especially low grade), ventricular tumors, epilepsy *(29)*, and complicated larger suprasellar pituitary tumors *(22)*. In addition, intraoperative MRI should be used to compensate for the effects of brain shift, if ongoing neuronavigational guidance is needed in complicated cases with major distortion of the surgical field *(30–33)*. Further indications, not investigated by our group, may be biopsy procedures with additional therapy control provided by the scanner, e.g., temperature monitoring in cryoablation or laser ablation *(27)*.

Operating Room Setup

All procedures were performed under general anesthesia. The local ethical committee approved the intraoperative MRI with intraoperative patient transport, and all patients signed an informed consent. Timing of intraoperative MRI was decided by the neurosurgeon. MRI was performed either when the neurosurgeon had the impression of complete tumor resection or, in case of incomplete tumor removal, when the neurosurgeon felt that no further tumor removal was possible, e.g., because of an infiltration of eloquent brain areas.

Intraoperative MRI was performed using a 0.2-T Magnetom Open MR scanner (Siemens Medical Solutions, Erlangen, Germany), which was located in the radiofrequency-shielded part of a twin operating theater *(12,34)*. Two operating sites were mainly used: either an adjacent conventional operating theater, necessitating intraoperative patient transport, or the extended table of the MR scanner at the 5-G line.

The concept of surgery in the fringe field of the scanner was first applied in transsphenoidal surgery, because in these cases no navigation microscope was needed, so that a conventional operating microscope could be used. The head of the patient was placed directly on the movable table of the MR scanner at the 5-G line. A standard flexible coil was attached around the head. For safety reasons, when working closer than 1.5 m from the magnet isocenter, MR-compatible instruments, especially developed for this purpose, were used *(35)*. Prior to imaging, an MR-compatible speculum was inserted. For intraoperative scanning the table was placed in the center of the magnet, and then data acquisition was started. In the routine setup coronal and sagittal T1-weighted spin-echo sequences were acquired (slice thickness 3 mm, TR 340 ms, TE 26 ms, bandwidth 39 Hz, FOV 200 mm, matrix 192 × 256). In selected cases, e.g., in cystic adenomas, T2-weighted turbo spin-echo sequences were used in addition (slice thickness 3 mm, TR 5700 ms, TE 117 ms, bandwidth 33 Hz, FOV 230 mm, matrix 224 × 256). For craniopharyngiomas, T1-weighted imaging was repeated after contrast media was applied (gadolinium-DTPA 0.2 mL/kg body weight IV).

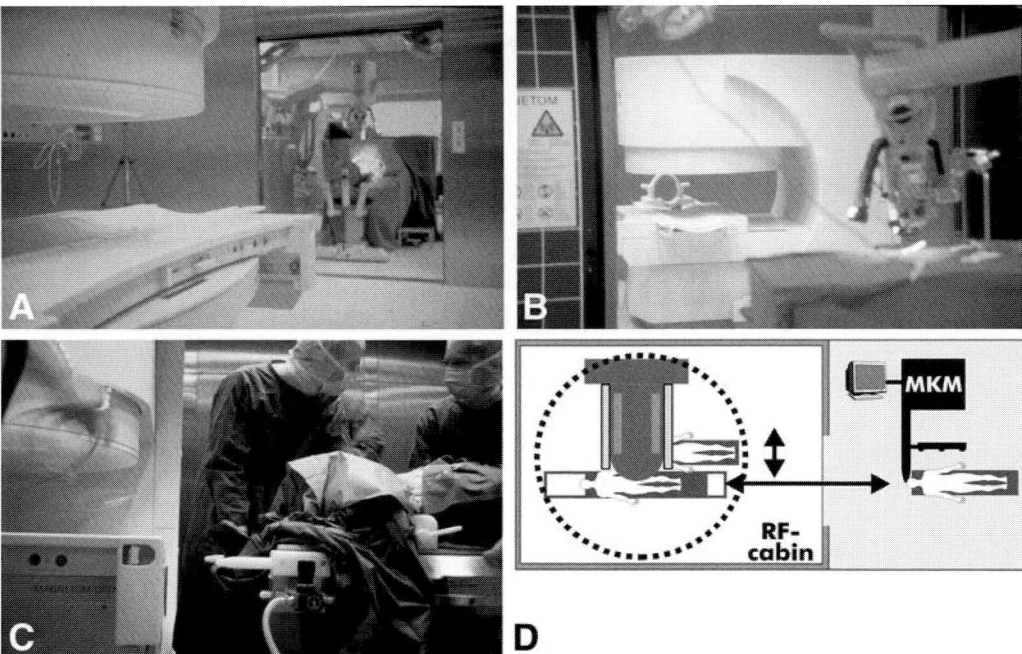

Fig. 1. Twin operating room setup: the initial concept combining microscope-based neuronavigation using the MKM microscope with intraoperative low-field imaging (0.2-T Magnetom Open). **(A)** View from the RF-cabin to the MKM microscope, which is placed in an adjacent operating room. **(B)** Opposite view. **(C)** Intraoperative patient transport, the draped patient, laying on an air-cushioned OR table has just been moved to the scanner. **(D)** Schematic drawing of the twin operating room setup.

For transcranial surgery of gliomas, other brain tumors, and drug-resistant epilepsy, the head was fixed in a ceramic, MR-compatible head holder. Using the MKM navigation microscope (Zeiss, Oberkochen, Germany), which was the only navigation microscope available in 1996, surgery was performed in an adjacent operating room (twin operating room concept). The patient was placed on an air-cushioned OR table, and the table was transported into the scanner during surgery over a distance of 5 m (Fig. 1) *(12,34)*. With the introduction of the NC4 navigation microscope (Zeiss), which consists of only a few magnetic parts, intraoperative patient transport could be abandoned, and all procedures could be performed in the same position as for transsphenoidal surgery (Fig. 2) *(21)*. For imaging, an experimental separable coil was used. The lower, nonsterile part was applied prior to surgery; the sterile upper part of the coil was placed onto sterile adapters just before the head was moved into the center of the scanner.

For glioma surgery, axial inversion recovery (slice thickness 6 mm, TR 6000 ms, TE 48 ms, TI 300 ms, bandwidth 65 Hz, FOV 250 mm, matrix 182 × 256) and dark fluid sequences (slice thickness 6 mm, TR 6000 ms, TE 93 ms, TI 1600 ms, bandwidth 65 Hz, FOV 230 mm, matrix 210 × 256) were measured. Additionally, volume data were obtained routinely using a T1-weighted 3D fast low-

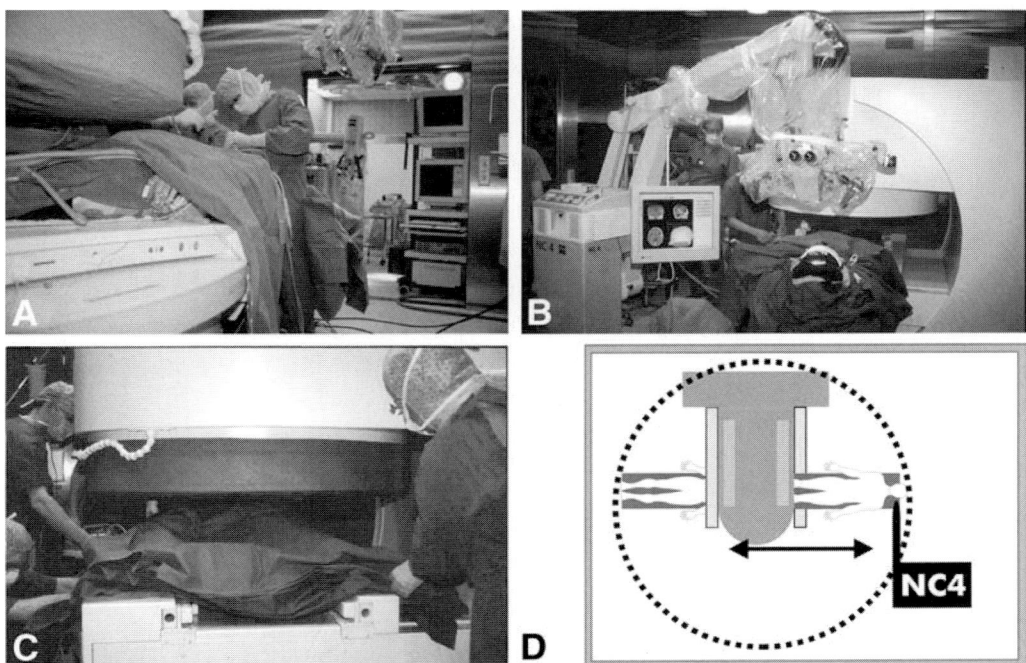

Fig. 2. Surgery at the fringe field, the NC4 microscope is placed at the 5-G line, so no long, time-consuming intraoperative patient transport is necessary. **(A)** Same view as in Fig. 1A. **(B)** Microscope position near the scanner, a flat screen depicts the navigational views with integrated functional data. **(C)** For scanning, the MR tray is moved into the center of the scanner. **(D)** Schematic drawing.

angle shot (FLASH) gradient-echo sequence (slice thickness 1.5 mm, TR 16.1 ms, TE 7 ms, bandwidth 98 Hz, FOV 250 mm, matrix 256 × 256). This sequence was used for multiplanar reformatting to obtain standard projections, which compensates for the fact that the head was fixed intraoperatively in variable angles. This sequence was also the prerequisite for an intraoperative update of neuronavigation. MR contrast agent (gadolinium-DTPA 0.2 mL/kg body weight, IV.) was administered just prior to scanning only if the tumor showed enhancement in the preoperative images. For resection control in cavernoma, other brain tumors, and nonlesional cases of epilepsy surgery, a reduced scanning protocol was used.

Each OR position allowed unlimited patient access and full use of standard neurosurgical microinstrumentation. Either pointer-based neuronavigation (Stealth, Medtronic, Broomfield, CO) or microscope-based neuronavigation (MKM or NC4 navigation microscopes, Zeiss) were used. In addition to anatomical neuronavigation, functional data from MEG or fMRI to identify eloquent brain areas were integrated. Functional data were measured with a MAGNES II biomagnetometer (BTI, San Diego, CA) and a 1.5-T Magnetom Symphony (Siemens Medical Solutions) *(13–15,36–38)*.

In case of a suspected tumor remnant, several MR-visible bone fiducials (Howmedica-Leibinger, Freiburg, Germany) were placed around the craniotomy opening prior to intraoperative scanning, allowing an intraoperative registration of the 3D image data to update neuronavigation. The 3D image data were then transferred to the navigation system via intranet, and the tumor remnant was segmented manually with the software of the respective neuronavigation systems (e.g., STP 4.0, Zeiss, Oberkochen, Germany). Then the neuronavigation system was reregistered with the intraoperative image data, allowing compensation for the effects of brain shift (31,32).

In case of further tumor removal, repeated imaging was performed either directly after removal of the tumor remnant or at the end of surgery, i.e., after craniotomy closure. Contrast media was not applied repeatedly.

Clinical Experience

Between March 1996 and July 2001, we performed intraoperative MRI in 330 patients. Histopathologic examination revealed pituitary adenoma in 61, craniopharyngioma in 26, glioma in 106, cavernoma in 18, and other diagnoses in 54 patients (including chordoma, gangliocytoma, germinoma, lymphoma, melanoma, meningioma, metastasis, neurocytoma, pinealoma, primitive neuroectodermal tumor, and subependymoma). For remaining 65 cases, either resective or disconnective epilepsy surgery was carried out for nonlesional conditions ($n = 40$), or procedures were performed in which intraoperative MRI was used as an online control during catheter or electrode placements ($n = 25$). Among the 330 procedures, there were 240 craniotomies, 59 transsphenoidal approaches, and 31 burr hole procedures.

We did not observe any adverse effects of intraoperative imaging on the postoperative course of the patients. Intraoperative patient transport (applied in 166 patients) did not cause any harm. On average, a delay of some 10 min occurred until imaging could start. The same time was necessary until surgery could be continued after imaging, so that intraoperative patient transport was felt to be time consuming and cumbersome. A further time delay occurred when only an anesthesiology team without experience in intraoperative patient transport was available, since all anesthesia lines had to be switched twice for intraoperative imaging. In the patients who were operated on directly on the MR table at the 5-G line ($n = 164$), scanning started on average after 20 s to 1 min. The overall complication rate with respect to wound infection ($n = 3$) and rebleeding ($n = 1$) was a bit lower than the average in our department.

Transsphenoidal Procedures

Among 59 patients who underwent transsphenoidal pituitary surgery (52 pituitary adenomas, 7 craniopharyngiomas), image evaluation was limited in only 16, either because drilling artifacts from metal debris disturbed image interpretation in the sella region, or because blood in the resection cavity mimicked tumor remnants. With increasing experience in image interpretation, as well as repeated intraoperative scanning and the application of T2-weighted sequences, further evaluation was possible in most of the patients. In 30 patients a repeat inspection of the surgical field was performed. This led to further tumor removal in 17 out of the total 59 patients. Among a subgroup ($n = 44$) of resectable pituitary macroadenomas with a distinct suprasellar extension, the further resection of tumor increased the rate of complete removal from 45% (21/44) to 75% (33/44). In the remaining patients, an extensive supra- and parasellar tumor extension did not allow complete transsphenoidal removal, necessitating surveillance, secondary transcranial surgery, or radiation therapy. In only one patient was there a transient postoperative visual impairment, caused by a secondary empty sella after complete tumor removal. In none of the 59 patients was endocrine function disturbed owing to the surgical intervention (22).

In transsphenoidal pituitary surgery, intraoperative MRI provides a possibility for further tumor removal in the case of residual tumor, thus increasing the rate of complete tumor removals significantly (39,40). Removal of the suprasellar tumor portion could be evaluated reliably. However, low-field MRI did not seem to be suitable for evaluation of the removal of intrasellar microadenomas. Also, interpretation of the extent of removal of parasellar, i.e., intracavernous, tumor parts was limited. Image artifacts caused by metal debris from drilling or by blood accumulation in the resection cavity were further challenges. In case of incomplete tumor removal intraoperative MRI allowed additional therapy planning at a much earlier state; usually further diagnostics have to be delayed for 2–3 mo after surgery, to obtain artifact-free postoperative images (22).

Glioma Surgery

For glioma surgery, intraoperative MRI showed remaining tumor in a high percentage (63%). In 42% of these patients we continued tumor resection and tried to remove as much tumor as possible; in more than 50%, neuronavigation was updated by the intraoperative image data to localize the tumor remnants. Further tumor removal increased the gross total removal rate, especially for low-grade gliomas; however, in some patients, despite further tumor removal, complete resection was not performed since some tumor remnants invaded eloquent brain areas, which were identified by functional neuronavigation.

Intraoperative MRI in glioma surgery ($n = 106$) revealed incomplete tumor removal in 67 (63%); in one additional case intraoperative imaging did not allow a clear distinction between artifacts and tumor remnants. In 34 patients, i.e., 51% (34 of 67) of the patients with incomplete resection, the resection cavity was inspected again. In 28 patients (42% of the patients with tumor remnants, i.e., 26% of all glioma patients), the extent of resection could be expanded based on the results of intraoperative MR scanning. This increased the rate of gross total removal in World Health Organization (WHO) grade I tumors ($n = 15$) from 87 to 100%. In grade II tumors ($n = 37$) further tumor removal was performed in 19 patients. In 10 of them, complete tumor removal was finally achieved. Thus, the gross total removal rate in the grade II tumors increased from 27 to 54%. In the remaining nine patients, despite further tumor removal, complete resection was not possible because small tumor remnants had infiltrated eloquent brain areas. In the high-grade astrocytomas, the extent of resection was enlarged in seven patients only. This resulted in an increased gross total removal of 55% vs 41% in the grade III and 22% vs 19% in the grade IV patients.

In eight of the low grade gliomas (WHO grade II), the resection could not be extended primarily, because eloquent brain areas were infiltrated. In the majority (82%: 32 out of 39) of the high-grade gliomas (grades III and IV), for which intraoperative imaging had depicted incomplete removal, it was the policy above all to avoid new neurological deficits.

Forty-five glioma patients had preoperative neurological deficits, which resolved at least partially in 32 and worsened in only 2 patients. In the group of patients without preoperative neurological deficits ($n = 61$), three developed a postoperative neurological deterioration (two pareses, and one aphasia). In five glioma patients (4.7%), a neurological postoperative deficit occurred; in only two of them had functional neuronavigation been applied.

We used functional neuronavigation if the tumor was located near eloquent areas to preserve neurological function *(14,15,36,37)*, as a limitation for total resection. In addition to anatomical data, functional data from MEG ($n = 64$) or fMRI ($n = 15$), identifying either motor, sensory, or language-related cortex in 66 patients, were integrated into the neuronavigation, which allowed identification and avoided damage to eloquent brain areas during surgery. The identification of these cortical areas at the beginning of tumor removal was not affected by brain shift, since the functional markers from MEG or fMRI were used to identify the eloquent cortex just after dural opening. The application of functional neuronavigation was associated with low postoperative morbidity. In only two of the 66 patients (3%) in whom functional neuronavigation was applied did a persistent neurological deterioration occur, which in both patients fortunately improved in the further postoperative course. Anatomical and functional neuronavigation were used as guidance to identify relevant structures. Intraoperative MRI allowed a delineation of the extent of resection, so the combination of both allowed a maximum possible resection with the least neurological deficits, while taking incomplete tumor removal into account, when eloquent brain areas were infiltrated.

Besides the possibility of evaluating the completeness of a tumor resection, intraoperative MRI not only allowed us to delineate and visualize the extent of brain shift, which results in great inaccuracies of neuronavigation systems in an ongoing operation, but also offered the possibility of compensating for the effects of brain shift. This could be achieved reliably by an intraoperative update of the neuronavigation system with the intraoperative 3D image data *(31–33)*. Of the 28 patients in whom resection was continued after intraoperative imaging, an intraoperative update of neuronavigation was performed in 18 (64%; 17% of the total 106 gliomas). The update procedure was performed only when it was difficult to localize the remaining tumor in the surgical field. In all these cases the intraoperative update of neuronavigation was technically successful. Image transfer, new segmentation, and rereferencing added another 15–20 min to the whole procedure. The registration error, calculated as the root mean square error, was low (mean 0.85 mm, standard deviation 0.44 mm, maximum error 2.3 mm), resulting in a reliable navigation with high accuracy that quickly led to the suspicious areas *(31,32)*. In three patients the histopathological examination revealed no tumor in the tissue that was removed additionally because of intraoperative imaging. Complete tumor removal was confirmed by early scanning in all three of them.

One of the general limitations of glioma surgery is that by histological definition a 100% tumor removal is not possible. Furthermore, the extension of the tumor into eloquent brain areas will also result in only partial removal. According to our experience with intraoperative MR evaluation of glioma removal, we still doubt the long-term benefit of intraoperative MRI in surgery of high-grade gliomas, although the first reports published on this topic claim a benefit even in high-grade tumors *(16,18,41)*. In the high-grade tumors, differentiation among tumor remnants, surgically induced imaging changes, edema, and normal brain may be very difficult. Controversial reports on life expectancy in high-grade gliomas emphasize that life expectancy depends more on low postoperative deficits than on "macroscopic" total tumor removal *(42)*. In the low-grade gliomas *(43)*, at a microscopic level complete resection also will not be possible, but since survival of patients seems to be correlated with the extent of tumor resection *(44)*, we believe that surgery of these tumors will benefit more from intraoperative imaging *(45)*. It is still too early to determine the effects on life expectancy in these patients, but it can be stated that more radical resections are possible without increasing morbidity, especially when intraoperative imaging is supported by the use of functional neuronavigation *(14,15)*. Long-term survival studies are still needed.

Other Procedures

Epilepsy surgery is another indication for intraoperative MRI; it has led to reliable evaluation of the extent of resection or disconnection procedure. Not only did it allow us to evaluate completeness of resection in the lesional cases (e.g., glioma, cavernoma), but also in the nonlesional cases the exact extent of a callosotomy ($n = 6$) or the size and shape of a tailored temporal lobe resection ($n = 34$) in its neocortical and hippocampal extent could be documented *(29)*. Increased knowledge of structure–function relationships as partially defined by intraoperative imaging may reduce adverse neuropsychological sequels of epilepsy surgery in the future *(29,46,47)*.

Besides the application of intraoperative MRI in epilepsy surgery, the extent of tumor resection was also evaluated in transcranial pituitary tumor surgery and in various other nongliomatous brain tumors. Furthermore, intraoperative MR resection control of ventricular tumors ($n = 8$) in particular proved helpful. In surgery of ventricular tumors, the cerebrospinal fluid CSF loss quickly resulted in inaccurate neuronavigation. Intraoperative imaging, with the possibility of an update of the neuronavigation system, allowed us to obtain a good orientation in the surgical field and to evaluate the extent of the resection. Catheter and electrode placements, as well as cyst punctures (craniopharyngiomas and other cysts), were reliably controlled by intraoperative MRI in all cases ($n = 31$). We did not encounter problems in visualizing the catheters and electrodes. In only one case was an electrode not easily visualized. Intraoperative X-ray showed that in this patient the depth electrode deviated considerably from the preplanned path into the subdural space.

HIGH-FIELD INTRAOPERATIVE MRI

Parallel to the investigation of intraoperative low-field MRI in several centers, two pioneering groups applied high-field scanners in the operating room environment. The major concepts are similar to those of low-field MR. For high-field scanning, a dedicated system for intraoperative use was designed, the ceiling-mounted movable 1.5-T IMRIS scanner, in Calgary by Sutherland *(48–50)*. Hall and Truwit in Minneapolis adapted a standard 1.5-T Philips scanner to the operating room *(51–54)*.

High-field MR systems offer not only the possibility of shorter scanning times and better image quality but also a broader spectrum of sequences, as well as the application of further intraoperative MRI modalities. High-field systems provide MR angiography, diffusion- and perfusion-weighted imaging, and functional and spectroscopic imaging *(49–53,55)*. Whether all these modalities can be applied during surgery remains to be investigated.

Since intraoperative image quality and sequence spectra of the low-field scanners could not compete with the routine pre- or postoperative imaging quality, being performed with high-Tesla machines, we decided to develop a new concept to adapt a high-field MR scanner to our operating environment, preserving the benefits of standard microsurgical equipment and microscope-based neuronavigational guidance with integrated functional data. Active magnetic shielding of modern high-field MR systems results in a steep decrease in the magnetic field, so that the 5-G line is close to the scanner, facilitating the intraoperative application of these high-field MR scanners. Thus, our concept of surgery in the fringe field *(21,23)* can also be applied for high-field scanners. In close cooperation with the Siemens Corporation, we evolved this concept further. A rotating MR-compatible operating table was adapted to a 1.5-T high-field scanner. For surgery, the patient's head is placed at the 5-G line; for scanning, the table is rotated and the head is moved into the center of the scanner. This allows microsurgery with fully integrated microscope-based neuronavigational support in combination with intraoperative high-field MRI. Between August 2001 and March 2002, our intraoperative MR operating room was reconstructed. The first patients were operated on at the end of April 2002.

Operating Room Setup

A 1.5-T Magnetom Sonata Maestro Class scanner (Siemens) is placed in a radiofrequency (RF)-shielded operating theater (Fig. 3) equipped with a laminar air-flow field ensuring optimal hygiene requirements. MR-compatible anesthesia monitoring (wireless 2.4-GHz monitoring by Invivo Research, Orlando, FL) and respirator equipment (Servo 900 C, Siemens) are provided as well; all standard gaseous support is available in the RF-shielded cabin. Glass fiber adapters allow Ethernet connections to the intra- and internet at various points

Imaging Guidance

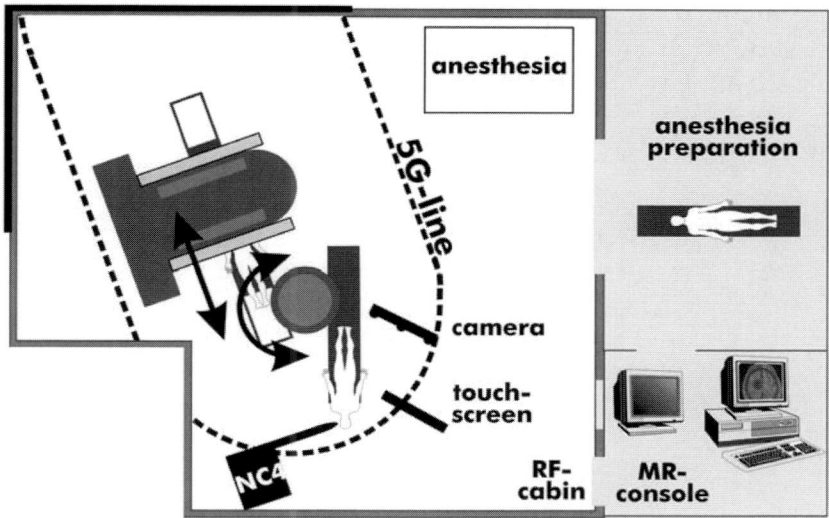

Fig. 3. Operating room setup for intraoperative high-field MR imaging: a rotating table, which is locked at the 160° position, allows surgery in the fringe field, where the NC4 microscope is placed, and a ceiling-mounted neuronavigation system (VectorVision Sky) with a camera and touch screen is integrated into the RF cabin.

of the operating theatre. Electrical support is adjustable from outside so that in case of artifacts during measurements, designated equipment can be shut off.

A rotating OR table (Trumpf, Saalfeld, Germany) is adapted to the 1.5-T scanner serving as operating table and MR tray. It permits free adjustments of the head position; elevation and side rotation are also possible. During surgery the head is placed at the 5-G line, and the table is fixed at the 160° position; for scanning, the table can be turned around and the patient placed in the center of the scanner in less than 2 min (Fig. 4). The head can be fixed in an MR-compatible head holder, which is integrated into the standard head coil (Siemens) *(56)*. The NC4-Multivision microscope (Zeiss) is placed on the patient's left side in the fringe field. Extensive testing at the Siemens labs showed no artifacts generated by the microscope during scanning, and navigation was not influenced at the 5-G line by the magnetic field. For scanning, the microscope is switched off. Neuronavigational guidance is provided by the VectorVisionSky navigation system (BrainLab, Heimstetten, Germany). The camera tracking the position of the microscope in space and the touch-screen to operate the navigation system are ceiling mounted (Ondal, Hünfeld, Germany). Neuronavigational accuracy is not impeded by the fringe field. At the main operating position, functional microscope-based neuronavigation with integrated data from MEG or fMRI is available.

An alternative operating position, with the patient placed in the scanner during surgery, is possible. Stereotactic burr hole procedures using full MR-compatible operating equipment can be performed, while intraoperative MRI allows online monitoring of the stereotactic procedure. Two ceiling-mounted

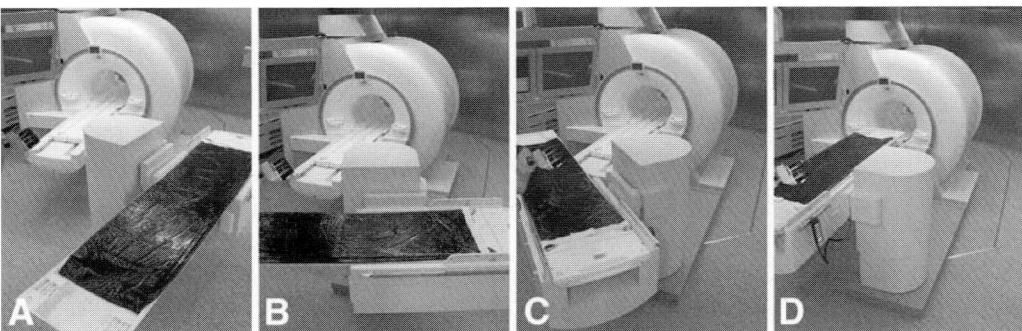

Fig. 4. **(A–D)** A rotating OR table, which allows elevation and side rotation, is attached to the scanner (1.5-T Magnetom Sonata), and the table is turned from the operating position **(A)** to the scanning position **(D)**, allowing scanning in less than 2 min after surgery is stopped.

17.4-inch flat screens (AS4431D, Iiyama, Nagano-shi, Japan) display the MR console and the microscope video. A remote console is placed in the RF-shielded operating theater, allowing operation of various PC hardware from inside the operating room, e.g., for intraoperative functional measurements or neuroelectrophysiological monitoring *(57)*.

First Clinical Experiences

From the end of April 2002, more than 30 patients were investigated over 3 mo, mostly glioma and pituitary tumor cases. The new design with the adapted rotating OR table prooved to be very convenient; intraoperative imaging could start in less than 2 min after completion of surgery. Since all anesthesia lines go over the pivoting axis of the table, no time-consuming rearrangement is necessary. When the patient is placed inside the scanner, biopsy procedures can be monitored online.

In transsphenoidal surgery a standard large flex coil is taped around the head, so surgery is not impeded. Figure 5 displays the OR setup in transsphenoidal surgery. A typical example for evaluation of pituitary adenoma surgery is depicted in Fig. 6; complete adenoma removal was confirmed by intraoperative high-field MRI. Figure 7 illustrates the high intraoperative image quality, with clear delineation of the pituitary stalk and the optic chiasm.

In transcranial surgery, the patient could be placed supine and prone, so the head could be fixed at various angles without major problems (Fig. 8). Refinements of the combination of head coil and head fixation, which will allow more flexibility, must be developed. Figure 9 depicts the intraoperative imaging of a typical glioma case, with various sequences revealing complete tumor removal.

The imaging quality is clearly superior to that of the low-field system (Fig. 10). In contrast to our low-field experience, the comparison between pre- and intraoperative image quality does not show major differences. Besides increased image quality with better image resolution and contrast, the high-field system allows much shorter scanning times, e.g., in evaluation of pituitary

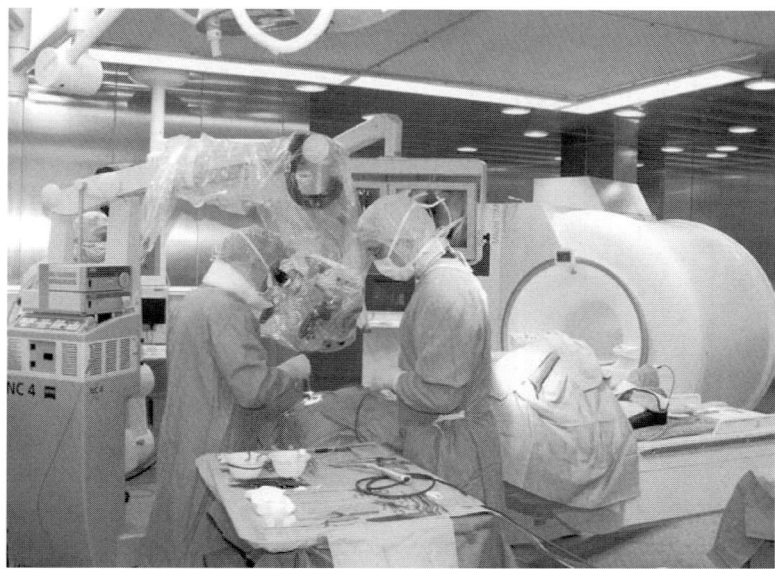

Fig. 5. Intraoperative setup during transsphenoidal surgery. The neurosurgeon is standing behind the patient's head.

adenoma removal T2-weighted half-Fourier single-shot turbo spin-echo (HASTE) sequences give a reliable impression of the extent of removal after 5 s (Fig. 6A and C). Shorter overall scanning times allow the measurement of more detailed protocols in an acceptable time frame. In contrast to our former 0.2-T system, the high-field system offers a wide range of different sequences, including spectroscopy, echoplanar imaging, and diffusion-weighted imaging, which additionally will all be integrated into the navigational setup.

The navigation system VectorVision Sky, which is ceiling mounted and integrated into the RF cabin, was used without any problems. Intraoperative updating of the navigation data was easy, so the effects of brain shift could be compensated for.

PERSPECTIVE

MRI was introduced in the neurosurgical operating room in the mid 1990s *(10–12)*. We now face the transition from its first experimental application to routine use. The first reports on larger patient series have been published now *(16–18)*.

We have investigated low-field intraoperative MRI using a 0.2-T Magnetom Open scanner for 5½ yr in 330 patients. Without doubt it can be stated that intraoperative MRI allows a reliable evaluation of the extent of tumor removal in most cases. Advances in scanner design, e.g., active magnetic shielding, allowed us to adapt a high-field system to the operating room environment. Even though our experience in intraoperative high-field MRI is preliminary, involving more than 30 patients, it can be stated that intraoperative high-field

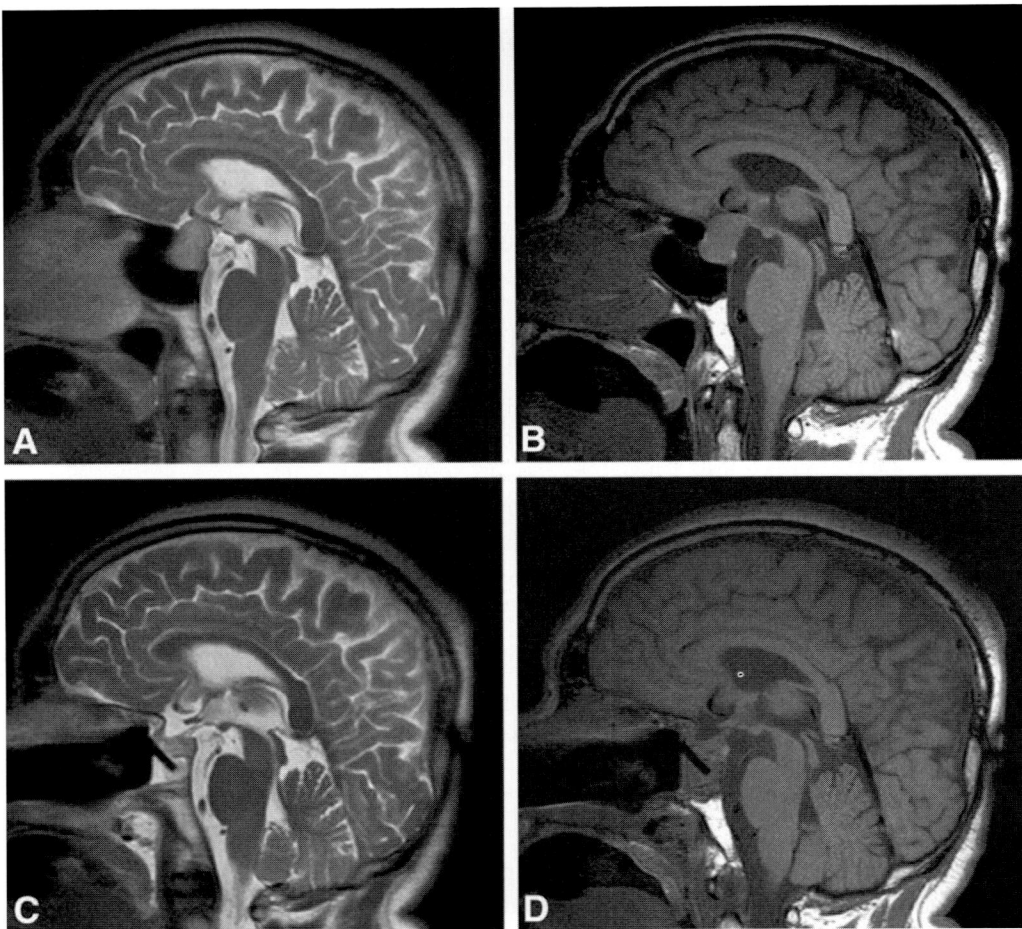

Fig. 6. A 57-yr-old male patient with a large intra- and suprasellar, hormonally inactive pituitary adenoma. (A,B) Preoperative sagittal scans. (C,D) Intraoperative images, depicting complete removal. (A,C) Images are available after 5 s, measured with a HASTE sequence. (B,D) T1-weighted.

imaging is clearly superior to low-field imaging. We expect that this excellent intraoperative image quality will result in a higher validity of intraoperative diagnostic evaluation of the extent of tumor resection. There is increasing consensus that achieving gross total resection of brain tumors can make a big difference *(58)*, so intraoperative imaging for quality control gains increasing importance. Up to now, high-field intraoperative MRI seems to be the most advanced possibility to give the neurosurgeon an intraoperative tool, for reliabe evaluation of intraoperative actions permitting immediate modification, i.e., further resection of the tumor during the same operation.

Besides enhanced image quality compared with low-field intraoperative systems, intraoperative high-field MRI offers further modalities, such as functional imaging, angiography, spectroscopy, and diffusion-weighted imaging,

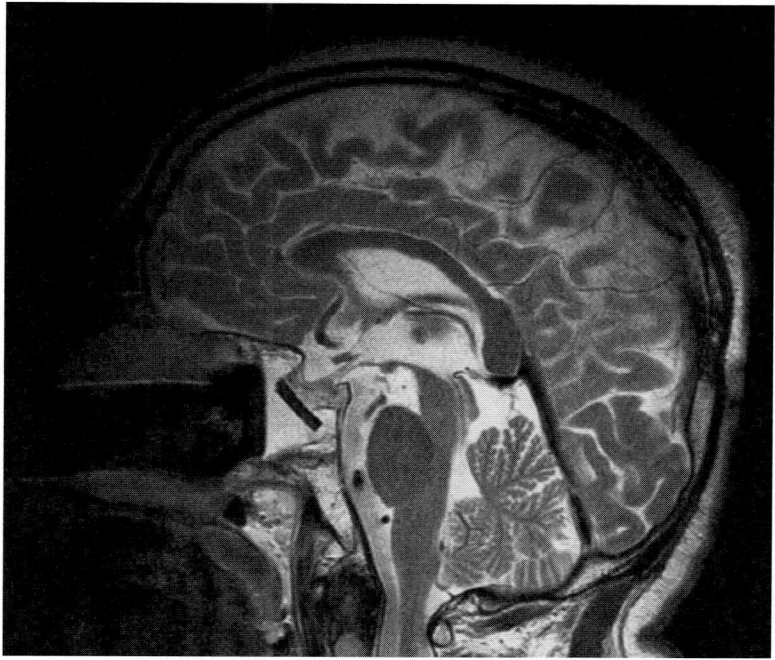

Fig. 7. Same patient as in Fig. 6. Intraoperative T2-weighted image, illustrating the high image quality. The floor of the sella is covered with a wax plate to give a good contrast.

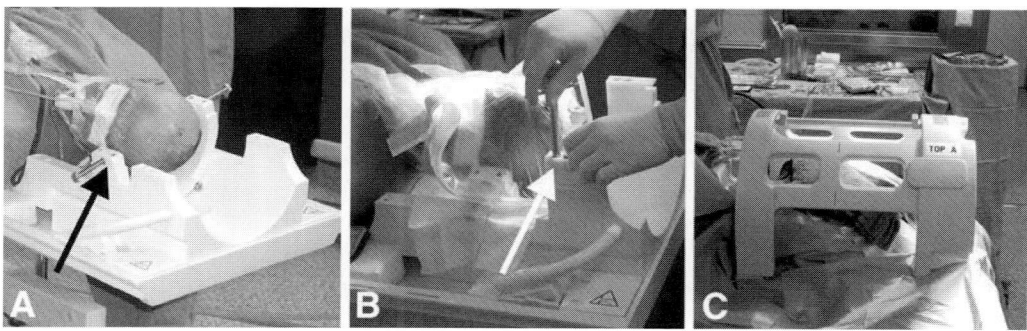

Fig. 8. In glioma surgery the head is fixed in an MR-compatible four-pin head holder (black arrow in **A**), which is integrated into the standard head coil. **(B)** Sterile adapters (white arrow) are placed on the lower part of the head coil before sterile draping. **(C)** After tumor removal, the sterile upper part of the head coil is placed on the adapters, and then imaging can start.

all contributing to an advanced neuronavigational setup. All these modalities have to be integrated into the navigational setup, providing not only functional neuronavigation but also multimodality neuronavigation. Progress in navigation technologies such as laser scanning *(59)* or automatic registration of

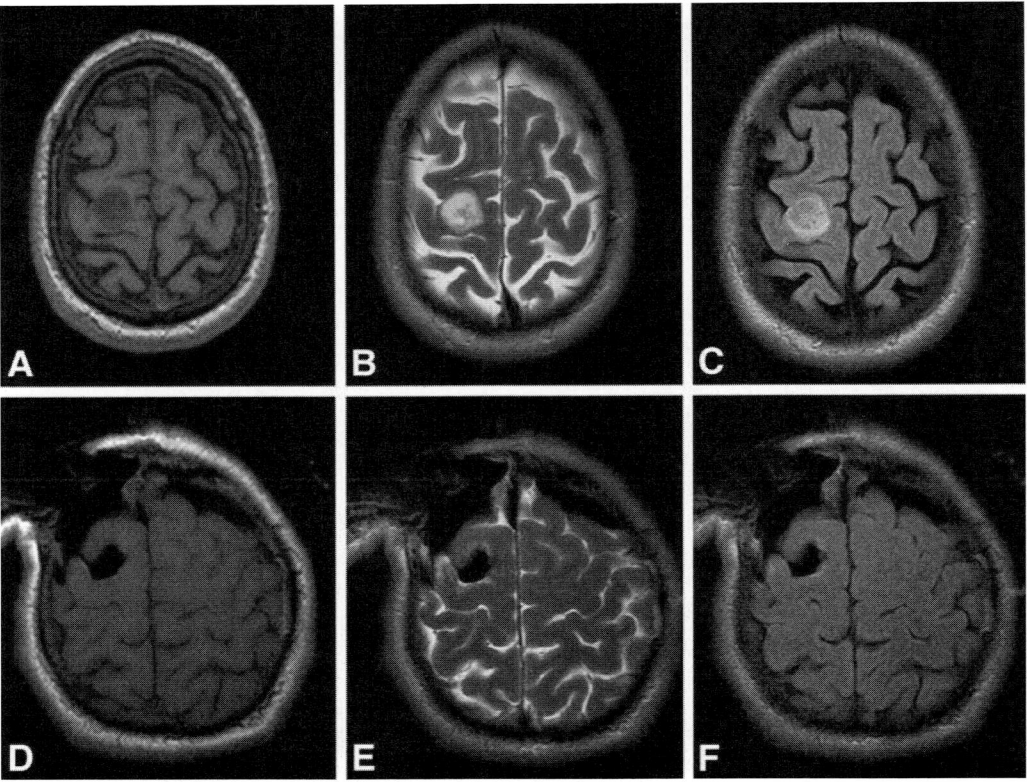

Fig. 9. A 34-yr-old male patient with a right precentral WHO grade II astrocytoma. (A–C) Preoperative axial images. (D–F) Corresponding intraoperative images. (A,D) T1-weighted images. (B,E) T2-weighted images. (C,F) FLAIR images.

intraoperative MR images, on which we are working, will improve registration accuracy, leading to more reliable ongoing neuronavigational application accuracy, especially if the navigation data are updated during critical steps of the overall procedure.

The application of MR spectroscopy to delineate normal brain vs pathological tissue (60–63) and to delineate the tumor border, its integration into the navigational setup, and intraoperative spectroscopic measurements are important projects, which will open new avenues in the treatment of brain tumors. Furthermore, the integration of information on pathways, such as the pyramidal tract, is an important and challenging task (64). Updated intraoperative compensation for brain shift, not only concerning the standard anatomical information, but also including pathways and functional data has to be established (32,65). Mathematical models describing the brain shift phenomenon, based mainly on finite element technology, will aid in this process (66,67). Intraoperative high-field MRI may also have indications beyond resection control in tumor surgery, e.g., intraoperative MRI with MR angiography in combination with perfusion imaging to monitor surgical effects in angioma and

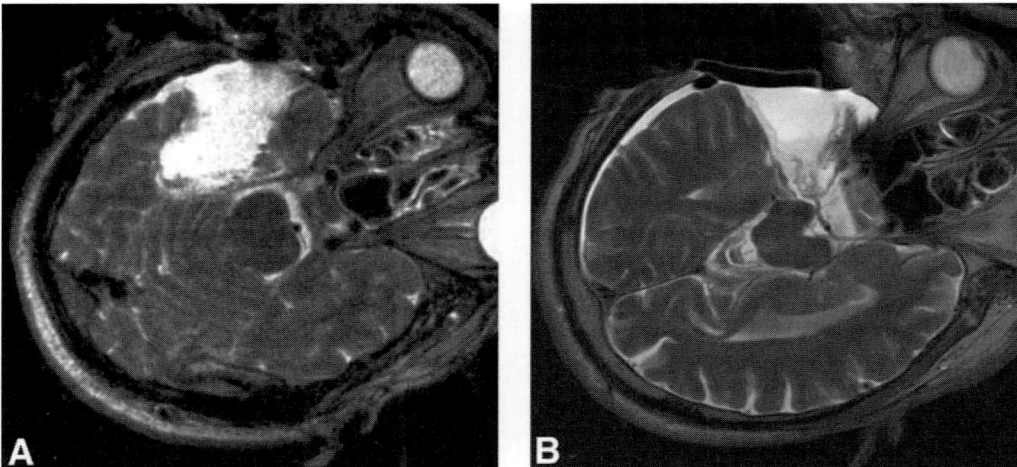

Fig. 10. The intraoperative image quality of the high-field system is clearly superior to that of the low-field system. Similar cases with right temporal lobe tumors, which were investigated by T2-weighted imaging with the 0.2-T **(A)** or the 1.5-T system **(B)**.

aneurysm surgery opens a new field of immediate intraoperative therapy control *(55)*.

Even now, it seems obvious that the patient investigated by intraoperative MRI is profiting from it. For a large group of patients, intraoperative imaging can replace early postoperative controls; when a tumor is completely removed with the aid of intraoperative imaging, the costs of repeated postoperative imaging and a potential second operation are saved. Of course, the cost of intraoperative MRI are high for a neurosurgical department; considering the beneficial effects, they may not be high when seen from the perspective of the national economy. Prospective cost–benefit studies for intraoperative MRI must be performed.

Today the intraoperative application of high-field MR with the integration of all kinds of functional and anatomical data, including sophisticated brain atlases, seems to be the major challenge for intraoperative imaging. Furthermore, robotic devices, assisting and improving the mechanical skills of the neurosurgeon, will be integrated. In the future, major advances may be also new developments in MR technology, such as extremely low-field MRI with magnetic field strengths of 10 mT. These techniques, relying on the so-called Overhauser effect *(68)*, may result in the realization of small, nearly invisible MR scanners, which will not impair surgical maneuvers. The advanced operating room of the future will include continuous and immediate imaging with integrated display of anatomy and function in a cartesian room, supporting the neurosurgeon without interfering with the surgical workflow.

ACKNOWLEDGMENTS

We are grateful to Dr. Ralf Steinmeier for his extensive efforts in the implementation and setup of the initial twin operating theater and to Dr. Oliver

Ganslandt for his ongoing support in intraoperative imaging and functional imaging. We are grateful to Dr. Helmut Kober for his outstanding work in functional imaging. We also acknowledge continuing support from Dr. A. Oppelt and Dr. T. Vetter (Siemens), and N. Ehrke and A. Dombay (BrainLab), as well as the Deutsche Forschungsgemeinschaft.

REFERENCES

1. Hammoud MA, Ligon BL, elSouki R, Shi WM, Schomer DF, Sawaya R. Use of intraoperative ultrasound for localizing tumors and determining the extent of resection: a comparative study with magnetic resonance imaging. *J Neurosurg* 1996; 84:737–741.
2. LeRoux PD, Winter TC, Berger MS, Mack LA, Wang K, Elliott JP. A comparison between preoperative magnetic resonance and intraoperative ultrasound tumor volumes and margins. *J Clin Ultrasound* 1994;22:29–36.
3. Woydt M, Krone A, Becker G, Schmidt K, Roggendorf W, Roosen K. Correlation of intra-operative ultrasound with histopathologic findings after tumour resection in supratentorial gliomas. A method to improve gross total tumour resection. *Acta Neurochir* 1996;138:1391–1398.
4. Butler WE, Piaggio CM, Constantinou C, et al. A mobile computed tomographic scanner with intraoperative and intensive care unit applications. *Neurosurgery* 1998;42:1304–1311.
5. Grunert P, Muller-Forell W, Darabi K, et al. Basic principles and clinical applications of neuronavigation and intraoperative computed tomography. *Comput Aided Surg* 1998;3:166–173.
6. Kabuto M, Kubota T, Kobayashi H, et al. Intraoperative CT imaging system using a mobile CT scanner gantry mounted on floor-embedded rails for neurosurgery. *No To Shinkei* 1998;50:1003–1008.
7. Lunsford LD, Rosenbaum AE, Perry J. Stereotactic surgery using the "therapeutic" CT scanner. *Surg Neurol* 1982;18:116–122.
8. Lunsford LD, Parrish R, Albright L. Intraoperative imaging with a therapeutic computed tomographic scanner. *Neurosurgery* 1984;15:559–561.
9. Okudera H, Kyoshima K, Kobayashi S, Sugita K. Intraoperative CT scan findings during resection of glial tumours. *Neurol Res* 1994;16:265–267.
10. Black PM, Moriarty T, Alexander E III, et al. Development and implementation of intraoperative magnetic resonance imaging and its neurosurgical applications. *Neurosurgery* 1997;41:831–845.
11. Tronnier VM, Wirtz CR, Knauth M, et al. Intraoperative diagnostic and interventional magnetic resonance imaging in neurosurgery. *Neurosurgery* 1997;40:891–902.
12. Steinmeier R, Fahlbusch R, Ganslandt O, et al. Intraoperative magnetic resonance imaging with the magnetom open scanner: concepts, neurosurgical indications, and procedures. A preliminary report. *Neurosurgery* 1998;43:739–748.
13. Ganslandt O, Steinmeier R, Kober H, et al. Magnetic source imaging combined with image-guided frameless stereotaxy: a new method in surgery around the motor strip. *Neurosurgery* 1997;41:621–628.
14. Ganslandt O, Fahlbusch R, Nimsky C, et al. Functional neuronavigation with magnetoencephalography: outcome in 50 patients with lesions around the motor cortex. *J Neurosurg* 1999;91:73–79.
15. Nimsky C, Ganslandt O, Kober H, et al. Integration of functional magnetic resonance imaging supported by magnetoencephalography in functional neuronavigation. *Neurosurgery* 1999;44:1249–1256.

16. Black PM, Alexander E III, Martin C, et al. Craniotomy for tumor treatment in an intraoperative magnetic resonance imaging unit. *Neurosurgery* 1999;45:423–433.
17. Schwartz RB, Hsu L, Wong TZ, et al. Intraoperative MRI guidance for intracranial neurosurgery: experience with the first 200 cases. *Radiology* 1999;211:477–488.
18. Knauth M, Wirtz CR, Tronnier VM, Aras N, Kunze S, Sartor K. Intraoperative MRI increases the extent of tumor resection in patients with high-grade gliomas. *AJNR Am J Neuroradiol* 1999;20:1642–1646.
19. Seifert V, Zimmermann M, Trantakis C, et al. Open MRI-guided neurosurgery. *Acta Neurochir* 1999;141:455–464.
20. Tronnier V, Staubert A, Wirtz R, Knauth M, Bonsanto M, Kunze S. MRI-guided brain biopsies using a 0.2 Tesla open magnet. *Minim Invasive Neurosurg* 1999;42:118–122.
21. Nimsky C, Ganslandt O, Kober H, Buchfelder M, Fahlbusch R. Intraoperative magnetic resonance imaging combined with neuronavigation: a new concept. *Neurosurgery* 2001;48:1082–1091.
22. Fahlbusch R, Ganslandt O, Buchfelder M, Schott W, Nimsky C. Intraoperative magnetic resonance imaging during transsphenoidal surgery. *J Neurosurg* 2001;95:381–390.
23. Rubino GJ, Farahani K, McGill D, Van De Wiele B, Villablanca JP, Wang-Mathieson A. Magnetic resonance imaging-guided neurosurgery in the magnetic fringe fields: the next step in neuronavigation. *Neurosurgery* 2000;46:643–654.
24. Bernstein M, Al-Anazi AR, Kucharczyk W, Manninen P, Bronskill M, Henkelman M. Brain tumor surgery with the Toronto open magnetic resonance imaging system: preliminary results for 36 patients and analysis of advantages, disadvantages, and future prospects. *Neurosurgery* 2000;46:900–909.
25. Hadani M, Spiegelman R, Feldman Z, Berkenstadt H, Ram Z. Novel, compact, intraoperative magnetic resonance imaging-guided system for conventional neurosurgical operating rooms. *Neurosurgery* 2001;48:799–809.
26. Schulder M, Liang D, Carmel PW. Cranial surgery navigation aided by a compact intraoperative magnetic resonance imager. *J Neurosurg* 2001;94:936–945.
27. Lewin JS. Interventional MRI: concepts, systems, and applications in neuroradiology. *AJNR Am J Neuroradiol* 1999;20:735–748.
28. Bohinski RJ, Kokkino AK, Warnick RE, et al. Glioma resection in a shared-resource magnetic resonance operating room after optimal image-guided frameless stereotactic resection. *Neurosurgery* 2001;48:731–744.
29. Buchfelder M, Ganslandt O, Fahlbusch R, Nimsky C. Intraoperative magnetic resonance imaging in epilepsy surgery. *J Magn Reson Imaging* 2000;12:547–555.
30. Nabavi A, Black PM, Gering DT, et al. Serial intraoperative magnetic resonance imaging of brain shift. *Neurosurgery* 2001;48:787–798.
31. Nimsky C, Ganslandt O, Cerny S, Hastreiter P, Greiner G, Fahlbusch R. Quantification of, visualization of, and compensation for brain shift using intraoperative magnetic resonance imaging. *Neurosurgery* 2000;47:1070–1080.
32. Nimsky C, Ganslandt O, Hastreiter P, Fahlbusch R. Intraoperative compensation for brain shift. *Surg Neurol* 2001;56:357–364.
33. Wirtz CR, Bonsanto MM, Knauth M, et al. Intraoperative magnetic resonance imaging to update interactive navigation in neurosurgery: method and preliminary experience. *Comput Aided Surg* 1997;2:172–179.
34. Fahlbusch R, Nimsky C, Ganslandt O, Steinmeier R, Buchfelder M, Huk W. The Erlangen concept of image guided surgery, in *CAR'98* (Lemke H, Vannier M, Inamura K, Farman A, eds.), Elsevier, Amsterdam, 1998, pp. 583–588.
35. Fahlbusch R, Heigl T, Huk W, Steinmeier R. The role of endoscopy and intraoperative MRI in transsphenoidal pituitary surgery, in *Pituitary Adenomas. From Basic*

Research to Fiagnosis and Therapy (Werder v K, Fahlbusch R, eds.), Elsevier, Amsterdam, 1996, pp. 237–241.

36. Kober H, Möller M, Nimsky C, Vieth J, Fahlbusch R, Ganslandt O. New approach to localize speech relevant brain areas and hemispheric dominance using spatially filtered magnetoencephalography. *Hum Brain Mapp* 2001;14:236–250.
37. Kober H, Nimsky C, Möller M, Hastreiter P, Fahlbusch R, Ganslandt O. Correlation of sensorimotor activation with functional magnetic resonance imaging and magnetoencephalography in presurgical functional imaging: a spatial analysis. *Neuroimage* 2001;14:1214–1228.
38. Möller M, Kober H, Ganslandt O, Nimsky C, Vieth J, Fahlbusch R. Functional mapping of speech evoked brain activity by magnetoencephalography and its clinical application. *Biomed Tech (Berl)* 1999;44:159–161.
39. Pergolizzi RS Jr, Nabavi A, Schwartz RB, et al. Intra-operative MR guidance during trans-sphenoidal pituitary resection: preliminary results. *J Magn Reson Imaging* 2001;13:136–141.
40. Martin CH, Schwartz R, Jolesz F, Black PM. Transsphenoidal resection of pituitary adenomas in an intraoperative MRI unit. *Pituitary* 1999;2:155–162.
41. Wirtz CR, Knauth M, Staubert A, et al. Clinical evaluation and follow-up results for intraoperative magnetic resonance imaging in neurosurgery. *Neurosurgery* 2000;46:1112–1122.
42. Kowalczuk A, Macdonald RL, Amidei C, et al. Quantitative imaging study of extent of surgical resection and prognosis of malignant astrocytomas. *Neurosurgery* 1997;41:1028–1038.
43. Keles GE, Lamborn KR, Berger MS. Low-grade hemispheric gliomas in adults: a critical review of extent of resection as a factor influencing outcome. *J Neurosurg* 2001;95:735–745.
44. Nicolato A, Gerosa MA, Fina P, Iuzzolino P, Giorgiutti F, Bricolo A. Prognostic factors in low-grade supratentorial astrocytomas: a uni-multivariate statistical analysis in 76 surgically treated adult patients. *Surg Neurol* 1995;44:208–223.
45. Schneider JP, Schulz T, Schmidt F, et al. Gross-total surgery of supratentorial low-grade gliomas under intraoperative MR guidance. *AJNR Am J Neuroradiol* 2001;22:89–98.
46. Schwartz TH, Marks D, Pak J, et al. Standardization of amygdalohippocampectomy with intraoperative magnetic resonance imaging: preliminary experience. *Epilepsia* 2002;43:430–436.
47. Kaibara T, Myles ST, Lee MA, Sutherland GR. Optimizing epilepsy surgery with intraoperative MRI. *Epilepsia* 2002;43:425–429.
48. Hoult DI, Saunders JK, Sutherland GR, et al. The engineering of an interventional MRI with a movable 1.5-T magnet. *J Magn Reson Imaging* 2001;13:78–86.
49. Kaibara T, Saunders JK, Sutherland GR. Advances in mobile intraoperative magnetic resonance imaging. *Neurosurgery* 2000;47:131–138.
50. Sutherland GR, Kaibara T, Louw D, Hoult DI, Tomanek B, Saunders J. A mobile high-field magnetic resonance system for neurosurgery. *J Neurosurg* 1999;91:804–813.
51. Hall WA, Liu H, Martin AJ, Pozza CH, Maxwell RE, Truwit CL. Safety, efficacy, and functionality of high-field strength interventional magnetic resonance imaging for neurosurgery. *Neurosurgery* 2000;46:632–642.
52. Hall WA, Martin AJ, Liu H, et al. High-field strength interventional magnetic resonance imaging for pediatric neurosurgery. *Pediatr Neurosurg* 1998;29:253–259.
53. Hall WA, Martin AJ, Liu H, Nussbaum ES, Maxwell RE, Truwit CL. Brain biopsy using high-field strength interventional magnetic resonance imaging. *Neurosurgery* 1999;44:807–814.

54. Hall WA, Liu H, Martin AJ, Maxwell RE, Truwit CL. Brain biopsy sampling by using prospective stereotaxis and a trajectory guide. *J Neurosurg* 2001;94:67–71.
55. Sutherland GR, Kaibara T, Wallace C, Tomanek B, Richter M. Intraoperative assessment of aneurysm clipping using magnetic resonance angiography and diffusion-weighted imaging: technical case report. *Neurosurgery* 2002;50:893–898.
56. Nimsky C, Ganslandt O, Fischer H, et al. Kombination aus Kopffixation und Kopfspule für neurochirurgische Operationen. *Siemens Tech Rep* 2000;3:64–65.
57. Romstöck J, Fahlbusch R, Ganslandt O, Nimsky C, Strauss C. Localisation of the sensorimotor cortex during surgery for brain tumours: feasibility and waveform patterns of somatosensory evoked potentials. *J Neurol Neurosurg Psychiatry* 2002;72:221–229.
58. Bradley WG. Achieving gross total resection of brain tumors: intraoperative MR imaging can make a big difference. *AJNR Am J Neuroradiol* 2002;23:348–349.
59. Raabe A, Krishnan R, Wolff R, Hermann E, Zimmermann M, Seifert V. Laser surface scanning for patient registration in intracranial image-guided surgery. *Neurosurgery* 2002;50:797–803.
60. Tzika AA, Cheng LL, Goumnerova L, et al. Biochemical characterization of pediatric brain tumors by using in vivo and ex vivo magnetic resonance spectroscopy. *J Neurosurg* 2002;96:1023–1031.
61. Tzika AA, Zarifi MK, Goumnerova L, et al. Neuroimaging in pediatric brain tumors: Gd-DTPA-enhanced, hemodynamic, and diffusion MRI compared with MR spectroscopic imaging. *AJNR Am J Neuroradiol* 2002;23:322–333.
62. Hall WA, Martin A, Liu H, Truwit CL. Improving diagnostic yield in brain biopsy: coupling spectroscopic targeting with real-time needle placement. *J Magn Reson Imaging* 2001;13:12–15.
63. Dowling C, Bollen AW, Noworolski SM, et al. Preoperative proton MR spectroscopic imaging of brain tumors: correlation with histopathologic analysis of resection specimens. *AJNR Am J Neuroradiol* 2001;22:604–612.
64. Coenen VA, Krings T, Mayfrank L, et al. Three-dimensional visualization of the pyramidal tract in a neuronavigation system during brain tumor surgery: first experiences and technical note. *Neurosurgery* 2001;49:86–93.
65. Hastreiter P, Engel K, Soza G, et al. Remote analysis for brain shift compensation, in *Medical image computing and computer assisted intervention* (Niessen W, Viergever M, eds.), 4th International Conference. Lecture Notes in Computer Science, vol 2208. Springer, Berlin, 2001, pp. 1248–1249.
66. Miga MI, Paulsen KD, Hoopes PJ, Kennedy FE, Hartov A, Roberts DW. In vivo modeling of interstitial pressure in the brain under surgical load using finite elements. *J Biomech Eng* 2000;122:354–363.
67. Ferrant M, Warfield SK, Nabavi A, Jolesz F, Kikinis R. Registration of 3D intraoperative MR images of the brain using a finite element biomechanical model, in *Medical Image Computing and Computer-Assisted Intervention* (Delp SL, DiGioia AM, Jaramaz B, eds.), Springer, Berlin, 2000, pp. 19–28.
68. Katscher U, Petersson S. Kernspintomographie unter Nutzung des Overhauser-Effekts. *Phys Bl* 2000;56:51–54.

7
Endovascular Treatment of Intracranial Aneurysms

Christos Gkogkas, MD, John Baker, MD, Alexander M. Norbash, MD, and Kai U. Frerichs, MD

INTRODUCTION

Historical Perspectives

Endovascular treatment of intracranial aneurysms was first described in the early 1970s in the pioneering paper of Serbinenko. He treated aneurysms with detachable balloons that were positioned in the parent artery or in the aneurysm lumen itself through a microcatheter *(1,2)*. In 1991, Guglielmi et al. *(3,4)* described the endovascular occlusion of intracranial aneurysms using electrolytic detachable platinum coils (Target Therapeutics/Boston Scientific). The Guglielmi detachable coils (GDCs) could be introduced through a microcatheter into the aneurysm lumen and detached from a stainless steel microwire by an electrical current. In 1995 the device was approved by the Food and Drug Administration (FDA) and has become widely used in patients with ruptured and unruptured intracranial aneurysms. The GDC technology has evolved ever since, and as clinical experience with this technique has accumulated, it has become the method of choice for the endovascular treatment of intracranial aneurysms. Improved microcatheter and microwire designs have greatly facilitated intracranial intravascular navigation, allowing catheterization of distal aneurysms. Until recently, endovascular treatment in the Unites States was reserved for aneurysms not amenable to surgical clipping. In August 2003, the FDA granted approval to market GDC for the treatment of all brain aneurysms. Continuous technical advances and increasing clinical experience with endovascular techniques as well as its minimal invasiveness have made endovascular treatment an attractive alternative, even in patients who could be treated by conventional neurosurgical clipping.

COMPARISON OF ENDOVASCULAR COILING WITH NEUROSURGICAL CLIPPING

Endovascular aneurysm treatment strategies are now challenging neurosurgical clipping as the standard approach to treatment of cerebral aneurysms. In some institutions, GDC coiling is even considered the first-line treatment in

From: *Minimally Invasive Neurosurgery*, edited by: M.R. Proctor and P.M. Black © Humana Press Inc., Totowa, NJ

these patients *(5–7)*. It was estimated that in August 2002, 100,000 patients with intracranial aneurysms had been treated with GDCs worldwide *(8)*. Considering these large and increasing numbers, a comparison of the efficacy and risk of morbidity and mortality of the two treatment strategies must be made. Comparisons between surgical and endovascular series should be made with caution because of the heterogeneity in study design, patients, and aneurysms *(9)*.

A small randomized single-institution trial compared the outcomes of surgical clipping and endovascular treatment in 109 patients with ruptured intracranial aneurysms. The basic characteristics of the patients in both treatment groups were similar in terms of aneurysm location and size, severity of subarachnoid bleeding, and clinical grade. Surgery- and coiling procedure-related mortality was similar in both groups, and there was no difference in the short-term clinical outcome. One-year clinical and neuropsychological outcomes were comparable *(10,11)*.

The International Subarachnoid Aneurysm Trial (ISAT) is a multicenter, randomized clinical trial comparing a policy of neurosurgical clipping with a policy of endovascular treatment with detachable platinum coils in patients with ruptured intracranial aneurysms considered suitable for either treatment *(12)*. In all, 9278 patients were evaluated for eligibility, and finally clinical equipoise was observed in 2143 patients who were enrolled in the study and randomly assigned to endovascular treatment ($n = 1073$) or neurosurgical clipping ($n = 1070$). Almost all (97.3%) lesions were located in the anterior circulation, 50.5% in the anterior cerebral artery (ACA), 32.5% in the internal cerebral artery (ICA), and 14.1% in the middle cerebral artery (MCA), with only 2.7% of lesions in the posterior circulation. The great majority of the aneurysms were 10 mm or smaller in size. At 1 yr, 23.7% of patients allocated to endovascular treatment were dead or dependent compared with 30.6% in the surgical group. The relative risk of dependence or death was reduced by 22.6% in patients treated with endovascular coiling, with an absolute risk reduction of 6.9%. Trial recruitment was stopped by the steering committee after a planned interim analysis, but follow-up will continue.

In a retrospective observational study, Johnston et al. *(13)* compared the risks of endovascular and surgical treatment in 130 patients with unruptured cerebral aneurysms, who were considered candidates for either procedure on blinded review, and overall anticipated procedure risk was rated as identical. Surgery was found to be associated with greater rates of early and persistent disability, more procedure-related major complications, and longer delays in return of function. Length of stay was longer, and hospital charges were greater for the surgical group.

A permanent complication rate of 7% was shown on metaanalysis of 1383 patients with intracranial aneurysms, treated with endovascular GDC embolization *(9)*.

In a recent review on surgery of unruptured aneurysms in 2460 patients, the morbidity was 11% and mortality 3% *(14)*. The International Study of Unruptured Intracranial Aneurysms (ISUIA) showed an unexpectedly high rate of neurological deficits, cognitive impairment, and mortality after surgical clipping of unruptured intracranial aneurysms *(15)*. At 30 d after surgery, cognitive impairements were evident in 5.5% of patients, neurologic disabilities in 3.6%, and both in 6.1% in the subgroup of patients without previous surgery or subarachnoid hemorrhage (SAH). Furthermore, the cognitive deficits failed to improve during the next year.

The available studies indicate that the complications in the endovascular series are lower than in the surgical series. This difference is accentuated by the fact that aneurysm treatment by endovascular methods is usually reserved for sicker patients with more difficult aneurysms *(16)*. The lower procedural mortality and morbidity rates of endovascular aneurysm treatment, compared with those of surgical clipping, have to be weighed against a higher rate of incomplete aneurysm obliteration and aneurysm recurrence following aneurysm coiling. Several studies attest to the protective effect of coiling in the acute phase of SAH . On metaanalysis, a rerupture rate of 0.9% per yr is estimated after coil embolization of ruptured aneurysms in various locations in an average follow-up of up to 1.8 yr *(17)*. Vinuela et al. *(18)* reported a 6-mo rebleeding rate of 2.2% in 403 patients with acute SAH treated with GDCs. Rerupture after surgical clipping does also occur *(11,12,19,20)*.

In the ISAT study, the long-term risks of further bleeding from the treated aneurysm were low with either therapy, although somewhat more frequent with endovascular coiling. Within 1 yr, 2.4% of endovascular cases (26/1048) and 1% (10/994) of surgical cases rebled *(12)*. It is hoped that the ongoing follow-up of these patients will shed some light on the long-term efficacy of endovascular therapy.

ANEURYSM LOCATION

Surgical accessibility of the aneurysm is the most important factor predicting treatment failure in patients undergoing microsurgical aneurysm clipping. Unlike surgical aneurysm treatment, endovascular treatment is less dependent on the location of the aneurysm. The morphologic aneurysm characteristics, as delineated by cerebral angiography, are the major determinants of endovascular treatment outcome (Fig. 1). The impact of aneurysm location in the selection of the treatment modality is reflected in the ISAT study. Patients with ruptured posterior circulation aneurysms (and to a lesser degree patients with middle cerebral artery aneurysms) are underrepresented *(12)*.

Posterior Circulation

The basilar apex aneurysms are technically challenging to treat microsurgically because of their deep location and their intimate relationship to the thalamoperforating arteries. On the other hand, in a review study, the endovascular treatment results and complications in patients with basilar bifurcation aneurysms were in the same range as those in patients with an aneurysm located elsewhere.

Lempert et al. *(21)* reported a morbidity of 2.8% and a procedure-related mortality of 0% in 109 patients with ruptured posterior circulation aneurysms treated with coiling. Nearly one-half of these aneurysms (49%) were located in

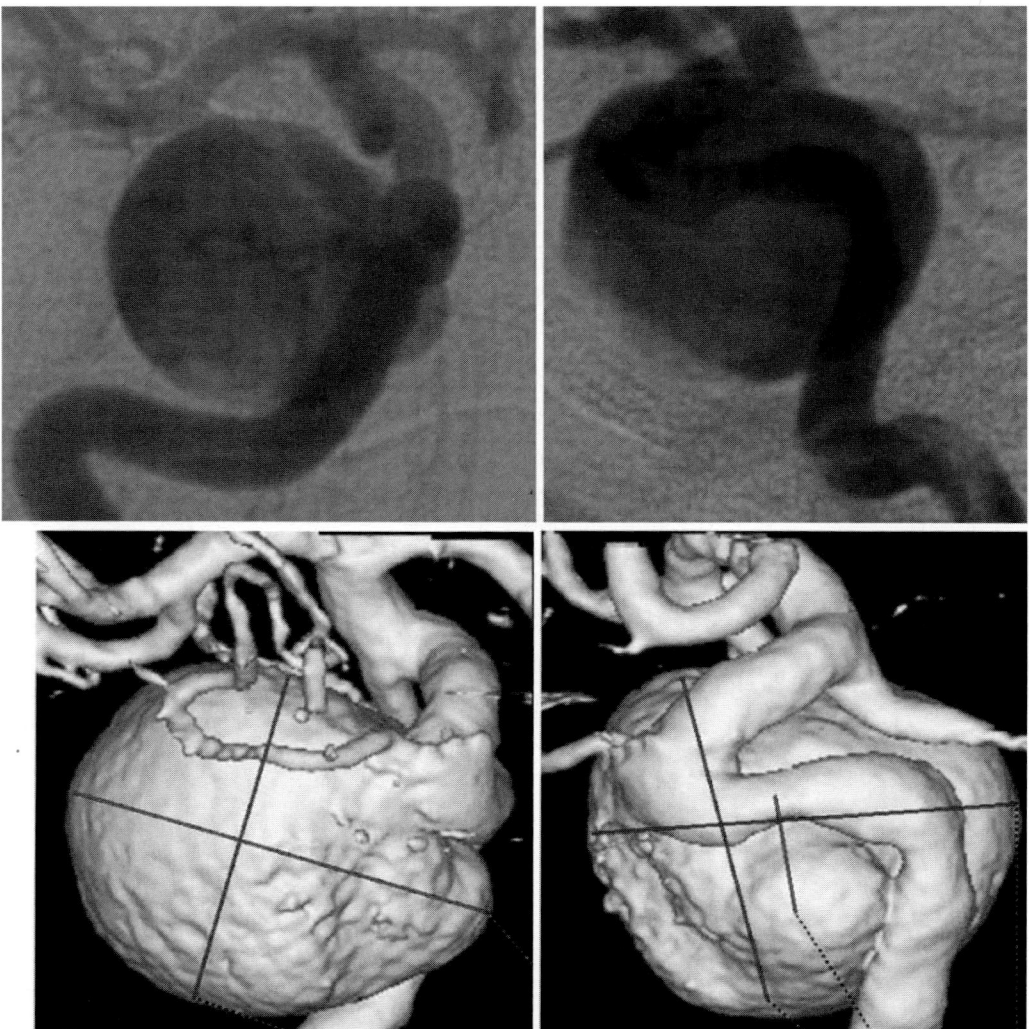

Fig. 1. Three-dimensional rotational angiography (3D RA) can help elucidate aneurysm characteristics that will guide the choice of intervention. (Top) From 2D angiography this right internal carotid artery (ICA) giant aneurysm causing right cranial nerve III palsy and V1–2, discomfort was initially felt to have a very wide neck originating from the cavernous segment. (Bottom) Three-dimensional RA showed that it originated from the clinoidal segment with a favorable dome-to-neck ratio. Thus treatment was changed to coiling without assist. Previously the plan was open neurosurgical takedown of the right ICA. The patient had experienced right hemisphere hypoperfusion during balloon occlusion testing of the right ICA. This precluded endovascular takedown of the right ICA, as bypass to the right middle cerebral artery from the right superficial temporal artery would have been required to maintain right hemisphere perfusion.

the basilar bifurcation. Late rebleeding was seen in one patient (0.9%) with a partially treated aneurysm. Mean duration of clinical follow-up was 13.1 mo. A 22.4% recanalization rate was reported, at a mean angiographic follow-up 7.1 mo *(21)*.

Bavinzski et al. *(22)* reported mortality and permanent morbidity rates directly related to the intervention of 2.2 and 4.4%, respectively, in 45 basilar artery aneurysms treated with GDCs, 35 of which were ruptured. A single rerupture was observed during 74.8 patient years of follow-up, corresponding to a rate of 1.3% per yr *(22)*. An annual rerupture rate of 2.9% was reported by Eskridge et al. *(23)* for 61 patients with basilar tip aneurysms, on a mean follow-up of 1.1 yr. Samson et al. *(24)* reported the results of surgical clipping in a series of 303 basilar apex aneurysms, one-third of which were unruptured. At 6-mo follow-up, 81% of patients were neurologically intact or had minor deficits, 10% were dead, and 9% had a poor outcome. No recurrent SAH was seen at a mean follow-up of 8 yr. Residual aneurysm was observed in 6% on follow-up angiography. Lawton et al. *(25)* reported a surgical mortality rate of 9% and a permanent neurologic morbidity associated with treatment in 5% in a series of 57 basilar apex aneurysms, 47% of which were large or giant in size.

In a retrospective comparative study, endovascular treatment demonstrated a 50% combined morbidity/mortality rate in the surgical group compared with 10% in the endovascular group in a cohort of ruptured and unruptured basilar artery apex aneurysms. There were no reruptures during approx 24 patient-years of follow-up *(26)*.

Middle Cerebral Artery Aneurysms

MCA aneurysms are often wide based and tend to incorporate the proximal segment of the M2 branches. This unfavorable angioanatomy poses a challenge to the endovascular surgeon and renders most aneurysms in this location unsuitable for coiling *(27)*. In a prospective study, coiling of ruptured MCA aneurysms was found to be associated with a poorer outcome than coiling of aneurysms located elsewhere in the anterior circulation *(5)*.

TISSUE RESPONSE TO GDC: HISTOPATHOLOGICAL FINDINGS

In contrast to surgical clipping, which results in immediate apposition of the intima surfaces across the aneurysmal neck, endovascular coiling induces a sequential intraaneurysmal cellular response to the coil material. The tissue response to endovascular coils is variable. Tenjin et al. *(28)* studied the temporal sequence of histopathological events induced by GDC placement on carotid artery aneurysms in primates. Thrombus formation occurred immediately after coil placement. Two weeks after placement, neoendothelialization of the orifice of the aneurysm was observed. At 3 mo a thick membrane resembling vascular media was covering this site. Mawad et al. *(29)* showed similar results at 6 months in canine aneurysms treated with GDC.

Histologic studies in embolized human cerebral aneurysms with platinum coils are limited. The presence of a thin fibrin membrane across the aneurysm

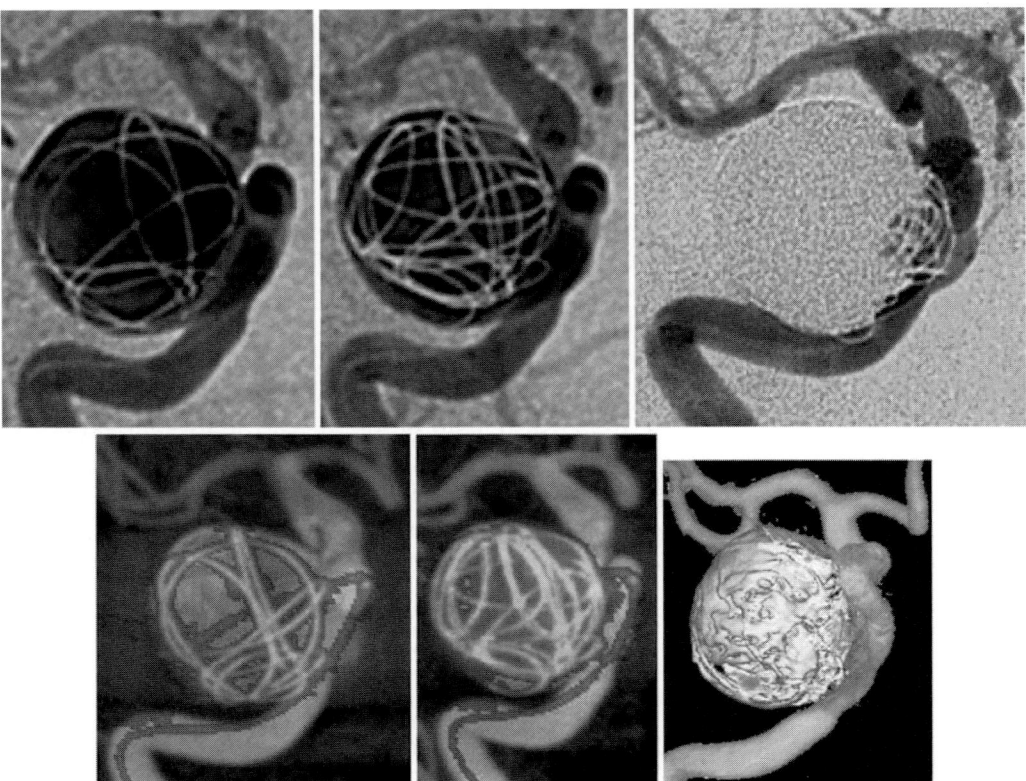

Fig. 2. Complete exclusion of an aneurysm from the circulation is not usually from the coil mass alone. An unruptured right middle cerebral artery (MCA) anterior temporal branch aneurysm before and 6 mo after coiling in a patient found to have multiple cerebral aneurysms after presenting with subarachnoid hemorrhage. The left and center panels are 2D angiograms with right internal carotid artery (ICA) injection. The 3D rendering in the right panel shows that the radiodense coil mass is separated from the contrast within the artery by a layer of radiolucent material probably representing fibrosis of the aneurysm neck.

neck has been demonstrated as early as 36 h after coiling and has been suggested to serve as a substrate for endothelialization *(30)*. Complete isolation of the aneurysm from the parent vessel can promote scar formation and stabilization of the thrombus (Fig. 2). Ishihara et al. *(31)* showed endothelialization of platinum coils at the orifice of human cerebral aneurysms at 2 wk and at 20 mo after embolization in five cases of small neck aneurysms. Bavinzski et al. *(32)* studied the histopathological changes in 18 human cerebral aneurysms treated with GDC and concluded that endothelialization of the aneurysm orifice after coiling can occur but seems to be the exception rather than the rule. They found tiny gaps between the coils at the aneurysm neck in 50% of densely packed aneurysms that appeared completely occluded on angiography. Small neck size and dense coil packing across the aneurysm neck are important factors to induce endothelialization, which excludes the aneurysm from the parent vessel.

Shimizu et al. *(33)* showed the presence of organized thrombus at the periphery of a small, broad-necked aneurysm 6 wk after loose coil application in the absence of neck neoendothelium. They suggested that this could provide reinforcement of the aneurysmal wall despite the absence of exclusion from the parent vessel.

HEMODYNAMIC EFFECTS

Hemodynamic stress has been implicated in the formation, growth, and rupture of intracranial aneurysms. GDC treatment of aneurysms is effective in reducing the rebleeding rate. Animal studies have shown that coiling of intracranial aneurysms does not reduce the mean intraaneurysmal pressure *(34,35)*. However, GDC treatment was shown to dampen the pressure amplitude and delayed pressure increases during locally induced hypertension *(36)*. Moreover, the intraaneurysmal flow was significantly reduced even after incomplete treatment with GDC *(37)*. Graves et al. *(38)* investigated the flow dynamics of lateral carotid aneurysms and their effects on coils and balloons in an experimental canine model. They found that the inflow zone at the distal aspect of the aneurysm ostium is a major determining factor in the placement and stability of coils in aneurysms. Modification of the inflow zone can be used to promote aneurysmal thrombosis. The distal neck of the aneurysm is exposed to the highest shear stress pressures, and its obliteration is crucial whether the aneurysm is being surgically or endovascularly treated *(39)*.

The 3D angiography (3DA) data can be used as the basis for computational simulation of intraaneurysmal flow in order to elucidate the patient-specific aneurysm hemodynamic information *(40)*. It is hoped that in the future it will be possible to use these simulations for patient triage to therapy.

PROCEDURE

Anticoagulation

For endovascular procedures in unruptured aneurysms, systemic anticoagulation with heparin should be administered during the procedure to minimize thromboembolic complications. Intravenous aspirin is also administered. Some groups elect to give heparin to patients with ruptured aneurysms from the start of the procedure. Our approach with regard to coiling of ruptured aneurysms is to withhold the administration of heparin until the first coil is placed. Heparin is sometimes continued for 1–2 d after the procedure.

The GDC System

The GDC system consists of a platinum coil attached to a stainless steel delivery wire. The coil has a circular memory, which it assumes once it is advanced past the microcatheter tip. Application of electric current results in dissolution of the solder joint between the delivery wire and the platinum coil. Several sizes, shapes, and softness grades are available to conform to the diverse aneurysm morphology.

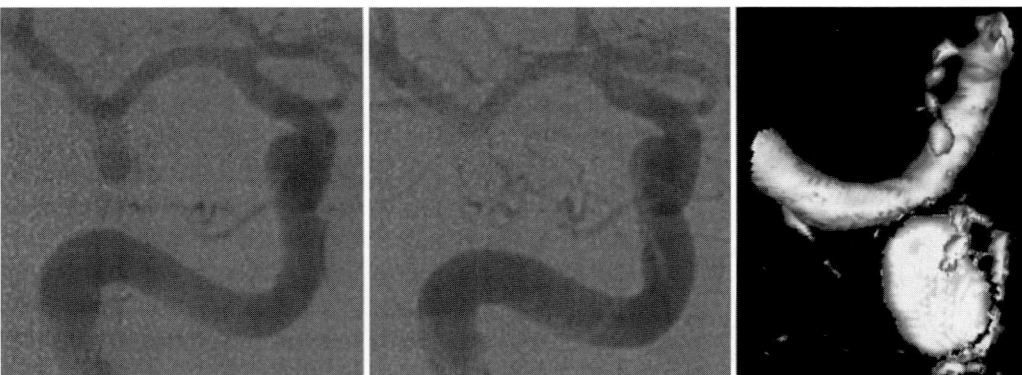

Fig. 3. Sequential coiling of a right internal carotid artery (ICA) giant aneurysm. Angiograms in 2D (top) and/or 3D (bottom) are performed after a coil has been positioned but not detached. From left to right are angiograms after 1 coil, 3 coils, and 22 coils have been placed. The pushwire within the microcatheter is also visible in the right ICA. The angiogram is evaluated for coil position, residual aneurysm, and patency of parent and daughter arteries. The coil can then be detached, repositioned, or removed.

Technique

The microcatheter is advanced into the aneurysm lumen over the microguidewire. The microguidewire is then removed, and the coil is then introduced into the aneurysm (Fig. 3). The largest coil is used first, to form the initial basket. Subsequently, smaller coils are used to increase the packing density. The sequential coil placement continues until resistance is felt. The goal should be to achieve as dense a packing as possible (*see* Aneurysm Remnant section following). During the coil delivery, proximal and distal radiopaque markers on the microcatheter are used to maintain its position. It is crucial to avoid forward migration of the microcatheter and impingement on the thin aneurysm wall. Control angiography is performed prior to each coil detachment to assess patency of the parent vessel and coil position stability. The microcatheter can be repositioned within the aneurysm if it is felt that there are loosely filled or unfilled regions of its lumen, and further coils can be delivered.

PROCEDURE COMPLICATIONS

Aneurysm Rupture During Coiling

Vinuela et al. *(41)* reported a rupture rate of 2% in a series of 700 aneurysms treated with GDCs. This complication was more common in small aneurysms. In a reported series of 128 aneurysms, Valavanis et al. *(42)* observed aneurysmal perforation only in previously ruptured small aneurysms. The most common cause is forward migration of the micocatheter. Therefore, tension within the microcatheter has to be minimized *(43)*. The guidewire should be removed very slowly under fluoroscopic visualization *(44)*. Perforations also commonly occur during the first coil placement *(45)*. The strategy for managing this serious and potentially fatal complication includes immediate reversal of heparin anticoagulation with protamine sulfate. The coil delivery should be completed in an attempt to achieve dense packing and sealing of the perforation site. Some neurointerventionalists suggest leaving the initial microcatheter in place across the perforation and using a second microcatheter to access the aneurysm and coil its lumen *(46)*. The blood pressure should be pharmacologically reduced. Emergency ventriculostomy placement in the angiography suite should also be considered to decrease the intracranial pressure.

Thromboembolic Complications

Thromboembolic events are the commonest complication of endovascular treatment of aneurysms. A rate of up to 28% clinically evident thromboembolic events has been reported, with a 3.4% rate of permanent neurologic deficit *(47)*. The anticoagulation regimen, the aneurysm size, location, and neck morphology, the number of guiding catheters and microcatheters, the patient's clinical status, and the operator's experience are important determining variables of the frequency of these events *(48)*. Intraarterial fibrinolysis or mechanical clot fragmentation can be used to restore vascular patency *(49)*. In cases of ruptured aneurysms, the administration of fibrinolytic drugs should be avoided. The platelet glycogen receptor IIb/IIIa antagonist abciximab has been used successfully in the treatment of acute arterial intracranial thrombosis, resulting in prompt clot dissolution *(50)*. The shorter half-life platelet glycogen receptor IIb/IIIa antagonists eptifibatide and tirofiban may be a better choice in this setting.

Coil Herniation into the Parent Vessel

Coil protrusion into the parent artery is more common in aneurysms with a wide neck, which is less likely to contain the coil loops, and in aneurysms located at complex branching points incorporating outflow arteries into the aneurysm base or walls such as the MCA bifurcation. It can potentially lead to occlusion of the parent vessel or serve as a source of distal emboli. These are more common in small arteries, such as the M1 segments of the MCA, the P1 segments of the posterior cerebral arteries and the anterior communicating arteries *(41)*. Attempts can be made to push the herniated coil part back into the aneurysm lumen with a microwire or by inflating a balloon at the ostium of the aneurysm. If these prove unsuccessful, we elect to use long-term antithrombotic therapy with aspirin. 3DA delineates the exact relationship of the aneurysmal sac to the parent vessel and helps to minimize the risk of parent vessel occlusion. 3D imaging is particularly useful in MCA and anterior communicating artery aneurysms. In a study of the added value of 3DA in the endovascular management of cerebral aneurysms, it was found that 3DA facilitated coiling, modified treatment, eliminated the need for treatment, and predicted potential complications by providing additional morphological information *(51)* (Fig. 1).

ANATOMIC RESULTS

The goal of aneurysm treatment, whether it is microsurgical or endovascular, is the complete exclusion of the aneurysm sac and neck from the cerebral circulation. The size of the aneurysm neck and its relationship to the body of the aneurysm are probably the most important determinants of the endovascular treatment result *(52)*. Zubilaga et al. *(53)* demonstrated a complete occlusion rate of 85% for small neck aneurysms with a neck less than 4 mm, but only 15% for aneurysms with a neck 4mm or greater. Studying the predictors of the immediate outcome of aneurysm occlusion, Turjman et al. *(54)* found that large aneurysmal diameter and volume and large neck size, as well as increasingly obtuse angulation between the long axis of aneurysm and the parent artery, correlated with unsatisfactory treatment result. Besides the morphological aneurysm characteristics, the operator experience was associated with higher occlusion rates.

Aneurysm Remnant

Endovascular treatment is often incomplete. A metaanalysis of 1383 patients showed that are more than 90% occlusion rate could be achieved in 90% of treated aneurysms and a complete occlusion rate in 54% *(9)*. Small aneurysm neck remnants are frequently seen after endovascular GDC embolization. Vinuela et al. *(18)* reported aneurysm neck remnants in 21.4% of small aneurysms with small necks, 41.6% of small aneurysms, with wide necks, 57.1% of large aneurysms and 50% of giant aneurysms.

The evolution of the aneurysm rest is unclear. It may undergo thrombosis and disappear, or it may enlarge as a result of coil compaction or aneurysm regrowth. The water hammer effect of blood flow in the aneurysm inflow zone may result in aneurysm recanalization. Broad-necked aneurysms are exposed to higher intensity hemodynamic shear forces than small-neck aneurysms *(55)*. Besides the pulsatile blood flow, scar contraction of the connective tissue that forms on the coil surface may contribute to the coil compaction *(32)*. Large neck size and large aneurysm size were found to be associated with higher recanalization rates. Hayakawa et al. *(56)* found that denser packing of the aneurysm significantly reduces the recanalization rate. They studied the natural history of 73 coiled aneurysms with residual necks for a period of 3–71 mo (mean 17.3 mo): 25% exhibited progressive thrombosis, 26% remained unchanged, and 49% displayed recanalization on postembolization angiography.

It is not known whether the aneurysm remnants following endovascular treatment differ from surgical remnants. Malish et al. *(57)* demonstrated a bleeding rate of postembolization aneurysm remnants of 0% in patients with small aneurysms, 4% in large aneurysms, and 33% in giant aneurysms in a follow-up of 2–6 yr (mean 3.5 yr). Long-term observational studies are needed to assess the evolution of the postembolization aneurysm remnants and compare it with the surgical remnants.

The reported rate of aneurysm remnants after surgical clipping ranges between 3.9 and 26% *(10,58)*. The lack of a standardized definition for residual postoperative angiographic aneurysm filling and the differences in patient populations in different studies may partially explain these differences. In a recent metaanalysis, residual filling on postoperative angiography was found in 5.2% of 1370 surgically treated patients *(59)*. Two large studies have investigated the natural history of surgical aneurysm remnants. David et al. *(20)* demonstrated a rehemorrhage rate of 1.9% per yr from aneurysm residua. Feuerberg et al. *(58)* reported an annual rehemorrhage rate from aneurysmal residua of up to 0.8%. Reoperation of the remnant was shown to carry a morbidity of 7% and a mortality of 5.2% *(60)*. Endovascular treatment of aneurysm remnants is effective and can be performed without significant morbidity *(61)*.

Aneurysm Recurrence

Aneurysm recanalization owing to coil compaction or continuous aneurysm growth can also occur in completely occluded aneurysms. Cognard et al. *(62)* reported a recurrence in 20 of 148 *(14%)* completely occluded aneurysms in an angiographic follow-up of 3–40 mo. The recurrences were more common in ruptured *(17%)* than in unruptured (7%) aneurysms. Intraaneurysmal thrombus may lead to coil migration and recanalization *(41,62)*. David et al. *(20)* reported a 0.52% annual regrowth rate for completely clipped aneurysms and an 1.8% annual rate of *de novo* aneurysm formation. Tsutsumi et al. *(63)* found an 8% rate of de novo aneurysm formation and a 2.9% aneurysm regrowth rate at 9 yr, in a series of 220 patients with SAH, who underwent complete surgical aneurysm clipping confirmed by postoperative angiography. Rebleeding has been reported to affect 2.7% of patients cumulatively in 10 yr, even after complete aneurysm clipping *(19)*.

All patients treated with coil embolization should have angiographic follow-up studies to assess the temporal evolution of the initial treatment result (Figs. 2 and 4).

MASS EFFECT

Intracerebral aneurysms occasionally present with symptoms of compression of the adjacent parenchyma or cranial nerves. Endovascular coiling has been shown to result in complete resolution of symptoms in 32% of patients, improvement in 42%, and worsening of symptoms in 5%. In 21% it showed no effect *(64)*. Smaller aneurysms and those with shorter pretreatment duration of symptoms showed a more favorable symptom response to coiling than giant aneurysms. Intraaneurysmal thrombosis is thought to eliminate the expansile pressure and result in aneurysm shrinkage owing to clot retraction *(65)*.

ENDOVASCULAR TREATMENT OF WIDE NECK ANEURYSMS

Broad neck aneurysms are more difficult to treat with the traditional coiling technique. Debrun et al. *(52)* reported an 80% total occlusion rate in aneurysms with a dome-to-neck ratio of 2 or larger and only 58% for a dome-to-neck ratio of less than 2. A variety of devices and adjunct techniques have been developed to allow successful endovascular treatment of aneurysms that are otherwise difficult or impossible to treat. 3DA is key to define the aneurysm geometry and thereby choose an appropriate treatment option.

Balloon Remodeling

This technique utilizes a nondetachable balloon as a mechanical barrier to prevent coil herniation through the aneurysm neck into the parent artery *(66)*

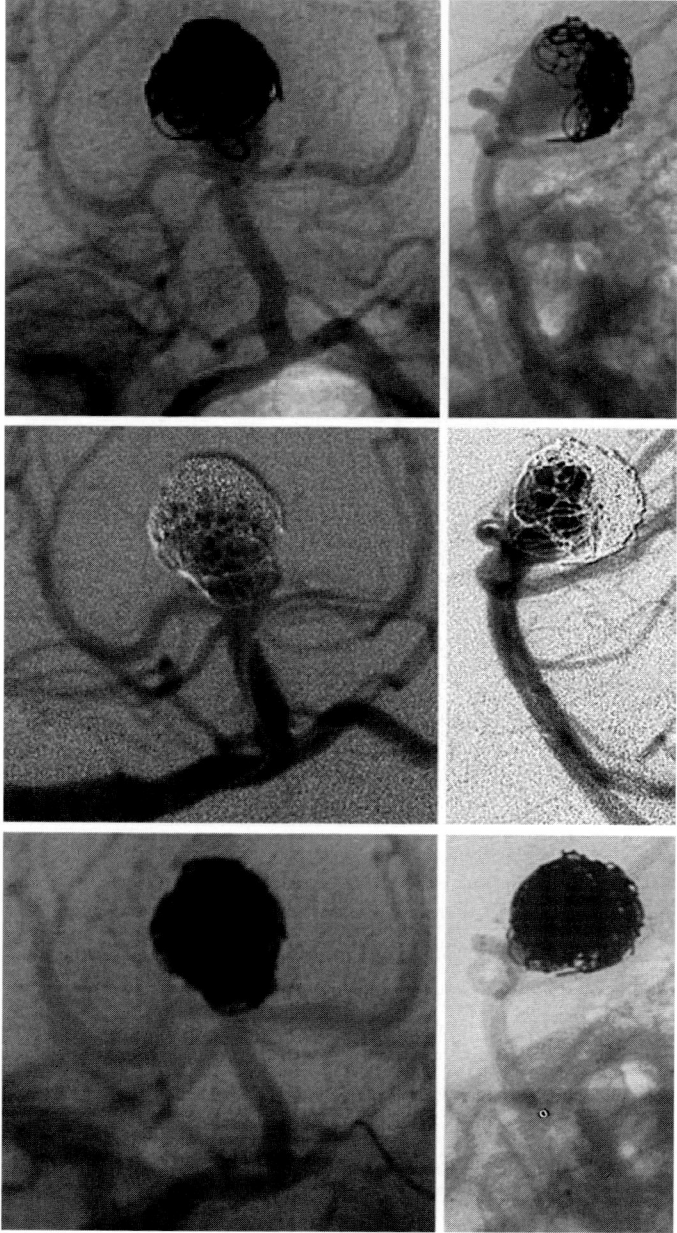

Fig. 4. Balloon-assisted coil embolization of a previously ruptured and treated basilar artery apex aneurysm. The top panels show coil compaction and aneurysm regrowth 6 mo after initial treatment. The aneurysm neck is broad, extending into both posterior cerebral arteries (PCAs). The middle panels show a soft microballoon (deflated) positioned in the distal basilar artery and proximal left P1 from the right vertebral artery. A coil that unfolds to form a 3D basket is being delivered via the microcatheter within the aneurysm from the left vertebral artery. The microballoon is only briefly inflated to keep the coil basket in the aneurysm as the coil is placed. The initial 3D coil basket provides a scaffold to help hold subsequent coils in place. For an unrup-

(Fig. 4). It involves the placement of a second microcatheter with a microballoon tip placed across the aneurysm orifice. Coil delivery is performed while the balloon is temporarily inflated. The balloon is then deflated, and the coil stability is assessed prior to coil detachment. The support of the balloon helps retain the coils within the aneurysm and allows for denser coil packing by compressing the coil meshwork. Potential risks are associated with balloon inflation in the intracranial arteries. There is an increased risk for thromboembolism owing to the use of a second microcatheter *(67)*. Ischemia from prolonged vascular occlusion can also complicate the procedure. Therefore, care should be taken to minimize the duration of the flow occlusion. Rupture of the parent vessel can be caused by overinflation of the balloon. Sealing of the aneurysm with the inflated balloon during continuous flushing of the microcatheter can potentially increase the tensile stress in the aneurysm wall. To minimize the aneurysm rupture risk, the distal inflow zone can be left open while the proximal inflow zone is sealed. Alternatively, the balloon is incompletely inflated or the microcatheter flushing is temporarily discontinued *(68)*.

Stent-Assisted Coil Embolization

The technique involves deployment of a stent across the aneurysm neck prior to the placement of coils into the aneurysm. The placement of an endovascular stent across the aneurysm neck can act as a scaffold to prevent coil herniation into the parent vessel *(69,70)* (Fig. 5). Unlike the temporary coil support provided by the balloon remodeling technique, the intravascular stent provides permanent support to the coil mesh. Aneurysms may also spontaneously thrombose following stent placement only, even without GDC packing *(71–73)*. The stent mesh probably causes alterations in the flow in the aneurysmal lumen that induce gradual thrombosis. Less porous stents could provide tighter aneurysmal coil packing. This has to be weighed against an increased risk for side branch obstruction.

Antithrombotic medication is necessary following stent deployment to prevent stent thrombosis and distal emboli. Stents induce neointimal proliferation, which may result in hemodynamically significant stenosis. Heparin-coated stents have been tested in animals and showed decreased proliferative changes *(74)*. Another limitation of stent placement is the potential for occlusion of the ostia of side branches, resulting in infarction. This, however is rarely encountered. Experimental evidence in dogs showed that side branches remain patent if less than 50% of their ostia are covered by the stent struts *(75)*.

Further improvements in stent design are expected to facilitate navigation in the intracranial vessels. Our initial experience with a new flexible intravascular

---

tured aneurysm, heparin is given intravenously throughout the procedure to help decrease the risk of emboli; for a ruptured aneurysm, it is given once the rupture site is felt to be secure usually after two or three coils have been placed. The bottom panels show the final angiogram after placement of an additional 24 coils. On the lateral view note that the density of the newly placed coils is higher than the previously placed coils even after compaction.

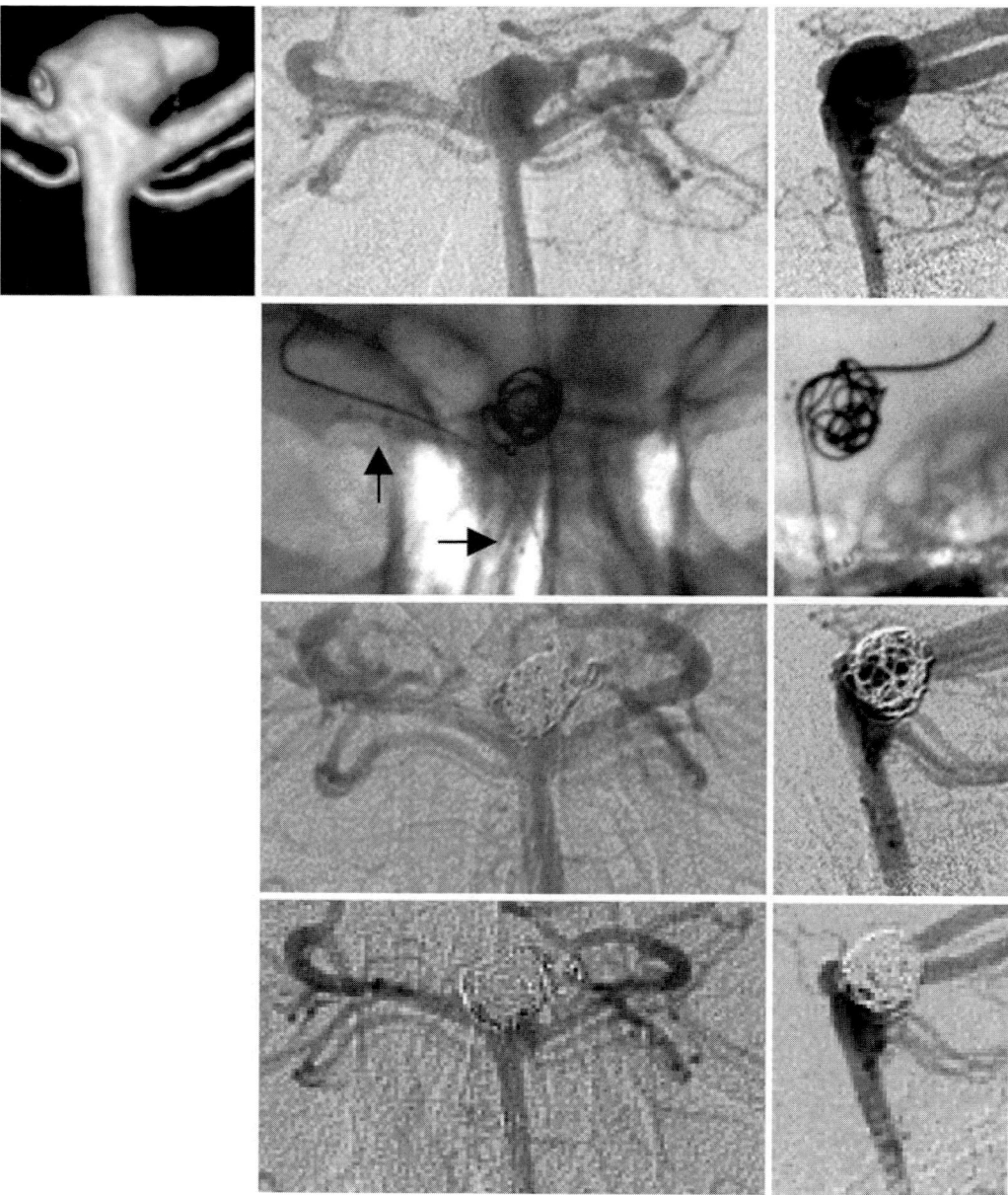

Fig. 5. Stent-assisted coil embolization of a large ruptured basilar apex aneurysm. The top row shows a daughter dome pointing to the left, which was the presumed rupture site. This dome could be secured by balloon-assisted coiling, but treating the neck of the aneurysm would probably compromise flow in the distal basilar artery or posterior cerebral arteries (PCAs). A soft stent was placed from the distal basilar artery extending into the right PI prior to coil placement. This supports the coil mass, as shown in the second row. Arrows point to markers on the stent strut tips. The third row shows the result after placement of 13 coils. A small region of inflow remains at the right edge during intravenous anticoagulation and antiplatelet therapy, which were started after the second and third coils, respectively. In the fourth row this region has throm-

stent, specifically designed for the intracranial vasculature (Neuroform stent, Boston Scientific) has been very encouraging.

Three-Dimensional GDC

3D-GDC is designed for endovascular treatment of wide-neck aneurysms. It is made of large and small loops that alternate at 90° angles. After deployment, the coil assumes a 3D spherical shape, with coil loops bridging the aneurysm neck. It is used as the first coil to form the basket multiplanar framework (76). It can be used in conjunction with balloon and stent assist techniques (Figs. 4 and 5). The 3D- GDCs are more rigid than the standard GDCs; therefore they should be used with caution in small aneurysms and in acutely ruptured aneurysms.

Trispan Device

The Trispan device (Target Therapeutics) is a new tool designed for treatment of wide-neck aneurysms. It consists of three nitinol loops that form a scaffold at the ostium. The disadvantage of this technique is the need to use two microcatheters (77). The device is not available in the United States.

PARENT VESSEL SACRIFICE

Parent vessel occlusion is still an acceptable treatment for aneurysms that are not amenable to endovascular coiling or surgical clipping. Broad-necked and fusiform aneurysms are often not amenable to endovascular treatment unless parent vessel sacrifice is an option. This procedure is mainly reserved for large or giant aneurysms that lack a definable neck.

Balloon test occlusion of the parent vessel to assess tolerance to the occlusion should always precede balloon detachment. If the test is not tolerated, an extracranial–intracranial bypass procedure can be considered. Following a successful balloon occlusion test, detachable balloons are placed proximal to or at the aneurysm neck. Fox et al. (78) reported a 0% mortality in a series of 65 patients with cerebral aneurysms treated with proximal artery occlusion with detachable latex balloons. Of the treated patients, 37 had aneurysms in the cavernous or petrous ICA, 21 had aneurysms in the supraclinoid ICA, 6 had aneurysms of the proximal basilar artery, and 1 had an aneurysm of the vertebral artery. Delayed ischemic symptoms developed in 13.2% of the patients, with a 1.5% permanent morbidity. In a large series of 87 patients with cavernous carotid artery aneurysms treated with detachable silicone balloons, proximal occlusion was performed in 68 patients, and intraaneurysmal balloon placement in 19 patients, followed by filling of the balloon with liquid polymerizing permanent embolic material to ensure lasting results (79). The permanent morbidity in this series was 4.6%. Three of the 68 patients (4.4%) with a proxi-

---

bosed, with no residual inflow after 4 d on oral antiplatelet therapy. There is a small neck remnant above the left P1. An additional stent from the distal basilar artery to the left P1 could be considered to help support coil reconstruction of this remnant if indicated.

mal occlusion and 1 of 19 patients (5%) with direct balloon occlusion of the aneurysms developed a stroke. The physical properties of silicone balloons are more favorable for endovascular use compared with the latex balloons. Silicone balloons are more pliable and are thought to carry a lower risk of vessel rupture *(80,81)*. Moreover, the silicone shell does not degrade over time as latex does *(81,82)*. These results compare favorably with those of surgical ligation of the common carotid artery or the proximal ICA, which carry a high procedural morbidity and mortality and are associated with a substantial permanent neurologic deficits *(83)*.

Occlusion of the parent vessel can also be performed with coils *(84,85)* (Fig. 6). The procedure can be combined with temporary proximal flow arrest with a nondetachable balloon in cases in which the arterial anatomy or disease process precludes the safe delivery and deployment of detachable balloons *(86)*. Hughes et al. *(87)* showed in an experimental canine model that the use of proximal flow arrest during coil placement eliminated the risk of distal embolic events and reduced the risk of distal coil migration. The precise coil placement was facilitated with this technique.

NEW TECHNOLOGICAL ADVANCEMENTS

The rapid evolution and refinement of the endovascular aneurysm techniques is fueled by continued technologic advancements that facilitate the endovascular aneurysm treatment and improve the final outcome. Several new devices and a new embolic agent are currently being tested.

Onyx

A liquid embolic agent (Onyx, Micro Therapeutics) has been tested in a European multicenter study for aneurysm embolization *(88)*. Onyx is a mixture of ethylene vinyl alcohol, dimethyl sulfoxide, and tantalum that appears to offer good aneurysm occlusion rates at acceptable morbidity rates. Long-term results of this alternative treatment have not yet been published.

New Coil Devices

Technical innovations, such as coating of coils with proteins as well as the development of endovascular bioabsorbable bioactive embolic implants (Matrix, Target/Boston Scientific) are promising methods that may improve the anatomic results of endovascular aneurysm embolization by inducing an accelerated cellular reaction *(89–91)*. The development of polymer-coated coils (Hydrocoil, MicroVention) that expand shortly after they come in contact with blood and conform to the aneurysm shape is currently being tested. In the canine model, it has been shown to yield a higher volume of packing compared with GDC, with less coil compaction *(92)*.

LEARNING CURVE

Aneurysm coiling is a complex procedure that can be improved with practice. Malish et al. *(57)* showed a steep learning curve by comparing the complication rate of coiling of their first 100 patients with ruptured aneurysms with

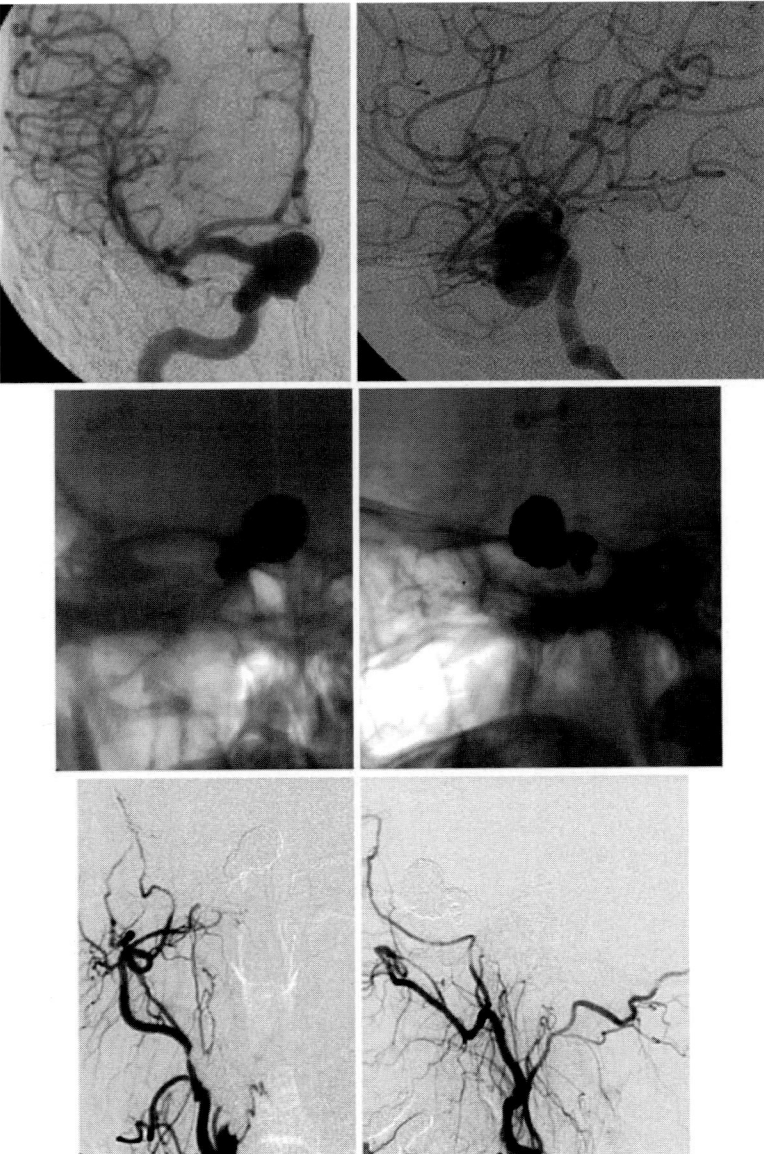

Fig. 6. Sacrifice of the parent vessel to obliterate a large right internal carotid artery (ICA) aneurysm with an indistinct neck. After a previous attempt at microsurgical trapping was unsuccessful, it was decided to perform coil takedown of the parent vessel. The patient did well during balloon occlusion testing of the right ICA prior to permanent occlusion with coils. Followup angiography (bottom panel) confirmed no flow into the aneurysm and parent vessel after 2 yr.

the next 100 patients. The procedure-related complications rate dropped from 14% in the first 100 patients to 7% in the next 100 patients. A dramatic decrease of the complication risk with increasing experience was also shown for coiling of unruptured aneurysms (93).

CONCLUSIONS

Endovascular aneurysm coiling has gained acceptance as an attractive and valuable alternative to neurosurgical aneurysm clipping. It is of paramount importance to realize that both treatment options are complementary and that multiple factors must be considered in the decision about management of patients with intracranial aneurysms. Multidisciplinary patient assessment is the safest strategy to select the best treatment option for the particular patient.

Future developments are expected to improve the endovascular treatment results and render more lesions amenable to coil embolization.

SUMMARY

Endovascular aneurysm treatment has been integrated into the management of patients with intracranial aneurysms. Evolving technical refinements have dramatically improved the technique of endovascular coil embolization during the past decade. Aneurysm geometry is playing a key role in the selction of patients for endovascular aneurysm coiling. The lower morbidity compared with neurosurgical clipping has to be weighed against a higher rate of incomplete occlusion and recanalization. Therefore angiographic follow-up of patients with coiled aneurysms is necessary. Continuous technical developments may improve the anatomic results.

REFERENCES

1. Serbinenko FA. [Catheterization, and occlusion of major cerebral vessels and prospects for the development of vascular neurosurgery. *Neirokhir* 1971;35:17–27.
2. Serbinenko FA. Balloon catheterization and occlusion of major cerebral vessels. *J Neurosurg* 1974;41:125–145.
3. Guglielmi G, Vinuela F, Sepetka I, Macellari V. Electrothrombosis of saccular aneurysms via endovascular approach, part 1:electrochemical basis, technique, and experimental results. *J Neurosurg* 1991;75:1–7.
4. Guglielmi G, Vinuela F, Dion J, Duckwiler G. Electrothrombosis of saccular aneurysms via endovascular approach. Part 2: Preliminary clinical experience. *J Neurosurg* 1991;75:8–14.
5. Raftopoulos C, Mathurin P, Boscherini D, Billa RF, Van Boven M, Hantson P. Prospective analysis of aneurysm treatment in a series of 103 consecutive patients when endovascular embolization is considered the first option. *J Neurosurg* 2000; 93:175–182.
6. Moret J, Pierot L, Boulin A, Castaings L, Rey A. Endovascular treatment of anterior communicating artery aneurysms using Guglielmi detachable coils. *Neuroradiology* 1996;38:800–805.
7. Cognard C, Pierot L, Boulin A, et al. Intracranial aneurysms: endovascular treatment with mechanical detachable spirals in 60 aneurysms. *Radiology* 1997;202:783–792.
8. Hopkins LN, Lanzino G, Guterman LR. Treating complex nervous system vascular disorders through a "needle stick": origins, evolution, and future of neuroendovascular therapy. *Neurosurgery* 2001;48:463–475.
9. Brilstra EH, Rinkel GJE, van der Graaf Y, van Rooij WJJ, Algra A. Treatment of intracranial aneurysms by embolization with coils: a systematic review. *Stroke* 1999;30:470–476.

10. Vanninen R, Koivisto T, Saari T, Hernesniemi J, Vapalahti M. Ruptured intracranial aneurysms: acute endovascular treatment with electrolytically detachable coil: a prospective randomized study. *Radiology* 1999;211:325–336.
11. Koivisto T, Vanninen R, Hurskainen H, Saari T, Hernesniemi J, Vapalahti M. Outcomes of early endovascular versus surgical treatment of ruptured cerebral aneurysms: a prospective randomized study. *Stroke* 2000;31:2369–2377.
12. Molyneux A, Kerr R, Stratton I, et al. International Subarachnoid Aneurysm Trial (ISAT) Collaborative Group. International Subarachnoid Aneurysm Trial (ISAT) of neurosurgical clipping versus endovascular coiling in 2143 patients with ruptured intracranial aneurysms: a randomised trial. *Lancet* 2002;360:1267–1274.
13. Johnston SC, Wilson CB, Halbach VV, et al. Endovascular and surgical treatment of unruptured cerebral aneurysms: comparison of risks. *Ann Neurol* 2000;48:11–19.
14. Raaymakers TWM, Rinkel GJE, Algra A. Morbidity and mortality of operation of unruptured intracranial aneurysms: a meta-analysis. *Stroke* 1998;29:1531–1538.
15. International Study of Unruptured Intracranial Aneurysms Investigators. Unruptured intracranial aneurysms: risk of rupture and risks of surgical intervention. *N Engl J Med* 1998;339:1725–1733.
16. Latchaw RE. Acutely ruptured intracranial aneurysm: should we treat with endovascular coils or with surgical clipping? *Radiology* 1999;211:306–308.
17. Johnston SC, Higashida RT, Barrow DL, et al. Committee on Cerebrovascular Imaging of the American Heart Association Council on Cardiovascular Radiology. Recommendations for the endovascular treatment of intracranial aneurysms: a statement for healthcare professionals from the Committee on Cerebrovascular Imaging of the American Heart Association Council on Cardiovascular Radiology. *Stroke* 2002;33:2536–2544.
18. Vinuela F, Duckwiler G, Mawad M. Guglielmi detachable coil embolization of acute intracranial aneurysm: perioperative anatomical and clinical outcome in 403 patients. *J Neurosurg* 1997;86:475–482.
19. Tsutsumi K, Ueki K, Usui M, Kwak S, Kirino T. Risk of recurrent subarachnoid hemorrhage after complete obliteration of cerebral aneurysms. *Stroke* 1998;29:2511–2513.
20. David CA, Vishteh AG, Spetzler RF, Lemole M, Lawton MT, Partovi S. Late angiographic follow-up review of surgically treated aneurysms. *J Neurosurg* 1999;91:396–401.
21. Lempert TE, Malek AM, Halbach VV, et al. Endovascular treatment of ruptured posterior circulation cerebral aneurysms: clinical and angiographic outcomes. *Stroke* 2000;31:100–110.
22. Bavinzski G, Killer M, Gruber A, Reinprecht A, Gross CE, Richling B. Treatment of basilar artery bifurcation aneurysms by using Guglielmi detachable coils: a 6-year experience. *J Neurosurg* 1999;90:843–852.
23. Eskridge JM, Song JK. Endovascular embolization of 150 basilar tip aneurysms with Guglielmi detachable coils: results of the Food and Drug Administration multicenter clinical trial. *J Neurosurg* 1998;89:81–86.
24. Samson D, Batjer HH, Kopitnik TA Jr. Current results of the surgical management of aneurysms of the basilar apex. *Neurosurgery* 1999;44:697–702.
25. Lawton MT. Basilar apex aneurysms: surgical results and perspectives from an initial experience. *Neurosurgery* 2002;50:1–8.
26. Gruber DP, Zimmerman GA, Tomsick TA, van Loveren HR, Link MJ, Tew JM Jr. A comparison between endovascular and surgical management of basilar artery apex aneurysms. *J Neurosurg* 1999;90:868–874.

27. Regli L, Dehdashti AR, Uske A, de Tribolet N. Endovascular coiling compared with surgical clipping for the treatment of unruptured middle cerebral artery aneurysms: an update. *Acta Neurochir Suppl* 2002;82:41–46.
28. Tenjin H, Fushiki S, Nakahara Y, et al. Effect of Guglielmi detachable coils on experimental carotid artery aneurysms in primates. *Stroke* 1995;26:2075–2080.
29. Mawad ME, Mawad JK, Cartwright J Jr, Gokaslan Z. Long-term histopathologic changes in canine aneurysms embolized with Guglielmi detachable coils.*AJNR Am J Neuroradiol* 1995;16:7–13.
30. Stiver SI, Porter PJ, Willinsky RA, Wallace MC. Acute human histopathology of an intracranial aneurysm treated using Guglielmi detachable coils: case report and review of the literature. *Neurosurgery* 1998;43:1203–1208.
31. Ishihara S, Mawad ME, Ogata K, et al. Histopathologic findings in human cerebral aneurysms embolized with platinum coils: report of two cases and review of the literature. *AJNR Am J Neuroradiol* 2002;23:970–974.
32. Bavinzski G, Talazoglu V, Killer M, et al. Gross and microscopic histopathological findings in aneurysms of the human brain treated with Guglielmi detachable coils. *J Neurosurg* 1999;91:284–293.
33. Shimizu S, Kurata A, Takano M, et al. Tissue response of a small saccular aneurysm after incomplete occlusion with a Guglielmi detachable coil. *AJNR Am J Neuroradiol* 1999;20:546–548.
34. Novak P, Glikstein R, Mohr G. Pulsation-pressure relationship in experimental aneurysms: observation of aneurysmal hysteresis. *Neurol Res* 1996;18:377–382.
35. Boecher-Schwarz HG, Ringel K, Kopacz L, Heimann A, Kempski O. Ex vivo study of the physical effect of coils on pressure and flow dynamics in experimental aneurysms. *AJNR Am J Neuroradiol* 2000;21:1532–1536.
36. Sorteberg A, Sorteberg W, Turk AS, Rappe A, Nakstad PH, Strother CM. Effect of Guglielmi detachable coil placement on intraaneurysmal pressure: experimental study in canines. *AJNR Am J Neuroradiol* 2001;22:1750–1756.
37. Sorteberg A, Sorteberg W, Rappe A, Strother CM. Effect of Guglielmi detachable coils on intraaneurysmal flow: experimental study in canines. *AJNR Am J Neuroradiol* 2002;23:288–294.
38. Graves VB, Strother CM, Partington CR, Rappe A. Flow dynamics of lateral carotid artery aneurysms and their effects on coils and balloons: an experimental study in dogs. *AJNR Am J Neuroradiol* 1992;13:189–196.
39. Gonzalez CF, Cho YI, Ortega HV, Moret J. Intracranial aneurysms: flow analysis of their origin and progression. *AJNR Am J Neuroradiol* 1992;13:181–188.
40. Steinman DA, Milner JS, Norley CJ, Lownie SP, Holdsworth DW. Image-based computational simulation of flow dynamics in a giant intracranial aneurysm. *AJNR Am J Neuroradiol* 2003;24:559–566.
41. Vinuela F, Murayama Y, Duckwiler GR, Gobin YP. Present and future technical developments on aneurysm embolization. Impact on indications and anatomic results. *Clin Neurosurg* 2000;47:221–241.
42. Valavanis A, Machado E, Chen JJ. Aneurysm rupture during GDC treatment: incidence, management and outcome. *Neuroradiology Suppl 2* 1996;38:45.
43. Malisch TW. Aneurysm rupture during GDC treatment: optimizing the rescue strategy. *AJNR Am J Neuroradiol* 2000;21:1372–1373.
44. McDougall CG, Halbach VV, Dowd CF, Higashida RT, Larsen DW, Hieshima GB. Causes and management of aneurysmal hemorrhage occurring during embolization with Guglielmi detachable coils. *J Neurosurg* 1998;89:87–92.
45. Ricolfi F, Le Guerinel C, Blustajn J, et al. Rupture during treatment of recently ruptured aneurysms with Guglielmi electrodetachable coils. *AJNR Am J Neuroradiol* 1998;19:1653–1658.

46. Willinsky R, terBrugge K. Use of a second microcatheter in the management of a perforation during endovascular treatment of a cerebral aneurysm. *AJNR Am J Neuroradiol* 2000;21:1537–1539.
47. Pelz DM, Lownie SP, Fox AJ. Thromboembolic events associated with the treatment of cerebral aneurysms with Guglielmi detachable coils. *AJNR Am J Neuroradiol* 1998;19:1541–1547.
48. Nichols DA. Thromboembolic events during endovascular coil occlusion of cerebral aneurysms. *AJNR Am J Neuroradiol* 2001;22:1–2.
49. Cronqvist M, Pierot L, Boulin A, Cognard C, Castaings L, Moret J. Local intraarterial fibrinolysis of thromboemboli occurring during endovascular treatment of intracerebral aneurysm: a comparison of anatomic results and clinical outcome. *AJNR Am J Neuroradiol* 1998;19:157–165.
50. Alexander MJ, Duckwiler GR, Gobin YP, Vinuela F. Management of intraprocedural arterial thrombus in cerebral aneurysm embolization with abciximab: technical case report. *Neurosurgery* 2002;50:899–901.
51. Albuquerque FC, Spetzler RF, Zabramski JM, McDougall CG. Effects of three-dimensional angiography on the coiling of cerebral aneurysms. *Neurosurgery* 2002;51:597–605.
52. Debrun GM, Aletich VA, Kehrli P, Misra M, Ausman JI, Charbel F. Selection of cerebral aneurysms for treatment using Guglielmi detachable coils: the preliminary University of Illinois at Chicago experience. *Neurosurgery* 1998;43:1281–1295.
53. Fernandez Zubillaga A, Guglielmi G, Vinuela F, Duckwiler GR. Endovascular occlusion of intracranial aneurysms with electrically detachable coils: correlation of aneurysm neck size and treatment results. *AJNR Am J Neuroradiol* 1994;15:815–820.
54. Turjman F, Massoud TF, Sayre J, Vinuela F. Predictors of aneurysmal occlusion in the period immediately after endovascular treatment with detachable coils: a multivariate analysis. *AJNR Am J Neuroradiol* 1998;19:1645–1651.
55. Burleson AC, Strother CM, Turitto VT. Computer modeling of intracranial saccular and lateral aneurysms for the study of their hemodynamics. *Neurosurgery* 1995;37:774–782
56. Hayakawa M, Murayama Y, Duckwiler GR, Gobin YP, Guglielmi G, Vinuela F. Natural history of the neck remnant of a cerebral aneurysm treated with the Guglielmi detachable coil system. *J Neurosurg* 2000;93:561–568.
57. Malisch TW, Guglielmi G, Vinuela F, et al. Intracranial aneurysms treated with the Guglielmi detachable coil: midterm clinical results in a consecutive series of 100 patients. *J Neurosurg* 1997;87:176–183.
58. Feuerberg I, Lindquist C, Lindqvist M, Steiner L. Natural history of postoperative aneurysm rests. *J Neurosurg* 1987;66:30–34.
59. Thornton J, Bashir Q, Aletich VA, Debrun GM, Ausman JI, Charbel FT. What percentage of surgically clipped intracranial aneurysms have residual necks? *Neurosurgery* 2000;46:1294–1298.
60. Drake CG, Friedman AH, Peerless SJ. Failed aneurysm surgery. Reoperation in 115 cases. *J Neurosurg* 1984;61:848–856.
61. Rabinstein AA, Nichols DA. Endovascular coil embolization of cerebral aneurysm remnants after incomplete surgical obliteration. *Stroke* 2002;33:1809–1815.
62. Cognard C, Weill A, Spelle L, et al. Long-term angiographic follow-up of 169 intracranial berry aneurysms occluded with detachable coils. *Radiology* 1999;212:348–356.
63. Tsutsumi K, Ueki K, Morita A, Usui M, Kirino T. Risk of aneurysm recurrence in patients with clipped cerebral aneurysms: results of long-term follow-up angiography. *Stroke* 2001;32:1191–1194.

64. Malisch TW, Guglielmi G, Vinuela F, et al. Unruptured aneurysms presenting with mass effect symptoms: response to endosaccular treatment with Guglielmi detachable coils. Part I. Symptoms of cranial nerve dysfunction. *J Neurosurg* 1998;89: 956–961.
65. Halbach VV, Higashida RT, Dowd CF, et al. The efficacy of endosaccular aneurysm occlusion in alleviating neurological deficits produced by mass effect. *J Neurosurg* 1994;80:659–666.
66. Moret J, Cognard C, Weill A, Castaings L, Rey A. [Reconstruction technic in the treatment of wide-neck intracranial aneurysms: long-term angiographic and clinical results: apropos of 56 cases.] *J Neuroradiol* 1997;24:30–44.
67. Levy DI, Ku A. Balloon-assisted coil placement in wide-necked aneurysms. Technical note. *J Neurosurg* 1997;86:724–727.
68. Malek AM, Halbach VV, Phatouros CC, et al. Balloon-assist technique for endovascular coil embolization of geometrically difficult intracranial aneurysms. *Neurosurgery* 2000;46:1397–1406.
69. Szikora I, Guterman LR, Wells KM, Hopkins LN. Combined use of stents and coils to treat experimental wide-necked carotid aneurysms: preliminary results. *AJNR Am J Neuroradiol* 1994;15:1091–1102.
70. Massoud TF, Turjman F, Ji C, et al. Endovascular treatment of fusiform aneurysms with stents and coils: technical feasibility in a swine model. *AJNR Am J Neuroradiol* 1995;16:1953–1963.
71. Vanninen R, Manninen H, Ronkainen A. Broad-based intracranial aneurysms: thrombosis induced by stent placement. *AJNR Am J Neuroradiol* 2003;24:263–266.
72. Marks MP, Dake MD, Steinberg GK, Norbash AM, Lane B. Stent placement for arterial and venous cerebrovascular disease: preliminary experience. *Radiology* 1994;191:441–446.
73. Manninen HI, Koivisto T, Saari T, et al. Dissecting aneurysms of all four cervicocranial arteries in fibromuscular dysplasia: treatment with self-expanding endovascular stents, coil embolization, and surgical ligation. *AJNR Am J Neuroradiol* 1997;18:1216–1220.
74. Levy EI, Boulos AS, Hanel RA, et al. In vivo model of intracranial stent implantation: a pilot study to examine the histological response of cerebral vessels after randomized implantation of heparin-coated and uncoated endoluminal stents in a blinded fashion. *J Neurosurg* 2003;98:544–553.
75. Wakhloo AK, Tio FO, Lieber BB, Schellhammer F, Graf M, Hopkins LN. Self-expanding nitinol stents in canine vertebral arteries: hemodynamics and tissue response. *AJNR Am J Neuroradiol* 1995;16:1043–1051.
76. Cloft HJ, Joseph GJ, Tong FC, Goldstein JH, Dion JE. Use of three-dimensional Guglielmi detachable coils in the treatment of wide-necked cerebral aneurysms. *AJNR Am J Neuroradiol* 2000;21:1312–1314.
77. Raymond J, Salazkin I, Georganos S, et al. Neck-bridge device for endovascular treatment of wide-neck bifurcation aneurysms: initial experience. *Radiology* 2001; 221:318–326.
78. Fox AJ, Vinuela F, Pelz DM, Peerless SJ, Ferguson GG, Drake CG, Debrun G. Use of detachable balloons for proximal artery occlusion in the treatment of unclippable cerebral aneurysms. *J Neurosurg* 1987;66:40–46.
79. Higashida RT, Halbach VV, Dowd C, et al. Endovascular detachable balloon embolization therapy of cavernous carotid artery aneurysms: results in 87 cases. *J Neurosurg* 1990;72:857–863.
80. Miller F. Elastomers in medicine. *Elastomerics* 1985;117:15–20.
81. Ranney MW. Silicones, vol 1: *Rubber, Electrical Molding Resins and Functional Fluids.* Noyes Data, Parks Ridge, NJ, 1977.

82. Arkley B, Redinger P. Silicones in biomedical applications, in *Biocompatible Polymers, Metals, and Composites* (Szycher M, ed.), Technonomic, Lancaster, PA, 1983, pp. 749–768.
83. Scott M, Skwarok E. The treatment of cerebral aneurysms by ligation of the common carotid artery. *Surg Gynecol Obstet* 1961;113:54–61.
84. Braun IF, Hoffman JC Jr, Casarella WJ, Davis PC. Use of coils for transcatheter carotid occlusion. *AJNR Am J Neuroradiol* 1985;6:953–956.
85. Rossi P, Passariello R, Simonetti G. Control of a traumatic vertebral arteriovenous fistula by a modified Gianturco coli embolus system. *AJR Am J Roentgenol* 1978;131:331–333.
86. Graves VB, Perl J 2nd, Strother CM, Wallace RC, Kesava PP, Masaryk TJ. Endovascular occlusion of the carotid or vertebral artery with temporary proximal flow arrest and microcoils: clinical results. *AJNR Am J Neuroradiol* 1997;18:1201–1206.
87. Hughes SR, Graves VB, Kesava PP, Rappe AH. The effect of flow arrest on distal embolic events during arterial occlusion with detachable coils: a canine study. *AJNR Am J Neuroradiol* 1996;17:685–691.
88. Molyneux AJ, Cekirge S, Gal G. Onyx liquid embolic system in the treatment of intracranial aneurysms: final results of the European multicenter study: Cerebral Aneurysm Multicenter European Registry (CAMEO), in *Proceedings of the 41st Annual Meeting of the American Society of Neuroradiology*, Washington DC 2003, p. 207.
89. Bavinzski G, Richling B, Binder BR, et al. Histopathological findings in experimental aneurysms embolized with conventional and thrombogenic/antithrombolytic Guglielmi coils. *Minim Invasive Neurosurg* 1999;42:167–174.
90. Murayama Y, Vinuela F, Suzuki Y, et al. Development of the biologically active Guglielmi detachable coil for the treatment of cerebral aneurysms. Part II: An experimental study in a swine aneurysm model. *AJNR Am J Neuroradiol* 1999;20:1992–1999.
91. Murayama Y, Tateshima S, Gonzalez NR, Vinuela F. Matrix and bioabsorbable polymeric coils accelerate healing of intracranial aneurysms: long-term experimental study. *Stroke* 2003;34:2031–2037.
92. Aagaard BDL, Strother CM, Rappe AH, Consigny DW. Larger hydrocoil embolization volumes result in more stable aneurysm occlusion in the canine bifurcation aneurysm model, in *Proceedings Book Additions of the 41st Annual Meeting of the American Society of Neuroradiology*, Washington DC, 2003, p. 6.
93. Singh V, Gress DR, Higashida RT, Dowd CF, Halbach VV, Johnston SC. The learning curve for coil embolization of unruptured intracranial aneurysms. *AJNR Am J Neuroradiol* 2002;23:768–771.

8
Stent Angioplasty for Treatment of Intracranial Cerebrovascular Disease

Adel M. Malek, MD, PhD and Clemens M. Schirmer, MD

INTRODUCTION

Advances in the design and manufacturing of balloon and stent catheters made in the last decade have improved the operator's ability to negotiate the tortuous anatomy of the high cervical and intracranial carotid and vertebral arteries *(1–3)*. These technical developments have led to the endovascular treatment of cerebrovascular pathologies previously considered unapproachable from a percutaneous approach. The ability to reach and treat intracranial stenotic lesions using miniature balloon-mounted microstents has provided a promising form of therapy for well-selected patients who have failed medical therapy and for those who are not candidates for surgical bypass grafting *(4,5)*. Similarly, the availability of improved low-profile microstents has expanded the spectrum of intracranial aneurysms that are amenable to endovascular therapy to include the wide-necked and fusiform morphology *(6,7)*.

STENT ANGIOPLASTY FOR INTRACRANIAL ATHEROSCLEROSIS

Severe intracranial atherosclerotic disease accounts for an 8–12% yearly risk of stroke *(8–10)* and can be associated with recurrent neurological symptoms despite maximal medical therapy. These neurological events can result from either thromboembolism or hemodynamic insufficiency. Medical therapy with antiplatelet and anticoagulant therapy is only partially effective against thromboembolic phenomena and largely futile in cases of insufficiency *(9)*. Although surgical bypass grafting from the extracranial to intracranial circulation is technically feasible and effective in carefully selected cases, it was found to be not effective in the cooperative study for anterior circulation intracranial disease, possibly because of poor patient selection and study bias *(11–14)*. In addition, a large proportion of intracranial posterior circulation stenoses are not suitable for bypass grafting because of lesion location in and around the brainstem or because of poor tolerance to temporary occlusion.

Intracranial atherosclerosis risk factors include age, hypertension, smoking, diabetes, and ethnic origin *(8)*. Intracranial atherosclerotic lesions most commonly

From: *Minimally Invasive Neurosurgery*, edited by: M.R. Proctor and P.M. Black © Humana Press Inc., Totowa, NJ

involve the following locations: the distal V4 segment of the vertebral artery (VA), the basilar artery (BA), the petrous, cavernous, and paraclinoid segments of the intracranial internal carotid artery (ICA), and the M1 segment of the middle cerebral artery (MCA). Intracranial atherosclerotic lesions have a dynamic natural history showing progression and regression in certain cases *(15)*. More distal lesions with poor collateral circulation are associated with a higher risk of stroke. Lesions of the MCA have a significantly higher risk of stroke compared with more proximal ICA lesions *(16)*, and only one-third of patients with symptomatic intracranial ICA stenoses remained alive and free of strokes at 30 mo of follow-up *(17)* (Fig. 1). In the posterior circulation, the outcome of acute BA occlusion is almost invariably fatal *(18–22)*, and a lesion in the BA has been shown to imply a 22% risk of a stroke over a 1-yr period *(9)*. Although oral anticoagulation has been postulated to offer greater protection than antiplatelet therapy, the WASID trial will shortly yield outcome data comparing warfarin with aspirin in patients with intracranial atherosclerosis *(23)*. However, patients remaining symptomatic despite warfarin or aspirin therapy have been increasingly treated with endovascular revascularization with an acceptable risk profile *(5,7,24–26)*.

Percutaneous balloon angioplasty without stenting has been reported intracranially for the past two decades, but its efficacy has been hampered by a high incidence of iatrogenic intimal dissection, as well as vessel recoil *(24–26)*. More recently long-term clinical follow-up of patients treated with primary balloon angioplasty *(27)* has shown encouraging results despite a relatively high residual stenosis. This can be partially attributed to the fact that resistance across a vessel is estimated to be inversely proportional to the fourth power of the radius according to Poiseuille's equation; accordingly, a small improvement in luminal caliber can significantly decrease resistance to flow. Technological advances and increased operator expertise have resulted in improved success rates and fewer complications over the last decade *(27–30)*.

Rationale for Stent Angioplasty

The potential advantages of balloon angioplasty followed by stenting compared with angioplasty alone include a lower risk of intimal dissection with consequent thromboembolism or acute vessel closure and improved short-term patency rates. The main limiting factor for the use of stenting to treat intracranial lesions has been the lack of flexible low-profile stents that could be navigated into and deployed within the intracranial vasculature. The early attempts at intracranial stent deployment employed manually crimped Palmaz-Schatz coronary stents that were mounted on coronary balloon angioplasty microcatheters *(2)*. These hand-mounted stents had a high rate of slippage off the balloon microcatheter when the surgeon was navigating the sharp confines of intracranial vessels. A significant hurdle was overcome with the introduction of next-generation premounted coronary stents such as the GFX (Arterial Vascular Engineering, Santa Rosa, CA) in 1998; these coronary stents were significantly better suited for high cervical and intracranial navigation *(31,32)*. More recent generations of coronary stents, including heparin-coated variants such as the Cordis Bx Velocity (Johnson & Johnson, New Brunswick, NJ) and lower pro-

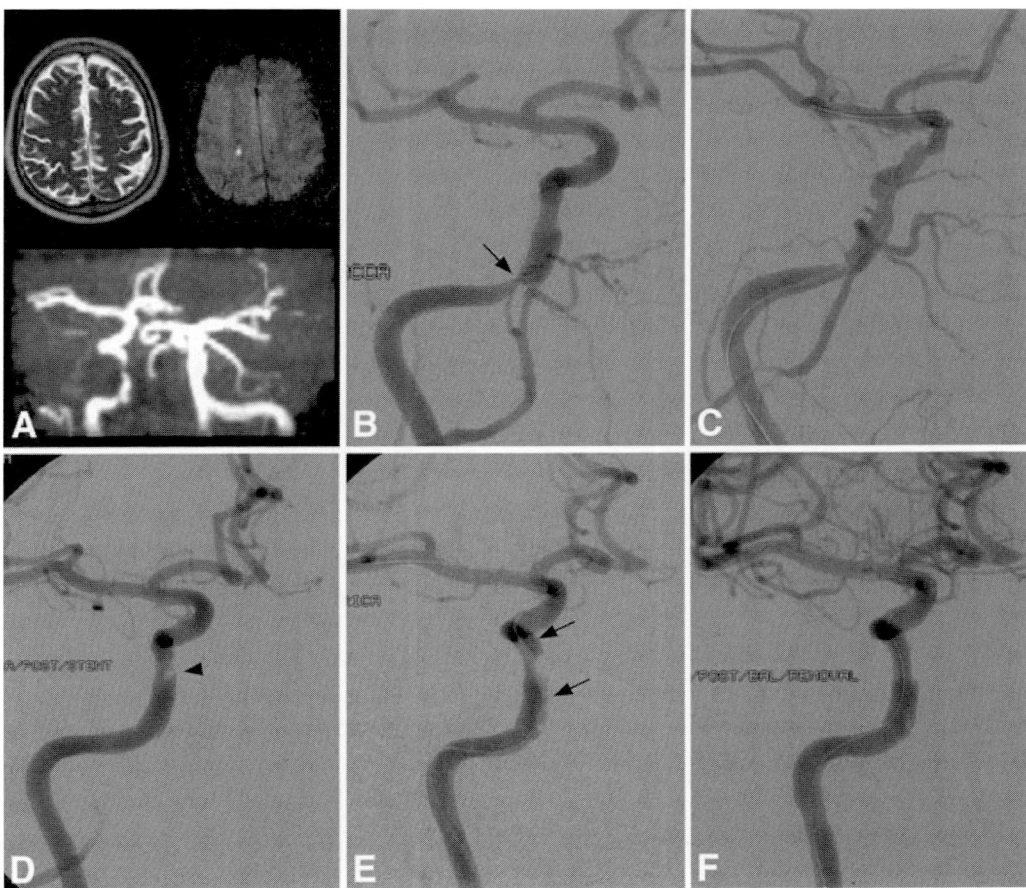

Fig. 1. Stent angioplasty of a petrous internal carotid artery stenosis. A 69-yr-old man with coronary artery disease was noted to have postoperative blood pressure-dependent episodes of confusion and dysphasia. **(A)** MRI revealed a subacute infarct associated with a focal stenosis in the petrous segment of a dominant right internal carotid artery (arrow). **(B)** Angiography revealed a focal 80% stenosis with a poststenotic dilation (arrow). **(C)** A Medtronic-AVE S7 4 × 15-mm coronary stent was used to cross the stenosis primarily over a hydrophilic microwire whose tip is parked in the right M1 segment of the middle cerebral artery. **(D)** The stent was centered over the lesion and deployed successfully, but delayed angiography showed the *de novo* appearance of a postangioplasty dissection flap noted distal to the stent (arrowhead). **(E)** This was treated by traversing the first stent and positioning a second Medtronic-AVE S7 3.5 × 9-mm coronary stent in tandem fashion (arrows). **(F)** The final result shows a patent right petrous ICA with postprocedural resolution of the patient's symptoms.

file designs have been used. In addition, balloon-mounted stent designs have been developed specifically for use in the intracranial circulation such as the INX stent (Medtronic-AVE, Santa Rosa, CA) and the Neurolink (Guidant, Indianapolis, IN) *(33)*; these designs feature easier tracking and more compliant balloons better suited to intracranial vascular characteristics.

The potential for endovascular therapy of a lesion reflects the heterogeneity of intracranial stenosis encountered in the workup of cerebrovascular disease. The treatment of lesions in the petrous and cavernous portions of the ICA at present represents a simple technical challenge compared with the ability to track the available stents beyond the carotid artery siphon into the paraclinoid portion of the carotid, or even into the MCA *(34)*. Stenting of the intracranial portions of the vertebrobasilar system, namely, the V3 and V4 portions of the VA and the BA, has also been shown to be feasible and relatively safe *(31,34–40)*, and this has proved to be an easier vascular territory to work in than the supraclinoid anterior circulation. The ability to reach the intracranial stenosis is highly dependent on the proximal cervical and great vessel anatomy, tortuosity, and degree of calcification. Although newer stents have better tracking and flexibility characteristics, they can be thwarted by tortuous vessel loops and sharp angulations.

Procedural and Technical Description

Patients are pretreated with aspirin (325 mg qd) and ticlopidine (150 mg bid) or clopidogrel (75 mg qd) for at least 3 d prior to the procedure. Although aspirin is rapidly absorbed, clopidogrel and ticlopidine require at least 3 d to achieve full effect; both antiplatelet regimens are continued indefinitely in cases of intracranial stenting for atherosclerosis. Most procedures are performed under general anesthesia in order to have the best possible imaging quality and to minimize motion artifact, given the small size of the target vessels. A complete four-vessel diagnostic angiogram is obtained (unless contraindicated) to assess the available collateral pathways in a dynamic fashion. Intravenous heparin is administered to achieve an activated clotting time between 250 and 300 s. The parent vessel is then accessed via a 6- or 7-Fr guiding catheter, which is positioned sufficiently distal in the cervical carotid or vertebral artery so as to form a stable delivery platform while maintaining flow downstream and avoiding iatrogenic vasospasm. The lesion can then be crossed either primarily using the stent delivery microcatheter over an exchange-length (260–300 cm) microwire (0.014 inch), or, in the case of more challenging and critically narrowed lesions by using a microcatheter as an intermediate step.

Once the stenosis has been traversed in a controlled fashion, the tip of the exchange wire is parked in a sufficiently distal location to allow tracking of the stent or balloon delivery. In cases of a proximal lesion of the VA or of the petrous segment of the ICA, the requirement for distal wire placement is less stringent than for a midbasilar or supraclinoid carotid stenosis, in which the tip of the wire is parked in a P2 (PCA) or M2 (MCA) branch, respectively. The microcatheter is then exchanged for the stent microcatheter catheter (for primary stent angioplasty) or a balloon microcatheter (in the case of secondary stent angioplasty). In cases of more proximal lesions of the petro-cavernous segment of the ICA or V4 segment of the VA, it may be possible and preferable to cross the lesion primarily with the stent or balloon delivery microcatheter to spare an exchange procedure. It is critical, however, to use exchange-length microwires in order to maintain access to the true lumen until after angioplasty and stent deployment have been performed successfully, to avoid the risk of irretrievable target vessel closure in the case of intimal dissection. Only after high-resolution control angiography has been performed with satisfactory results can the exchange wire be removed safely.

A number of obstacles can hinder successful intracranial stenting. The first impediment is the inability to obtain a secure platform using the guide catheter in the cervical region, either because of critical proximal stenosis or because of aortic arch or proximal vessel tortuosity. The former can often be solved by performing proximal angioplasty to allow passage of the guider; the latter can often be solved by opting for a larger bore guide catheter, by using a coaxial proximal long sheath-type shuttle to stiffen the assembly proximally, or by using a stabilizing wire *(41)*. Alternatively, a nonfemoral percutaneous approach may be employed such as the radial or brachial artery *(42)*, or in extreme cases direct carotid puncture, although the latter carries an associated higher risk of dissection or pseudoaneurysm *(43)*.

Once a satisfactory proximal platform has been achieved, the next limiting factor will be the presence of any acute curvature or looping vascular segments of the proximal parent vessel, since these usually result in loss of distal microwire control, which will impede the ability to advance the microstent delivery catheter by compromising proximal guide catheter position. Great care needs to be taken to evaluate blood flow periodically in the parent vessel and detect any signs of proximal vasospasm and/or dissection that may result from the occasionally high frictional forces exerted on the intima by the guide catheteter or stent microcatheter in cases of difficult anatomy. When the lesion cannot be traversed by the balloon-mounted stent catheter, primary angioplasty can be performed using a miniature (1.5-mm-diameter) angioplasty balloon, which can then exchanged for a stent to be deployed in secondary fashion. In cases of acute thrombotic occlusion, the procedure is preceded or accompanied by intraarterial superselective infusion of a fibrinolytic agent (urokinase or tissue plasminogen activator). The emergence of contrast defect or haziness near the stent interstices after deployment is usually the result of exuberant platelet activation, which can proceed rapidly to complete vessel occlusion and formation of organized thrombus. Patients demonstrating *de novo* thrombus formation are administered a glycoprotein IIb/IIIa inhibitor intravenously, such as abciximab or eptifibatide, concomitantly.

The risks of deploying stents intracranially include vessel rupture during angioplasty, hemodynamically significant intimal dissection, and occlusion of target vessel perforating branches. The risk of vessel rupture can be decreased by a slight undersizing of the stent compared with the affected vessel and slow balloon inflation. Intimal dissection is a largely inevitable consequence of angioplasty and is tolerable unless a hemodynamically significant plaque develops, which can subsequently lead to thrombosis or vessel occlusion. Despite reports to the contrary, perforating vessel occlusion remains a risk of intracranial stent angioplasty and can lead to stroke *(1,31,32,34–38,44–47)*. Postoperatively, patients are observed in the neurointensive care setting until they are deemed neurologically stable (Fig. 2).

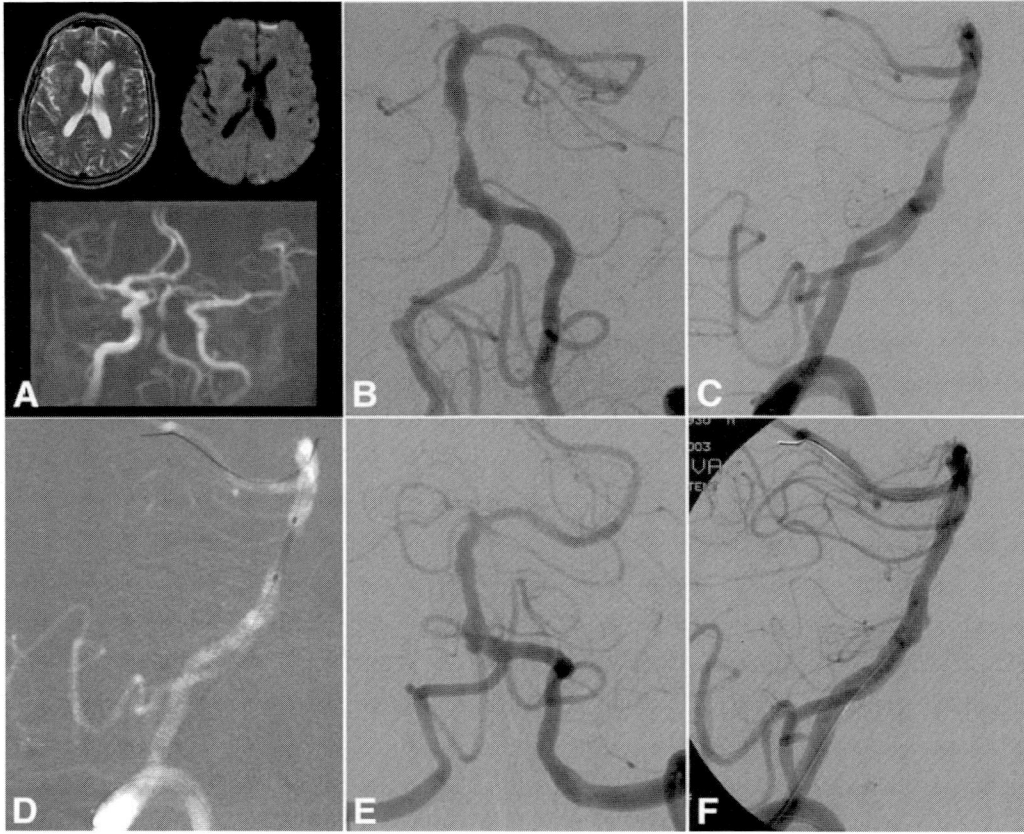

Fig. 2. Stent angioplasty of a hemodynamically symptomatic basilar artery stenosis despite medical therapy. A 73-yr-old man presented with transient left-sided hemiplegia and hemianesthesia, episodes of lightheadedness, and vertical diplopia, which were persistent despite warfarin therapy. MRI revealed a severe midbasilar stenosis (**A**), which was confirmed to be greater than 85% with biplane digital subtraction angiography (**B**, anteroposterior; **C**, lateral). A Medtronic-AVE S670 3 × 9-mm stent was chosen, deliberately undersized to prevent angioplasty-induced intimal dissection or vessel rupture. It positioned across the stenosis and inflated. (**D**) The final result shows significant improvement in the basilar lumen (**E,F**); the patient has remained asymptomatic on antiplatelet therapy with aspirin and clopidogrel.

Clinical Results and Patient Selection

Preliminary results of the University of California at San Francisco experience point to a statistically significant higher risk of postoperative intracranial and reperfusion hemorrhage in patients who were administered glycoprotein IIb/IIIa inhibitors *(48)*. In addition, symptomatic patients who underwent endovascular revascularization in the setting of a stroke or who were neurologically unstable had a significantly worse outcome compared with symptomatic patients treated in a preemptive fashion *(48)*.

The intracranial stenting series in the literature have reported somewhat better results than those on primary unassisted balloon angioplasty despite the limitations inherent in stent navigation above the skull base *(34,40,45,49)*. The rates of immediate postprocedure residual stenosis following stent angioplasty are between 0% and 18% *(50)*, which compares favorably with 41–47% residual from angioplasty alone *(24,27)*. Other reports demonstrate neurological complication rates of around 4.2–25% and mortality rates of 0–13% *(24,27,49–51)*. More recent data, which included mostly neurologically unstable patients undergoing intracranial stenting emergently, showed a high rate of complication including postprocedural intracranial hemorrhage (17%) and stroke (11%) *(4)*. Recent results from the Stenting of Symptomatic Atherosclerotic Lesions in the Vertebral or Intracranial Arteries (SSYLVIA) study indicated a 0% risk of death and a 6.6% risk of stroke in the 30-d periprocedural period. Angiographic follow-up indicated a 30% risk of more than 50% restenosis in the intracranial treatment subset at the 6-mo follow-up mark.

Angioplasty and stenting of selected atherosclerotic lesions should be considered as a treatment option when maximal medical management has failed because symptomatic intracranial stenosis carries a relatively high risk for stroke. Our current practice limits intracranial stent angioplasty to symptomatic patients who have already failed current optimal medical therapy consisting either of oral warfarin or of a combination of aspirin and clopidogrel. In this subset of patients, we recommend proceeding with stent angioplasty, and if the latter is not technically feasible, then unassisted angioplasty is indicated in an attempt to improve distal perfusion. A lower threshold for intervention is used in patients who clearly suffer from hemodynamic insufficiency rather than thromboembolism from an embologenic intracranial stenosis. The rate of technical complications and postprocedural stroke in intracranial stent angioplasty is undoubtedly higher than for extracranial carotid revascularization such as carotid endarterectomy or stenting. This is not surprising considering the size and fragile wall of the intracerebral vessel wall. Accordingly, this procedure should be reserved for cases of emergency or medically refractory ischemia and not used as a primary modality of treatment until a randomized trial can be performed comparing short- and long-term outcomes from best medical therapy and endovascular stenting *(52–54)*.

INTRACRANIAL STENTING FOR ANEURYSM THERAPY

Intracranial stent placement has also allowed the endovascular treatment of wide-necked aneurysms, which were previously not amenable to endovascular treatment despite the use of adjunctive techniques such as the balloon-assist method *(55)* (Fig. 3). In this mode of use, the stent is deployed as a scaffold across the neck of the aneurysm to effectively decrease the neck width and allow deployment of embolic coils through the stent interstices into the aneurysm dome *(1,2,7)*. This can be performed in at least two ways; in the first, the stent is deployed, and then a microcatheter is used separately to navigate into an open cell of the stent, thereby gaining access to the aneurysm dome where coiling can proceed. In the other technique, the microcatheter is first used

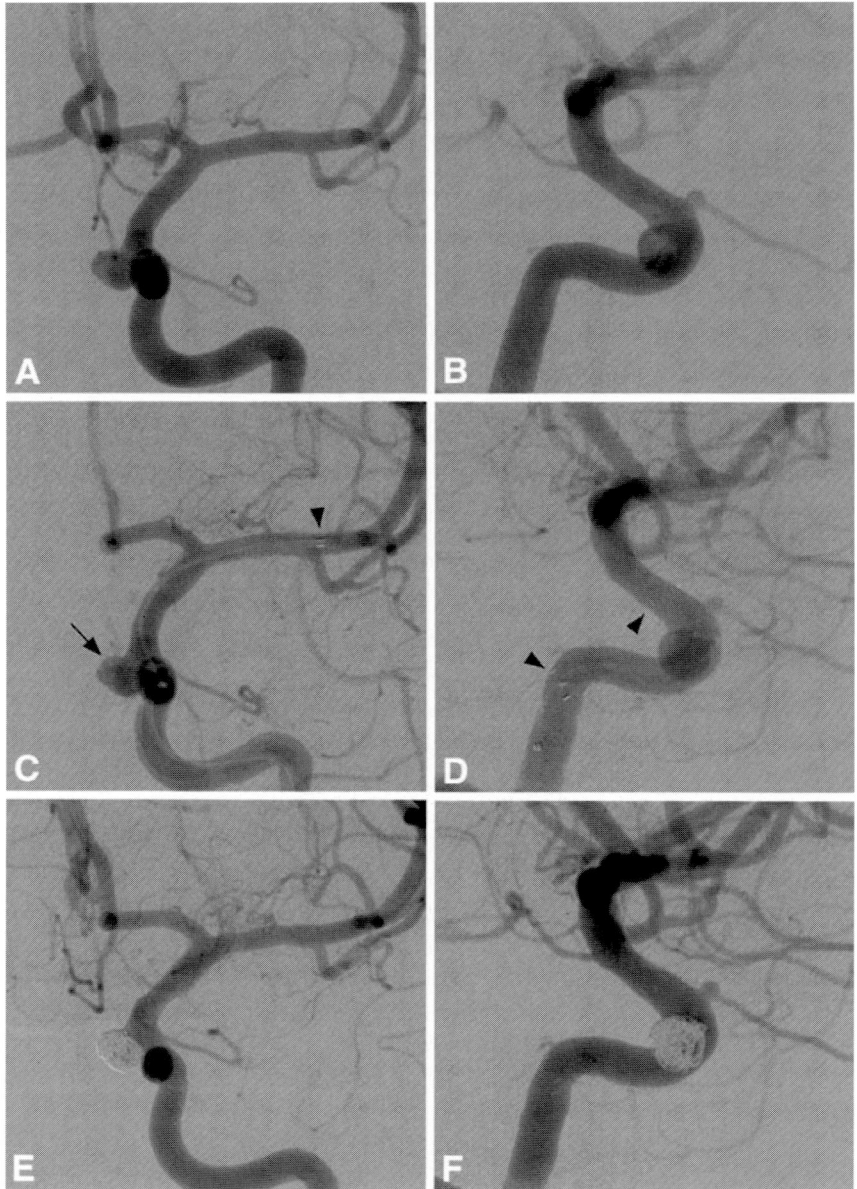

Fig. 3. Treatment of a carotid siphon wide-necked aneurysm using the self-expanding microcatheter-contained Neuroform stent. A 52-yr-old woman with a medially pointing left internal carotid siphon aneurysm measuring 5 mm in diameter with a 4-mm neck failed conventional coiling (**A**, anteroposterior; **B**, lateral). (**C**) Using a bifemoral approach, a microcatheter is seen within the aneurysm dome (arrow); the microcatheter constraining the undeployed Neuroform stent has been advanced into the left middle cerebral artery (arrowhead) in preparation for final positioning and deployment. The Neuroform stent is deployed while the coiling microcatheter remains inside the aneurysm dome; note that the stent interstices are not visible even using high-resolution imaging; opaque radiomarkers (**D**, arrowheads) outline the proximal and distal ends of the stent. Final angiographic result and (**E**, anteroposterior; **F**, lateral).

to access the dome, and then the stent is deployed submaximally while the coils are being delivered, thereby avoiding the occasionally difficult task of passing the microcatheter through the stent interstices after deployment. The latter technique is invaluable in cases of aneurysms on the inner curvatures because of the difficult geometry. There have been reports of benchtop hemodynamic evaluations that have highlighted the important role of the stent placement itself in decreasing the velocity of blood flow inside sidewall aneurysms *(56)* and a few case reports of clinical progression to thrombosis after stent placement alone without coiling *(57)*. In addition, the use of a double stent technique whereby a porous stent is placed within another porous stent can act together to decrease overall inflow into the aneurysm dome and alter the fluid boundary layer enough so as to yield progressive thrombosis *(58)*. This phenomenon, is not, however readily predictable at the current time since others have reported recanalization of previously stented aneurysms of the dissecting type *(59)*.

More recently, the purpose-built self-expanding low-profile Neuroform microstent (Smart Therapeutics/Boston Scientific, San Leandro, CA) has become available, which is more maneuverable than the balloon-expandable coronary-type devices *(6)*. The Neuroform stent is a shape-memory alloy nitinol stent that is constrained inside a high-flow microcatheter containing a coaxial stent pusher. After the high-flow microcatheter containing the stent is advanced beyond the aneurysm neck, the stent is deployed by unsheathing by pushing it out of the delivery microcatheter while the latter is being withdrawn over the stabilized central exchange microwire. The stent has shown great promise but has also been noted to have a relatively low radial force, which makes it unsuitable for use in rescue treatment of herniated coil loops or for treating wide-necked large aneurysms in which its lower radial strength prevents it from providing a strong enough scaffold to counter coil prolapse without stent compression and vessel caliber compromise *(60)*. In addition, it is difficult to traverse the stent once it is deployed in a vessel bend without inadvertently engaging one of the stent cross-members, which are so radiolucent as to be invisible, even in high-resolution digital subtraction angiography units. These problems can be overcome with careful preparation and by ensuring the maintenance of an exchange wire through the true lumen to enable tandem or overlapping stent placement if necessary. Another approach may include the staged deployment of the Neuroform stent, allowing it to be covered by intima and incorporated into the wall prior to attempting to embolize the aneurysm with coils. Purpose-designed stents for intracranial aneurysm treatment are expected to evolve rapidly in the next few years.

CONCLUSIONS

Intracranial stent angioplasty has emerged as a technically feasible and useful adjunct to treatment of both severe intracranial atherosclerosis and geometrically challenging aneurysms. Newer stent designs specifically tailored for the treatment of intracranial lesions have been developed and are in current clinical trials. The current data available from a growing number of retrospective series and case reports continue to highlight the high risk of these procedures. These same reports have also illustrated significant clinical successes in well-selected cases that would not have been achievable using alternate therapies. Consequently, intracranial stent angioplasty should be limited to the treatment of patients who have failed conventional modes of therapy in select centers with high caseloads and expertise until results from randomized trials become available. The continued improvement of the currently available microstent designs will undoubtedly lead to improved clinical outcomes in the future.

REFERENCES

1. Lanzino G, et al. Efficacy and current limitations of intravascular stents for intracranial internal carotid, vertebral, and basilar artery aneurysms. *J Neurosurg* 1999;91:538–546.
2. Higashida RT, et al. Intravascular stent and endovascular coil placement for a ruptured fusiform aneurysm of the basilar artery. Case report and review of the literature. *J Neurosurg* 1997;87:944–949.
3. Phatouros CC, et al. Endovascular stenting of an acutely thrombosed basilar artery: technical case report and review of the literature. *Neurosurgery* 1999;44:667–673.
4. Gupta R, et al. Urgent endovascular revascularization for symptomatic intracranial atherosclerotic stenosis. *Neurology* 2003;61:1729–1735.
5. Levy EI, et al. Transluminal stent-assisted angioplasty of the intracranial vertebrobasilar system for medically refractory, posterior circulation ischemia: early results. *Neurosurgery* 2001;48:1215–1221; discussion 1221–1223.
6. Fiorella D, et al. Preliminary experience using the Neuroform stent for the treatment of cerebral aneurysms. *Neurosurgery* 2004;54:6–16; discussion 16–17.
7. Lylyk P, et al. Endovascular reconstruction of intracranial arteries by stent placement and combined techniques. *J Neurosurg* 2002;97:1306–1313.
8. Sacco RL, et al. Race-ethnicity and determinants of intracranial atherosclerotic cerebral infarction. The Northern Manhattan Stroke Study. *Stroke* 1995;26:14–20.
9. Prognosis of patients with symptomatic vertebral or basilar artery stenosis. The Warfarin-Aspirin Symptomatic Intracranial Disease (WASID) Study Group. *Stroke* 1998;29:1389–1392.
10. Bogousslavsky J, et al. Atherosclerotic disease of the middle cerebral artery. *Stroke* 1986;17:1112–1120.
11. The International Cooperative Study of Extracranial/Intracranial Arterial Anastomosis (EC/IC Bypass Study): methodology and entry characteristics. The EC/IC Bypass Study Group. *Stroke* 1985;16:397–406.
12. Ausman JI, Diaz FG. Critique of the extracranial-intracranial bypass study. *Surg Neurol* 1986;26:218–221.
13. Bogousslavsky J, et al. Bilateral occlusion of the trunk of the middle cerebral artery. Results of an international randomized trial. The EC/IC Bypass Study Group. *Stroke* 1986;17:1107–1111.
14. Awad IA, Spetzler RF. Extracranial-intracranial bypass surgery: a critical analysis in light of the International Cooperative Study. *Neurosurgery* 1986;19:655–664.
15. Akins PT, et al. Natural history of stenosis from intracranial atherosclerosis by serial angiography. *Stroke* 1998;29:433–438.
16. Caplan L, et al. Occlusive disease of the middle cerebral artery. *Neurology* 1985;35:975–982.
17. Craig DR, et al. Intracranial internal carotid artery stenosis. *Stroke* 1982;13:825–828.

18. Kubik C, Adams R. Occlusion of the basilar artery: a clinical and pathological study. *Brain* 1946;59:73–121.
19. Archer CR, Horenstein S. Basilar artery occlusion: clinical and radiological correlation. *Stroke* 1977;8:383–390.
20. Bruckmann H, et al. Acute vertebral-basilar thrombosis. Angiologic-clinical comparison and therapeutic implications. *Acta Radiol Suppl* 1986;369:38–42.
21. Hacke W, et al. Intra-arterial thrombolytic therapy improves outcome in patients with acute vertebrobasilar occlusive disease. *Stroke* 1988;19:1216–1222.
22. Caplan LR, Vertebrobasilar embolism. *Clin Exp Neurol* 1991;28:1–22.
23. Benesch CG, Chimowitz MI. Best treatment for intracranial arterial stenosis? 50 years of uncertainty. The WASID Investigators. *Neurology* 2000;55:465–466.
24. Clark WM, et al. Safety and efficacy of percutaneous transluminal angioplasty for intracranial atherosclerotic stenosis. *Stroke* 1995;26:1200–1204.
25. Terada T, et al. Transluminal angioplasty for arteriosclerotic disease of the distal vertebral and basilar arteries. *J Neurol Neurosurg Psychiatry* 1996;60:377–381.
26. Gress DR, et al. Angioplasty for intracranial symptomatic vertebrobasilar ischemia. *Neurosurgery* 2002;51:23–27; discussion 27–29.
27. Marks MP, et al. Outcome of angioplasty for atherosclerotic intracranial stenosis. *Stroke* 1999;30:1065–1069.
28. Connors JJ 3rd, Wojak JC. Percutaneous transluminal angioplasty for intracranial atherosclerotic lesions: evolution of technique and short-term results. *J Neurosurg* 1999;91:415–423.
29. Mori T, et al. Follow-up study after intracranial percutaneous transluminal cerebral balloon angioplasty. *AJNR Am J Neuroradiol* 1998;19:1525–1533.
30. Nahser HC, et al. Intracranial vertebrobasilar stenosis: angioplasty and follow-up. *AJNR Am J Neuroradiol* 2000;21:1293–1301.
31. Lanzino G, et al. Angioplasty and stenting of basilar artery stenosis: technical case report. *Neurosurgery* 1999;45:404–407; discussion 407–408.
32. Malek AM, et al. Tandem intracranial stent deployment for treatment of an iatrogenic, flow-limiting, basilar artery dissection: technical case report. *Neurosurgery* 1999;45:919–924.
33. Lutsep HL, et al. Stenting of Symptomatic Atherosclerotic Lesions in the Vertebral or Intracranial Arteries (SSYLVIA): Study Results. *Stroke* 2003;34:253, abstract.
34. Gomez CR, et al. Elective stenting of symptomatic middle cerebral artery stenosis. *AJNR Am J Neuroradiol* 2000;21:971–973.
35. Fessler RD, et al. Improved cerebral perfusion after stenting of a petrous carotid stenosis: technical case report. *Neurosurgery* 1999;45:638–642.
36. Horowitz MB, et al. Percutaneous transluminal angioplasty and stenting of midbasilar stenoses: three technical case reports and literature review. *Neurosurgery* 1999;45:925–930; discussion 930–931.
37. Morris PP, et al. Intracranial deployment of coronary stents for symptomatic atherosclerotic disease. *AJNR Am J Neuroradiol* 1999;20:1688–1694.
38. Phatouros CC, et al. Primary stenting for high-grade basilar artery stenosis. *AJNR Am J Neuroradiol* 2000;21:1744–1749.
39. Gahn G, et al. Cerebrovascular reserve before and after vertebral artery angioplasty. *AJNR Am J Neuroradiol* 1999;20:785–786.
40. Mori T, et al. Short-term arteriographic and clinical outcome after cerebral angioplasty and stenting for intracranial vertebrobasilar and carotid atherosclerotic occlusive disease. *AJNR Am J Neuroradiol* 2000;21:249–254.
41. Eckard DA, et al. Stiff guide technique: technical report and illustrative case. *AJNR Am J Neuroradiol* 2003;24:275–278.

42. Fessler RD, et al. Transradial approach for vertebral artery stenting: technical case report. *Neurosurgery* 2000;46:1524–1527; discussion 1527–1528.
43. Blanc R, et al. Hemostatic closure device after carotid puncture for stent and coil placement in an intracranial aneurysm: technical note. *AJNR Am J Neuroradiol* 2002; 23:978–981.
44. Mori T, Kazita K, Mori K. Cerebral angioplasty and stenting for intracranial vertebral atherosclerotic stenosis. *AJNR Am J Neuroradiol* 1999;20:787–789.
45. Ramee SR, et al. Provisional stenting for symptomatic intracranial stenosis using a multidisciplinary approach: acute results, unexpected benefit, and one-year outcome. *Catheter Cardiovasc Interv* 2001;52:457–467.
46. Al-Mubarak N, et al. Stenting of symptomatic stenosis of the intracranial internal carotid artery. *AJNR Am J Neuroradiol* 1998;19:1949–951.
47. Dorros G, Cohn JM, Palmer LE. Stent deployment resolves a petrous carotid artery angioplasty dissection. *AJNR Am J Neuroradiol* 1998;19:392–394.
48. Malek AM, et al. Intracranial stent angioplasty for the treatment of symptomatic intracranial atherosclerotic disease. *CV Joint Section AANS/CNS/ASITN* 2001, abstract.
49. Rasmussen PA, et al. Stent-assisted angioplasty of intracranial vertebrobasilar atherosclerosis: an initial experience. *J Neurosurg* 2000;92:771–778.
50. Lylyk P, et al. Angioplasty and stent placement in intracranial atherosclerotic stenoses and dissections. *AJNR Am J Neuroradiol* 2002;23:430–436.
51. Terada T, et al. Endovascular therapy for stenosis of the petrous or cavernous portion of the internal carotid artery: percutaneous transluminal angioplasty compared with stent placement. *J Neurosurg* 2003;98:491–497.
52. Chimowitz MI. Angioplasty or stenting is not appropriate as first-line treatment of intracranial stenosis. *Arch Neurol* 2001;58:1690–1692.
53. Gomez CR, Orr SC. Angioplasty and stenting for primary treatment of intracranial arterial stenoses. *Arch Neurol* 2001;58:1687–1690.
54. Chaturvedi, S. and L.R. Caplan, *Angioplasty for intracranial atherosclerosis: is the treatment worse than the disease? Neurology* 2003;61:1647–1648.
55. Moret J, et al. (Reconstruction technic in the treatment of wide-neck intracranial aneurysms. Long-term angiographic and clinical results. Apropos of 56 cases). *J Neuroradiol* 1997;24:30–44.
56. Lieber BB, Stancampiano AP, Wakhloo AK. Alteration of hemodynamics in aneurysm models by stenting: influence of stent porosity. *Ann Biomed Eng* 1997;25:460–469.
57. Vanninen R, Manninen H. Ronkainen A. Broad-based intracranial aneurysms: thrombosis induced by stent placement. *AJNR Am J Neuroradiol* 2003;24:263–266.
58. Benndorf G, et al. Treatment of a ruptured dissecting vertebral artery aneurysm with double stent placement: case report. *AJNR Am J Neuroradiol* 2001;22:1844–1848.
59. MacKay CI, et al. Recurrence of a vertebral artery dissecting pseudoaneurysm after successful stent-supported coil embolization: case report. *Neurosurgery* 2003;53:754–759; discussion 760–761.
60. Broadbent LP, et al. Management of neuroform stent dislodgement and misplacement. *AJNR Am J Neuroradiol* 2003;24:1819–1822.

9
The Role of Embolic Agents in Endovascular Treatment of Intracranial Arteriovenous Malformations and Tumors

Ricardo A. Hanel, MD, Bernard R. Bendok, MD, Jay U. Howington, MD, Elad I. Levy, MD, Lee R. Guterman, PhD, MD, and L. Nelson Hopkins, MD

INTRODUCTION

Advances in microneurosurgery, neurocritical care, and endovascular techniques have greatly improved outcomes for patients with complex neurosurgical disorders. The neurosurgeons of today have become involved in the application of high-technology solutions and have welcomed contributions from other disciplines. Less invasive approaches resulting in improved patient outcomes have helped to shift the focus of neurosurgery toward minimally invasive procedures. Currently, this trend is reflected in all aspects of the specialty. One of the most influenced areas is neuroendovascular surgery. With improvement and broad application of refined microsurgery, skull base techniques, computerized surgical guidance, and new catheter technology and embolic agents, this field has advanced quickly, with an ever increasing safety and effectiveness profile.

In this chapter, the role of endovascular treatment options in the overall management of intracranial arteriovenous malformations (AVMs) and tumors in clinical practice is reviewed. Drawing from our experience and the opinions of leading neurointerventionists, techniques and applications of current technology are highlighted, with a focus on the use of glues and other chemical agents used for embolization of these lesions.

EMBOLIC AGENTS FOR THE TREATMENT OF AVMS

Overview

The aim of endovascular therapy is to obliterate the AVM or reduce its size with little or no increased medical or neurological risk to the patient. As with any intervention, the overall goal is to enhance the patient's outcome.

In 1960 Luessenhop and Spence (1) performed the first embolization of an AVM by injecting Silastic spheres through surgical exposure of the cervical carotid artery. Forty years of advances brought new embolic agents to the scene,

From: *Minimally Invasive Neurosurgery,* edited by: M.R. Proctor and P.M. Black © Humana Press Inc., Totowa, NJ

including polyvinyl alcohol (PVA), *N*-butyl cyanoacrylate (NBCA), Onyx (Micro Therapeutics, Irvine, CA), and neuracryl M (Provasis Therapeutics, El Cajon, CA); novel microcatheters and microwires; and endovascular operative techniques altering the approach to this entity.

The endovascular treatment strategy for an AVM is significantly influenced by the overall treatment plan and is tailored to the patient and the malformation. Endovascular embolization strategies can be considered within the following categories of goals and issues: (1) embolization as a preoperative tool, (2) embolization as a pre-Gamma-Knife radiosurgery tool, (3) embolization alone as a curative modality, (4) embolization for palliation of symptoms, and (5) embolization of associated aneurysms.

Embolization reduces the amount of blood loss that is associated with the resection of an AVM by decreasing the vascularity of the nidus *(2)*. In a study by Jafar et al. *(2)*, the amount of blood loss during the resection of large AVMs embolized with NBCA (an adhesive liquid polymer) was similar to that for nonembolized small AVMs. Many authors have noted that NBCA embolization increases the ease of the operation *(2,3)*. For large AVMs, embolization can serve the purpose of gradually decreasing flow through the AVM, hence decreasing the risk of hemorrhage associated with "normal perfusion pressure breakthrough" *(4,5)*. Normal perfusion pressure breakthrough can occur when embolization or resection of a high-flow AVM directs blood from the AVM to surrounding vascular beds that have been chronically hypoperfused. Chronic hypoperfusion leads to a loss of the autoregulatory ability of the vascular beds. When blood flow is redirected into these vascular territories, hemorrhage can occur as a result of the normal perfusion pressure breakthrough phenomenon, even at a patient's "normal" systemic blood pressure. Embolized AVM vessels can also serve as a roadmap during surgical resection by helping the surgeon to define the anatomy of the feeding pedicles and the nidus.

Despite these advantages, AVM embolization carries considerable risk. Only patients with AVMs who will significantly benefit from embolization before surgery should undergo this treatment. For example, a small AVM in the right frontal lobe with limited feeders that are easily accessible by surgery probably does not warrant embolization, unless the embolization may be curative (*see* Case Illustration section on p. 204). In presurgical planning of AVM embolization, the authors embolize those pedicles felt to be the most technically challenging for surgery. If lenticulostriate and other deep feeding vessels appear to be easy to embolize but difficult to access surgically, we attempt these feeders first. Alternatively, if the deep feeders appear too difficult to access, the larger, more superficial feeders are embolized first. After the occlusion of superficial feeders, deep feeders may recruit additional blood supply and become enlarged. The enlarged vessels may be more accessible during a second embolization session several weeks later. It is extremely important to coordinate with the operating surgeon as to the goals and timing of treatment.

For the patient in whom the management plan involves radiosurgery, embolization strategies have been used to reduce the volume of an AVM and to eliminate associated pedicle and proximal aneurysms when possible. The size of an AVM nidus influences the success of radiosurgery *(6)*. Therefore, reducing the size of an AVM with embolization may increase the success rate of radiosurgery and help avoid use of the higher radiation doses needed to treat a larger AVM. Circumferential embolization of the AVM, rather than fragmentation of the nidus, is the preferred strategy here since a fragmented nidus may result in multiple targets for radiation dosing, which could make radiosurgery planning difficult, thereby negating the benefits of embolization. Some limited evidence exists to support the embolization of large AVMs to a size that is amenable to radiosurgery *(7,8)*. The long-term results of this strategy have not yet been adequately documented. The authors' results with this strategy in select AVMs is encouraging thus far (unpublished data).

Endovascular treatment alone is rarely curative *(8)*. In general, this strategy works for some small AVMs with limited arterial feeders and draining veins. Rarely, a medium-size AVM can be embolized in one or multiple sessions and a cure can be achieved (*see* Case Illustration section on p. 204).

Some high-grade AVMs may be too dangerous to treat by any method, and pure observation may be indicated. Embolization solely for palliation of symptoms is rarely indicated. An AVM may be responsible for debilitating symptoms such as severe headaches or ischemia related to steal phenomena. In these situations, partial embolization may help reduce flow through the AVM and lead to an improvement in the patient's symptoms. The embolization of dural feeders may be particularly helpful for amelioration of headaches. Steal symptoms can be reduced by embolizing large "incurable" AVMs *(9)*. Adhesive embolic agents (such as NBCA) should be used for these types of indications. It has been suggested that partial embolization of an AVM may yield a worse prognosis than no treatment, so this strategy should be practiced with caution *(8,10,11)*.

Embolization techniques can be used to treat associated aneurysms. Owing to the risk of rupture of proximal aneurysms during AVM embolization or excision, treatment of these lesions should precede AVM treatment when possible. If the aneurysm appears to be appropriate for coiling, it can potentially be occluded during the first embolization session before the AVM nidus is approached. If the aneurysm appears to be better suited for surgery, surgical clipping can be performed before AVM embolization. Aneurysms on feeding pedicles of the AVM (flow-related aneurysms) can be occluded primarily using detachable coils. Alternatively, an aneurysm that is close to the AVM nidus can often be occluded by embolization of the pedicle harboring that aneurysm while glue is injected from the microcatheter (the glue refluxes from the nidus into the pedicle and aneurysm). This occlusion can result from infiltration of glue into the aneurysm sac or secondarily as the feeding pedicle becomes occluded. Pedicle aneurysms can be embolized with detachable coils before glue is injected into the pedicle. If the pedicle aneurysm is distal enough from the AVM, it can be treated with the same glue injection used to embolize the nidus. Attention should be paid to intranidal aneurysms during embolization. If a hemorrhage has occurred, an intranidal aneurysm should be suspected as a rupture site. When possible, the pedicle feeding the nidus harboring the aneurysm should be treated first.

Tools for Embolization

Embolic Agents

Embolic agents can be classified as solid or liquid (Table 1). Each agent requires a significant learning curve. Earlier agents with low safety or high recanalization profiles have been abandoned for newer and safer agents. Our discussion will focus not only on the most commonly used agents, NBCA and PVA particles, but also on promising new agents, Onyx and neuracryl M.

PVA

Before refinements were made in microcatheter technology, particulate agents such as PVA were the mainstay of preoperative embolic therapy for AVMs. First reported by Porstmann et al. *(12)*, PVA particles are currently used only for those cases in which the AVM will be resected within several days or to slow the flow in a high-flow pedicle before NBCA embolization is performed. Slowing the flow in a high-flow pedicle with PVA may allow more NBCA to penetrate the AVM nidus, rather than escaping through the draining vein. As AVM obliteration caused by PVA embolization is the result of thrombosis, embolization with PVA particles results in slower occlusion of the nidus (compared with NBCA), and because the thrombus is broken down over the course of time, a relatively high rate of recanalization is associated with PVA embolization *(13)*. Concerns regarding recanalization and recruitment of new feeders have made particle embolization fall out of favor at most centers except for the previously mentioned circumstances. In addition, PVA particles are not radiopaque.

NBCA

The agent used most commonly for AVM embolization over the past several years has been NBCA. Introduced in the late 1980s, NBCA is an attractive embolic agent because of its associated low rate of recanalization. Although a steep learning curve is involved in its use, many authors have reported successful use and low morbidity in recent years *(2,14)*. Gluing the catheter intracranially and embolizing the draining vein, causing hemorrhage or infarction, are the two most common complications associated with NBCA *(14)*. The technique of NBCA embolization involves subjectively assessing the AVM angioarchitecture, which is seen by use of superselective angiography. Particular attention must be paid to the anatomy of the nidus and veins.

ONYX

Unlike NBCA, Onyx is a nonadhesive, liquid embolic agent *(15)*. Onyx is a biocompatible polymer (ethylene-vinyl alcohol copolymer) dissolved in an organic solvent (dimethyl sulfoxide [DMSO]). Its nonadhesive nature eliminates the risk of gluing the catheter intracranially. Onyx allows for greater variability in injection force, volume, and duration. These characteristics may allow for a more controlled embolization of the nidus. The ability to administer the Onyx slowly allows the interventionist to stop the injection easily before this material penetrates the draining veins. Early animal studies showed that the DMSO component of the Onyx can cause severe vasospasm and angionecrosis

Table 1
Classification of Embolic Agents

Solid agents
    Gelfoam (Upjohn, Kalamazoo, MI)
    Polyvinyl alcohol particles
    Avitene (microfibrillar collagen)
    Silk sutures
    Balloons
    Coils
    Microspheres (EmboGold Microspheres,
        Biosphere Medical, Rockland, MA)
Liquid agents
    Cyanoacrylates (NBCA, neuracryl M, others)
    Onyx (Micro Therapeutics, Irvine, CA)
    Polyvinyl acetate
    Pure ethanol
    Cellulose acetate polymer

(16). In more recent studies, this angiotoxic effect has been attributed to the amount of the DMSO injected and the velocity of the Onyx injection, with larger volumes of DMSO and faster injection rates being related to angiotoxicity *(17)*. Chaloupka et al. *(17)* showed that slow injections in the swine rete mirabile (between 30 and 90 s of small volumes of DMSO [0.5 or 0.8 mL]) are well tolerated in terms of less angiotoxicity.

The neurointerventional team at the University of California at Los Angeles has reported encouraging data on 23 patients who underwent Onyx embolization of AVMs *(15)*. A 63% reduction in AVM volume was observed after a total of 129 arterial feeders were embolized. There was a 4% permanent morbidity. Of these 23 patients, 12 underwent subsequent radiosurgery, and 11 had operations that resulted in complete resection of the AVM. Histopathologic examination of the resected specimens was performed. Specimens resected 1 d after embolization showed mild inflammatory changes. Those resected more than 4 d after embolization showed chronic inflammatory changes. Angionecrosis of the embolized vessels was noted in two of the 11 patients who underwent operations. The authors emphasize the need to inject Onyx slowly and to avoid reflux. They also emphasize the need to mix tantalum powder thoroughly with the compound to ensure optimal visualization under fluoroscopy. DMSO compatibility with currently used catheters is also a concern. The solvent has been shown to damage some of the catheters used for its delivery in the past *(15,17)*. The introduction of new catheter designs, including coated catheters, and minor changes in the composition of the agent will solve this issue.

Akin et al. *(18)* recently compared the surgical handling characteristics of Onyx and NBCA for embolization of vessels in an AVM resection model in swine. They reported better handling of specimens after Onyx embolization, with a tendency toward less blood loss in surgery. On the basis of these reports and our laboratory experience with Onyx, we believe that this agent holds great promise for the treatment of cerebral AVMs and aneurysms (A.S. Boulos and L.R. Guterman, personal communication, 2001). No long-term angiographic follow-up analyses of patients treated with Onyx have been conducted, so the long-term recanalization rate is unknown.

NEURACRYL M

In an effort to avoid the inconsistent polymerization rates, the premature beading and breakup, and the inadvertent gluing of the catheter to the vessel wall associated with NBCA as well as the lack of angionecrosis and associated recanalization potential seen with Onyx, Kerber and colleagues began work on neuracryl M (C.W. Kerber et al., personal communication). They sought to develop a radiopaque, injectable embolic agent composed primarily of the basic cyanoacrylate monomer that would stay together as much as possible when exposed to rapidly flowing blood and cause the inflammatory reaction necessary to result in permanent occlusion. The new agent, once polymerized, had to have a soft consistency so that surgeons could easily manipulate embolized vessels. After working with many different amalgamations, they produced a cyanoacrylate-based polymer named neuracryl M.

Initial studies comparing the behavioral characteristics of neuracryl M and NBCA were done using porcine blood in four different settings (19). Drops of the two substances were placed on and beneath the surface of stagnant blood and were also injected into a linear flow model as well as a standardized AVM model. In the stagnant models, NBCA and neuracryl M had equivalent polymerization times, but when placed beneath the surface of the blood, the neuracryl formed a rubbery mass, which remained at the tip of the needle, whereas the NBCA dropped to the bottom of the beaker, forming a friable mass. When injected in the flow models, the neuracryl remained as a cohesive mass that filled the entire linear flow model and yielded better penetration of the AVM model than did the NBCA. In the linear flow model, the NBCA formed small droplets that embolized downstream in the tubing. Unfortunately, neuracryl M is a cyanoacrylate derivative and as such has the potential to glue the catheter to the vessel wall. As with NBCA, a significant learning curve accompanies the use of neuracryl M. Inadvertent adherence to the vessel wall can be largely avoided by mastering the technique of using cyanoacrylates in the treatment of AVMs and taking the proper precautions.

A randomized clinical trial was undertaken to compare neuracryl M with PVA for the treatment of AVMs (20). Among 10 patients receiving neuracryl M, five lesions were totally obliterated. Of the lesions in the remaining five patients, nidus size was reduced by 50–99% in two, and by less than 50% in two others and was felt to have increased slightly in one. This study was an angiographic study and did not focus on the histopathologic changes induced by the neuracryl M. Chopko et al. (21) reported the first human histopathologic results in a 34-yr-old man who was treated with neuracryl M 4 d before surgical resection. Histopathologic examination showed scattered foci of neuracryl M that filled the lumen and did not breach the vessel wall. A profound acute inflammatory response surrounding many of the AVM vessels, a giant-cell foreign-body reaction, and angionecrosis were noted. The results obtained with neuracryl M embolization are promising. Further studies are needed to prove the safety and efficacy of this agent.

Catheters

Dramatic improvements in microcatheter and microguidewire designs over the past several years have allowed for safer, more effective AVM embolization. Flow-directed and wire-directed catheters are used for AVM embolization. In general, wire-directed catheters are used to access low-flow pedicles and flow-directed catheters to access high-flow pedicles. Positioning a flow-directed microcatheter into the distal cerebral circulation is a relatively atraumatic event. It can be difficult to get the catheter to travel distally into low-flow vessels, which can be easily accessed with a wire-directed catheter. Great care is required, however, when positioning a wire-directed catheter to avoid perforating the nidus or pedicle with the microwire. An advantage of flow-guided microcatheters is the lack of a wire and, therefore, a decreased risk of intracerebral hemorrhage. A disadvantage is the inability to select precisely which pedicle to embolize because this type of catheter is directed mostly by the flow and not by the operator. For wire-directed catheters, the authors commonly use the Transcend platinum tip wire (Boston Scientific Scimed, Maple Grove, MN) or the PVS Synchro wire (Precision Vascular Systems, West Valley City, UT). Either flow- or wire-directed catheters can be used to deliver liquid embolic agents, such as cyanoacrylate, Onyx, and pure ethanol, as well as liquid coils. For particulate agents such as PVA, larger lumen wire-directed microcatheters are needed.

Over the last few years, guidewires have been developed that can be passed through flow-directed catheters. Initially, these wires were used only to bolster the proximal segment of the microcatheter, hence, giving it some "pushability." With time, some interventionists have begun to use flow-directed catheters like over-the-wire systems. Using this technique, perforation of the target vessels and breach of the catheter wall are possible, so caution is advised when attempting this approach. Perforation of vessels can occur because flow-directed catheters can be navigated more distally toward the nidus, where the vessels can be more fragile. Moreover, extreme caution is required when passing wires thorough these catheters to avoid damage to the wall of the catheter (The walls of a flow-directed catheter are relatively thin compared with those of a wire-directed catheter.) Improving wire technology (less traumatic tips) has caused the authors to shift gradually toward using wire-directed microcatheters more often for AVM embolization. Wire-directed catheters are braided and are less likely to be perforated or to burst during glue injection than are flow-directed catheters.

When using cyanoacrylates, the tip of the catheter selected for embolization should be advanced as far into the pedicle as possible. In this way, a controlled injection can be performed, thus minimizing the risk of reflux into normal vessels. With precipitates, like Onyx, the catheter tip can be positioned more proximally within the pedicle. When one pedicle is filled, injection can continue until more pedicles on the same feeding branch are filled.

Flow-directed microcatheters can be navigated up to the nidus without the risk of wire perforation. These catheters should be checked for small leaks by injecting saline into them before use to prevent complications related to extravasation of embolic material in unwanted areas.

Technical Strategies and Nuances

In this section, technical strategies applied by the authors in most cases of NBCA embolization and nuances oriented toward goals for the management of a given AVM in a given patient are addressed. After the decision has been made to treat an AVM, the need for embolization is carefully assessed. Angiographic and magnetic resonance images are scrutinized to gain a better understanding of the hemodynamics of the lesion and its periphery. Special attention is paid to the proximity of the AVM to eloquent cortex, the presence of associated aneurysms, the pattern of venous drainage, and the presence or absence of venous outflow obstruction. A strategy is devised that is based on the patient's needs. In general, three arterial pedicles or less are embolized in a given session. The rationale here is to allow a gradual readjustment of the regional hemodynamics to occur. If a pedicle is large, embolizing that pedicle alone may be prudent and sufficient. If there are several small pedicles, more than three pedicles can be embolized. Aneurysms associated with the AVM are treated first by clipping or endovascular embolization (either on a separate occasion or during the same procedure). If a pseudoaneurysm or an intranidal aneurysm appears to be the source of hemorrhage, the feeder that contributes to this compartment of the nidus is embolized. In addition, embolization of any arterial feeder supplying a compartment drained by ectatic or stenosed veins is attempted. Otherwise, the pedicle that is easiest to access and provides the best route to the nidus is selected for embolization. Care should be taken to avoid vessels en passage (those vessels feeding not only the AVM but also normal brain tissue). Patients are allowed to recover for several weeks between embolization sessions. A single session may be required for embolization of a small AVM with two to three pedicles, whereas two to four sessions may be necessary for a large AVM.

General Anesthesia vs Awake Testing During AVM Embolization

AVM embolization is carried out after the administration of sedative and analgesic agents or the induction of general anesthesia. When embolization is performed in an awake patient, the patient can be monitored for the duration of the procedure, which allows for provocative pharmacologic test injection of the pedicle or pedicles selected for embolization with a barbiturate (amobarbital or methohexital) or lidocaine (i.e., if the AVM is dural based or intimately involved with the cranial nerves or has supply from the external circulation) in an effort to evaluate better the territory supplied by that vessel or vessels. In addition, the medical complications associated with general anesthesia can be avoided. The authors prefer to have the patient awake whenever possible during embolization. Exceptions are patients who are unwilling or those who cannot cooperate because of age, decreased mental status, or claustrophobia.

Preparation for Embolization

After the patient is positioned on the angiography table and ready for treatment, a cerebral angiogram is performed that includes the external carotid arteries. The treatment strategy is assessed according to current angiographic findings about the hemodynamics of the AVM. A bolus of heparin (60–70 U/kg) is administered to achieve an activated coagulation time in the range of 250–300 s. After the target feeding vessel has been selected, a 5- or 6-French guide catheter, which is connected to a heparinized saline drip, is placed in the brachiocephalic vessel of choice using over-the-wire and road-map techniques. A microcatheter (either wire- or flow-directed) is connected to the heparinized saline drip. Vigilant attention is paid to avoiding air bubbles and blood clots in the catheters. After treating any proximal aneurysms with coils, attention is directed to the chosen pedicle. Using road-map techniques, a wire-directed catheter can be navigated close to the AVM nidus, with a soft-tip guidewire used to avoid vessel perforation. Flow-directed catheters follow high flow and can be pushed forward by injecting small amounts of saline with a 3-mL syringe. Care must be taken to ensure that the microcatheter is as close as possible to the nidus without entering and perforating the fragile vessels of the nidus. With the microcatheter in position, provocative testing of the feeding pedicle is carried out.

Neurological examinations are conducted before and after test injection. Typically, an injection of 20 mg of lidocaine will effectively produce symptoms referable to a peripheral nerve within that vessel's distribution. If the vessel anastomoses to the external carotid artery, we are especially careful to administer lidocaine and perform a detailed cranial nerve examination (Table 2 lists possible dangerous anastomoses between the extracranial and intracranial circulation.) Symptoms referable to the retina can also be detected with lidocaine if the pedicle is in close proximity to the ophthalmic artery. If lidocaine administration is tolerated without symptoms, 10 mg of methohexital or amobarbital is injected through the microcatheter. The methohexital or amobarbital will depress the cerebral activity in the brain within that vessel's distribution. A detailed neurological examination is then performed to ascertain whether any new neurological symptoms have resulted. The authors have found this combination of tests to be very useful before permanent sacrifice of AVM feeding pedicles *(22,23)*. Even when the examination is unchanged, caution with NBCA embolization is recommended. Flow patterns through the microcatheter and pedicle will change while the glue is being injected, so glue may begin to embolize to eloquent branches that the methohexital did not reach because it was injected when the malformation was fully patent.

NBCA Embolization

After the microcatheter is in position, the NBCA (Trufill NBCA Liquid Embolic Treatment System, Cordis, Miami Lakes, FL) is prepared. The Trufill system includes glue, ethiodized oil, and tantalum powder. After confirming that the pedicle is safe to embolize, ethiodized oil is mixed with the NBCA and

Table 2
Possible Dangerous Anastomoses Between the Extracranial and Intracranial Circulation

Extracranial Arteries
    Anterior branch of middle meningeal
    Anterior meningeal
    Petrosquamosal branch of middle meningeal
    Occipital
    Neuromeningeal branch of ascending pharyngeal

Intracranial Arteries
    Ophthalmic (ethmoidal)
    Anterior cerebral
    Petrous internal carotid (cranial nerve VII)
    Vertebral
    Posterior inferior cerebellar/anterior inferior cerebral (cranial nerves IX–XI)

Adapted from Standard SC, Hopkins LN. Principles of neuroendovascular intervention, in *Endovascular Neurological Intervention* (Maciunas RJ, ed.), The American Association of Neurological Surgeons, Park Ridge, IL, 1995, p. 16.

tantalum powder for radiopacity. Moreover, modifying the ratio of ethiodized oil and NBCA will vary the polymerization time. For direct arteriovenous fistulae and high-flow regions, the ratio of NBCA to ethiodized oil should be higher than for low-flow areas. High-speed (30 frames/s) angiographic images are obtained through the microcatheter to measure the transit time and degree of flow before embolizing the pedicle. For most situations (moderate-to-low flow), the authors use an ethiodized oil to NBCA ratio of 3:1. Changes in the speed of compound injection alter its embolization properties. In our opinion, altering the injection rate is probably better than altering the mixture for different microangiographic patterns. Furthermore, ethiodized oil is more viscous than NBCA. Therefore, changing the ratio has more of an effect than simply changing the polymerization time. Alternatively, detachable coils can be used to reduce the flow through the fistula. Because the NBCA polymerizes on contact with blood or saline, the preparation must take place in a sterile, ion-free environment to prevent the occurrence of premature polymerization. The interventionist changes gown and gloves and prepares the glue on a sterile table with sterile instruments. The tantalum powder is first mixed with the appropriate volume of ethiodized oil in a 3-mL syringe. NBCA is then added. The syringe is then well shaken for 2–3 min to ensure complete mixing.

While the operator mixes the glue, the assistant isolates the tip of the microcatheter with clean towels and flushes the microcatheter with a sterile dextrose solution (D5W). The assistant then creates a negative roadmap using the previously determined optimal angiographic projection. Alternatively, fluoroscopy can be used without a roadmap on one screen while an image of the pedicle and nidus obtained from the most recent angiographic imaging (and the same projection as will be used for the injection) is projected on the adjacent screen. After the glue is well mixed, the operator injects it and observes filling of the nidus. Following the injection, the microcatheter is removed while suction is applied by the operator, and the assistant quickly withdraws the microcatheter from the guide catheter. An angiographic run is then obtained through the guide catheter to assess the effects of the embolization. If the patient's condition is unchanged neurologically and if another pedicle requires embolization concurrently, the new pedicle is accessed and embolized as above; otherwise, the procedure is terminated. Patients are observed in the intensive care unit for one night and discharged the following day if they are neurologically stable and without a severe headache. The authors allow a 3- to 4-wk interval between embolization sessions.

Complication Management

Acute complications of embolization that require special attention in the endovascular suite include but are not limited to vessel perforation with intraparenchymal hemorrhage, intraventricular hemorrhage, gluing of the catheter to the nidus, and occlusion of draining vein(s). Intraparenchymal or intraventricular hemorrhage can be detected by a contrast blush observed on angiography or by a change in the patient's neurological exam. An intubated patient who experiences unexplained bradycardia and hypertension (Cushing's reflex) should be suspected of having an intracranial hemorrhage. If a hemorrhage is suspected, the procedure should be aborted, anticoagulation reversed, and a computed tomographic scan obtained. If a neurosurgeon is not a member of the endovascular team, one should be contacted immediately. An awake patient who becomes unresponsive should be intubated for intracranial pressure management and airway protection. An external ventricular drain may be indicated to monitor and control intracranial pressure. When a catheter is glued to the nidus, the catheter should be cut at the groin region. If surgical excision of the AVM is possible, excision with removal of the catheter during AVM resection may be possible. If the AVM is not surgically accessible, anticoagulation therapy (when it can be administered safely) should be considered to prevent the formation of clot on the catheter.

Occlusion of draining veins by NBCA is a feared complication. Occlusion of a draining vein can result in or predispose the patient to intraparenchymal hemorrhage. When a major draining vein has been occluded, immediate embolization of all possible arterial feeders, in conjunction with lowering of the patient's arterial blood pressure, should be considered. If additional pedicles are not accessible, the procedure should be aborted. A computed tomographic scan should be obtained promptly. If a hemorrhage has occurred, prompt neurosurgical evaluation is essential. If no hemorrhage has occurred, the management is controversial. Some clinicians have advocated prompt surgical excision if a significant portion of venous drainage has been occluded and if the AVM is surgically accessible. This idea arises from the observation that occluding the

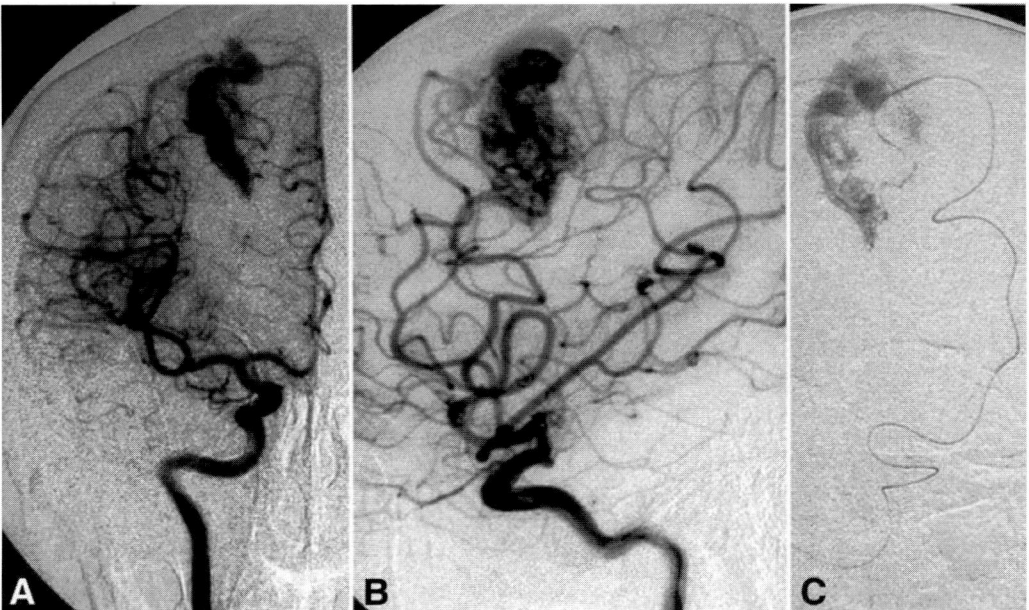

Fig. 1. Anteroposterior **(A)** and lateral **(B)** projection angiograms of the right hemisphere demonstrate an arteriovenous malformation (AVM) fed by anterior cerebral artery (ACA) and middle cerebral artery (MCA) branches. Superselective angiography **(C)** via an ACA pedicle shows the AVM angioarchitecture with no evidence of vessels en passage.

draining veins in surgery before isolating the nidus can lead to hemorrhage. If only a small amount of venous drainage has been compromised, close observation in the intensive care unit with blood pressure control is an option.

Results

The safety and effectiveness of AVM embolization with NBCA has been reported in multiple series *(2,14,24–26)*. Embolization resulted in 50% or more reduction in AVM size in most patients in these series. Surgeons have reported greater ease during the excision of embolized versus nonembolized AVMs *(2)*. In a recent report on the effectiveness of combining Gamma-Knife radiosurgery and endovascular embolization, AVM obliteration was achieved in 46% of patients *(8)*. Complication rates ranging from 3 to 25% have been reported *(15)*.

Case Illustration

A 41-yr-old woman was diagnosed with a right frontal AVM during head trauma evaluation (Spetzler-Martin grade II). The AVM was fed by branches of the right anterior communicating artery (ACA) and right middle cerebral artery (MCA) (Fig. 1A,B). Both the ACA and the MCA pedicles were embolized with NBCA during the same session, with complete AVM obliteration achieved. A follow-up angiogram 12 mo after the procedure showed no recurrence of the lesion (Fig. 2A,B).

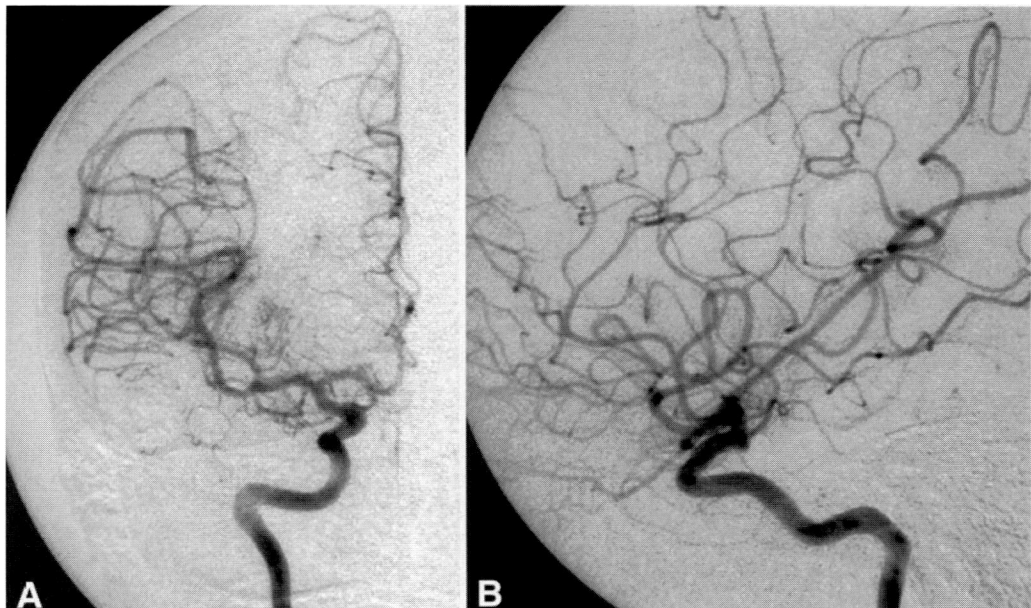

Fig. 2. Anteroposterior (A) and lateral (B) projection angiograms of the right anterior circulation demonstrate no residual AVM.

EMBOLIC AGENTS FOR THE TREATMENT OF TUMORS

Overview

Endovascular treatment of benign and malignant intracranial tumors is focused on superselective intraarterial delivery of chemotherapeutic agents and pedicle embolization for tumor devascularization. Endovascular techniques are particularly valuable in the preoperative embolization of tumors that are highly vascular as well as those involving difficult surgical exposures, such as skull base neoplasms. Vascular metastatic lesions, such as renal cell carcinoma, are also routinely referred for preoperative embolization. In select cases of advanced stage medical illness or inoperable tumors, endovascular therapy may be used alone as a palliative option.

Superselective Delivery of Chemotherapy

The intraarterial delivery of chemotherapeutic agents to treat central nervous system disorders dates back to the 1940s when direct injection of drugs into the carotid artery was attempted for the treatment of syphilis. Several more contemporary studies have demonstrated that the uptake of antitumoral agents by neoplastic cells depends on many factors including pharmacologic properties of the agent, integrity of the blood–brain barrier, intravascular concentration of the agent, and the presence of arterial flow *(27,28)*. Under appropriate conditions, tumor uptake is nearly 50 times higher when chemotherapeutic agents are administered intraarterially rather than intravenously *(29)*. The local nature of brain tumors should theoretically permit local chemotherapy *(30)*.

Previous intraarterial regimens used nitrosoureas, but these have generally been abandoned because the side effects outweighed the benefits of treatment *(31–33)*. Shapiro et al. *(32)* reported a randomized study of intracarotid infusion of chemotherapy (1,3-bis(2-chloroethyl)-1-nitrosourea [BCNU]) for newly diagnosed malignant gliomas. Their results showed a reduced rate of survival among patients receiving intraarterial chemotherapy, especially those with anaplastic astrocytoma. The presence of BCNU-induced necrosis on white matter and the ocular toxicity of the drug explained these results. Other agents such as cisplatin have also been tried, but their neurological and retinal toxicity limits the dosage that can be safely administered locally *(34,35)*.

Qureshi et al. *(36)* reported their experience with intraarterial infusions in a series of patients with intracranial neoplasms that had demonstrated a poor response to radiation, intravenous chemotherapy, and/or surgical removal. In some treatment sessions, RMP-7, a bradykinin analog, was infused concomitantly with carboplatin in an attempt to manipulate blood–brain barrier permeability and increase the transport of chemotherapeutic agents into the tumor. Owing to the retrospective characteristic of the study and the variety of tumors treated, these authors could only conclude that intraarterial administration of carboplatin with or without RMP-7 appeared to be safe and feasible.

Although it is an appealing approach, local intraarterial delivery has not yet contributed to any significant improvement in the length of survival of patients with central nervous system diseases *(37)*. Further investigation is necessary to evaluate the long-term survival and effects of intraarterial administration of carboplatin and other chemotherapeutic drugs.

Pedicle Embolization for Tumor Devascularization

Preoperative occlusion of vascular pedicles is feasible for certain types of tumors including extraaxial and primary bone tumors and for some intraaxial tumors as well *(38,39)* (Table 3). The goal of embolization with these neoplastic disorders is to devascularize the tumor capillary bed while preserving the normal arterial circulation. Before the injection of any embolic material, the interventionist should carefully reexamine the anatomy and hemodynamics of the vessel to be embolized, with special attention paid to possible dangerous anastomoses, caliber and pattern of tumor vessels, blood flow characteristics, and circulation to adjacent territories *(39)*.

Preoperative assessment of the tumor is of particular importance in planning the embolization and assessing the risk that may apply to a certain tumor. In particular, anatomic localization will determine the vascular supply that will provide access for embolization. The neuroendovascular surgeon must be thoroughly familiar with the blood supply to the skull base and meninges to obtain adequate angiographic images of the tumor. Preoperative assessment must also include a detailed examination of the neurological territory adjacent to the tumor and the vascular territory at risk during the embolization *(40)*.

Preoperative magnetic resonance imaging provides important information regarding the growth pattern and compartmentalization of the tumor. Rela-

**Table 3
Most Commonly Embolized
Tumors According to Location**

Extraaxial Tumors
    Meningioma
       (embolized most often)
    Hemangiopericytoma
    Neurogenic tumor
    Paraganglioma
    Esthesioneuroblastoma
    Malignant bone tumors

Intraaxial Tumors
    Hemangioblastoma
    Glioblastoma
    Metastatic tumors

Primary Bone Tumors
    Aneurysmal bone cyst
    Hemangioma
    Chordoma
    Chondrosarcoma
    Osteogenic sarcoma

tionships to bony landmarks, such as the petrous apex and basal foramina, are critical aspects of any evaluation. The relationship of the tumor to major vascular structures, such as the petrous or cavernous carotid artery, will suggest whether vessel sacrifice is an option. If it is a possibility, a balloon test occlusion should be performed to determine the patient's tolerance to such a procedure. In cases of failure to pass the balloon test occlusion, a major revascularization procedure (bypass) should be considered before definitive vessel occlusion.

Superselective angiography often demonstrates a vascular blush that was inapparent on routine angiography. Of particular interest are dangerous anastomoses that may exist between vascular territories (Table 2). Angiographic visualization must not be relied on exclusively, however; provocative testing with lidocaine can be used to demonstrate risk to the cranial nerve blood supply. Additional provocative testing with methohexital or amobarbital may demonstrate the presence of parenchymal anastomoses.

The selection of an embolic agent for preoperative tumor embolization depends on which vessel the interventionist can access, and the neurosurgeon must be involved in this determination. NBCA, PVA, and microspheres (EmboGold Microspheres, Biosphere Medical, Rockland, MA) are most widely used; however, Gelfoam (Upjohn, Kalamazoo, MI) and Avitene (microfibrillar collagen) are used as well. Absolute ethanol is an excellent liquid agent that produces intense angionecrosis and liquefaction of the tumor. However, pericapsular extravasation may occur, and the neurotoxicity of this agent raises the level of

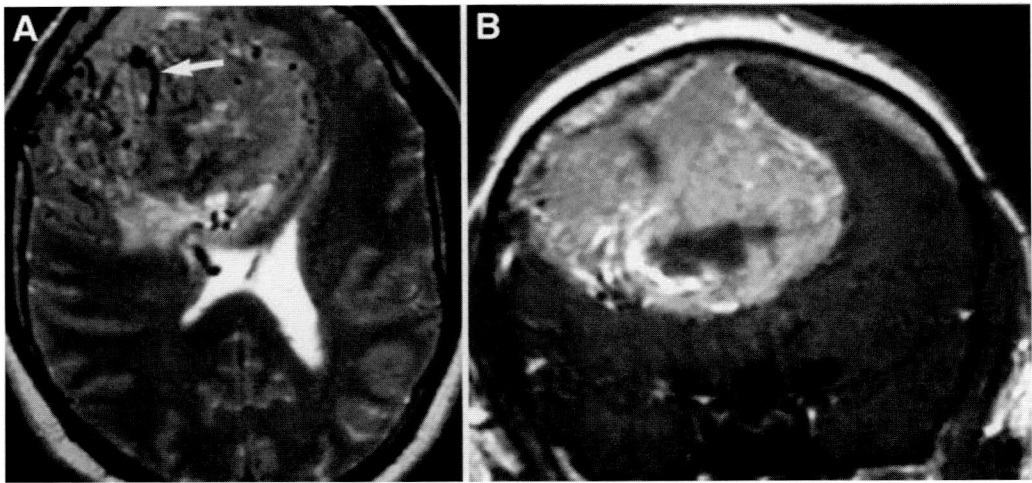

Fig. 3. Contrast-enhanced magnetic resonance images, axial T2-weighted (A) and coronal T1-weighted (B), demonstrate a right frontal lesion, with diffuse contrast enhancement exerting a mass effect on the right frontal lobe and right lateral ventricle. These findings are suggestive of a meningioma. Several flow void signals are observed on the T2 image (arrow), denoting intense neovascularization of the lesion.

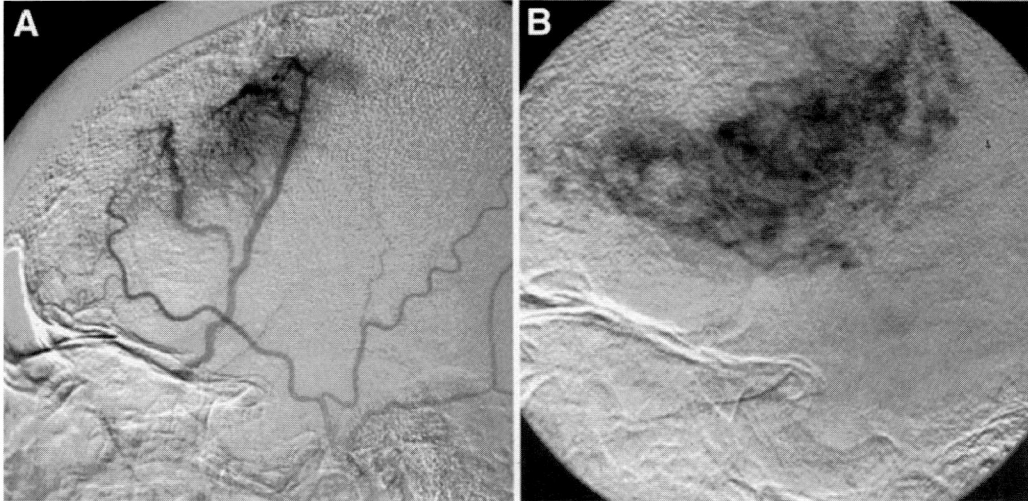

Fig. 4. Selective right external carotid artery (A) and selective right internal carotid artery (B) lateral projection angiograms demonstrate tumoral blush.

concern regarding its use. Reflux of absolute ethanol should be assiduously avoided. Each embolic agent has advantages and disadvantages. The discussion of the suitability of each agent for a particular situation is beyond the scope of this chapter.

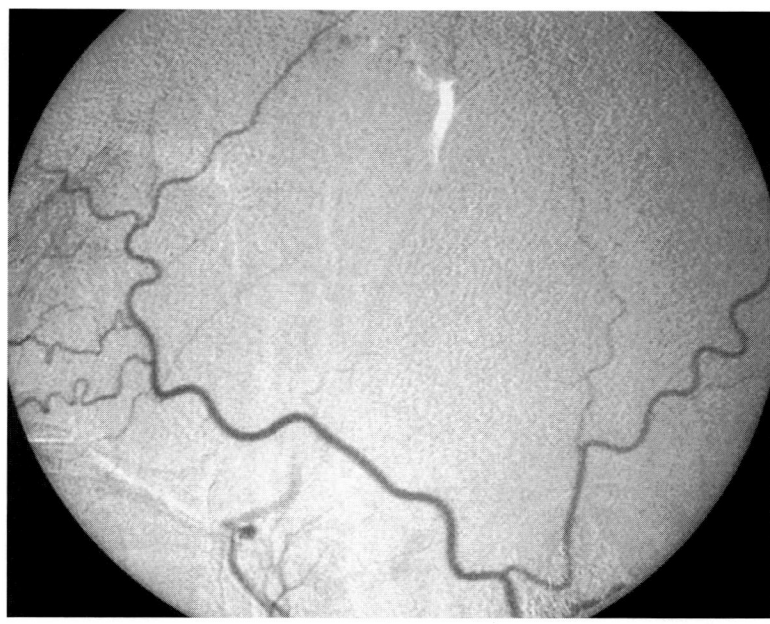

Fig. 5. Lateral projection angiogram of the right external carotid artery demonstrates obliteration of the tumors feeders after selective Gelfoam powder injection.

The tumors most commonly embolized are meningiomas (see Case Illustration section next). These benign tumors can be extremely vascular and may be associated with extensive blood loss during surgery. Although radical surgical removal remains the gold standard of treatment for meningiomas, the endovascular occlusion of nourishing vessels facilitates and shortens the length of the surgical procedure. Jungreis (41) described a significant reduction in intraoperative blood loss after endovascular pedicle occlusion.

Direct percutaneous puncture with intratumoral injection of embolic agent may be another effective treatment for selected vascular tumors. Casasco et al. (42,43) used direct puncture of vascular intracranial and head and neck tumors with intratumoral injection of NBCA. Complete angiographic filling of the tumor volume was achieved with regression of the tumors in 80% of cases.

Some controversy remains concerning the ideal timing for surgery after tumor embolization. Embolization is usually accomplished in one session. Intervals of 1 d to several weeks have been suggested; however, the optimum interval still needs to be determined (39,44,45). In the authors' experience, delays of more than 6–12 wk are associated with tumor revascularization (39). Surgical resection 1–4 wk after embolization is recommended to allow for maximal devascularization, as well as minimal cerebral edema and tumor swelling.

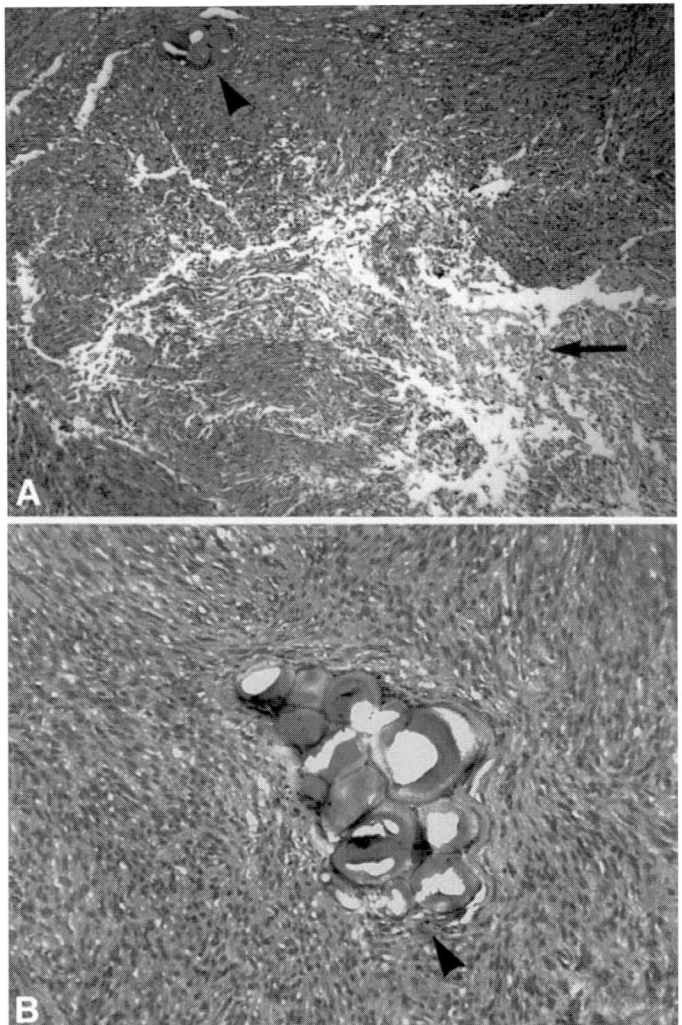

Fig. 6. Photomicrographs of the tumor (**A**, H&E ×60; **B**, H&E ×120) demonstrate a hypercellular lesion with densely packed cells and areas of necrosis (arrow in A), compatible with an atypical meningioma. Note the presence of embolic material inside some of the vessels (arrowheads).

Case Illustration

A 41-yr-old man was admitted with new onset of seizures, blurred vision, and headaches. Magnetic resonance images of the brain showed a right frontal dura-based mass consistent with a meningioma (Fig. 3A,B). The preoperative angiogram demonstrated intense tumoral blushing from the right internal and external carotid arteries (Fig. 4A,B). Embolization with Gelfoam powder, performed via superselective catheterization of branches of the right middle meningeal artery, resulted in good obliteration of the tumoral vascular bed (Fig. 5). Twenty-four hours later, the patient underwent a right frontoparietal craniotomy, with gross total tumoral resection. The histological diagnosis was compatible with an atypical meningioma with areas of necrosis related to embolic material (Fig. 6A,B) and evidence of Gelfoam inside the vessels.

CONCLUSIONS

The embolization of cerebral AVMs and tumors must be approached strategically with a clear and logical plan in mind. This plan should ideally be discussed in a multidisciplinary environment that includes neurosurgeons, neuroendovascular specialists, neuroradiologists, and radiosurgeons. As discussed in this chapter, the goals of therapy should dictate the approach to embolization.

Several areas of embolization are likely to improve over the next several years. Catheter and wire technology will continue to improve, thereby allowing safer, more effective treatment of vascular pedicles. Better embolic agents are likely to emerge, allowing safer, easier, and more effective treatment.

ACKNOWLEDGMENTS

We thank Paul H. Dressel for preparation of the illustrations.

REFERENCES

1. Luessenhop AJ, Spence WT. Artificial embolization of cerebral arteries: report of use in a case of arteriovenous malformation. *JAMA* 1960;172:1153–1155.
2. Jafar JJ, Davis AJ, Berenstein A, Choi IS, Kupersmith MJ. The effect of embolization with N-butyl cyanoacrylate prior to surgical resection of cerebral arteriovenous malformations. *J Neurosurg* 1993;78:60–69.
3. de Oliveira E, Tedeschi H, Raso J. Comprehensive management of arteriovenous malformations. *Neurol Res* 1998;20:673–683.
4. Batjer HH, Devous MD, Sr., Meyer YJ, Purdy PD, Samson DS. Cerebrovascular hemodynamics in arteriovenous malformation complicated by normal perfusion pressure breakthrough. *Neurosurgery* 1988;22:503–509.
5. Spetzler RF, Wilson CB, Weinstein P, Mehdorn M, Townsend J, Telles D. Normal perfusion pressure breakthrough theory. *Clin Neurosurg* 1978;25:651–672.
6. Flickinger JC, Pollock BE, Kondziolka D, Lunsford LD. A dose-response analysis of arteriovenous malformation obliteration after radiosurgery. *Int J Radiat Oncol Biol Phys* 1996;36:873–879.
7. Gobin YP, Laurent A, Merienne L, et al. Treatment of brain arteriovenous malformations by embolization and radiosurgery. *J Neurosurg* 1996;85:19–28.
8. Wikholm G, Lundqvist C, Svendsen P. The Goteberg cohort of embolized cerebral arteriovenous malformations: a 6-year follow-up. *Neurosurgery* 2001;49:799–806.
9. Batjer HH, Purdy PD, Giller CA, Samson DS. Evidence of redistribution of cerebral blood flow during treatment for an intracranial arteriovenous malformation. *Neurosurgery* 1989;25:599–605.
10. Han PP, Ponce FA, Spetzler RF. Intention-to-treat analysis of Spetzler-Martin grades IV and V arteriovenous malformations: natural history and treatment paradigm. *J Neurosurg* 2003;98:3–7.
11. Heros RC. Spetzler-Martin grades IV and V arteriovenous malformations. *J Neurosurg* 2003;98:1–2.

12. Porstmann W, Wierny L, Warnke H, Gerstberger G, Romaniuk PA. Catheter closure of patent ductus arteriosus. 62 cases treated without thoracotomy. *Radiol Clin North Am* 1971;9:203–218.
13. Standard SC, Guterman LR, Chavis TD, Hopkins LN. Delayed recanalization of a cerebral arteriovenous malformation following angiographic obliteration with polyvinyl alcohol embolization. *Surg Neurol* 1995;44:109–113.
14. Debrun GM, Aletich V, Ausman JI, Charbel F, Dujovny M. Embolization of the nidus of brain arteriovenous malformations with n-butyl cyanoacrylate. *Neurosurgery* 1997;40:112–121.
15. Jahan R, Murayama Y, Gobin YP, Duckwiler GR, Vinters HV, Vinuela F. Embolization of arteriovenous malformations with Onyx: clinicopathological experience in 23 patients. *Neurosurgery* 2001;48:984–997.
16. Sampei K, Hashimoto N, Kazekawa K, Tsukahara T, Iwata H, Takaichi S. Histological changes in brain tissue and vasculature after intracarotid infusion of organic solvents in rats. *Neuroradiology* 1996;38:291–294.
17. Chaloupka JC, Huddle DC, Alderman J, Fink S, Hammond R, Vinters HV. A reexamination of the angiotoxicity of superselective injection of DMSO in the swine rete embolization model. *AJNR Am J Neuroradiol* 1999;20:401–410.
18. Akin ED, Perkins E, Ross IB. Surgical handling characteristics of an ethylene vinyl alcohol copolymer compared with N-butyl cyanoacrylate use for embolization of vessels in an arteriovenous malformation resection model in swine. *J Neurosurg* 2003;98:366–370.
19. Kerber C, Connors J, III, Knox K. The behavior of a new liquid embolic agent, neuracryl M, in blood. AANS/CNS Section on *Cerebrovascular Surgery and American Society of Interventional and Therapeutic Neuroradiology Meeting*, Nashville, TN, 1999 (oral presentation).
20. Kerber CW, Wong W, Knox K, et al. Neuracryl M, a new liquid embolic agent: initial clinical results (abstract). *J Neurosurg* 2000;92:196.
21. Chopko BW, Kerber C, Wong W, Knox K, Krall R. Initial neuropathologic observations after treatment of a human arteriovenous malformation with a novel liquid embolic agent, neuracryl-M, American Association of Neurological Surgery/Congress of Neurological Surgeons Section on *Cerebrovascular Surgery and American Society of Interventional and Therapeutic Neuroradiology Meeting*, New Orleans, LA, 2000 (poster presentation).
22. Horton JA, Kerber CW. Lidocaine injection into external carotid branches: provocative test to preserve cranial nerve function in therapeutic embolization. *AJNR Am J Neuroradiol* 1986;7:105–108.
23. Peters KR, Quisling RG, Gilmore R, Mickle P, Kuperus JH. Intraarterial use of sodium methohexital for provocative testing during brain embolotherapy. *AJNR Am J Neuroradiol* 1993;14:171–174.
24. Fournier D, TerBrugge KG, Willinsky R, Lasjaunias P, Montanera W. Endovascular treatment of intracerebral arteriovenous malformations: experience in 49 cases. *J Neurosurg* 1991;75:228–233.
25. Fox AJ, Pelz DM, Lee DH. Arteriovenous malformations of the brain: recent results of endovascular therapy. *Radiology* 1990;177:51–57.
26. Vinuela F, Dion JE, Duckwiler G, et al. Combined endovascular embolization and surgery in the management of cerebral arteriovenous malformations: experience with 101 cases. *J Neurosurg* 1991;75:856–864.
27. Bullard DE, Bigner SH, Bigner DD. Comparison of intravenous versus intracarotid therapy with 1,3-bis(2-chloroethyl)-1-nitrosourea in a rat brain tumor model. *Cancer Res* 1985;45:5240–5245.

28. Chiras J. Intra-arterial chemotherapy for the central nervous system, in *Interventional Neuroradiology,* 1st ed. (Connors J, Wojak J, eds.), WB Saunders, Philadelphia, 1999, pp. 368–371.
29. Theron J, Villemure JG, Worthington C, Tyler JL. Superselective intracerebral chemotherapy of malignant tumours with BCNU. Neuroradiological considerations. *Neuroradiology* 1986;28:118–125.
30. Collins JM. Pharmacologic rationale for regional drug delivery. *J Clin Oncol* 1984;2: 498–504.
31. Defer G, Fauchon F, Schaison M, Chiras J, Brunet P. Visual toxicity following intraarterial chemotherapy with hydroxyethyl-CNU in patients with malignant gliomas. A prospective study with statistical analysis. *Neuroradiology* 1991;33:432–437.
32. Shapiro WR, Green SB, Burger PC, et al. A randomized comparison of intraarterial versus intravenous BCNU, with or without intravenous 5-fluorouracil, for newly diagnosed patients with malignant glioma. *J Neurosurg* 1992;76:772–781.
33. Stewart DJ, Grahovac Z, Russel NA, et al. Phase I study of intracarotid PCNU. *J Neurooncol* 1987;5:245–250.
34. Maiese K, Walker RW, Gargan R, Victor JD. Intra-arterial cisplatin-associated optic and otic toxicity. *Arch Neurol* 1992;49:83–86.
35. Tfayli A, Hentschel P, Madajewicz S, et al. Toxicities related to intraarterial infusion of cisplatin and etoposide in patients with brain tumors. *J Neurooncol* 1999;42: 73–77.
36. Qureshi AI, Suri MF, Khan J, et al. Superselective intraarterial carboplatin for treatment of intracranial neoplasms: experience in 100 procedures. *J Neurooncol* 2001;51: 151–158.
37. Hopkins LN, Lanzino G, Guterman LR. Treating complex nervous system vascular disorders through a "needle stick": origins, evolution, and future of neuroendovascular therapy. *Neurosurgery* 2001;48:463–475.
38. Choi IS, Tantivatana J. Neuroendovascular management of intracranial and spinal tumors. *Neurosurg Clin N Am* 2000;11:167–185.
39. Standard SC, Hopkins LN. Principles of neuroendovascular intervention, in *Endovascular Neurological Intervention* (Maciunas RJ, ed.), The American Association of Neurological Surgeons, Park Ridge, IL, 1995, pp. 1–34.
40. Ahn HS, Kerber CW, Deeb ZL. Extra- to intracranial arterial anastomoses in therapeutic embolization: recognition and role. *AJNR Am J Neuroradiol* 1980;1:71–75.
41. Jungreis CA. Skull-base tumors: ethanol embolization of the cavernous carotid artery. *Radiology* 1991;181:741–743.
42. Casasco A, Herbreteau D, Houdart E, et al. Devascularization of craniofacial tumors by percutaneous tumor puncture. *AJNR Am J Neuroradiol* 1994;15:1233–1239.
43. Casasco A, Houdart E, Biondi A, et al. Major complications of percutaneous embolization of skull-base tumors. *AJNR Am J Neuroradiol* 1999;20:179–181.
44. Manelfe C, Lasjaunias P, Ruscalleda J. Preoperative embolization of intracranial meningiomas. *AJNR Am J Neuroradiol* 1986;7:963–972.
45. Richter HP, Schachenmayr W. Preoperative embolization of intracranial meningiomas. *Neurosurgery* 1983;13:261–268.

10
Radiofrequency Lesioning

Michael Petr, MD, PhD and John M. Tew, Jr., MD

INTRODUCTION

Radiofrequency lesioning (RFL) is a time-proven, safe method of long-term pain relief. It provides successful treatment for trigeminal neuralgia and has been explored as a tool for symptomatic relief of many other neurologic conditions including Parkinson's disease, oncologic pain, spinal pain syndromes, facial spasm, facial pain of multiple sclerosis, vagoglossopharyngeal neuralgia, and (rarely) atypical facial pain *(1–5)*. Originally the RFL method was poorly controlled; a 1-cm noninsulated electrode tip placed in the gasserian ganglion was guided with a stereotactic frame *(6)*. Although this technique successfully relieved symptoms of tic douloureux, a high incidence of complications occurred including anesthesia dolorosa, cranial nerve palsies, corneal ulcers, and blindness. Attempts to improve outcomes and reduce complications led to the practice of creating small serial lesions and intervening neurologic exams while titrating the lesion to the desired effect *(7)*. Many published series of RFL for trigeminal neuralgia accumulated over decades have demonstrated its relative safety and efficacy for select patient populations.

Typical treatment options for trigeminal neuralgia include microvascular decompression (MVD), glycerol rhizolysis, peripheral nerve rhizotomy, radiosurgery, and peripheral nerve block. When the risks and benefits are weighed, RFL is a reasonable option for pain relief in many elderly patients who have complex health problems and in whom medical therapy has failed. Young healthy patients may undergo open surgical decompression, thus avoiding the neurologic complication risks of percutaneous procedures. Criteria for percutaneous procedures include stereotypical pain, failure of medical treatment, advanced physiologic age, poor medical condition, multiple sclerosis, and patient preference. For patients with pain in the V_1 division, MVD is recommended to avoid corneal anesthesia.

PHYSICAL CHARACTERISTICS OF RADIOFREQUENCY

RFL generates heat in a controlled and minimally invasive manner to damage nerve fibers selectively with the goals of attaining asymptomatic relief and minimizing the risk of complications. Key elements of successful RFL include

From: *Minimally Invasive Neurosurgery*, edited by: M.R. Proctor and P.M. Black © Humana Press Inc., Totowa, NJ

heat control and localization in the lesion process. Clinical observations support the physical principles of RFL that small δ and poorly myelinated c-fibers are more susceptible to heat than are heavily myelinated α- and β-fibers (8). Regarding the concept of selective sensitivity of fiber types to heat, however, in vivo animal experiments have demonstrated no difference in heat sensitivity among fiber types and equal destruction of all fiber types within a lesion (9). In temperature-controlled studies in dogs using a 2-min duration and range of 45–85°C in 10° increments, histological studies found no differential effect in lesioning between unmyelinated and myelinated fibers (10).

The RFL technique relies on controlled thermocoagulation of tissues to create a predictable and reproducible size without boiling or carbonization (11–13). Variables in controlling the lesion include tissue impedance, electrode type (i.e., unipolar, monopolar), temperature, and time interval of coagulation. In vitro and in vivo studies have characterized the methods of lesion production by radiofrequency techniques. Monopolar electrodes generate lesions that enlarge in direct relation to temperature increases; bipolar electrodes generate lesions that plateau in size at 85°C (14). In relation to time, lesion size stabilizes at 60-s durations (15). Lesion size increases in direct proportion to electrode size (14,15). The most significant control parameter is temperature monitoring in real time. Real-time temperature monitoring at the electrode tip eliminates the variable of tissue impedance and maintains constant temperature with continual feedback that produces reliable, predictable lesions without boiling or carbonization (15). In summary, radiofrequency ablation is a form of thermocoagulation controlled by electrode size, duration of coagulation, and constant temperature control that allows the optimal tissue lesioning.

TECHNIQUE OF PERCUTANEOUS RFL FOR TRIGEMINAL NEURALGIA

Patients can undergo radiofrequency rhizotomy in the radiology department, except for patients with pulmonary or cardiac issues that require precise control of anesthesia parameters. In most cases, neither is general anesthesia required nor must an anesthesiologist be present. The equipment list typically includes X-ray fluoroscopey, sterile drapes, sponges and skin prep, ruler and marking pen to delineate landmarks, sterile spinal tray with syringe for methohexital anesthetic (Brevital 500 mg 10:1 dilution), intravenous tubing with side injection port to alternate between Brevital and 5% dextrose, atropine 0.4 mg, pins and cotton for sensory testing, and Nipride. Additionally, the Radionics TIC and Tew kits are used. Various electrodes (e.g., straight 7-mm temperature monitoring electrode, curved temperature monitoring Tew electrode, angled 3-mm cordotomy electrode) (16) and generator systems are available; our experience in 1500 cases was with Radionics equipment. The Radionics RFG-3C lesion generator system provides the necessary power output of 15 W or higher and a radiofrequency exceeding 250 kH/s. The electrode tip should include features to monitor voltage, current, radiofrequency, and temperature. A built-in timer and stimulator are essential. Another useful feature of the Radionics RFG-3C model includes the capability for continuous impedance monitoring during

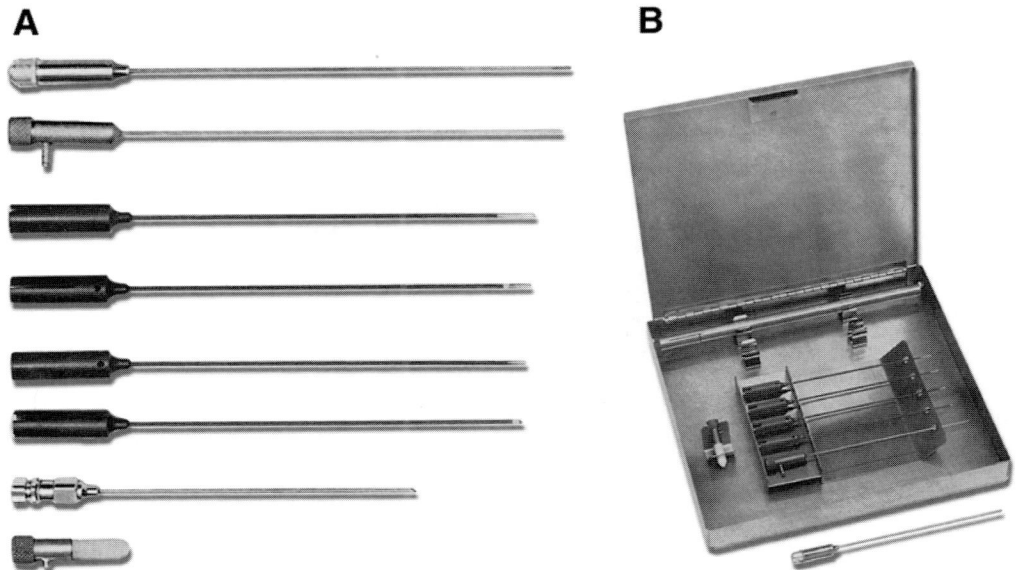

Fig. 1. Components of a Type TIC Kit. (A) Top to bottom: TIC-TM temperature monitoring electrode; TIC-SS solid stylet; TIC-C10 10-mm tip cannula; TIC-7 7-mm-tip cannula; TIC-C5 5-mm-tip cannula; TIC-C2 2-mm-tip cannula; TIC-IE 19-gage TW indifferent electrode; and TIC-FA flushing adaptor. (B) Kit includes a stainless steel storage case and a sterilizing metal tube containing the TM electrode. (Courtesy of the Mayfield Clinic.)

electrocoagulation. The TIC kit includes a 19-gage Teflon-insulated cannula with 2-, 5-, 7-, and 10-mm tips to create a variety of lesion sizes (Fig. 1).

Patient Preparation

After admission as an outpatient the morning of the procedure, the patient undergoes preoperative laboratory tests, electrocardiogram, and chest X-ray; no food or drink is permitted for 5 h before the procedure. With the patient positioned supine, the surgeon is on the right side regardless of pain location. The fluoroscopy is placed for convenient viewing by the surgeon. Lateral fluoroscopic images should show overlapping orbits and clinoids and should include the sella turcica, clivus, and petrous apex. The radiofrequency generator is placed for easy access by the surgeon. An adhesive grounding pad or stainless steel plate completes the electric circuit; without a grounding pad, the electrode can monitor temperature but cannot deliver a stimulus or generate a lesion.

Standing opposite the surgeon on the patient's left, an assistant can manage the intravenous, anesthesia, vital, and lesion parameters. The skin is prepared with Betadine and the field is draped with sterile towels. Anatomic landmarks are mapped as described by Hartel *(17)*. Three points are marked on the skin for guidance. The first reference point is 3 cm anterior to the external auditory meatus. The second point is beneath the medial aspect of the pupil on the lower lid

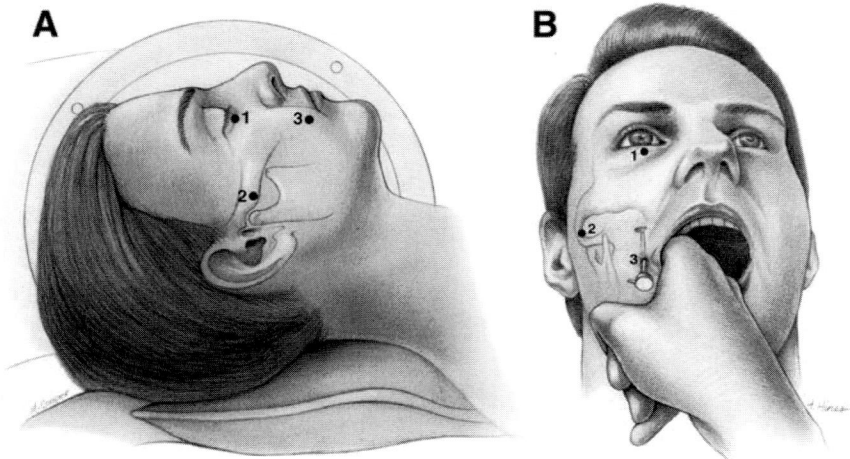

Fig. 2. Anatomic landmarks described by Hartel shown in two views. **(A)** The target foramen is at the intersection of three planes. **(B)** Surgeon's finger guides placement to the lateral pterygoid wing. 1, beneath the medial aspect of the pupil on the lower end; 2, 3 cm anterior to the external auditory canal; and 3, 2.5 cm lateral to the oral commissure. (Courtesy of the Mayfield Clinic.)

when the eye is in neutral position. The third point is 2.5 cm lateral to the oral commissure (Fig. 2A).

Insertion of the Electrode

The needle is placed in the retrogasserian ganglion portion of the trigeminal nerve by free-hand manipulation based on the Hartel reference points. After the patient is anesthetized with an intravenous injection of 30–50 mg of methohexital (Brevital), a 100-mm-long, 20-gage cannula with a stylet penetrates the skin 2.5 cm lateral to the oral commissure. An oral airway may be placed to prevent closure of the jaw during the procedure. Atropine (0.4 mg) may be given to reduce oral secretions. The surgeon's index finger, placed in the patient's mouth inferior to the lateral pterygoid wing, guides insertion without penetrating mucosa. The needle is aimed toward the intersection of the coronal plane 3 cm anterior to the auditory meatus and the sagittal plane medial to midpupillary line (Fig. 2B). The cannula is advanced based on cine or serial true lateral fluoroscopic images; it then rests 5–10 mm below the sella floor (Fig. 3). Penetration of the foramen ovale by the cannula is signaled by a wince and contraction of the ipsilateral masseter muscle because of contact irritation to the sensory and motor fibers.

Successful access to the retrogasserian ganglion usually produces a free flow of cerebrospinal fluid when the stylet is removed. Spinal fluid may also be obtained from the distal nerve if the dural sleeve extends extracranially along the nerve, or from the infratemporal subarachnoid if the electrode is distal or proximal to the target. Malposition of the cannula poses a risk of carotid artery

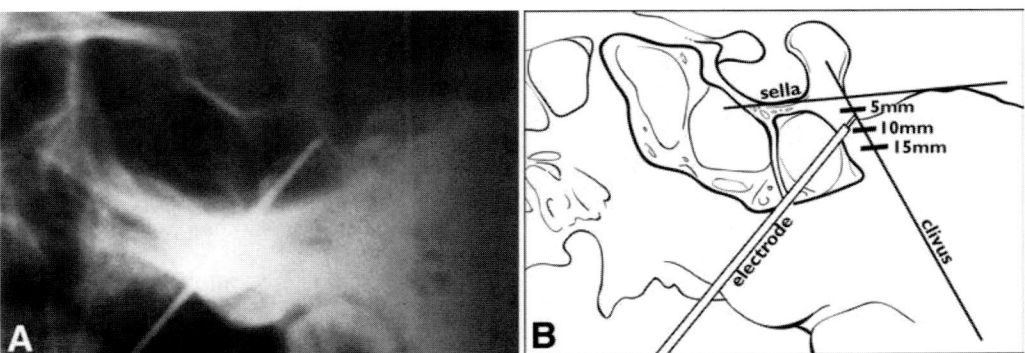

Fig. 3. Electrode trajectory. **(A)** Lateral radiograph. **(B)** Illustration shows ideal trajectory (5–10 mm below the floor of the sella turcica). (Courtesy of the Mayfield Clinic.)

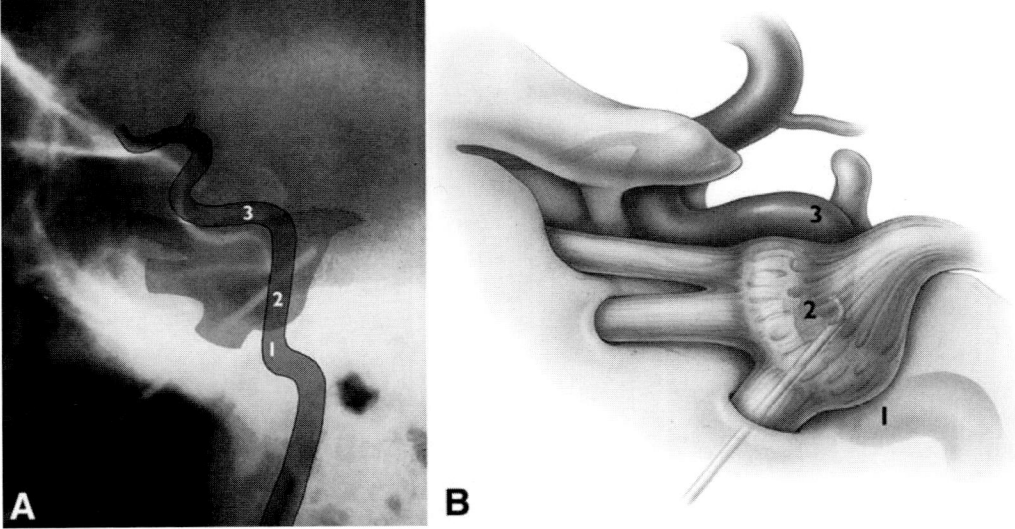

Fig. 4. Relationship of the electrode tip and surgical anatomy. Lateral radiograph **(A)** and composite illustration **(B)** shows the (1) relationship of the electrode tip and its trajectory to the mandibular nerve; (2) carotid artery in Meckel's cave; and (3) cavernous carotid artery. (Courtesy of the Mayfield Clinic.)

injury. The herald of carotid artery puncture is pulsatile blood from the cannula when the stylet is removed or when rhythmic fluctuation of temperature occurs during monitoring *(18)*. The carotid artery is vulnerable to injury at three sites: the foramen lacerum posteromedially, posterolaterally in Meckel's cave, and the cephalad cavernous sinus *(18)* (Fig. 4). In the foramen lacerum, the cannula may penetrate the cartilaginous floor; however, Meckel's cave below V_3 may lack a barrier of petrous bone. In the event of carotid artery violation, pressure should be applied manually, and the procedure should be postponed for 48 h. Complications of carotid artery injury include hemiparesis from ischemia and carotid cavernous fistula *(19)*. Additional risks include damage to other anatomic structures of the skull base, such as the superior orbital fissure anteriorly and the jugular foramen posteriorly or aberrant foramen near the foramen ovale. Complications of electrode advancement beyond 5 mm proximal to the clivus may include ocular nerve damage or abducens palsy. Cavernous sinus violation may result in trochlear or oculomotor palsy.

Localization

Confirmation of electrode localization is based on physiological and radiographic evidence. Physiological confirmation is the free flow of cerebrospinal fluid from the cannula and the lack of pulsatile blood flow. The patient should experience facial pain and masseter contraction when the electrode enters the foramen ovale. Facial paroxysms of pain should occur with electrical stimulation between 0.3 and 0.5 V. Impedance measurements of the electrode tip also serve as a localizing data point. Impedance of 150–350 Ω is typical of cerebrospinal fluid bathing the retrogasserian nerve roots, whereas impedance exceeding 1000 Ω is characteristic of solid tissue.

Radiographic confirmation includes the anterior/posterior projection of a target site 9 mm medial to the lateral wall of the internal auditory meatus, which coincides with the medial dip in the petrous ridge *(20)*. A true lateral projection is useful when one is advancing the electrode until the needle is 5–10 mm below the intersection of a line drawn from the floor of the sella turcica to the clival line. The final target is the intersection of the petrous ridge with the clival line *(18)*. Selective targeting of isolated divisions of the trigeminal nerve root is further defined by radiographic positioning. Division 1 is isolated with a curved electrode directed anteriorly and 5 mm above the clival petrous junction. Division 2 is best isolated with a straight electrode placed at the clival petrous junction. Division 3 may be isolated by placing a posteriorly curved electrode 5 mm below the clival line (Fig. 5).

Stimulation Procedures

Before connection of the cables for stimulation, the generator is either turned off or inactive. A reference dispersive electrode of 150 cm^2 or more is recommended. Needle electrodes for reference or ground purposes are avoided because of the possibility of tissue burns at the insertion site. When cables are connected and generators are unplugged, patients occasionally feel a benign stimulus, which is caused by small galvanic charges between electrodes. When one is ready to initiate stimulation, the voltage range is set to 0.0 with a pulse rate of 50 pulses/s and a 1-ms duration. During stimulation, voltage output is slowly increased. Unless a patient has undergone previous treatment with alcohol or compression therapy, typical values of 0.2–0.5 V generate paresthesias in the trigeminal division of the trigger zone. If paroxysmal pain at low threshold stimulation is not produced, the electrode is repositioned. During stimulation, contraction of the masseter muscle or eye movement also indicates the need to reposition the electrode. Eye movement may indicate that the electrode is near or in the cavernous sinus; such placement may result in damage to cranial

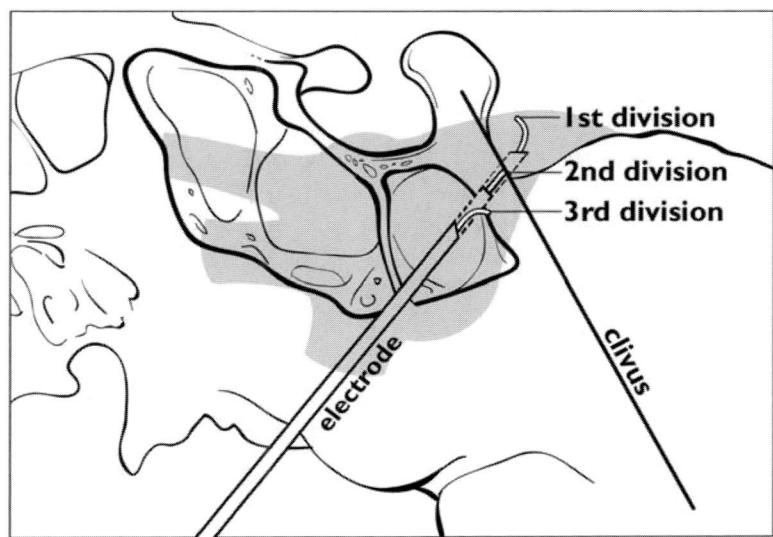

Fig. 5. Composite illustration shows the relationship of the trigeminal rootlets to the clivus. When the electrode tip is −5 mm beneath the clivus, the third division is stimulated: at 0, the second division is stimulated; and at +5 mm above the clivus, the first division fibers are stimulated. (Courtesy of the Mayfield Clinic.)

nerves III, IV, and VI. During repositioning, the curved electrode is retracted to prevent mechanical damage to nerves. After its retraction, it may be rotated to a new position that is confirmed by fluoroscopy.

Radiofrequency Lesion Procedure

After confirmation of electrode physiologic and radiographic localization, the creation of the lesion begins. Anesthesia, administered in 30–50 mg boluses with the short-acting barbiturate methohexital (Brevital), induces somnolence and amnesia without compromise of the airway. The patient's blood pressure is closely monitored from the time of electrode insertion. Nipride is available in case of a hypertensive induced by nerve manipulation, stimulation, or ablation. An initial lesion temperature of 60°C for 90 s is sufficient for patients who have not undergone treatment by other means. If stimulation thresholds are high, initial temperature requirements may be elevated.

After the effects of methohexital resolve, within 2 to 3 min, sensory testing is performed. The goal of sensory testing, which includes pinprick and light touch, is preservation of corneal reflex and touch while inducing analgesia in the trigger zone. Additionally, corneal reflexes and extraocular muscle, pterygoid, and masseter strength may be checked between lesioning intervals. Every precaution is taken to preserve corneal sensation. If the first lesion results in sensory deficit but not analgesia, further lesion production performed in awakened patients provides the most reliable sensory evaluations. Another lesion-localizing sign is erythema in the trigeminal distribution of coagulation; this occurs in fewer than 50% of patients. Although this physiologic mechanism is not understood, it is a valuable sign that the division is being destroyed.

Constant-temperature RFL depends on the heat-conducting properties of the surrounding milieu. The electrode tip may be placed in the retrogasserian ganglion, rootlets, or cerebrospinal fluid. As impedance and stimulation intensities vary, so do fluctuations of current, voltage, and heat to maintain the appropriate temperature. Cerebrospinal fluid is a heat sink, so that as heat disperses, increases in radiofrequency current are needed. Close monitoring of current and voltage aids in resolution of this issue and in the identification of tissue boiling characterized by a rapid rise in volts and sudden drop in current.

Postoperative care includes the gradual discontinuation of neurogenic pain medication except for long-term use. Medications are tapered slowly to prevent withdrawal symptoms. Postoperative pain can be alleviated by a mild narcotic and by periodic application of an ice pack to the jaw. The patient is observed in recovery and typically discharged that same day. If oral sensation is diminished, a soft diet is temporarily recommended. Postoperative instructions include meticulous eye care and mandatory use of artificial tears (methylcellulose) if corneal sensation is compromised.

RESULTS

Using percutaneous radiofrequency rhizotomy, the senior author has treated more than 2000 patients who had trigeminal neuralgia *(21)*. The initial 700 cases were performed with a straight electrode and the last 1300 cases with the curved electrode. Pain, which averaged 8 yr in duration, was treated with medical and procedural interventions. Medications included carbamazepine (Tegretol), baclofen (Lioresal), and diphenylhydantoin (Dilantin). Interventions included nerve avulsion, alcohol injection, subtotal intracranial rhizotomy, ganglionectomy, microvascular decompression, and percutaneous RFL.

Although medical treatment provided initial relief, pain recurred in 75% of patients. In this series, 35% of patients had undergone a previous surgical procedure; this group was characterized by a 2:1 ratio of women to men, with an overwhelming occurrence in the right trigeminal nerves. The afflicted divisions were as follows: the first in 1%, the second in 16%, the third in 16%, the first and second in 15%, the second and third in 39%, and all three divisions in 13% (Table 1). Early outcomes were graded on pain relief and levels of dysesthesia and paresthesia (Table 2). The vast majority of patients reported good pain relief, absent or minor dysesthesias, and absent or minor paresthesias *(21)*. Compared with a straight electrode, a curved electrode reduced complications by more than 50%, including dysesthesias, anesthesia dolorosa, absent corneal reflexes, trigeminal pain, keratitis, diplopia, and masseter weakness (Table 3). There were no deaths and no intracranial hemorrhages. There was a 0.1% incidence of carotid cavernous fistula, 0.2% meningitis, 2% keratitis, 1.2% diplopia, 6% absent corneal reflex, and 1% anesthesia dolorosa (Table 4). Motor weakness decreased from 24 to 7% when a curved electrode was used.

Ophthalmologic complications include diplopia caused by damage to the abducens, trochlear, and oculomotor nerves; these motor nerve injuries were

Table 1
Characteristics of 1200 Patients Who Underwent Percutaneous Radiofrequency Rhizotomy [a]

Characteristic	%
Sex	
Female	63
Male	37
Side of coagulation	
Right	60
Bilateral	5
Division of trigeminal nerve involved	
First	1
Second	16
Third	16
First and second	15
Second and third	39
First, second, and third	13

[a] Patients (mean age 65 yr) with multiple sclerosis excluded.
From ref. 21, copyright 1995 W. B. Saunders.

Table 2
Early Results of Percutaneous Radiofrequency Rhizotomy in 1200 Patients [a]

Result	Description	%
Excellent	No tic pain, dysesthesia, or troublesome paresthesia	72
Good	No tic pain, minor dysesthesia/paresthesia	21
Fair	No tic pain, moderate dysesthesia/paresthesia	4
Poor	No tic pain, major dysesthesia/paresthesia	1
Failure	Immediate	2

[a] Patients with multiple sclerosis excluded.
From ref. 21, copyright 1995 W. B. Saunders.

self-limiting and resolved within months. Although corneal anesthesia can cause keratitis and blindness, this complication is rare. Blindness from loss of corneal sensation may be prevented by the use of soft contact lenses, early ophthalmologic treatment, eye care, and tarsorrhaphy when necessary.

Motor Paresis

The use of electrical stimulation as a localizing technique may prevent injury to the motor division of the trigeminal nerve. Motor weakness, which occurred in 16% of patients treated with RFL, was reduced with stimulation tests and manipulation of electrode placement *(18)*. The motor division rootlets are located rostral and medial to the sensory roots and cross under the ganglion *(22)*. When stimulation testing results in masseter contraction, the electrode should be repositioned. Lateral rotation of the electrode reduces the occurrence of motor deficits. Motor losses are usually partial and recover over time.

Table 3
Percentage of Patients Suffering Complications After Percutaneous
Radiofrequency Rhizotomy: Comparison of Curved vs Straight Electrode

	% of patients	
Complication	Curved electrode ($n = 500$)	Straight electrode ($n = 700$)
Dysesthesia	11	27
Minor	9	22
Major	2	5
Anesthesia dolorosa	0.2	1.6
Absent corneal reflex	3	8
First division pain	8	20
Second division pain	2	8
Third division pain	0.3	2
Keratitis	0.6	4
Diplopia	0.5	2
Masseter weakness	7	24

From ref. 21, copyright 1995 W. B. Saunders.

Table 4
Complications in 1200 Cases
of Percutaneous Radiofrequency Rhizotomy [a]

Complications	%
Masseter weakness	16
Pterygoid weakness	7
Dysesthesia/paresthesia (minor)	17
Dysesthesia/paresthesia (major)	3
Anesthesia dolorosa	1
Absent corneal reflex	6
With first division pain	15
With second division pain	5
With third division pain	1
Keratitis	2
Diplopia[b]	1.2
Oculomotor	0.1
Trochlear	0.5
Abducens	0.6
Meningitis	0.2
Carotid cavernous fistula	0.1
Intracranial hemorrhage	0
Death	0

[a] Includes patients undergoing multiple percutaneous rhizotomies.
[b] Nearly all nerve palsies (motor root and extraocular) represented axonotmesis and resolved within 6 mo.
From ref. 21, copyright 1995 W. B. Saunders.

Muscles affected most often include the masseter, temporalis, pterygoid and, less often, the tensor veli palatini and tensor tympany (18). Symptoms of motor paresis include difficulty chewing, jaw deviation, tinnitus, and auditory white noise.

Recurrence

Trigeminal neuralgia pain relief may be temporary after RFL. The goal of treatment is dense hypalgesia in the most affected division with moderate hypalgesia in trigger divisions. The degree of lesioning depends in part on the patient's tolerance to numbness. Initial conservative lesions provide relief with a trial of mild sensory loss. Over time, tic pain may return. Based on the experience of the earlier treatment, patients may choose denser lesions if reoperation is needed. More aggressive lesions may result in numbness that is intolerable to some patients. In the event that pain recurs, the surgeon determines how much of the nerve should be treated based on the amount of numbness that the patient can tolerate.

VAGOGLOSSOPHARYNGEAL NEURALGIA

Vagoglossopharyngeal neuralgia is described as pain in the ear, tonsillar fossa, throat, larynx, pharynx, or tongue, typically with periods of long remissions. Pain is triggered by swallowing and by other movements of the face or mouth (e.g., chewing, sneezing, coughing) (23). Vagoglossopharyngeal neuralgia occurs for many reasons, mostly compression or irritation of the nervous tissue by surrounding structures that include abscess, tumor, aneurysm, tonsillitis, arachnoiditis, styloid process, styloid ligament, vertebral artery, or trauma (24,25).

Primary treatment, as for other neuralgias, includes medications such as baclofen, carbamazepine, and phenyl hydantoin. When medical therapy fails, surgical options are considered. Patient selection may be instrumental in predicting pain relief with RFL. Evaluation of vagoglossopharyngeal neuralgia includes clinical history and radiographic imaging to exclude a more critical pathology (i.e., tumor, abscess, aneurysm). Test dosing of local anesthetics to the tonsillar fossa during pain attacks is a reliable diagnostic test for glossopharyngeal neuralgia. Pain relief with anesthetics to the pyriform fossa or jugular foramen is more likely diagnostic of vagal neuralgia (26).

RFL of the glossopharyngeal nerve in the nervous portion of the jugular canal is possible using techniques similar to treatment of trigeminal pain. During the senior author's early experience with trigeminal neuralgia rhizotomy (5), safe penetration of the jugular foramen was performed inadvertently. As with trigeminal neuralgia, percutaneous RFL for vagoglossopharyngeal neuralgia is performed in the radiographic suite. The target of the electrode is the pars nervosa of the jugular foramen. The pars nervosa (glossopharyngeal nerve) is isolated from the larger lateral pars venosa (jugular bulb, vagal nerve, accessory nerve) by a fibrous band. The patient receives small doses of methohexital for pain. The surgeon performs RFL with free-hand electrode placement and confirms the trajectory with a lateral fluoroscopic view. The needle is inserted

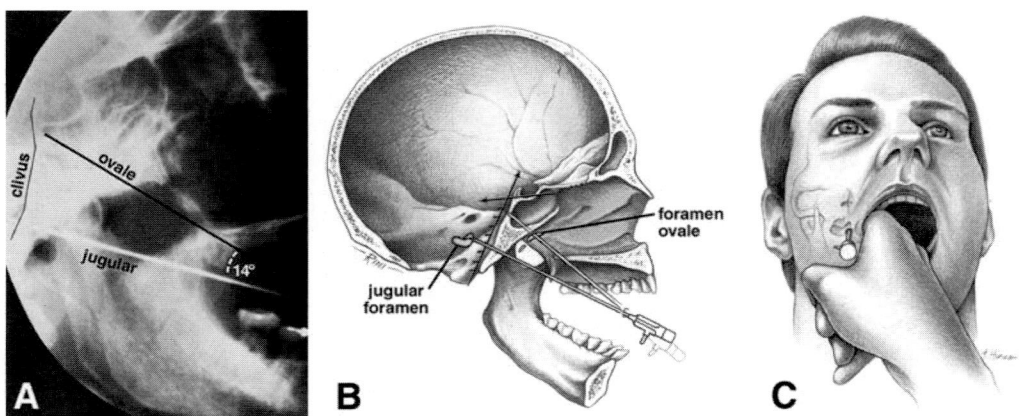

Fig. 6. Various projections show the approach trajectories to the foramen ovale and jugular foramen. **(A)** Composite illustration shows that the sagittal plane is identical for both targets. **(B)** Illustration of a lateral projection of the head shows that the needle is inserted 27–33 mm below the sella floor; it lies posterior to the temporomandibular joint and anterior to the occipital condyle. **(C)** Illustration shows the needle insertion into the anteromedial pars nervosa of the jugular foramen; this foramen is in a direct line with and 2–2.5 cm inferior to the foramen ovale. (A,C: courtesy of the Mayfield Clinic. B, from Tew JM Jr, Taha JM: Surgical management of glossopharyngeal and other uncommon facial neuralgias, in *The Practice of Neurosurgery* (Tindall GT, Cooper PR, Barrow DL, eds.), Williams & Wilkins, Baltimore, 1995. Reprinted by permission.)

2.5 cm lateral to the oral commissure using the same sagittal trajectory necessary for the foramen ovale. The pars nervosa is in direct sagittal alignment with the foramen ovale. An angle of 14° caudal to the trigeminal target is sufficient to obtain access to the pars nervosa. The jugular foramen is posterior to the temporomandibular joint and anterior to the occipital condyle 30 mm below the sella (Fig. 6). This trajectory passes below the hard palate, medial to the ramus of the mandible, and medial to the carotid canal. Although lateral approaches have been described, their use during RFL may result in vagal nerve injury *(27)*.

Electrophysiologic localization is accomplished by 1-ms-duration stimulations at 10–75 pulses/s with 100–300 mV current. Resulting pain in the throat and ear identifies the correct location. Stimulation with higher currents may cause coughing or contraction of the sternocleidomastoid. Creation of thermal lesions begins at 60°C for 90 s, increasing in increments of 5°C until the pharynx is analgesic and triggers no longer cause pain *(18)*.

Immediate risks of vagoglossopharyngeal neuralgia include procedural hypotension, hypertension, bradycardia, syncope, or cardiac arrest related to injury to vagal nerve or nerve of herding *(28,29)*. Complications or procedural side effects also include vocal cord dysfunction that results in hoarseness and sensory losses with a decreased gag reflex and dysphagia. Physiologic monitoring, including electrical stimulation or heating tests, allows accurate localization and electrode position testing before the creation of a permanent lesion *(30–32)*. Stimulation causing hypotension, bradycardia, coughing, or sternocleidomastoid contraction is an indication to reposition the electrode. Lesion production of the glossopharyngeal rootlets requires less heat than trigeminal lesions because of anatomic differences, that is, glossopharyngeal rootlets are not located in a spinal-fluid filled cistern *(33)*. Because of reduced heat dissipation, lesions are successfully created with repetitive low energy trials of shorter duration and intervening neurological exams.

Glossopharyngeal RFL has been successful in 70% of cervicofacial pain from neoplastic processes and 90% of idiopathic neuralgias *(31–35)*. Opinions vary considerably about the appropriate use of glossopharyngeal RFL. Arguments against RFL include the possibility of serious and frequent side effects and recommend its restriction for patients with neoplastic disease. Advocates of RFL for the treatment of idiopathic glossopharyngeal neuralgia suggest its safety when used conservatively, that is, avoiding the creation of dense lesions and reducing the risks of serious complications by careful localization.

HEMIFACIAL SPASM

Hemifacial spasm was first described as an aneurysmal compression of the facial nerve on postmortem examination of subjects with a known history of facial spasm *(36)*. Typical hemifacial spasm involves the orbicularis oculi, may progress in a caudal direction, and may extend to the buccal muscles and platysma. Symptoms include contraction of the facial muscles, eye closure, and pulling at the corner of the mouth. Prolonged twitching or tonus results in temporary weakness. A typical hemifacial spasm originates with symptoms in the buccal muscles and progresses rostrally to include the frontalis muscle.

Medical treatment (e.g., carbamazepine, baclofen, phenytoin, clonazepam) is ineffective *(37–39)*. Most early treatments included destruction of nerve tissue that resulted in facial weakness. Microvascular decompression is considered safe and effective for the treatment of facial spasm in adults and children *(40,41)*.

An alternative minimally invasive technique introduced for hemifacial spasm initially included RFL *(42)* and was further refined by combined use of fluoroscopic guidance and stimulation *(43)*. The fluoroscopic view requires placement of the patient's head supine and extended 45° with the X-ray tube 15° caudal; the total angle in the anterior–posterior view is 60°. The electrode insertion point is 2–3 cm caudal to the tip of the mastoid process. The ring of the styloid foramen is the end target on fluoroscopy. Other bone landmarks include the styloid process (anteromedial to the foramen), and the medial border of the mandibular condyle (same sagittal plane as foramen). Lesions are made with 0.1–0.3 V starting at 55°C and rising to 65°C until the patient develops mild weakness. Complications of facial weakness quickly resolve. RFL is a reasonable alternative when open microvascular decompression fails or for those who are not strong surgical candidates because of medical issues.

CONCLUSIONS

Additional applications for RFL include selective RFL rhizotomy for extremity spasticity, dorsal root entry zone or dorsal root ganglion for chronic neck pain, intradiscal electrothermal therapy for back pain, and deep brain lesions for Parkinson's disease. Each of these applications deserves detailed discussion and analysis beyond the scope of this chapter. Radiofrequency lesioning is a safe, effective, selective, and noninvasive treatment whose initial success was relief of trigeminal pain. This technology is applied to ablate nerve tissue selectively for a variety of motor and sensory symptoms. The adoption of radiofrequency as a power source for lesion production is partly owing to the precision of power control through temperature and impedance monitoring. The predictability of lesion morphology shape and size is a feature not shared by other noninvasive means, such as glycerol rhizolysis. RFL applications offer safe and effective minimally invasive treatment options for medically aged or medically unstable patients.

REFERENCES

1. Laitinen LV, Bergenheim AT, Hariz MI. Ventralposterolateral pallidotomy can abolish all parkinsonian symptoms. *Stereotact Neurosurg* 1992;58:14–21.
2. Hassenbusch SJ, Pillay PK, Barnett GH. Radiofrequency cingulotomy for intractable cancer pain using stereotaxis guided by magnetic resonance imaging. *Neurosurgery* 1990;27:220–223.
3. Saal JS, Saal JA. Management of chronic discogenic low back pain with thermal intradiscal catheter: a preliminary report. *Spine* 2000;25:382–388.
4. Hori T, Fukushima T, Terao H, et al. Percutaneous radiofrequency facial nerve coagulation in the management of facial spasm. *J Neurosurg* 1981;54:655–658.
5. Tew JM Jr. Percutaneous rhizotomy in the treatment of intractable facial pain (trigeminal, glossopharyngeal, and vagal nerves), in *Current Techniques in Operative Neurosurgery* (Schmidek HH, Sweet WH, eds.), Grune & Stratton, New York, 1977, pp. 409–426.
6. Kirschner M. Elektrocoagulation des ganglion gasseri. *Zentralbl Chir* 1932;47: 2841–2843.
7. Sweet WH, Wepsic JG. Controlled thermocoagulation of trigeminal ganglion and rootlets for differential destruction of pain fibers. *J Neurosurg* 1974;39:143–156.
8. Letcher FS, Goldring S. The effect of radiofrequency current and heat on peripheral nerve action potential in the cat. *J Neurosurg* 1968;29:42–47.
9. Uematsu S. Percutaneous electrothermal coagulation of spinal nerve trunk, ganglion, and rootlets, in *Current Techniques in Operative Neurosurgery* (Schmidek HH, Sweet WS, eds.), Grune & Stratton, New York, 1977, pp. 469–490.
10. Smith HP, Mcwhorter JM, Challa VR. Radiofrequency neurolysis in a clinical model. *J Neurosurg* 1988;55:246–253.
11. Alberts WW, Wright EW, Feinstein B, et al. Experimental radiofrequency brain lesion size as a function of physical parameters. *J Neurosurg* 1966;25:421–423.
12. Bonin GV, Alberts WW, Wright EW J, et al. Radiofrequency brain lesions: size as a function of physical parameters. *Arch Neurol (Chicago)* 1965;12:25–29.
13. Dickman G, Gabriel E, Hassler R. Size, form and structural peculiarities of experimental brain lesions obtained by thermocontrolled radiofrequency. *Confin Neurol* 1965;26:134–142.
14. Moringlane JR, Koch R, Schafer H, et al. Experimental radiofrequency coagulation with computer-based on line monitoring of temperature and power. *Acta Neurochir* 1989;96:126–131.

15. Vinas FC, Zamorano L, Dujovny M, et al. In vivo and in vitro study of the lesions produced with a computerized radiofrequency system. *Stereotact Funct Neurosurg* 1992;58:121–133.
16. Nugent GR. Percutaneous techniques for trigeminal neuralgia, in *Operative Neurosurgery* (Kaye HA, Black PM, eds.), Harcourt, London, 2000, pp. 1615–1633.
17. Hartel F. Uber die intracranielle injektionsbehandlung der trigeminusneuralgie. *Med Klin* 1914;10:582.
18. Taha JM and Tew JM Jr. Treatment of trigeminal and other facial neuralgias by percutaneous techniques, in *Neurological Surgery*, 4th ed. (Youmans JR, ed.) WB Saunders, Philadelphia, 1996, pp. 3386–3403.
19. Rish BL. Cerebrovascular accident after percutaneous thermocoagulation of the trigeminal ganglion. *J Neurosurg* 1976;44:376–377.
20. Sweet WH. Trigeminal neuralgia: problems as to cause and consequent conclusions regarding treatment, in *Neurosurgery*, 2nd ed. (Wilkins RF, Rengachary SS, eds.), McGraw-Hill, New York, 1996, pp. 3931–3943.
21. Tew JM Jr, Taha JM. Percutaneous rhizotomy in the treatment of intractable pain (trigeminal, glossopharyngeal and vagal nerves), in *Operative Neurosurgical Techniques* (Schmidek HH, Sweet WH, eds.), WB Saunders, Philadelphia, 1995, pp. 1469–1484.
22. Rhoton AL. The cerebellopontine angle and posterior fossa cranial nerves by the retrosigmoid approach. *Neurosurgery* 2000;47:S93-S129.
23. King J. Glossopharyngeal neuralgia. *Clin Exp Neurol* 1987;24:113–121.
24. Rushton J, Stevens C, Miller R. Glossopharyngeal neuralgia (vagoglossopharyngeal neuralgia): a study of 217 cases. *Arch Neurol* 1981;38:201–205.
25. Waga S and Kojima T. Glossopharyngeal neuralgia of traumatic origin. *Surg Neurol* 1982;17:77–79.
26. van Loveren HR, Tew JM Jr, Thomas G. Vagoglossopharyngeal and geniculate neuralgias, in *Neurological Surgery*, 3rd ed. (Youmans J, ed), WB Saunders, Philadelphia, 1990, pp. 3943–3949.
27. Saler G, Ori C, Baratto V, et al. Selective percutaneous thermolesions of the ninth cranial nerve by lateral cervical approach: report of eight cases. *Surg Neurol* 1983; 20:276–279.
28. Jannetta P. Cranial nerve vascular compression syndromes (other than tic douloureux and hemifacial spasm). *Clin Neurosurg* 1981;28:445–580.
29. Ori C, Salar G, Giron G. Percutaneous glossopharyngeal thermocoagulation complicated by syncope and seizures. *Neurosurgery* 1983;13:427–429.
30. Arias MJ. Percutaneous radiofrequency thermocoagulation with low temperature in the treatment of essential glossopharyngeal neuralgia. *Surg Neurol* 1986;25: 94–96.
31. Isamat F, Ferran E, Acebes JJ. Selective percutaneous thermocoagulation rhizotomy in essential glossopharyngeal neuralgia. *J Neurosurg* 1981;55:575–580.
32. Pagura J, Schnapp M, Passerelli P: Percutaneous radiofrequency glossopharyngeal rhizotomy for cancer pain. *Appl Neurophysiol* 1983;46:154–159.
33. Gybles JM. Sweet WH. Neurosurgical treatment of persistent pain: Physiological and pathological mechanisms of human pain, in *Pain and Headache* (Gildengberg PL, ed.), Karger, S Basel, 1988, pp. 70–103.
34. Giorgi C, Broggi G: Surgical treatment of glossopharyngeal neuralgia and pain from cancer of the nasopharynx: a 20 year experience. *J Neurosurg* 1984;61:952–955.
35. Lazorthes Y, Verdie J. Radiofrequency coagulation of the petrous ganglion in glossopharyngeal neuralgia. *Neurosurgery* 1979;4:512–516.

36. Schultze F. Linksseitiger facialiskrampf in folge eines aneurysma der arteria vertebralis sinistra. *Virchows Arch Pathol Anat Physiol Klin Med* 1875;65:385–391.
37. Alexander GE, Moses H. III. Carbamazepine for hemifacial spasm. *Neurology* 1982;32:286–287.
38. Herzberg L. Management of hemifacial spasm with clonazepam [Letter]. *Neurology* 1982;35:1676–1677.
39. Sandyk R, Gillman MA. Baclofen in hemifacial spasm. *Int J Neurosci* 1987;33:261–264.
40. Levy EL, Resnick DK, Jannetta PJ, et al. Pediatric hemifacial spasm. The efficacy of microvascular decompression. *Pediatr Neurosurg* 1997;27:238–241.
41. Levy EL, Jannetta PJ. Microvascular decompression for hemifacial spasm, in *Operative Neurosurgery* (Kaye AH, Black PM, eds.), Harcourt, London, 2000, pp. 1647–1653.
42. Kao MC, Hung CC, Chen RC, et al. Controlled thermocoagulation of the facial nerve in the treatment of hemifacial spasm. *Taiwan I Hsueh Hui Tsa Chih* 1978;7:226–233.
43. Hori T, Fukushima T, Terao H, et al. Percutaneous radiofrequency facial nerve coagulation in the management of facial spasm. *J Neurosurg* 1981;54:655–658.

11
Radiosurgery
Techniques and Applications

William A. Friedman, MD

INTRODUCTION

Stereotactic radiosurgery (SRS) is a minimally invasive treatment modality that delivers a large single dose of radiation to a specific intracranial target while sparing surrounding tissue. Unlike conventional fractionated radiotherapy, SRS does not rely on, or exploit, the higher radiosensitivity of neoplastic lesions relative to normal brain (therapeutic ratio). Its selective destruction is dependent mainly on sharply focused high-dose radiation. The biological effect is irreparable cellular damage and delayed vascular occlusion within the high-dose target volume. Because a therapeutic ratio is not required, traditionally radioresistant lesions can be treated. Since destructive doses are used, however, any normal structure included in the target volume is subject to damage.

The basis for SRS was conceived over 40 yr ago by Lars Leksell *(1)*. He proposed the technique of focusing multiple nonparallel beams of external radiation on a stereotactically defined intracranial target. The averaging of these intersecting beams results in very high doses of radiation to the target volume, but innocuously low doses to nontarget tissues along the path of any given beam. His team's implementation of this concept culminated in the development of the Gamma Knife. The modern Gamma Knife employs 201 fixed cobalt radiation sources in a fixed hemispherical array, such that all 201 photon beams are focused on a single point (Fig. 1). The patient is stereotactically positioned in the Gamma Knife so that the intracranial target coincides with the isocenter of radiation. Using variable collimation, beam blocking, and multiple isocenters, the radiation target volume is shaped to conform to the intracranial target.

Wilson *(2)*, a physicist, has been credited with first suggesting the medical usage of particle beams (in the 1940s). Early radiosurgical groups utilized the proton beam produced by synchrocyclotrons. Workers in Sweden employed high-energy intersecting proton beams, in a fashion analogous to the intersecting cobalt beams of the Gamma Knife. Groups in Boston and Berkeley, however, used the Bragg peak effect to maximize the radiosurgical effectiveness of the proton beam. Single-dose and fractionated treatments have been devised (Fig. 2). A 160-MeV proton beam, with a 10-mm-wide Bragg peak, is used in Boston *(3)*. Since 1980, 130-MeV

From: *Minimally Invasive Neurosurgery,* edited by: M.R. Proctor and P.M. Black © Humana Press Inc., Totowa, NJ

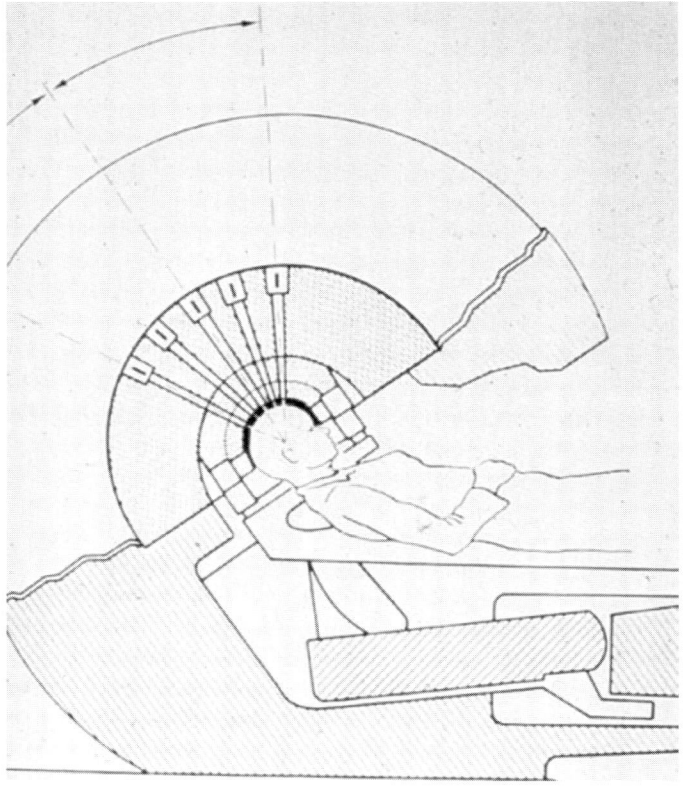

Fig. 1. The Gamma Knife contains 201 fixed cobalt sources, all focused on the target spot. Each beam takes a different path though the brain. They all converge at the target. This averaging process yields a high dose at target with a steep dose gradient.

helium ion beams have been used at the Berkeley installation *(4)*. The limiting factor on the utilization of particle beam radiosurgery appears to be the requirement for a synchrocyclotron to generate the radiation source. These facilities are currently available only at a small number of high-energy physics research institutes. Nonetheless, an extensive literature is extant on the clinical applications of proton radiosurgery, especially for pituitary adenomas *(5)*, arteriovenous malformations *(6,7)*, choroidal melanomas *(8)*, and chordomas *(9)*. Particle beam radiosurgery involves a very different technique than Gamma Knife or linear accelerator (LINAC) radiosurgery and will not be discussed further in this chapter.

An alternate radiosurgical solution using a LINAC was first described in 1984 by Betti et al. *(10)*. Colombo et al. *(11)* described such a system in 1985, and LINACs have subsequently been modified in various ways to achieve the precision and accuracy required for radiosurgical applications *(12–21)*. In 1986, a team composed of neurosurgeons, radiation physicists, and computer programmers began development of the University of Florida LINAC-based radiosurgery system *(22)*. This system has been used to treat more than 2000 patients at the University of Florida since May 1988 and is in use at multiple sites worldwide.

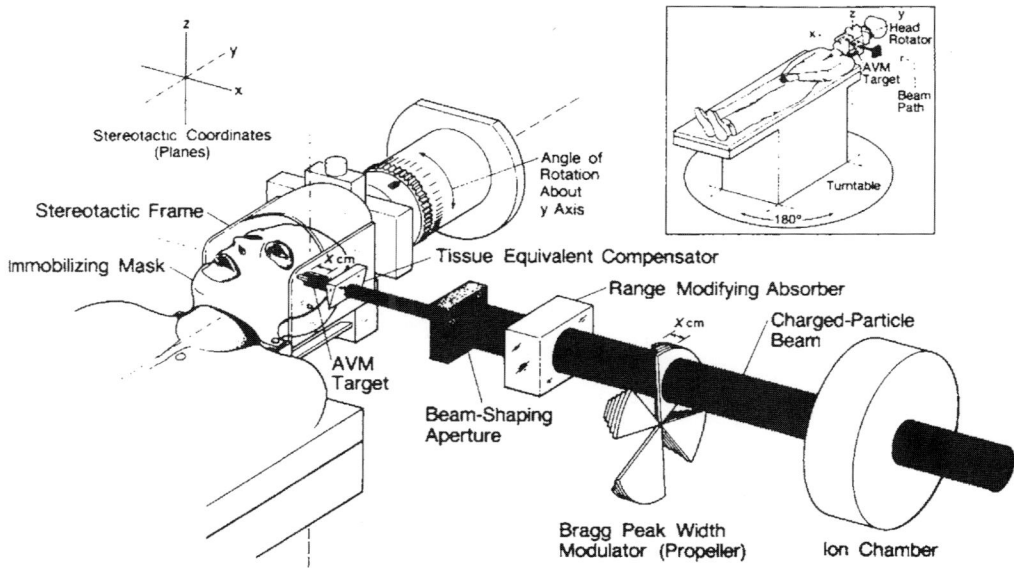

Fig. 2. Particle beam radiosurgery uses highly energetic protons or helium nuclei, which are produced in a cyclotron. The propeller modulator, tissue compensator, and beam shaping aperture are used to deposit the beam energy at the desired target point. Typically, four to six portals of radiation are used. AVM, arteriovenous malformation.

All LINAC radiosurgical systems rely on the same basic paradigm: a collimated X-ray beam is focused on a stereotactically identified intracranial target. The gantry of the LINAC rotates around the patient, producing an arc of radiation focused on the target (Fig. 3). The patient couch is then rotated in the horizontal plane, and another arc is performed. In this manner, multiple noncoplanar arcs of radiation intersect at the target volume and produce a high target dose, with minimal radiation to surrounding brain. This dose concentration method is exactly analogous to the multiple intersecting beams of cobalt radiation in the Gamma Knife.

The target dose distribution can be tailored by varying collimator sizes, eliminating undesirable arcs, manipulating arc angles, using multiple isocenters, and differentially weighting the isocenters (23). More recently, some LINAC systems have also started to employ advanced beam shaping techniques, using multileaf collimators and intensity modulation. Achievable dose distributions are similar for LINAC-based and Gamma Knife systems. With both systems, it is possible to achieve dose distributions that conform closely to the shape of the intracranial target, thus sparing the maximum amount of normal brain. Recent advances in stereotactic imaging and computer technology for dose planning, as well as refinements in radiation delivery systems have led to improved efficacy, fewer complications, and a remarkable amount of interest in the various applications of SRS. Perhaps of equal importance is the fact that increasing amounts of scientific evidence have persuaded the majority of the international neurosurgical

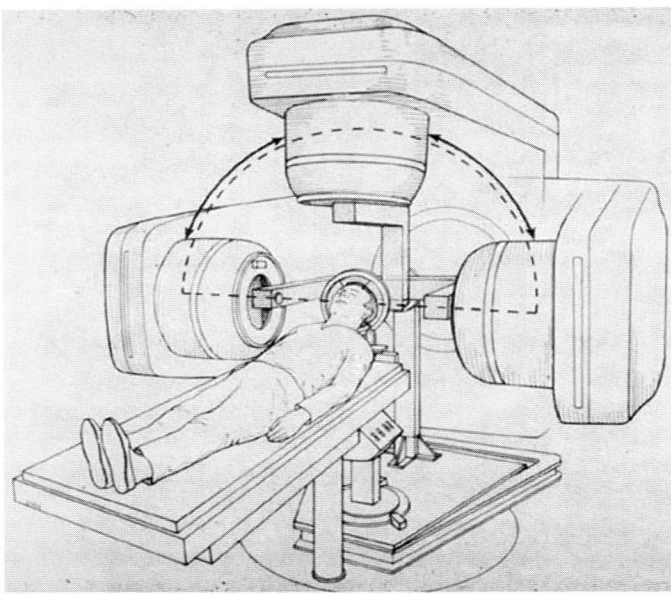

Fig. 3. A LINAC radiosurgery system. The head of the linear accelerator rotates around the patient. The highly collimated X-ray beam is always focused on the stereotactic target, which has been moved to the center of the arc. A removable floorstand has been added to this system (University of Florida) to improve the accuracy of beam delivery.

community that radiosurgery is a viable treatment option for selected patients suffering from a variety of challenging neurosurgical disorders.

This chapter presents a brief description of radiosurgical technique, followed by a review of the more common applications of stereotactic radiosurgery in the treatment of intracranial disease.

TECHNIQUE

Although the details of radiosurgical treatment techniques differ somewhat from system to system, the basic paradigm is quite similar everywhere. Below is a detailed description of a typical radiosurgical treatment at the University of Florida:

Almost all radiosurgical procedures in adults are performed on an outpatient basis. The patient reports to the neurosurgical clinic the day before treatment for a detailed history and physical, as well as an in-depth review of the treatment options. A team that can provide surgical or endovascular options should make the selection of radiosurgery as an appropriate treatment option as well. The fundamental elements of any successful radiosurgical treatment include the following: head ring application, stereotactic image acquisition, treatment planning, dose selection, radiation delivery, and follow-up. All these elements are critical, and poor performance of any step will result in suboptimal results.

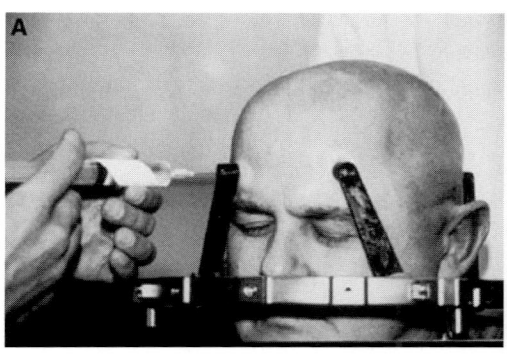 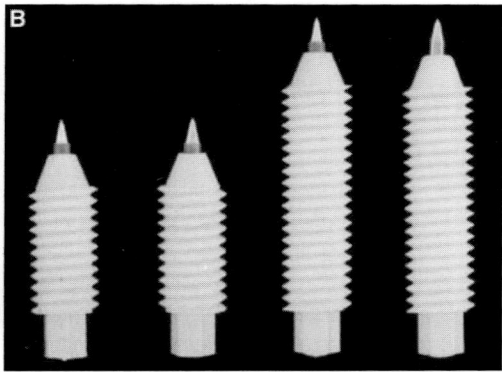

Fig. 4. **(A)** The stereotactic head ring hangs below the head via carbon fiber posts, which produce no artifact on CT scan. Local anesthetic is injected through each of the post holes. **(B)** These pins are used to secure the ring to the skull. The metal tips are composed of aluminum, which produces minimal artifact on CT.

Head Ring Application

The techniques for optimal head ring application for radiosurgery are no different from those for other target lesions and are described in detail elsewhere *(24)*. In general, patients 13 yr and older are able to tolerate head ring application under local anesthesia. We usually premedicate with oral Valium. Those younger are treated under general anesthesia. The head ring must be applied such that the metal ring falls below the plane of the target. In general, if the top of the head ring is below the external auditory canal, the entire head can be imaged. Most stereotactic frames are anchored to the skull with metal-tipped pins. It is important that these pins have tips that will not produce artifact on computer tomography (CT) scan (aluminum or ceramic vs steel; Fig. 4). Obviously caution must be utilized to avoid placing one of the pins over a previous craniotomy, burr hole, or shunt. In general, head ring application takes about 5 min.

Stereotactic Image Acquisition

Arteriovenous Malformations

The most problematic aspect of arteriovenous malformation (AVM) radiosurgery is target identification. In some series targeting error is listed as the most frequent cause of radiosurgical failure *(25,26)*. The problem lies with imaging. Although angiography very effectively defines blood flow (feeding arteries, nidus, and draining veins), it does so in only two dimensions. Using the 2D data from stereotactic angiography to represent the 3D target results in significant errors of both overestimation and underestimation of AVM nidus dimensions *(27–29)*. Underestimation of the nidus size may result in treatment failure, whereas overestimation results in the inclusion of normal brain within the treatment volume. This can cause radiation damage to normal brain, which—when affecting an eloquent area—may result in a neurological deficit. To avoid such targeting errors, a true 3D image database is required. Both contrast-enhanced CT and magnetic resonance imaging (MRI) are commonly used for this purpose.

Diagnostic (nonstereotactic) angiography is used to characterize the AVM, but because of its inherent inadequacies as a treatment-planning database, stereotactic angiography has been largely abandoned at our institution. We use contrast-enhanced, stereotactic CT as a targeting image database for the vast majority of AVMs. Our CT technique employs rapid infusion (1 mL/s) of contrast while scanning through the AVM nidus with 1-mm slices. The head ring is bolted to a bracket at the head of the CT table, ensuring that the head/ring/localizer complex remains immobile during the scan. This technique yields a very clear 3D picture of the nidus. Alternative approaches use MRI/magnetic resonance angiography (MRA), as opposed to CT. Attention to optimal image sequences in both CT and MRI is essential for effective AVM radiosurgical targeting.

Tumors

If a tumor is to be treated, the patient is sent to the radiology department for a volumetric MRI scan. The next morning, the patient arrives at 7:00 AM. After head ring application, stereotactic CT scanning is performed. One-millimeter slices are obtained throughout the entire head. The stereotactic CT scan is transferred via Ethernet to the treatment-planning computer. Image fusion technology is used to fuse the patient's stereotactic CT to the previously acquired MRI images (Fig. 5).

Treatment Planning

The primary goal of radiosurgery treatment planning is to develop a plan with a target volume that conforms closely to the surface of the target lesion, while maintaining a steep dose gradient (the rate of change in dose relative to position) away from the target surface in order to minimize the radiation dose to surrounding brain. A typical radiosurgical dose gradient will reduce the treatment dose to one-half the treatment dose over a 3-mm space. A number of treatment planning tools can be used to tailor the shape of the target volume to fit even highly irregular shapes (Fig. 6). Regardless of its shape, the entire lesion must lie within the target volume (the "prescription isodose shell"), with as little normal brain included as possible.

The volumetric MRI obtained the day before treatment is used to generate a preplan. This plan can be generated manually or via a completely automated program *(30)* that will place multiple isocenters in such a way as to generate an optimally conformal prescription isodose line. The preplan is carefully examined and, if necessary, adjusted to generate the actual treatment plan. The technical methods of radiosurgery have been described at length in other publications *(24)*.

A detailed discussion of dose planning is beyond the scope of this chapter. Suffice it to say that the radiosurgical team must develop considerable expertise using the available tools (multiple isocenters, beam weighting, intensity modulation, and so on) to be able to efficiently develop highly conformal radiosurgical plans.

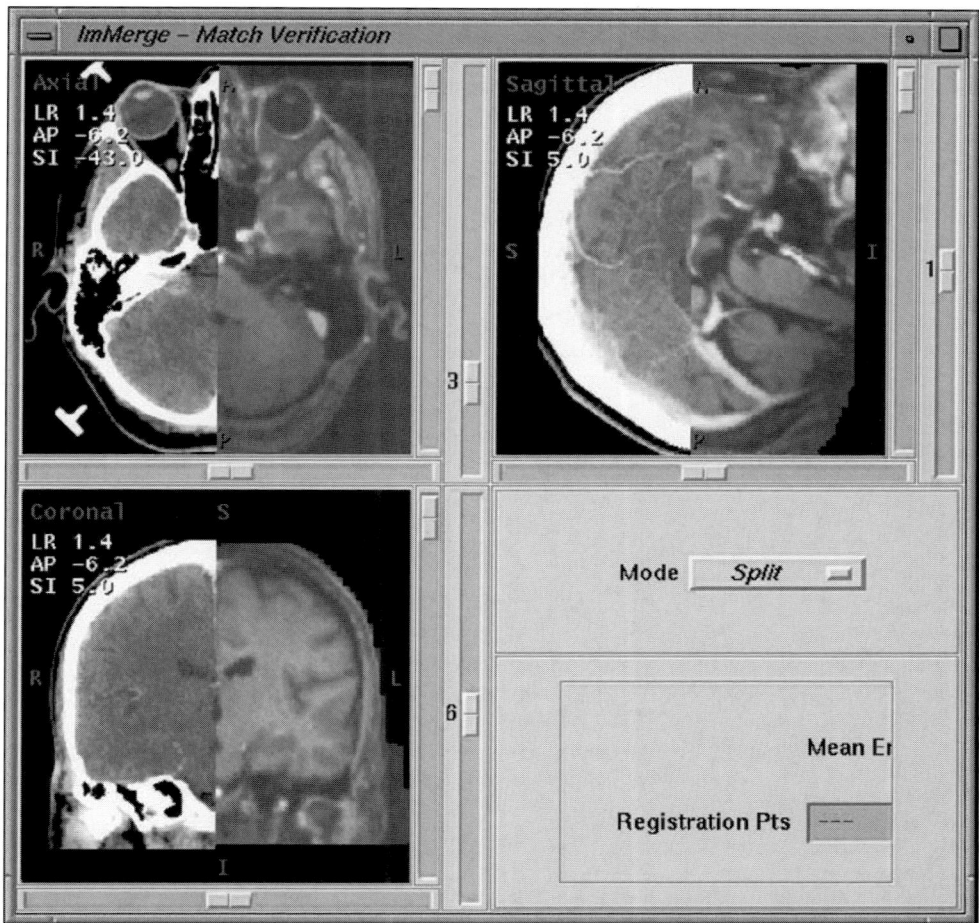

Fig. 5. This computer screen illustrates the process of image fusion. The previously acquired MR image is fused to the stereotactic CT image. Basically, the two image sets are translated and rotated until a pixel-for-pixel match is achieved. This can be verified by "sliding" back and forth from the CT image on the left to the MR image on the right.

Dose Selection

The radiosurgical literature is replete with suggestions regarding appropriate peripheral doses for a variety of lesions. The reader is referred to the references for a detailed exploration of these issues. At the University of Florida, the following doses are generally felt to be "optimal."

Arteriovenous malformations	20 Gy
Acoustic schwannomas	12.5 Gy
Meningiomas	12.5 Gy
Metastases	20 Gy
Gliomas	12.5–17.5 Gy (after conventional radiotherapy and highly dependent on tumor size and location)

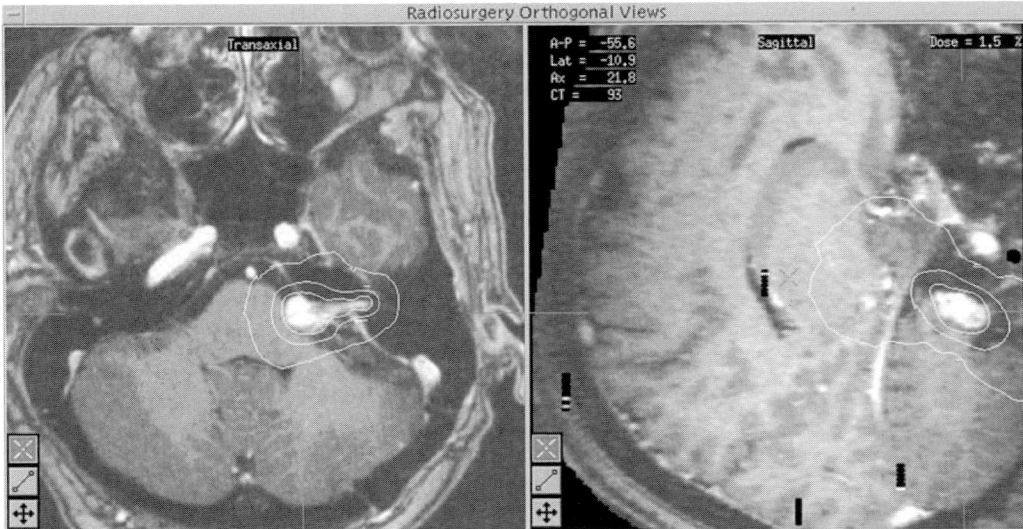

Fig. 6. Highly conformal dosimetry. An axial view of a vestibular schwannoma is shown with a six-isocenter treatment plan. The lines around the tumor, in centrifugal order, represent the 70, 35, and 14% isodose lines. The prescription dose is delivered to the 70% isodose shell, which has been constructed, using various computer dose-planning tools, to conform closely to the surface of the tumor. Note that the 35% isodose line (by definition, the boundary at which the radiation dose has fallen to half of the prescription dose) lies within millimeters of the tumor margin. This steep dose gradient allows a high dose of radiation to be delivered to the tumor, while exposing surrounding tissues to minimal radiation.

Radiation Delivery

The process of radiation delivery is the same for any radiosurgical target - careful attention to detail and the execution of various safety checks and redundancies are necessary to ensure that the prescribed treatment plan is accurately and safely delivered. When radiation delivery has been completed, the head ring is removed, the patient is observed for approx 30 min, and is then discharged to resume her/his normal activities.

Follow-Up

Standard follow-up after AVM radiosurgery typically consists of annual clinic visits with MRI/MRA to evaluate the effect of the procedure and monitor for neurological complications. If the patient's clinical status changes, she/he is followed more closely at clinically appropriate intervals.

Each patient is scheduled to undergo cerebral angiography at 3 yr after radiosurgery, and a definitive assessment of the success or failure of treatment is made based on the results of angiography. If no flow is observed through the AVM nidus, the patient is pronounced cured and is discharged from follow-up. If the AVM nidus is incompletely obliterated, appropriate further therapy (most commonly repeat radiosurgery on the day of angiography) is prescribed, and the treatment/follow-up cycle is repeated.

For benign tumors, yearly MRI scans and clinic evaluations are recommended. For malignant tumors, scans and exams are performed at 3-mo intervals.

APPLICATIONS TO CLINICAL NEUROSURGICAL PRACTICE
Radiosurgery for Arteriovenous Malformations

Steiner et al. *(31)* reported the first successful case of AVM radiosurgery in 1972. Their subsequent publications provided further strong evidence that radiosurgery, even without computerized dosimetry, could produce reasonable success rates in the treatment of carefully selected AVMs *(32–35)*. The Gamma Knife experience with radiosurgery for AVMs has been extensive and is well documented *(13,36–50)*.

Particle beam radiosurgery has also been employed successfully in the treatment of AVMs, as documented by another extensive literature *(51–64)*.

In 1987, Betti and his colleagues first reported the use of a linear accelerator radiosurgery system in the treatment of AVMs *(65,66)*. Again, an extensive literature has documented a generally successful experience *(24,67–82)*.

The University of Florida Experience

From 5/18/88 to 5/14/02, 495 patients with arteriovenous malformations were treated at the University of Florida. The mean age was 39 yr *(4–78)*. The mean treatment volume was 9 mL (0.2–45.3 mL). Many patients early in the series were treated with single isocenters *(254)*, but in recent years an effort has been made to produce highly conformal plans by employing multiple isocenters. The mean radiation dose to the periphery of the AVM was 1596 cGy, and the mean follow-up duration was 31 mo.

Presenting symptoms included the following: headache/incidental *(169)*, seizure *(197)*, hemorrhage *(165)*, and progressive neurological deficit *(20)*. Thirty patients had undergone prior surgery, and 49 had undergone prior embolization. Spetzler-Martin scores were as follows: I, 22; II, 173; III, 204; and IV, 86. AVMs were further delineated into four nidus volume categories: A, <1 mL; B = 1–4 mL; C=4–10 mL; and D= >10 mL.

Angiographic cure rates (Fig. 7) were as follows: A, 85%; B, 83%; C, 70%; and D, 44%. Ellis et al. *(25)* performed a detailed analysis of treatment failures in our series in 1998. He found that 26% of the failures were owing to targeting error, at least in part. Statistical predictors of failure were increasing AVM size, decreasing treatment dose, and increasing Spetzler-Martin score. Of particular interest were the "cutpoints" identified. There was a dramatic increase in cure rates when the peripheral dose was raised to a least 15 Gy. There was a dramatic decrease in cure rate when AVM size exceeded 10 mL (size D).

In a more recent analysis, a study was undertaken to determine which factors were statistically predictive of radiographic and clinical outcomes in the radiosurgical treatment of AVMs. The computerized dosimetry and clinical data on 269 patients were reviewed. The AVM nidus was hand-contoured on successive enhanced CT slices through the nidus, to allow detailed determination of nidus volume, target miss, normal brain treated, dose conformality, and dose gradient.

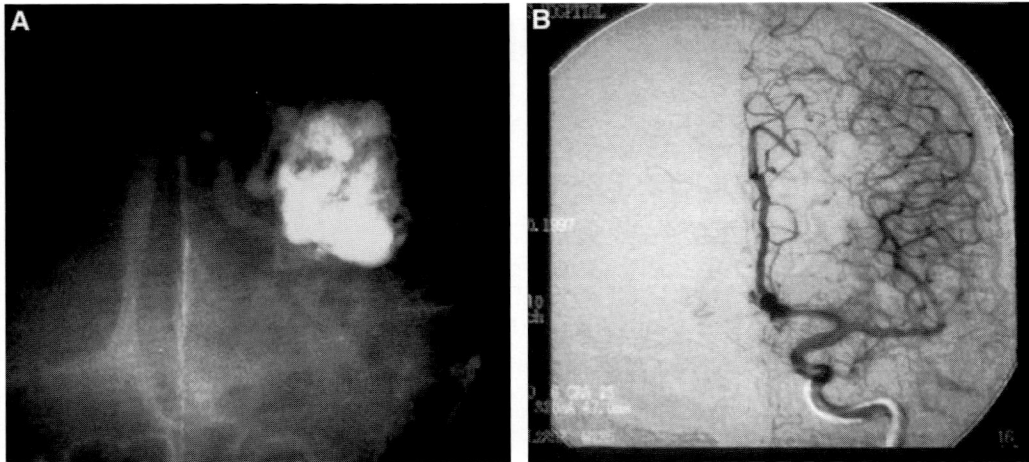

Fig. 7. **(A)** Anteroposterior angiogram shows an AVM nidus in the left parietal lobe. A dose of 1750 cGy was delivered to the 70% isodose line, using three isocenters. **(B)** Two years later, an anteroposterior angiogram shows complete resolution of the AVM, with preservation of normal middle cerebral vasculature in the same area.

In addition, a number of patient and treatment factors, including Spetzler-Martin score, presenting symptoms, dose, number of isocenters, radiographic outcome, and clinical outcome were subjected to multivariate analysis.

None of the analyzed factors were predictive of permanent radiation-induced complications or hemorrhage after radiosurgery in this study. Eloquent AVM location and 12-Gy volume correlated with the occurence of transient radiation-induced complications. Better conformality correlated with a reduced incidence of transient complications. Lower Spetzler-Martin scores, higher doses, and steeper dose gradients correlated with radiographic success.

When AVMs are not cured, current practice frequently involves a "retreatment," usually 3 yr after the original treatment. We reviewed the cases of 52 patients who underwent repeat radiosurgery for residual AVM at our institution between December 1991 and June 1998. In each case, residual arteriovenous shunting persisted beyond 36 mo after the initial treatment. The mean interval between the first and second treatments was 41 mo. Each AVM nidus was measured at the time of original treatment and again at the time of retreatment, and dosimetric parameters of the two treatments were compared. After retreatment, patients were followed and their outcomes evaluated according to our standard post-AVM radiosurgery protocol. Definitive end points included angiographic cure, radiosurgical failure (documented persistence of AVM flow 3 yr after retreatment), and death.

The mean original lesion volume was 13.8 mL, and the mean volume at retreatment was 4.7 mL, for an average volume reduction of 66% after the initial "failed" treatment. Only two AVMs (3.8%) failed to demonstrate size reduction after primary treatment. The median doses on initial and repeat treatment were 12.5 and 15 Gy, respectively. To date, 25 retreated patients have reached a definitive end point. These include 15 (60%) angiographically documented cures, 9 (36%) angiographically documented failures, and 1 fatal hemorrhage. A single permanent radiation-induced complication occurred among 52 patients (1.9%), and 1 patient experienced a transient deficit that resolved with steroid therapy. Two hemorrhages (one fatal) occurred during a total of 130 patient years at risk, resulting in a 1.5% annual incidence of posttreatment hemorrhage.

Four hundred sixty-six of the 495 patients were available for clinical followup. Eight patients (1.6%) sustained a permanent radiation-induced complication. Fifteen (3%) had a transient radiation-induced complication (Fig. 3). These problems usually resolved within several months of steroid therapy. Most importantly, 29 patients suffered hemorrhages after radiosurgical treatment and 7 were fatal.

The World Literature on Radiosurgery for AVMs

The results of other radiosurgery series are summarized in Table 1.

The overall angiographic cure rate in the University of Florida experience is 67%. Dose greater than or equal to 1500 cGy and AVM volume of <10 mL correlated with higher success rates (>80%). This experience is similar to that of other large radiosurgical series *(62,63,69,83)* in the literature. Radiation-induced complications were few. Of more import was the incidence of hemorrhage after radiosurgery *(84,85)* In 1996, our group investigated the incidence of hemorrhage after radiosurgery in our series *(86)*. Two hundred one consecutive patients were analyzed. Poisson and parametric survival statistics were used. No statistical alteration from the natural history hemorrhage rate of 4%/yr was identified at any time interval after radiosurgical treatment. In addition, all covariates that were predictive of hemorrhage correlated with increasing AVM size. Pretreatment hemorrhage did not lead to a higher incidence of posttreatment hemorrhage.

What about conservative followup? Assuming an annual hemorrhage rate of 3%/yr the chance of no hemorrhage is $1-0.97^n$, where n = number of years (Fig. 8). As documented by Kondziolka and McLaughlin *(87)*, using life insurance actuarial tables to predict number of years of remaining life at various ages, the cumulative risk of hemorrhage is quite high, even in the elderly. For example, an average 65-yr-old with an AVM has a 42% chance of hemorrhage from his AVM during the remaining expected life span. Consequently, conservative therapy (no treatment) is reserved for patients with AVMs that are too large for radiosurgery (and who are poor surgical candidates) or for patients whose medical infirmity predicts short life expectancy.

What about surgery vs radiosurgery? Let's assume that the following statements are true:

1. Based on what we know today, only surgery can immediately eliminate the risk of hemorrhage from AVMs.
2. The risk of hemorrhage until complete thrombosis occurs is approx 4%/yr.
3. Radiosurgery for AVMs <10 mL in volume has a >80% success rate.
4. It takes approx 2 yr for radiosurgery to produce thrombosis.
5. The risk of permanent radiation-induced complications after radiosurgery, using modern imaging and dosimetry techniques, is <2%.

Table 1
The Largest World Series of AVM Radiosurgical Cases

Parameter	Yamamoto et al., 1996 (83)	Pollock et al., 1998 (26)	Karlsson et al., (95)	Steinberg et al., 1990 (63)	Colombo et al., 1994 (69)	Friedman et al., 1995 (74)
Radiosurgical device	Gamma Knife	Gamma Knife	Gamma Knife	Proton beam	LINAC	LINAC
No. of patients	40	313	945	86	180	388
Agiographic cure rate (%)	65	61	56	92	80	67
Complications (Permanent, radiation induced)	3 patients (7.5%)	30 patients (9%)	5%	11%	4 patients (2%)	7 patients (2%)
Hemorrhage	None	8 fatal	55 patients	10 patients	15 patients, 5 fatal	25 patients, 5 fatal

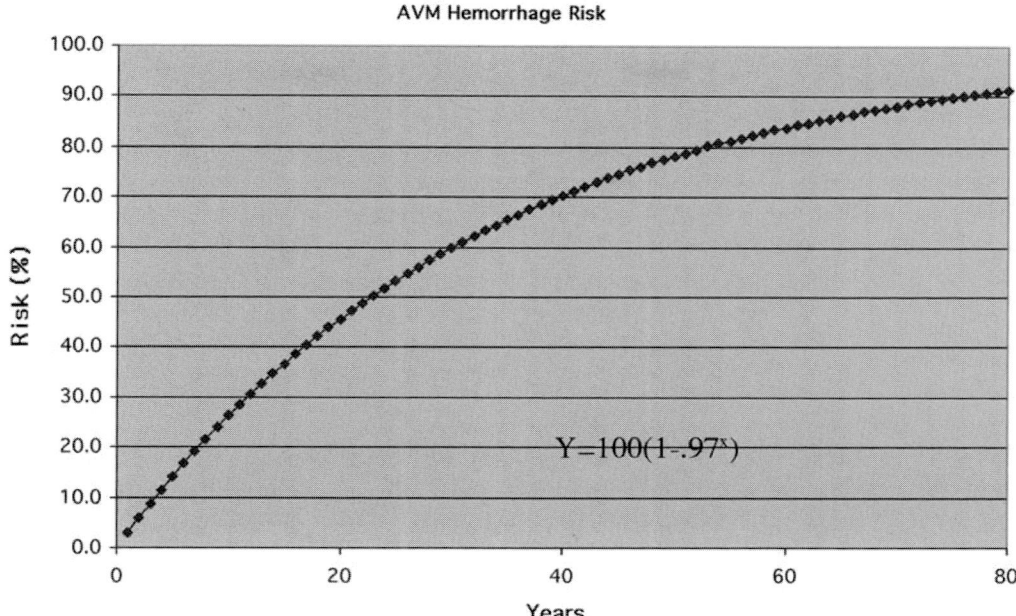

Fig. 8. Assuming a 3%/yr risk of AVM hemorrhage, this graph shows the cumulative risk of bleeding vs the number of years of projected life span.

Therefore, if surgery can be done with a risk less than that of radiosurgery (2% + 4% + 4%), and, if surgery can be done with an efficacy greater than 80%, the radiosurgeon should refer the patient for microsurgery. In other words, if surgery can be done "safely," it should be the first choice. The crux of the issue then is the definition of "safely." It is incumbent on the cerebrovascular surgeon to provide personal data that showing that his or her risk of mortality or serious morbidity is <10%.

Radiosurgery for Benign Tumors

SRS has proved useful for the treatment of a variety of benign intracranial neoplasms. These tumors commonly arise from the skull base, where their dramatic impact on quality of life belies their benign histology and small size. Despite progressive improvement in microsurgical techniques, outcomes for patients with these difficult tumors continue to be less than perfect (88,89). A significant amount of experience has been accumulated using SRS in the treatment of schwannomas and meningiomas. We will focus on each of these tumor types in turn.

Schwannomas

VESTIBULAR SCHWANNOMAS

Among benign intracranial tumors, vestibular schwannoma (acoustic neuroma) has to date been the most frequent target for stereotactic radiosurgery. This common tumor (representing approx 10% of all primary brain tumors) is a benign proliferation of Schwann cells arising from the myelin sheath of the vestibular branch of the eighth cranial nerve. These tumors are slightly more common in women, present at an average age of 50 yr, and occur bilaterally in patients with neurofibromatosis type II.

Leksell *(90)* first used stereotactic radiosurgery to treat a vestibular schwannoma in 1969. SRS is a logical alternative treatment modality for this tumor for several reasons. A vestibular schwannoma is typically well demarcated from surrounding tissues on neuroimaging studies. The sharp borders of this noninvasive tumor make it a convenient match for the characteristically steep dose gradient produced at the boundary of a radiosurgical target. This allows the radiosurgeon to minimize radiation of normal tissue. Excellent spatial resolution on gadolinium-enhanced MRI fused with stereotactic CT facilitates radiosurgical dose planning. These tumors typically occur in an older population that may be less fit for microsurgical resection under general anesthesia. Finally, as evidenced by the outcomes of surgery detailed above, the location of these tumors at the skull base in close proximity to multiple critical neurologic structures (i.e., cranial nerves, brainstem) leads to appreciable surgical morbidity and rare mortality even in expert hands. This makes the concept of an effective, less invasive, less morbid alternative treatment that could be performed in a single day under local anesthesia quite attractive. Whether or not radiosurgery fits this description has been extensively debated.

Certainly, the role of radiosurgery is limited by its inability to relieve mass effect expeditiously in patients for whom this is necessary. The radiobiology of SRS also requires lower, potentially less effective doses for higher target volumes in order to avoid complications. This limits the use of SRS to the treatment of smaller tumors. Despite these limitations, there is a growing body of literature substantiating the claim that radiosurgery is a safe and effective alternative therapy for acoustic schwannomas *(91)*.

The published experience using LINAC-based radiosurgery for the treatment of vestibular schwannomas is relatively limited compared with the Gamma Knife literature (Table 2). The University of Florida LINAC radiosurgery team has significant experience treating these tumors. Several reports documented our early experience with this issue *(92,93)*. Most recently, Foote et al. *(94)* performed an analysis of risk factors associated with radiosurgery for vestibular schwannoma at University of Florida. The aim of this study was to identify factors associated with delayed cranial neuropathy following radiosurgery for vestibular schwannoma (VS; or acoustic neuroma) and to determine how such factors may be manipulated to minimize the incidence of radiosurgical complications while maintaining high rates of tumor control. From July 1988 to June 1998, 149 cases of VS were treated using linear accelerator radiosurgery at the University of Florida. In each of these cases, the patient's tumor and brainstem were contoured in 1-mm slices on the original radiosurgical targeting images. Resulting tumor and brainstem volumes were coupled with the original radiosurgery plans to generate dose–volume histograms. Various tumor dimensions were also measured to estimate the length of cranial nerve that would be irradiated. Patient follow-up data, including evidence of cranial

Table 2
World's Literature Summary: Vestibular Schwannoma Radiosurgery

Study	System	n	Dose to tumor margin (Gy)	Median follow-up (range)	Tumor control (decreased or stable volume)	Delayed facial neuropathy	Delayed trigeminal neuropathy	Preserved functional hearing
Stockholm, 1993 (147)	Gamma Knife	254	18–20 (1969–88) 10–15 (1989–91)	(1–17 yr)	94% for unilateral 84% for NF2	17% overall (1.8% last 3 yr)	19% overall (0% last 3 yr)	22%
Stockholm, 1998 (148) (hearing preservation)	Gamma Knife	44	10–15	—	—	—	—	75% after 1 yr 71% after 2 yr
Pittsburgh, 1998 (149) (largest series)	Gamma Knife	402	17 early in series 12–14 recently	36 mo	93% (7% enlarged, but only 2% required surgery)	28% first 5 yr 8% last 5 yr	34% first 5 yr 8% last 5 yr	39% first 5 yr 68% last 5 yr
Pittsburgh, 1998 (150) (long-term f/u)	Gamma Knife	162	16.6 mean (12–20)	60% had >5 yr f/u	94% (6% enlarged, but only 2% required surgery)	21%	27%	51%
Pittsburgh, 2001 (4) (results with current methods)	Gamma Knife	190	11–18 (median 13)	30 mo (max. 85 mo)	91% (5-yr actuarial) 97% (freedom from resection)	1.1% (5 yr actuarial) (0 if dose <15 Gy)	2.6% (5 yr actuarial)	74% (7% improved)
U. of Virginia, 2000 (151)	Gamma Knife	153	9–20 (median 13)	52 mo	94% for primary radiosurgery 89% for previously operated	3.3%	2%	40%
Israel, 2001 (96)	LINAC	44	11–20 (median 14.6)	32 mo (12–60)	98%	24% (5.5% when dose <14 Gy)	18%	71%
U. of Florida, 2001 (current series)	LINAC	149	10–22.5 (mean 14)	36 mo (18–94)	93%	29% prior to 1994 5% since 1994	29% prior to 1994 2% since 1994	—

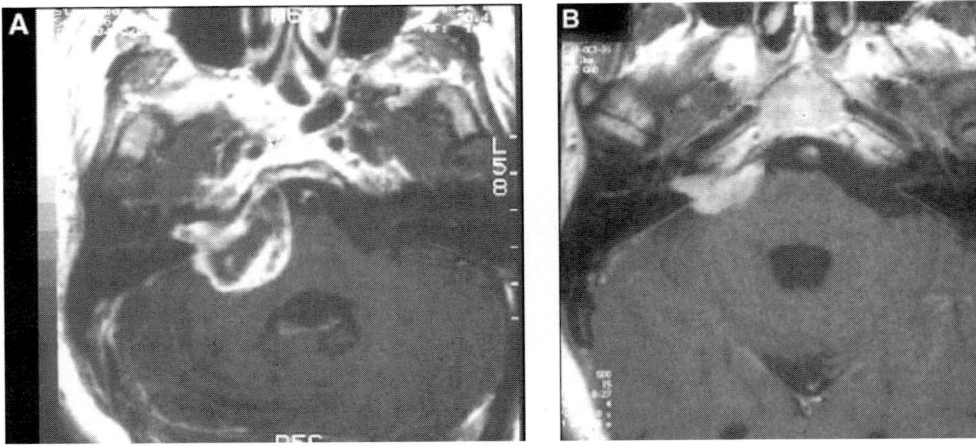

Fig. 9. (A) Contrast-enhanced MR image shows a 3-cm right vestibular schwannoma. (B) Enhanced MR image shows the same tumor, 2 yr later. Typically, tumors shrink slowly after radiosurgery. Although the MRI never normalizes, more than 90% of tumors so treated never grow again.

neuropathy and radiographic tumor control (Fig. 9), were obtained from a prospectively maintained, computerized database.

The authors performed statistical analyses to compare the incidence of posttreatment cranial neuropathies or tumor growth between patient strata defined by risk factors of interest. One hundred thirty-nine of the 149 patients were included in the analysis of complications. The median duration of clinical follow-up for this group was 36 mo (range 18–94 mo). The tumor control analysis included 133 patients. The median duration of radiological follow-up in this group was 34 mo (range 6–94 mo). The overall 2-yr actuarial incidences of facial and trigeminal neuropathies were 11.8 and 9.5%, respectively. In 41 patients treated before 1994, the incidences of facial and trigeminal neuropathies were both 29%, but in the 108 patients treated since January 1994, these rates declined to 5% and 2%, respectively. An evaluation of multiple risk factor models showed that maximum radiation dose to the brainstem, treatment era (pre-1994 compared with 1994 or later), and prior surgical resection were all simultaneously informative predictors of cranial neuropathy risk. The radiation dose prescribed to the tumor margin could be substituted for the maximum dose to the brainstem with a small loss in predictive strength. The overall radiological tumor control rate was 93% (59% tumors regressed, 34% remained stable, and 7.5% enlarged), and the 5-yr actuarial tumor control rate was 87% (95% confidence interval 76–98%). Based on this study, the authors currently recommend a peripheral dose of 12.5Gy for almost all acoustics, as the dose most likely to yield long-term tumor control without causing cranial neuropathy.

Spiegelmann et al. (95,96) recently reported their experience. They reviewed the methods and results of LINAC radiosurgery in 44 patients with acoustic neuromas who were treated between 1993 and 1997. CT scanning was selected as the stereotactic imaging modality for target definition. A single, conformally shaped isocenter was used in the treatment of 40 patients; two or three isocenters were used in four patients who harbored very irregular tumors. The radiation dose directed to the tumor border was the only parameter that changed during the study period: in the first 24 patients who were treated the dose was 15–20 Gy, whereas in the last 20 patients the dose was reduced to 11–14 Gy. After a mean follow-up period of 32 mo (range 12–60 mo), 98% of the tumors were controlled. The actuarial hearing preservation rate was 71%. New transient facial neuropathy developed in 24% of the patients and persisted to a mild degree in 8%. Radiation dose correlated significantly with the incidence of cranial neuropathy, particularly in large tumors (≥ 4 cm^3).

Several reports on smaller series of patients treated with linear accelerator-based radiosurgery for VS have been published in recent years. Martens et al. *(97)* reported on 14 patients with at least 1 yr of follow-up after radiosurgery in the LINAC unit in the University Hospital in Ghent, Belgium. A mean marginal dose of 19.4 Gy (range 16–20 Gy) was delivered to the 70% isodose line with a single isocenter. Mean follow-up duration was 19 mo (range 12–24 mo). During this relatively short follow-up interval, 100% radiographic tumor control has been achieved (29% regressed, 71% stable, zero enlarged). Rates of delayed facial and trigeminal neuropathy were 21 and 14%, respectively, and two of three facial nerve deficits resolved. Preoperative hearing was preserved 50% of the time.

Valentino and Raimondi *(98)* reported on 23 patients treated with LINAC radiosurgery in Rome. Five of these had neurofibromatosis, and seven (30%) had undergone previous surgery. Total radiation dose to the tumor margin ranged from 12 to 45 Gy (median 30 Gy) and was delivered in one to five sessions. One or two isocenters were used, and mean duration of follow-up was 40 mo (range 24–46 mo). Results using this less conventional method of multi-session radiosurgery were comparable to those of other radiosurgical techniques. Tumor control was achieved in 96% of patients (38% regressed, 58% stable, 4% enlarged), facial and trigeminal neuropathies each occurred at a rate of 4%, and "hearing was preserved at almost the same level as that prior to radiosurgery in all patients."

The use of LINAC radiosurgery for acoustics is briefly discussed in reports by Delaney et al. *(99)* and Barcia et al. *(100)*. In addition, fractionated stereotactic radiation therapy (SRT) has been used as an alternative management for VS *(101,102)* This method is proposed as a way of exploiting the precision of stereotactic radiation delivery to minimize dose to normal brain, while employing lower fractionated doses in an effort to minimize complications. Thus far, most radiosurgeons have felt that optimal results can be achieved with highly conformal single-fraction radiosurgery, while sparing the patient the inconvenience of a prolonged treatment course.

NONACOUSTIC SCHWANNOMAS

The vast majority of intracranial schwannomas arise from the myelin sheath of the vestibular branch of the eighth cranial nerve (VS), but nonacoustic schwannomas may originate from the sheaths of cranial nerves V, VII, IX, X, or XI. These are rare skull base tumors that, like their eighth nerve counterparts, are slow growing and noninvasive but frequently problematic owing to involvement of cranial nerves and extension throughout the skull base. They also share many of the characteristics cited for vestibular schwannomas that make them well suited for radiosurgery.

The standard treatment for nonacoustic schwannomas is microsurgical resection. Various surgical approaches have been advocated, and good local control rates are commonly achieved at the expense of significant cranial nerve injuries. Because of the significant morbidity associated with extensive skull base surgery (especially if the lower cranial nerves are involved), the existence of a subset of patients (elderly or medically infirm) in whom surgery is ill advised, and the frequent incidence of incomplete resection, the quest for a safe and effective alternative therapy for these tumors is warranted. Given its success in treating the closely related acoustic schwannoma, radiosurgery seems a natural possibility. Again, Gamma Knife groups have reported success (103,104)

Mabanta et al. (105) reported on 18 patients with nonacoustic schwannomas who were treated with LINAC radiosurgery at the University of Florida. Nine of the tumors were located in the jugular foramen region, seven on the trigeminal nerve, and two on the facial nerve. Half of these patients had undergone prior subtotal resection. Mean marginal dose was 13 Gy to the 80 or 70% isodose line. During a mean follow-up interval of 32 mo, tumor control was 100% (33% regressed, 67% remained stable, no tumor enlarged). Five patients had improvement of preexisting neurologic deficits. Four complications in three patients included one exacerbation of a preexisting facial palsy, two patients with new onset hearing loss, and one with ataxia. No surgical intervention or prolonged steroid use was necessary for any patient with complications.

Meningiomas

Meningiomas are common tumors that result from proliferation of meningothelial cells. They account for approx 20% of primary brain tumors, affect predominantly middle-aged patients, and have a 2:1 predilection for females (106). Like vestibular schwannomas, they are generally noninvasive and pathologically benign and tend to behave indolently, but the natural history of any particular case is unpredictable. Clinical presentation is variable, includes seizures, hemiparesis, visual field loss, aphasia, and other focal findings, and is determined in large part by the location of the tumor (107). Successful outcomes from radiosurgical treatment of vestibular schwannomas and the encouraging results of conventional radiotherapy for meningiomas have led to enthusiasm about radiosurgery as a possible alternative treatment for meningiomas. Gamma Knife reports have appeared in the literature documenting a successful experience (108,109) (Table 3).

Engenhart et al. (110) reported the first detailed series of meningiomas treated radiosurgically. In 1990, in that series, 17 patients were treated with a LINAC-based system (the Fishersystem), to a mean marginal dose of 23 Gy. One patient died from treatment-related complications (herniation from

Table 3
Gamma Knife (GK) Series of Meningioma Cases

Parameter	Kondziolka et al. (152) Pittsburgh 1991—GK	Subach et al. (108) Pittsburgh 1998—GK (petroclival)	Lunsford et al. (153) Pittsburgh 1998—GK	Nicolato et al. (154) Verona, Italy 1996—GK (skull base)	Pendl et al. (109) Austria 1997—GK (skull base)	Steiner et al. (155) Karolinska Institute 1998—GK
No. of patients	50	62	141	50	97	151
Mean tumor volume (cc)	6	13.7 (0.8–56.8)	8.6 (0.6–20)	13.7 (0.8–82)	(1–32)	
Mean marginal dose (Gy; range)	17 (10–25)	15 (11–20)	18 (10–28)	13.8 (7–25)	14 (10–20)	
Tumor control (%)	96	87 (8 yr, benign)	95	98	96	89
Complications [no. (%)]						
Transient	3 (6)	2 (3)		2 (4)		0
Permanent	0	3 (5)		1 (2)		0

swelling 8 mo after delivery of 35 Gy to a volume of 73.6 mL in the parasellar region). Of 13/17 patients followed for a mean of 40 mo, none had evidence of tumor relapse. Unfortunately, "late, severe" side effects occurred in five patients (including one patient with a recurrent optic canal meningioma who became blind 5 mo after a dose of 35 Gy to the optic nerve). The authors felt that the treatment dose needed to be lowered to reduce complications, and the doses delivered in this early series are, in fact, much higher than currently recommended.

Valentino et al. *(111)* reported on 72 meningioma patients treated with a mean marginal dose of 37 Gy (given over one to four sessions) (Table 4). Over a mean follow-up of 48 mo, 69% of the tumors regressed and 25% remained stable in size, for a local control rate of 94%. Three patients developed transient symptoms related to increased intracranial pressure, and one additional patient was noted on follow-up imaging to have asymptomatic transient peritumoral edema.

Chang and Adler *(112)* reported on 55 patients who were treated with LINAC radiosurgery for cranial base meningiomas at Stanford. Mean marginal dose was 18 Gy (range 12–25). Over a mean follow-up of 48 mo, only one tumor enlarged, resulting in a 2-yr actuarial local control rate of 98%. Ten patients experienced mild transient neurologic compromise, and four patients (7%) suffered the following persistent effects. Symptomatic radiation necrosis developed in two patients, with seizures in one and right hemiparesis in the other. One patient acquired vagal and hypoglossal palsies, and another suffered a persistent facial paresis. This group has also reported their experience with 24 cavernous sinus meningiomas *(113)*. The mean volume treated was 6.83 cm^3 (range 0.45–22.45 cm^3), covered with an average of 2.3 isocenters (range 1–5). Radiation dose averaged 17.7 Gy (range 14–20 Gy). Follow-up averaged 45.6 mo (range 19–80 mo). Tumor control (stabilization) following radiosurgery was noted in 15 *(63%)* and tumor shrinkage in 9 *(37%)*. Neurologic status was improved in 10 patients *(42%)* and unchanged in 12 patients *(50%)*. There was one case of symptomatic brain necrosis and one case of radiation edema (asymptomatic). The 2-yr actuarial tumor control rate was 100%.

Colombo and Francescon *(114)* reported their series of 74 cranial base meningiomas as part of a larger report detailing their entire experience at the LINAC radiosurgery unit at Vicenza City Hospital in Italy. After treatment with a mean marginal dose of 22 Gy (range 18–26 Gy) and follow-up for a mean duration of 33 mo, the 8-yr actuarial tumor control rate was calculated to be 75%. Two patients suffered delayed visual field reduction after irradiation of lesions impinging on the optic chiasm.

Hakim et al. *(115)* reported results of LINAC radiosurgery for 127 meningioma patients treated by the Harvard group. Eighty-three percent of patients had previous surgery. Mean marginal dose was 15 Gy and mean follow-up duration was 31 mo. Five-year actuarial survival for the benign subgroup was 89%. Complications included two treatment-related deaths (one case of edema-induced herniation and the other death secondary to edema and hypothalamic injury), as well as one case of (expected) monocular blindness, one incidence of

Table 4
LINAC Radiosurgery for Meningiomas

Parameter	Valentino (80) Rome 1993	Chang (113) Stanford 1997	Colombo (114) Vicenza, Italy 1998	Hakim (115) Harvard 1998	U of Florida (116) 1998
No of patients	72	55	74	127	70
Mean marginal dose (Gy) (range)	37 (1–4 fractions)	18.3 (12–25)	22.3 (18–26)	15 (9–20)	12.7 (10–20)
Tumor control	94%	98% (2 yr)	75% (8yr)	89% (5 yr, benign)	100%
Complications [no (%)]					
Transient	3 (4%)	10 (18%)			2 (3%)
Permanent	0	4 (7%)	2 (3%)	4 (3%)	0

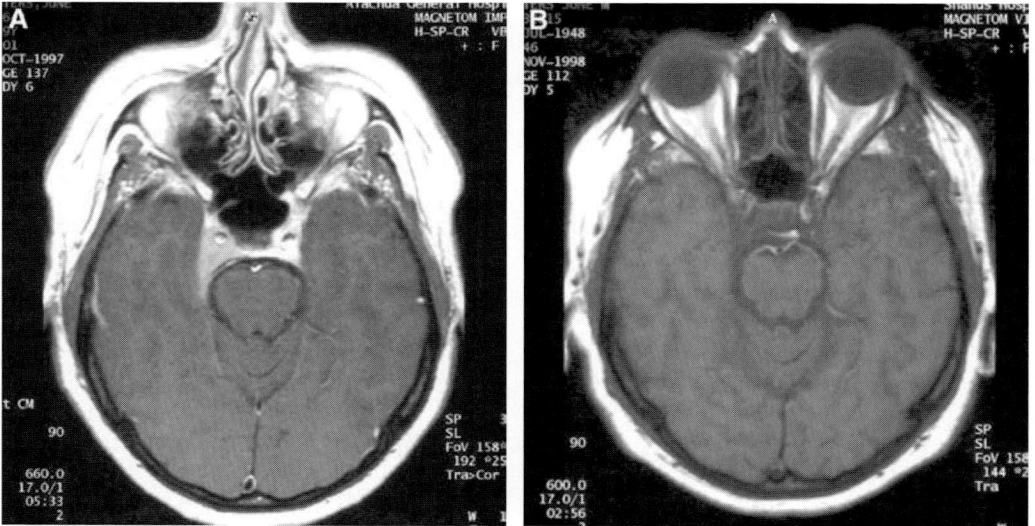

Fig. 10. (A) Enhanced MRI shows a right cavernous sinus lesion consistent with meningioma. It was treated with 12.5 Gy to the 70% isodose line, using eight isocenters. **(B)** Enhanced MRI shows the same lesion 3 yr later. The enhancement is gone and the lesion is barely visible.

delayed unilateral hearing loss, one case of left hemiparesis, and the development of leg weakness and hypoesthesia in another patient. This represents a treatment-related mortality of 1.6% and a morbidity of 3.1%.

Shafron et al. (116) reported on the University of Florida experience. The first 70 patients all followed for more than 2 yr, were analyzed. The group consisted of 54 women and 16 men. The average age was 58 (range 20–80 yr). Indications for radiosurgery were as follows: age > 60 yr (16), failed surgery (32), medical infirmity (1), and patient preference (21). One patient had undergone prior external beam radiotherapy. The mean tumor volume was 10 mL (range 0.6–29 mL), and the mean radiation dose was 12.7 Gy (range 10–20 Gy) applied to the 80% isodose line. Three isocenters (range 1–17) were used on average, and emphasis was placed on delivering dose distributions that conformed closely to the contour of the target lesion. Local control has been achieved in 100% of patients to date, with 44% of tumors displaying appreciable regression on follow-up imaging. Clinically, 7% of patients improved, 91% remained stable, and 2% had a worsening of neurological status.

Radiosurgery may well be the treatment of choice for cavernous sinus meningiomas (Fig. 10) and meningiomas in other locations where relatively high surgical morbidity may be accepted.

Radiosurgery for Malignant Tumors

Malignant tumors are radiobiologically more amenable to fractionated radiotherapy than benign lesions. Malignancies tend to infiltrate surrounding brain, resulting in poorly definable tumor margins. *A priori,* these two traits of cere-

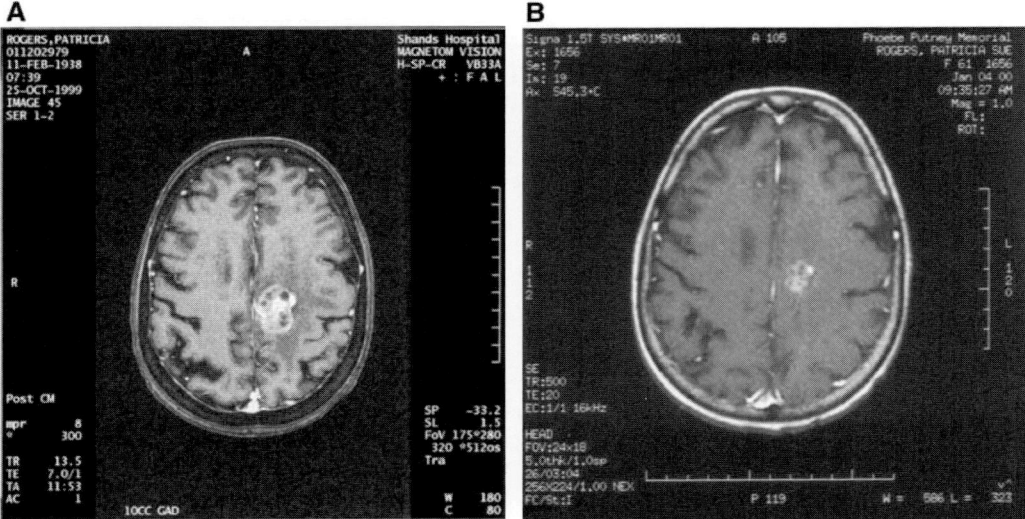

Fig. 11. (A) Enhanced MRI shows a solitary posterior left frontal metastatic brain tumor. This lesion was treated with 20 Gy to the 80% isodose line, using one isocenter. (B) Enhanced MRI shows the same lesion 9 mo later. Metastatic lesions are usually rapidly controlled with stereotactic radiosurgery.

bral malignancies would seem to make radiosurgery an unattractive treatment option. Nevertheless, SRS is proving to be a useful weapon in the armamentarium against malignant brain tumors. The most common applications of SRS to malignant tumors are the treatment of cerebral metastases and the delivery of an adjuvant focal radiation "boost" to malignant gliomas.

Cerebral Metastases

Unlike most cerebral malignancies, metastatic tumors tend to be pseudo-encapsulated, without substantial microscopic peripheral spread. This permits the use of the characteristically tight margins used in radiosurgery, without undo risk of marginal recurrence. Brain metastases also tend to be spherical and clearly delineated on gadolinium-enhanced MRI. This makes them convenient radiosurgical targets. Most importantly, a large body of literature supports the assertion that radiosurgery is a relatively inexpensive, minimally invasive, safe, and effective way to control local tumor progression and prolong survival in patients with cancers that have metastasized to the brain (Fig. 11).

Sturm et al. *(117)* published the first report on radiosurgical treatment of brain metastases in 1987. This group used a LINAC-based radiosurgery system to treat 12 patients with deep brain metastases and noted arrest of tumor growth, shrinkage of tumor, decreased enhancement, and loss of peritumoral edema in various patients. One patient, with a large posterior fossa metastasis, died shortly after treatment, but the remainder experienced no untoward side effects and a "marked, sometimes dramatic improvement of the clinical condition, beginning a few days after irradiation." The authors proposed that radiosurgery was a valuable tool in the treatment of inoperable, radioresistant brain metastases.

Since that time, many reports on LINAC and Gamma Knife radiosurgery for metastatic tumors have appeared in the literature *(118–124)*. A few of the larger series are reviewed here (Tables 5 and 6).

Alexander et al. *(125)* reported 1- and 2-yr actuarial local control rates of 85 and 65% for a series of 248 patients. The median tumor volume was 3 mL, and the median tumor dose was 15 Gy. The median survival was 9.4 mo.

A multiinstitutional analysis by Auchter et al. *(126)* retrospectively examined a group of 122 patients who had undergone SRS for single metastases. Patients were selected to match those enrolled in the earlier study of Patchell's et al. *(127)* of surgery vs surgery plus whole brain radiotherapy. Selected patients had single metastases, no prior surgery or whole body radiation therapy, age >18 yr, a surgically resectable lesion, Karnofsky performance scores ≥70, and nonradiosensitive histology. Treatment was carried out on a LINAC-based radiosurgery system, and the median dose to the tumor margin was 17 Gy (range 10–27 Gy). Nearly all patients also underwent whole body radiation therapy. Local control was 86%. Actuarial 1- and 2-yr survival was 53% and 30%.

Joseph et al. *(128)* reported on 120 patients treated with LINAC radiosurgery. Median survival was 32 wk. Patients with one or two metastases had equivalent survival times. Patients with three or more metastases had a significantly shorter survival time (14 wk). This group (Stanford) has published several other papers on this issue *(129,130)*.

Valentino et al.*(131)* reported on the treatment of 86 patients. Shrinkage or disappearance of lesions was seen in 80% of cases, but some required repeat radiosurgery. The median survival was 43 wk for patients treated with radiosurgery alone. Unpublished data from the University of Florida experience are reported in Table 2.

Malignant Gliomas

Malignant gliomas account for about 40% of the approx 17,000 new cases of primary central nervous system tumors in the United States every year, and an exceptionally high fatality rate makes their clinical impact dramatic. Glioblastoma multiforme (GBM) accounts for roughly 80% of malignant gliomas and has an annual incidence of over 5000 cases. The natural history of untreated GBM results in a median survival of 3 mo. With current standard therapy (resection plus conventional fractionated radiotherapy), median survival is typically 9–10 mo, with a 5-yr survival of about 5%. Similarly, 5-yr survival for anaplastic astrocytoma (AA) is typically under 20%.

Malignant gliomas rarely metastasize, and mortality is primarily attributed to nearly universal local failure. It has been demonstrated that more than 80% of failures occur within 2 cm of the primary tumor. Therefore, modern investigations are understandably focused on achieving local control in an attempt to improve the overall outcome in patients with malignant glioma. Various modalities, including radiation sensitizers, unconventional fractionation schemes, heavy particle radiotherapy, hyperthermia, interstitial brachytherapy,

Table 5
Gamma Knife (GK) Series: Metastatic Brain Tumors

Parameter	Kim (156) Pittsburgh GK 1997	Shiau (157) UCSF GK 1997	Rand (158) John Wayne Ca Inst GK 1995	Kida (159) Komaki, Japan GK 1995	Flickinger (160) Multi-institution GK 1994	Kihlström (161) Karolinska Inst, Sweden GK 1993
No. of patients	77 (lung cancer only)	100	63	20	116	160
No. of metastases	115	219	—	55	116	235
Local control (%)	88	77 (1 yr)	?	97	85	94
Median survival (post SRS) (mo)	10	12	?	6.4	11	7

Table 6
LINAC Radiosurgery for Metastases

Parameter	Breneman et al. (118) Cincinnati 1997	Joseph et al. (128) Stanford 1996	Alexander et al. (125) Harvard 1995	Valentino et al. (162) Rome, Italy 1995	Voges et al. (123) Germany 1994	Mehta et al. (121) Wisconsin 1992	University of Florida (116) 1998
No. of patients	84	120	248	139	46	40	166
No. of metastases	177	189	421	139	66	58	
WBRT %	96	83	100		30	100	>90%
Mean marginal dose (Gy) (range)	16 (10–22)	26.6 (10–35)	15	50 (15–80) (multi-fractions)	20 (10–25)	18.3 (12–37)	15 (10–17.5)
Local control (%)	25	96	85 (1 yr)	92	85	82	86%
Median survival (post SRS) (mo)	10	7.4	9.4	13.5	6	6.5	9.3

and stereotactic radiosurgical boost therapy have shown some promise, and continue to be investigated *(132)*.

The observation that local control and median survival can be extended through dose escalation is the basis for the application of brachytherapy and radiosurgery to malignant gliomas. Although achievable radiation doses with conventional external beam irradiation are limited by induced toxicity to around 70 Gy, the addition of a stereotactically focused boost of radiation allows total cumulative doses in excess of 100 Gy to be delivered to residual focal tumor. Brachytherapy and stereotactic radiosurgery offer similar abilities to deliver a focal radiation boost, but SRS may represent the better of the two solutions because it is noninvasive. SRS is an outpatient procedure that avoids the risks of hemorrhage, infection, and radiation exposure to personnel associated with brachytherapy.

Interpreting results of radiation boost treatments has been problematic because of the inherent selection bias toward smaller, more focal lesions. Shrieve et al. *(133)* compared radiosurgery boost and brachytherapy. Thirty-two patients were treated with brachytherapy and 86 with radiosurgery. Median survival after brachytherapy was 11.5 mo; after radiosurgery it was 10.2 mo. Fewer patients *(22%)* required reoperation after radiosurgery than after brachytherapy *(44%)*.

Mehta and colleagues *(134)* tried to eliminate selection bias using a technique called recursive-partitioning analysis (*see* next two paragraphs). They found that patients treated with radiosurgery had a 2-yr survival of 28%, when 9.7% would have been "expected."

A multicenter retrospective analysis was performed in an effort to control for prognostic factors and better evaluate the impact of SRS on the survival of patients with malignant gliomas *(135)*. The study evaluated 115 patients with malignant gliomas who were treated with a combination of surgery, external beam radiation therapy, and SRS boost at three different LINAC radiosurgery facilities under similar protocols. Patients were stratified into six prognostic classes based on the recursive partitioning analysis of multiple prognostic factors that had been previously reported by the Radiation Therapy Oncology Group (RTOG) *(136)*. This stratification is based on tumor pathology, patient age, patient's functional status (e.g., Karnofsky performance score-KPS), duration of symptoms, and extent of resection; it offers some control for the multitude of prognostic factors, allowing more direct comparison of results.

After a median follow-up of 91 wk, the 2-yr actuarial survival for the entire cohort of patients was 45%, with a median survival of 22 mo. AA patients had not reached median survival and had a 2-yr survival rate of 72%. The GBM patients had a median survival of 21 m and a 2-yr survival of 38%. When patients from the six different prognostic classes were evaluated, a significant difference in overall survival by class was confirmed ($p < 0.001$). Compared twitho published RTOG results for similarly stratified malignant glioma patients treated without a stereotactic radiation boost, radiosurgery resulted in longer median survival by 4–20 mo, depending on the prognostic class. This benefit was most pronounced for the patients in the moderate to poor prognostic classes; minimal benefit was observed for the patients in the more favorable prognostic classes. Although this strongly suggests that radiosurgical boost is advantageous for patients with GBM, little can be inferred from the study regarding the utility of SRS for AA.

Some caution is also indicated when interpreting the GBM results. RTOG results may be worse because much of the treatment was performed prior to the advent of quality neuroimaging. Also, postoperative tumor size, which was found to be highly prognostic in other studies, was not a factor in the RTOG stratification, and the average tumor size was greater for the RTOG patients compared with the SRS cohort. On univariate analysis, however, RTOG prognostic class and KPS were the only significant predictors of survival, excluding tumor size and extent of surgery among other potential factors. RTOG prognostic class was eliminated as an independent predictor of survival on multivariate analysis, leaving KPS as the only significant independent prognostic factor. In fact, patients with a KPS > 70 enjoyed a 2-yr actuarial survival rate of 51% with a median survival of 24 mo, compared with 2-yr and median survivals of 0 and 9 mo, respectively for patients with a KPS < 70. Overall, the study offers strong evidence that radiosurgical boost confers a survival advantage for patients with GBM. It also suggests that patients in poor prognostic classes (e.g., KPS < 70), who have been excluded as candidates for radiation boost in many series, actually may benefit significantly from this aggressive management.

Other Lesions

Many other brain tumors have been treated, in small numbers, by radiosurgery, including low-grade gliomas *(137,138)*, hemangioblastoma *(139,140)*, nasopharyngeal carcinomas *(141–143)*, germinoma *(144)*, medulloblastoma *(145)*, and pituitary tumors *(146)* A detailed discussion of these indications is beyond the limits of this chapter.

REFERENCES

1. Leksell L. The stereotaxic method and radiosurgery of the brain. *Acta Chir Scand* 1951;102:316–319.
2. Levy RP, Fabrikant JI, Frankel KA, et al. Charged-particle radiosurgery of the brain, in *Neurosurgical Clinics of North America: Stereotactic Surgery* (Friedman WA, ed.), WB Saunders, Philadelphia, 1990, pp. 955–990.
3. Kjellberg RN, Abbe M. Stereotactic Bragg peak proton beam therapy, in *Modern Stereotactic Neurosurgery,* 1st ed. (Lunsford LD, ed.), Martinus Nijhoff, Boston, 1988, pp. 463–470.
4. Lyman JT, Phillips MH, Frankel KA, Fabrikant JI. Stereotactic frame for neuroradiology and charged particle Bragg peak radiosurgery of intracranial disorders. *Int J Radiat Oncol Biol Phys* 1989;16:1615–1621.
5. Kjellberg RN, Kliman B. Lifetime effectiveness—a system of therapy for pituitary adenomas, emphasizing Bragg peak proton hypophysectomy, in *Recent Advances in the Diagnosis and Treatment of Pituitary Tumors* (Linfoot JA, ed.), Raven, New York, 1979, pp. 269–288.

6. Kjellberg RN, Davis KR, Lyons S, Butler W, Adams RD. Bragg peak proton beam therapy for arteriovenous malformations of the brain. *Clin Neurosurg* 1983;31:248–290.
7. Kjellberg RN, Hanamura T, Davis KR, Lyons SL, Adams RD. Bragg-peak proton-beam therapy for arteriovenous malformations of the brain. *N Engl J Med* 1983;309:269–274.
8. Munzenrider JE, Gragoudas ES, Seddon JM, et al. Conservative treatment of uveal melanoma: probability of eye retention after proton treatment. *Int J Radiat Oncol Biol Phys* 1988;15:553–558.
9. Castro JR, Linstadt DE, Bahary JP, et al. Experience in charged particle irradiation of tumors of the skull base: 1977–1992. *Int J Radiat Oncol Biol Phys* 1994;29:647–655.
10. Betti OO, Derechinsky VE. Hyperselective encephalic irradiation with a linear accelerator. *Acta Neurochir Suppl* 1984;33:385–930.
11. Colombo F, Benedetti A, Pozza F, et al. Stereotactic radiosurgery utilizing a linear accelerator. *Appl Neurophysiol* 1985;48:133–145.
12. Barrow DL, Bakay RA, Crocker I, McGinley P, Tindall GT. Stereotactic radiosurgery. *J Med Assoc Ga* 1990;79:667–676.
13. Coffey RJ, Nichols DA, Shaw EG. Stereotactic radiosurgical treatment of cerebral arteriovenous malformations. *Mayo Clin Proc* 1995;70:214–222.
14. Kooy HM, Dunbar SF, Tarbell NJ, et al. Adaptation and verification of the relocatable Gill-Thomas-Cosman frame in stereotactic radiotherapy. *Int J Radiat Oncol Biol Phys* 1994;30:685–691.
15. Kyuma Y, Hayashi A, Kitamura T, Yamashita K, Muranishi H, Hioki M. Stereotactic radiosurgery using a linear accelerator. *Neurol Med Chir* (Tokyo) 1992;32:572–577.
16. Lutz W, Winston KR, Maleki N. A system for stereotactic radiosurgery with a linear accelerator. *Int J Radiat Oncol Biol Phys* 1988;14:373–381.
17. Winston KR, Lutz W. Linear accelerator as a neurosurgical tool for stereotactic radiosurgery. *Neurosurgery* 1988;22:454–464.
18. Patil AA. Adaptation of linear accelerators to stereotactic systems, in *Modern Stereotactic Neurosurgery*, 1st ed. (Lunsford LD, ed.), Martinus Nijhoff, Boston, 1988, pp. 471–480.
19. Pastyr O, Hartmann GH, Schlegel W, et al. Stereotactically guided convergent beam irradiation with a linear accelerator: localization-technique. *Acta Neurochir* 1989;99:61–64.
20. Podgorsak EB, Olivier A, Pla M, Lefebvre PY, Hazel J. Dynamic stereotactic radiosurgery. *Int J Radiat Oncol Biol Phys* 1988;14:115–126.
21. Rocher FP, Sentenac I, Berger C, Marquis I, Romestaing P, Gerard JP. Stereotactic radiosurgery: the Lyon experience. *Acta Neurochir Suppl* 1995;63:109–114.
22. Friedman WA, Bova FJ. The University of Florida radiosurgery system. *Surg Neurol* 1989;32:334–342.
23. Friedman WA, Buatti JM, Bova FJ, et al. *LINAC Radiosurgery—A Practical Guide*. Springer-Verlag, Berlin, 1998.
24. Friedman WA, Buatti JM, Bova, FJ, et al. *LINAC Radiosurgery—A Practical Guide*. Springer-Verlag, Berlin, 1998.
25. Ellis TL, Friedman WA, Bova FJ, Kubilis PS, Buatti JM. Analysis of treatment failure after radiosurgery for arteriovenous malformations. *J Neurosurg* 1998;89:104–110.
26. Pollock BE, Flickinger JC, Lunsford LD, Maitz A, Kondziolka D. Factors associated with successful arteriovenous malformation radiosurgery. *Neurosurgery* 1998;42:1239–1244; discussion 1244–1247.

27. Bova FJ, Friedman WA. Stereotactic angiography: an inadequate database for radiosurgery? *Int J Radiat Oncol Biol Phys* 1991;20:891–895.
28. Blatt DL, Friedman WA, Bova FJ. Modifications in radiosurgical treatment planning of arteriovenous malformations based on CT imaging. *Neurosurgery* 1993;33: 588–596.
29. Spiegelmann R, Friedman WA, Bova FJ. Limitations of angiographic target localization in planning radiosurgical treatment. *Neurosurgery* 1992;30:619–624.
30. Wagner T. *Optimal Delivery Techniques for Intracranial Stereotactic Radiosurgery Using Circular and Multileaf Collimators* University of Florida, Gainesville, FL, 2000.
31. Steiner L, Leksell L, Greitz T, Forster DM, Backlund EO. Stereotaxic radiosurgery for cerebral arteriovenous malformations. Report of a case. *Acta Chir Scand* 1972; 138:459–464.
32. Steiner L, Leksell L, Forster DM, Greitz T, Backlund EO. Stereotactic radiosurgery in intracranial arterio-venous malformations. *Acta Neurochir* 1974;suppl 21:195–209.
33. Steiner L, Lindquist C, Adler JR, Torner JC, Alves W, Steiner M. Clinical outcome of radiosurgery for cerebral arteriovenous malformations. *J Neurosurg* 1992;77:1–8.
34. Steiner L. Treatment of arteriovenous malformations by radiosurgery, in *Intracranial Arteriovenous Malformations* (Wilson CB, Stein BM, eds.), Williams & Wilkins, Baltimore, 1984, pp. 295–313.
35. Steiner L. Radiosurgery in cerebral arteriovenous malformations, in *Cerebrovascular Surgery*, vol. 4 (Fein JM, Flamm ES, eds.), Springer-Verlag, New York, 1985, pp. 1161–1215.
36. Altschuler EM, Lunsford LD, Coffey RJ, Bissonette DJ, Flickinger JC. Gamma knife radiosurgery for intracranial arteriovenous malformations in childhood and adolescence. *Pediatr Neurosci* 1989;15:53–61.
37. Coffey RJ, Lunsford LD, Bissonette D, Flickinger JC. Stereotactic gamma radiosurgery for intracranial vascular malformations and tumors: report of the initial North American experience in 331 patients. *Acta Chir Scand* 1990;54–55:535–540.
38. Duma ChM, Lunsford LD, Kondziolka D, Bissonette DJ, Flickinger JC. Radiosurgery for vascular malformations of the brain stem. *Acta Neurochir* 1993;58:92–97.
39. Hadjipanayis CG, Levy EI, Niranjan A, et al. Stereotactic radiosurgery for motor cortex region arteriovenous malformations. *Neurosurgery* 2001;48:70–77.
40. Kemeny AA, Dias PS, Forster DM. Results of stereotactic radiosurgery of arteriovenous malformations: an analysis of 52 cases. *J Neurol Neurosurg Psychiatry* 1989; 52:554–558.
41. Kurita H, Kawamoto S, Sasaki T, et al. Results of radiosurgery for brain stem arteriovenous malformations. *J Neurol Neurosurg Psychiatry* 2000;68:563–570.
42. Levy EI, Niranjan A, Thompson TP, et al. Radiosurgery for childhood intrcranial arteriovenous malformation. *Neurosurgery* 2000;47:834–842.
43. Lindquist C, Steiner L. Stereotactic radiosurgical treatment of malformations of the brain, in *Modern Stereotactic Neurosurgery*, 1st ed. (Lunsford LD, ed.), Martinus Nijhoff, Boston, 1988, pp. 491–506.
44. Lindquist M, Karlsson B, Guo W-Y, Kihlstrom, Lippitz B, Yamamoto M. Angiographic long-term followup data for arteriovenous malformations previously proven to be obliterated after gamma knife radiosurgery. *Neurosurgery* 2000;46: 803–810.
45. Lunsford LD. Treatment of arteriovenous malformations by radiosurgery, in *Neurosurgical Topics: Intracranial Vascular Malformations* (Barrow DL, ed.), AANS, Park Ridge, IL, 1990, pp. 179–196.
46. Lunsford LD, Flickinger JC, Coffey RJ. Stereotactic gamma knife radiosurgery. Initial North American experience in 207 patients. *Arch Neurol* 1990;47:169–175.

47. Lunsford LD, Kondziolka D, Flickinger JC, et al. Stereotactic radiosurgery for arteriovenous malformations of the brain. *J Neurosurg* 1991;75:512–524.
48. Massager N, Regis J, Kondziolka D, Njee T, Levivier M. Gamma knife radiosurgery for brainstem arteriovenous malformations: preliminary results. *J Neurosurg* 2000; 93(suppl 3):102–103.
49. Pan DH-C, Guo W-Y, Chung W-Y, Shiau C-Y, Chang Y-C, Wang L-W. Gamma knife radiosurgery as a single treatment modality for large cerebral arteriovenous malformations. *J Neurosurg* 2000;(suppl 3):113–119.
50. Pollock BE, Lunsford LD, Kondziolka D, Maitz A, Flickinger JC. Patient outcomes after stereotactic radiosurgery for "operable" arteriovenous malformations. *Neurosurgery* 1994;35:1–8.
51. Fabrikant JI, Levy RP, Steinberg GK, Phillips MH, Frankel KA, Silverberg GD. Stereotactic charged-particle radiosurgery: clinical results of treatment of 1200 patients with intracranial arteriovenous malformations and pituitary disorders. *Clin Neurosurg* 1992;38:472–492.
52. Fabrikant JI, Lyman JT, Frankel KA. Heavy charged-particle Bragg peak radiosurgery for intracranial vascular disorders. *Radiat Res Suppl.* 1985;104:S244–S258.
53. Fabrikant JI, Lyman JT, Hosobuchi Y. Stereotactic heavy-ion Bragg peak radiosurgery for intra-cranial vascular disorders: method for treatment of deep arteriovenous malformations. *Br J Radiol* 1984;57:479–490.
54. Griffin BR, Warcola SH, Mayberg MR, Eenmaa J, Eskridge J, Winn HR. Stereotactic neutron radiosurgery for arteriovenous malformations of the brain. *Med Dosim* 1988;13:179–182.
55. Hosobuchi Y, Fabrikant JI, Lyman JT. Stereotactic heavy-particle irradiation of intracranial arteriovenous malformations. *Appl Neurophysiol* 1987;50:248–252.
56. Kjellberg RN. Stereotactic Bragg peak proton beam radiosurgery for cerebral arteriovenous malformations. *Ann Clin Res* 1986;18(suppl 47):17–19.
57. Kjellberg RN. Proton beam therapy for arteriovenous malformations of the brain, in *Operative Neurosurgical Techniques: Indications, Methods, and Results* 2nd ed. (Schmidek HH, Sweet WH, eds.), Grune & Stratton, Orlando, 1988, pp. 911–914.
58. Kjellberg RN, Davis KR, Lyons S, Butler W, Adams RD. Bragg peak proton beam therapy for arteriovenous malformations of the brain. *Clin Neurosurg* 1983;31: 248–290.
59. Kjellberg RN, Hanamura T, Davis KR, Lyons SL, Adams RD. Bragg-peak proton-beam therapy for arteriovenous malformations of the brain. *N Engl J Med* 1983;309: 269–274.
60. Kjellberg RN, Poletti CE, Roberson GH, Adams RD. Bragg-peak proton beam treatment of arteriovenous malformation of the brain. *Exc Med* 1977;433:181–186.
61. Levy RP, Fabrikant JI, Frankel KA, Phillips MH, Lyman JT. Stereotactic heavy-charged-particle Bragg peak radiosurgery for the treatment of intracranial arteriovenous malformations in childhood and adolescence. *Neurosurgery* 1989;24: 841–852.
62. Seifert V, Stolke D, Mehdorn HM, Hoffmann B. Clinical and radiological evaluation of long-term results of stereotactic proton beam radiosurgery in patients with cerebral arteriovneous malformations. *J Neurosurg* 1994;81:683–689.
63. Steinberg GK, Fabrikant JI, Marks MP, et al. Stereotactic heavy-charged particle Bragg peak radiation for intracranial arteriovenous malformations. *N Engl J Med* 1990;323:96–101.
64. Stelzer K, Griffin B, Eskridge J, et al. Results of neutron radiosurgery for inoperable arteriovenous malformations of the brain. *Med Dosim* 1992;16:137–141.

65. Betti OO. Treatment of arteriovenous malformations with the linear accelerator. *Appl Neurophysiol* 1987;50:262.
66. Betti OO, Munari C, Rosler R. Stereotactic radiosurgery with the linear accelerator: treatment of arteriovenous malformations. *Neurosurgery* 1989;24:311–321.
67. Colombo F, Benedetti A, Casentini L, Zanusso M, Pozza F. Linear accelerator radiosurgery of arteriovenous malformations. *Appl Neurophysiol* 1987;50:257–261.
68. Colombo F, Benedetti A, Pozza F, Marchetti C, Chierego G. Linear accelerator radiosurgery of cerebral arteriovenous malformations. *Neurosurgery* 1989;24:833–840.
69. Colombo F, Pozza F, Chierego G, Casentini L, De Luca G, Francescon P. Linear accelerator radiosurgery of cerebral arteriovenous malformations: an update. *Neurosurgery* 1994;34:14–21.
70. Croft MJ. Stereotactic radiosurgery of arteriovenous malformations. *Radiol Technol* 1990;61:375–379.
71. Friedman WA, Bova FJ. LINAC radiosurgery for arteriovenous malformations. *J Neurosurg* 1992;77:832–841.
72. Friedman WA, Bova FJ. Radiosurgery for arteriovenous malformations, in *Current Medicine* (Salcman M, ed.), Current Medicine, Philadelphia, 1993, pp. 1–14.
73. Friedman WA, Bova FJ. The University of Florida radiosurgery system. *Surg Neurol* 1989;32:334–342.
74. Friedman WA, Bova FJ, Mendenhall W. Linear accelerator radiosurgery for arteriovenous malformations: the relationship of size to outcome. *J Neurosurg* 1995;82:180–189.
75. Loeffler JS, Alexander EI, Siddon RL, Saunders WM, Coleman CN, Winston KR. Stereotactic radiosurgery for intracranial arteriovenous malformations using a standard linear accelerator. *Int J Radiat Oncol Biol Phys* 1989;17:673–677.
76. Saunders WM, Winston KR, Siddon RL, et al. Radiosurgery for arteriovenous malformations of the brain using a standard linear accelerator: rationale and technique. *Int J Radiat Oncol Biol Phys* 1988;15:441–447.
77. Schlienger M, Atlan D, Lefkopoulos D, et al. LINAC radiosurgery for cerebral arteriovenous malformations. *Int J Radiat Oncol Biol Phys* 2000;46:1135–1142.
78. Souhami L, Olivier A, Podgorsak EB, Hazel J, Pla M, Tampieri D. Dynamic stereotactic radiosurgery in arteriovenous malformation. Preliminary treatment results. *Cancer* 1990;66:15–20.
79. Souhami L, Olivier A, Podgorsak EB, Pla M, Pike GB. Radiosurgery of cerebral arteriovenous malformations with the dynamic stereotactic irradiation. *Int J Radiat Oncol Biol Phys* 1990;19:775–782.
80. Valentino V. Radiosurgery in cerebral tumours and AVM. *Acta Neurochir Suppl* 1988;42:193–197.
81. Young CS, Schwartz ML, O'Brien P, Ramaseshan R. Stereotactic radiotherapy for AVMs: the University of Toronto Experience. *Acta Neurochir Suppl* 1995;63:57–59.
82. Young C, Summerfield R, Schwartz M, O'Brien P, Ramani R. Radiosurgery for arteriovenous malformations: the University of Toronto experience. *Can J Neurol Sci* 1997;24:99–105.
83. Yamamoto M, Jimbo M, Hara M, Saito I, Mori K. Gamma knife radiosurgery for arteriovenous malformations: long-term follow-up results focusing on complications occurring more than 5 years after irradiation. *Neurosurgery* 1996;38:906–914.
84. Pollock BE, Flickinger JC, Lunsford LD, Bissonette DJ, Kondziolka D. Factors that predict the bleeding risk of cerebral arteriovenous malformations. *Str* 1996;27:1–6.
85. Karlsson B, Lax I, Soderman M. Risk for hemorrhage during the 2-year latency period following gamma knife radiosurgery for arteriovenous malformations. *Int J Radiat Oncol Biol Phys* 2001:1045–1051.

86. Friedman WA, Blatt DL, Bova FJ, Buatti JM, Mendenhall WM, Kubilis PS. The risk of hemorrhage after radiosurgery for arteriovenous malformations. *J Neurosurg* 1996;84:912–919.
87. Kondziolka D, McLaughlin MR. Simple risk predictions for arteriovenous malformation hemorrhage. *Neurosurgery* 1995;37:851–855.
88. Sekhar LN, Swamy KS, Jaiswal V. Surgical excision of meningiomas involving the clivus: preoperative and intraoperative features as predictors of postoperative functional deterioration. *J Neurosurg* 1994;81:860.
89. Sekhar LN, Altschuler EM. Meningiomas of the cavernous sinus, in *Meningiomas* (Al-Mefty O, ed.), Raven, New York 1991, pp. 445–460.
90. Leksell L. A note on the treatment of acoustic tumors. *Acta Chir Scand* 1971;137:763–765.
91. Pollock BE, Lunsford LD, Kondziolka D, et al. Outcome analysis of acoustic neuroma management: a comparison of microsurgery and stereotactic radiosurgery. *Neurosurgery* 1995;36:215–229.
92. Mendenhall WM, Friedman WA, Bova FJ. LINAC-based stereotactic radiosurgery for acoustic schwannomas. *Int J Radiat Oncol Biol Phys* 1994;28:803–810.
93. Mendenhall WM, Friedman WA, Buatti JM, Bova FJ. Preliminary results of linear accelerator radiosurgery for acoustic schwannoma. *J Neurosurg* 1996;85:1013–1019.
94. Foote KD, Friedman WA, Buatti JM, Meeks SL, Bova FJ, Kubilis PS. Analysis of risk factors associated with radiosurgery for vestibular schwannoma. *J Neurosurg* 2001;95:440–449.
95. Spiegelmann R, Gofman J, Alezra D, Pfeffer R. Radiosurgery for acoustic neurinomas (vestibular schwannomas). *Isr Med Assoc J* 1999;1:8–13.
96. Spiegelmann R, Lidar Z, Gofman J, Alezra D, Hadani M, Pfeffer R. Linear accelerator radiosurgery for vestibular schwannoma. J Neurosurg 2001;94:7–13.
97. Martens F, Verbeke L, Piessens M, Van Vyve M. Stereotactic radiosurgery of vestibular schwannomas with a linear accelerator. *Acta Neurochir* 1994;62(suppl):88–92.
98. Valentino V, Raimondi AJ. Tumour response and morphological changes of acoustic neurinomas after radiosurgery. *Acta Neurochir* 1995;133:157–163.
99. Delaney G, Matheson J, Smee R. Stereotactic radiosurgery: an alternative approach to the management of acoustic neuromas. *Med J Austral* 1992;156:440.
100. Barcia Salorio JL, Hernandez G, Ciudad J, Bordes V, Broseta J. Stereotactic radiosurgery in acoustic neurinoma. *Acta Neurochir Suppl* 1984;33:373–376.
101. Andrews DW, Suarez O, Goldman HW, et al. Stereotactic radiosurgery and fractionated stereotactic radiotherapy for the treatment of acoustic schwannomas: comparative observations of 125 patients treated at one institution. *Int J Radiat Oncol Biol Phys* 2001;50:1265–1278.
102. Bush DA, McAllister CJ, Loredo LN, Johnson WD, Slater JM, Slater JD. Fractionated proton beam radiotherapy for acoustic neuroma. *Neurosurgery* 2002;50:270–275.
103. Kida Y, Kobayashi T, Tanaka T. Radiosurgery of trigeminal neuroma, in *Radiosurgery 1997* (Kondziolka D, ed.), Karger, Basel, 1998, pp. 8–15.
104. Pollock BE, Kondziolka D, Flickinger JC, Maitz A, Lunsford LD. Preservation of cranial nerve function after radiosurgery for nonacoustic schwannomas. *Neurosurgery* 1993;33:597–601.
105. Mabanta SR, Buatti JM, Friedman WA, et al. Linear accelerator radiosurgery for nonacoustic schwannomas. *Int J Radiat Onol Biol hys* 1999;43:545–548.
106. McDermott MW, Wilson CB. Meningiomas, in *Neurological Surgery: A Comprehensive Reference Guide to the Diagnosis and Management of Neurosurgical Problems*, 4th ed. (Youmans JR, ed.), WB Saunders, Philadelphia, 1996, pp. 2782–2825.

107. Black PM. Meningiomas. *Neurosurgery* 1993;32:643–657.
108. Subach BR, Lunsford LD, Kondziolka D, Maitz AH, Flickinger JC. Management of petroclival meningiomas by stereotactic radiosurgery. *Neurosurgery* 1998;42:437–445.
109. Pendl G, Schrottner O, Eustacchio S, Feichtinger K, Ganz J. Stereotactic radiosurgery of skull base meningiomas. *Minim Invasive Neurosurg* 1997;40:87–90.
110. Engenhart R, Kimmig BN, Hover KH, et al. Stereotactic single high dose radiation therapy of benign intracranial meningiomas. *Int J Radiat Oncol Biol Phys* 1990;19:1021–1026.
111. Valentino V, Schinaia G, Raimondi AJ. The results of radiosurgical management of 72 middle fossa meningiomas. *Acta Neurochir* 1993;122:60–70.
112. Chang SD, Adler JR. Treatment of cranial base meningiomas with linear accelerator radiosurgery. *Neurosurgery* 1997;41:1019–1027.
113. Chang SD, Adler JR Jr, Martin DP. LINAC radiosurgery for cavernous sinus meningiomas. *Stereotact Funct Neurosurg* 1998;71:43–50.
114. Colombo F, Francescon P. Clinical linear accelerator radiosurgery, in *Textbook of Stereotactic and Functional Neurosurgery* (Gildenberg PL, Tasker RR, eds.), McGraw-Hill, New York, 1998, pp. 757–762.
115. Hakim R, Alexander III E, Loeffler JS, et al. Results of linear accelerator-based radiosurgery for inracranial meningiomas. *Neurosurgery* 1998;42:446–454.
116. Shafron DH, Friedman WA, Buatti JM, et al. LINAC radiosurgery for benign meningiomas. *Int J. Radiat Oncol Biol Phys* 1999;43:321–327.
117. Sturm V, Kober B, Hover KH, et al. Stereotactic percutaneous single dose irradiation of brain metastases with a linear accelerator. *Int J Radiat Oncol Biol Phys* 1987;13:279–282.
118. Breneman JC, Warnick RE, Albright RE, et al. Stereotactic radiosurgery for the treatment of brain metastases. *Cancer* 1997;79:551–557.
119. Caron J-L, Souhami L, Podgordak EB. Dynamic stereotactic radiosurgery in the palliative treatment of cerebral metastatic tumors. *J Neurooncol* 1992;12:173–179.
120. Mehta M, Noyes W, Craig B, et al. A cost-effectiveness and cost-utility analysis of radiosurgery vs. resection for single-brain metastases. *Int J Radiat Oncol Biol Phys* 1997;39:445–454.
121. Mehta MP. Radiosurgery of malignant brain tumors, in *Minimally Invasive Therapy of the Brain* (De Salles AAF, Lufkin RB, eds.), Thieme, New York, 1997, pp. 213–224.
122. Mehta MP, Rozental JM, Levin AB, et al. Defining the role of radiosurgery in the management of brain metastases. *Int J Radiat Oncol Biol Phys* 1992;24:619–625.
123. Voges J, Treuer H, Erdmann J, Schlegel W, Pastyr O, Müller RP, Sturm V. LINAC radiosurgery in brain metastases. *Acta Neurochir* 1994;62(suppl):72–76.
124. Buatti JM, Friedman WA, Bova FJ, Mendenhall WM. Treatment selection factors for stereotactic radiosurgery of intracranial metastases. *Int J Radiat Oncol Biol Phys* 1995;32:1161–1166.
125. Alexander E, Moriarty TM, Davis RB, et al. Stereotactic radiosurgery for the definitive, noninvasive treatment of brain metastases. *J Natl Cancer Inst* 1995;87:34–40.
126. Auchter RM, Lamond JP, Alexander E, et al. A multiinstitutional outcome and prognostic factor analysis of radiosurgery for resectable single brain metastasis. *Int J Radiat Oncol Biol Phys* 1996;35:27–35.
127. Patchell RA, Tibbs PA, Walsh JW, et al. A randomized trial of surgery in the treatment of single metastases to the brain. *N Engl J Med* 1990;322:494–500.
128. Joseph J, Adler JR, Cox RS, Hancock SL. Linear accelerator-based stereotaxic radisourgery for brain metastases: the influence of number of lesions on survival. *J Clin Oncol* 1996;14:1085–1092.

129. Adler JR, Cox RS, Kaplan I, Martin DP. Stereotactic radiosurgical treatment of brain metastases. *J Neurosurg* 1992;76:444–449.
130. Fuller BG, Kaplan ID, Adler J, Cox RS, Bagshaw MA. Stereotaxic radiosurgery for brain metastases: The importance of adjuvant whole brain irradiation. *Int J Radiat Oncol Biol Phys* 1992;23:413–418.
131. Valentino V, Mirri MA, Schinaia G, Ore GD. Linear accelerator and Greitz-Bergstrom's head fixation system in radiosurgery of single cerebral metastases. A report of 86 cases. *Acta Neurochir* 1993;121:140–145.
132. Colombo F, Pozza F, Chierego G, Casentini L, De Luca G, Francescon P. Linear accelerator radiosurgery of cerebral arteriovenous malformations: an update. *Neurosurgery* 1994;34:14–21.
133. Shrieve DC, Alexander E, Wen PY, et al. Comparison of stereotactic radiosurgery and brachytherapy in the treatment of recurrent glioblastoma multiforme. *Neurosurgery* 1995;36:275–284.
134. Mehta MP, Masciopinto J, Rozental J, et al. Stereotactic radiosurgery for glioblastoma multiforme: report of a prospective study evaluating prognostic factors and analyzing long-term survival advantage. *Int J Radiat Oncol Biol Phys* 1994;30:541–549.
135. Sarkaria JN, Mehta MP, Loeffler JS, et al. Radiosurgery in the initial management of malignant gliomas: survival comparison with the RTOG recursive partitioning analysis. *Int J Radiat Oncol Biol Phys* 1995;32:931–941.
136. Curran WJ, Scott CB, Horton J, et al. Recursive partitioning analysis of prognostic factors in three Radiation Therapy Oncology Group malignant glioma trials. *J Natl Cancer Inst* 1993;85:704–710.
137. Hodgson DC, Goumnerova LC, Loeffler JS, et al. Radiosurgery in the management of pediatric brain tumors. *Int J Radiat Oncol Biol Phys* 2001;50:929–935.
138. Souhami L, Olivier A, Podgorsak EB, Villemure J, Pla M, Sadikot AF. Fractionated stereotactic radiation therapy for intracranial tumors. *Cancer* 1991;68:2101–2108.
139. Chandler HC, Friedman WA. Radiosurgical treatment of a hemangioblastoma. *Neurosurgery* 1994;34:353–355.
140. Patrice SJ, Sneed PK, Flickinger JC, Shrieve DC, et al. Radiosurgery for hemangioblastoma: results of a multiinstitutional experience. *Int J Radiat Oncol Biol Phys* 1996;35:493–499.
141. Buatti JM, Friedman WA, Bova FJ, Mendenhall WM. LINAC radiosurgery for locally recurrent nasopharyngeal carcinoma: rationale and technique. *Head Neck* 1995;17:14–19.
142. Cmelak AJ, Cox RS, Adler JR, Fee WE, Goffinet DR. Radiosurgery for skull base malignancies and nasopharyngeal carcinoma. *Int J Radiat Oncol Biol Phys* 1997;37: 997–1003.
143. Kaplan ID, Adler JR, Hicks WL, Fee WE, Goffinet DR. Radiosurgery for palliation of base of skull recurrences from head and neck cancers. *Cancer* 1992;70:1980–1984.
144. Casentini L, Colombo F, Pozza F, Benedetti A. Combined radiosurgery and external radiotherapy of intracranial germinomas. *Surg Neurol* 1990;34:79–86.
145. Patrice SJ, Tarbell NJ, Goumnerova LC, Shrieve DC, Black PM, Loeffler JS. Results of radiosurgery in the management of recurrent and residual medulloblastoma. *Pediatr Neurosurg* 1995;22:197–203.
146. Voges J, Sturm V, Deub U, et al. LINAC-radiosurgery in pituitary adenomas: preliminary results. *Acta Neurochir Suppl* 1996;65:41–43.
147. Noren G, Greitz D, Hirsch A, Lax I. Gamma knife surgery in acoustic tumours. *Acta Neurochir* 1993;(suppl 58):104–107.
148. Norén G. Gamma knife radiosurgery for acoustic neurinomas, in *Textbook of Stereotactic and Functional Neurosurgery* (Gildenberg PL, Tasker RR, eds.), McGraw-Hill, New York, 1998, pp. 835–844.

149. Flickinger JC, Kondziolka D, Pollock BE, Lunsford LD. Radiosurgical management of intracranial vascular malformations. *Neuroimaging Clin N Am* 1998;8:483–492.
150. Kondziolka D, Lunsford LD, McLaughlin MR, Flickinger JC. Long-term outcomes after radiosurgery for acoustic neuromas. *N Engl J Med* 1998;339:1426–1433.
151. Prasad D, Steiner M, Steiner L. Gamma surgery for vestibular schwannoma. *J Neurosurg* 2000;92:745–759.
152. Kondziolka D, Lunsford LD, Coffey RJ, Flickinger JC. Stereotactic radiosurgery of meningiomas. *J Neurosurg* 1991;74:552–559.
153. Flickinger JC, Kondziolka D, Lunsford LD. Clinical applications of stereotactic radiosurgery. *Cancer Treat Res* 1998;93:283–297.
154. Nicolato A, Ferraresi P, Foroni R, et al. Gamma knife radiosurgery in skull base meningiomas. *Stereotact Funct Neurosurg* 1996;66:112–120.
155. Steiner L, Prasad D, Lindquist C, et al. Clinical aspects of gamma knife stereotactic radiosurgery, in *Textbook of Stereotactic and Functional Neurosurgery* (Gildenberg PL, Tasker RR, eds.), McGraw-Hill, New York, 1998, pp. 763–803.
156. Kim YS, Kondziolka D, Flickinger JC, Lunsford LD. Stereotactic radiosurgery for patients with nonsmall cell lung carcinoma metastatic to the brain. *Cancer* 1997;80:2075–2083.
157. Shiau C-Y, Sneed PK, Shu H-KG, et al. Radiosurgery for brain metastases: Relationship of dose and pattern of enhancement to local control. *Int J Radiat Oncol Biol Phys* 1997;37:375–383.
158. Rand RW, Jacques DB, Melbye RW, Copcutt BG, Irwin L. Gamma knife radiosurgery for metastatic brain tumors. *Acta Neurochir* 1995;63(suppl):85–88.
159. Kida Y, Kobayashi T, Tanaka T. Radiosurgery of the metastatic brain tumours with gamma-knife. *Acta Neurochir* 1995;63(suppl):89–94.
160. Flickinger JC, Kondziolka D, Lunsford LD, Coffey RJ, et al. A multi-institutional experience with stereotactic radiosurgery for solitary brain metastasis. *Int J Radiat Oncol Biol Phys* 1994;28:797–802.
161. Kihlström L, Karlsson B, Lindquist C. Gamma knife surgery for cerebral metastases. Implications for survival based on 16 years experience. *Stereotact Funct Neurosurg* 1993;61(suppl):45–50.
162. Valentino V. The results of radiosurgical management of 139 single cerebral metastases. *Acta Neurochir Suppl* 1995;63:95–100.

12
MRI-Guided Thermal Therapy for Brain Tumors

Ferenc A. Jolesz, MD and Ion-Florin Talos, MD

INTRODUCTION

Although the thermal therapy methods (interstitial laser therapy, radiofrequency therapy, and focused ultrasound therapy) are still in the experimental stage, mainly because of difficulties in accurately monitoring tissue temperature changes, they may develop into a minimally invasive alternative to open skull surgery for some brain tumors in the foreseeable future (1,2).

There is compelling physical and biological evidence that localized high-temperature thermal therapy is effective. If any tissue is heated beyond 57–60°C, protein denaturation and subsequent coagulation necrosis occurs. The thermal treatment results in irreversible cell damage in both normal and neoplastic tissues. Thermal energy is not selective, and both normal and neoplastic tissue is coagulated; therefore thermal ablation above the critical temperature is analogous to surgery and not to hyperthermia, which is performed around 41–42°C (3,4).

The magnitude and spatial distribution of temperature changes in the tissue depends on both the delivery parameters (i.e., intensity, duration) and the tissue properties, such as absorption, perfusion, and flow.

Optical characteristics and heat conductivity are variable even among tumors of the same grading (5). Both vascular distribution pattern and tissue perfusion rate have an influence on the spatial distribution of energy delivery and consequently on the volume of tissue affected by the treatment (6). Because of variable tissue properties, the outcome of such a treatment is difficult to predict.

The use of optical fibers for interstitial laser therapy (ILT) and the medical application of radiofrequency (RF) and microwave devices significantly advanced the ablation field by allowing percutaneous treatment. These are probe-delivered minimally invasive targeted heat deposition methods. Currently, high-energy focused ultrasound (HIFU) is a noninvasive extracorporeal alternative (1).

Thermal ablation methods have been known for decades, but their broader acceptance was restricted because of the lack of real-time volumetric "closed-

From: *Minimally Invasive Neurosurgery,* edited by: M.R. Proctor and P.M. Black © Humana Press Inc., Totowa, NJ

loop" feedback control of energy deposition. Without control of thermal energy spread in the tissue, safe and efficient thermal therapy cannot be carried out. This is especially true in the brain where not only is it important to achieve complete tumor treatment but injury of critical normal structures should be avoided.

Clinically applicable thermal coagulation has to be limited to the target volume and should not damage the surrounding normal tissue. This can be achieved by defining the exact 3D extent of the targeted tissue volume and the extent of heating within and outside the targeted tissue volume. Image guidance and image-guided therapy delivery control is necessary for thermal ablation of tumors. Accurate spatial and temporal temperature control is essential in the brain, where thermal damage must be limited to the target, especially if the targeted volume is close to critical structures (7).

MRI-BASED CONTROL OF ENERGY DELIVERY

With the introduction of magnetic resonance imaging (MRI) as a monitoring method for thermal therapies, a novel mechanism for controlling energy deposition became available (8). It was recognized that many MRI parameters are sensitive to temperature changes, which makes MRI suitable for monitoring thermal ablations by noninvasive means. Furthermore, one can take advantage of diffusion MRI, which detects changes in water mobility and compartmentalization, to identify reversible as well as irreversible thermally induced tissue changes (9,10). It became obvious, however, that MRI monitoring of thermal ablation is only feasible if the imaging and therapy delivering systems are integrated (2).

Most endogenous MRI parameters are temperature sensitive. The most commonly used parameters for temperature monitoring have been T1 (8,11–13), the diffusion coefficient (14,15), and the water proton resonant frequency (PRF) (16,17).

Having the highest temperature sensitivity and being independent of tissue type, the PRF method has been the most promising (18). However, it has the disadvantage of being very sensitive to movement.

The role of MRI during thermal ablations is to monitor temperature levels, to restrict the thermal coagulation to the targeted tissue volume, and to avoid heating of normal tissue. MRI can also detect irreversible tissue necrosis and demonstrate permanent changes within the treated tissue. Physiologic effects such as perfusion or metabolic response to elevated temperature can also be used for monitoring the ablation. Both flow and tissue perfusion can affect the rate and extent of energy delivery and the size of the treated tissue volumes (3). Monitoring can optimize treatment protocols.

Thus far, three approaches have been proposed for using MRI monitoring of thermal therapies: temperature threshold, thermal dose control, and imaging control. In the temperature control approach, the temperature threshold necessary to induce tissue damage is empirically determined from animal experiments and clinical experience. In some studies, temperature thresholds measured by MRI were used as indicators of tissue necrosis during thermal therapies *(19,20)*. Although there is a good correlation between temperature and tissue necrosis, experimental studies have shown that the exposure time also plays a significant role in achieving tissue damage.

In addition to temperature, the thermal dose approach also takes into account the exposure time. The thermal dose is a nonlinear function of the temperature and exposure time. This method is mainly indicated for monitoring thermal therapies that employ long heating times at constant temperatures *(4,21)*.

Whereas the temperature threshold method is useful, especially when the heating profile has the same shape and size, the dosimetry method is thought to be independent of these parameters. Control systems based on temperature threshold and thermal dosimetry have been described in *(22–24)*.

The third approach—imaging control—is based on T2- or T1- acquisitions with or without contrast agent during energy delivery *(13,25)*. The evolving lesions appear to correlate well or slightly underestimate the final lesion size. However, the specificity of this method may be too low in some cases, and differentiating between thermal lesion and viable tumor tissue/peritumoral edema is not always possible *(26)*.

Since thermal lesions may become visible on MRI with certain delays, this can result in underestimation of the extent of the thermal lesion.

INTERSTITIAL LASER THERAPY

ILT is a minimally invasive, high-temperature ablative technique designed for localized tumor tissue coagulation. The laser energy is delivered through optical fibers implanted interstitially. The treated volume "per fiber" is limited owing to the small penetration depth of the laser. Its extent also depends on the fiber tip, laser wavelength, and optical properties of the target tissue. The latter are highly variable even among tumors with the same histological grading *(5)* and also change during therapy. The difficulty presented by a limited treatment volume per fiber can be addressed by using multiple optical fibers or specially designed diffusing tips.

The laser-induced tissue damage follows a typical pattern, with a central necrosis zone and a shapely demarcated, reversible edema zone at the tumor periphery, containing viable tumor cells that represent the origin of recurrent tumor growth after treatment *(27,28)*. An effective method for separating the reversible and irreversible changes areas has still to be developed.

Since the original description of MRI monitoring and control of laser–tissue interactions *(8)*, MRI-guided tissue ablation has become a clinically tested and accepted minimally invasive treatment option. It is a relatively simple straightforward method, which can be well adapted to the interventional MRI environment.

After the original publication by Jolesz et al. *(8)*, Ascher et al. *(29)* performed the first ILT treatment under MRI. Later, this approach was further developed by Bettag et al. *(28)*, Kahn et al. *(30,31)*, and Jolesz et al. *(32–34)*.

Despite these early trials, the role of ILT as a therapeutic alternative for brain tumors has yet to be established. There are preliminary reports in the literature on this subject (5,30,35–37). All showed a low incidence of postoperative morbidity and no mortality. However, transient neurologic deficits are not uncommon in the early postoperative period due to perifocal edema, although full recovery is expected within a few weeks. One study also reported permanent neurologic deficits in glioblastoma patients, in whom administration of high-energy doses was attempted (36). Overall, these early results suggest that ILT is a safe therapy method. Although no definitive conclusion can be drawn based on the currently available data, it appears that ILT can be of benefit in patients with low-grade gliomas. In malignant gliomas, thermal therapy has been essentially unsuccessful, a predictable outcome, since such tumors extend far beyond the area of MRI contrast enhancement.

FOCUSED ULTRASOUND THERAPY

Among the currently developed thermal therapy methods, focused ultrasound (FUS) appears to be the most promising, since its use does not require any invasive intervention. The potential therapeutic use of ultrasound energy for intracranial pathology has long been acknowledged (38). There is no more convincing example for the FUS benefits than in the brain, where deep lesions can be induced without any associated damage along the path of the acoustic beam. In the brain, where most injuries have detectable functional consequences, it is extremely important to limit tissue damage to the targeted area. This necessitates the use of an imaging technique for localization, targeting, and real-time intraoperative monitoring and to control the spatial extent and intensity of the deposited energy.

MRI can be used for targeted and controlled image-guided FUS procedures. It can provide detection of tumor margins, functional mapping of the surrounding cortex, definition of the adjacent fiber tracts, and temperature-sensitive imaging during sonications. High resolution anatomic imaging and flow-, perfusion-, and diffusion-sensitive MRI methods are used for planning the procedures, and temperature-sensitive methods are used to monitor and control energy deposition. By combining FUS with MRI-based guidance and control, it may be possible to achieve complete tumor ablation without any associated structural injury or functional deficit.

Beyond thermal coagulation of tissue, FUS has various other effects that can be therapeutically exploited and thus open the way for potentially innovative vascular and functional neurosurgery applications and for targeted drug delivery to the central nervous system. Among the most important, the capability of occluding vessels could make FUS a therapeutic tool for the treatment of vascular malformations. Both arterial and venous occlusion can be achieved with FUS (39,40). Using averaged power levels two- to threefold lower than the levels necessary for tissue coagulation, FUS can be used to open the blood–brain barrier selectively without damaging the surrounding brain parenchyma (41). For this effect to be achieved, preformed gas bubbles must be introduced into the vasculature, as is routinely done with ultrasound contrast agents. The gas bubbles implode and release cavitation-related energy, which transiently inactivates the tight junctions. As a consequence, large molecules can pass through the artificially created "window" in the blood–brain barrier. These large molecules can be chemotherapeutic or neuropharmacological agents. FUS-based targeted selective drug delivery to the brain could result in novel therapeutic interventions for movement and psychiatric disorders.

Such MRI-guided focal opening of the blood–brain barrier, combined with ultrasound technology that permits sonications through the intact skull, will open the way for new, noninvasive, targeted therapies. Specifically, it would provide targeted access for chemothearapeutic and gene therapy agents (42), as well as monoclonal antibodies, and could even provide a vascular route for performing neurotransplantations.

Ultrasound has also proved useful in accelerating thrombolysis (43) and increasing cell membrane permeability.

Since the skull bone scatters and attenuates the propagation of the ultrasound beam, most clinical trials have been performed following craniotomy in order to provide an ultrasound window (44). However, the transcranial application of FUS, although challenging, is not impossible. Although bone scatters and absorbs most of the acoustic energy, a small fraction can penetrate through the skull.

Recent simulation (45) and experimental studies (46,47) have demonstrated the feasibility of accurately focusing ultrasound through the intact skull by using an array of multiple ultrasound transducers arranged over a large surface area. To correct for beam distortion, the driving signal for the transducer elements of the array is individually adjustable, either based on measurements obtained with an invasive hydrophone probe, or better, based on detailed MRI. Because of the large surface area, the ultrasound energy is distributed in such a manner as to avoid heating and consequent damage of skin, bone, meninges, or surrounding normal brain parenchyma, while at the same time being able to coagulate the tissue at the focus (47). The experimental data are extremely promising; it appears possible to coagulate brain tumors thermally through the intact skull under MRI thermometry control using MR-compatible arrays.

By applying multiple, smaller transducers around the skull in a helmet-like phased-array system, sufficient amounts of energy can be deposited in the target tissue. Unfortunately, the skull thickness is uneven, causing variable delays of the acoustic waves originating from individual phased array elements. Phase incoherence can be corrected, however, if the skull thickness is known from preoperative X-ray computed tomography scans. In an experimental setup, successful focusing through the skull was achieved and verified by MRI, thus providing the foundation for developing the first human MRI-guided FUS system for brain tumor treatment.

CONCLUSION

There is an ongoing effort to develop MRI-guided interventional radiology and intraoperative imaging-based endoscopic or open surgical applications. So far, neurosurgery has benefited most from intraoperative MRI guidance. The introduction of real-time volumetric image updates has improved localization, and targeting and, most importantly, has resulted in complete tumor resections. Following this success in neurosurgery, new MRI-guided applications have been introduced for tumor treatment in the breast, liver, and prostate, as well as in the musculoskeletal system. Several percutaneous treatment methods like prostate brachytherapy have emerged. Thermal ablations in the brain (laser, RF), liver (laser, RF, and cryotherapy), and pelvis (laser treatment of fibroids) have been performed at multiple institutions. Today, among the thermal ablation methods, noninvasive image-guided focused ultrasound treatment has the most potential for tumor ablation but is also applicable to occlusion of blood vessels and to targeted drug delivery and gene therapy.

REFERENCES

1. Jolesz, FA, Hynynen, K. Magnetic resonance image-guided focused ultrasound surgery. *Cancer J* 2002;8 Suppl 1:S100–S112.
2. Jolesz, FA. Interventional and intraoperative MRI: a general overview of the field. *J Magn Reson Imaging* 1998;8:3–7.
3. McDannold, NJ, Jolesz, FA. Magnetic resonance image-guided thermal ablations. *Top Magn Reson Imaging* 2000;11:191–202.
4. McDannold NJ, King R, Jolesz FA, Hynynen K. Usefulness of MR imaging-derived thermometry and dosimetry in determining the threshold for tissue damage induced by thermal surgery in rabbits. *Radiology* 2000;216:517–523.
5. Leonardi, MA, Lumenta, CB, Gumprecht, HK, von Einsiedel, GH, Wilhelm, T. Stereotactic guided laser-induced interstitial thermotherapy (SLITT) in gliomas with intraoperative morphologic monitoring in an open MR-unit. *Minim Invasive Neurosurg* 2001;44:37–42.
6. Craciunescu, OI, Raaymakers, BW, Kotte, AN, Das, SK, Samulski, TV, Lagendijk, JJ. Discretizing large traceable vessels and using DE-MRI perfusion maps yields numerical temperature contours that match the MR noninvasive measurements. *Med Phys* 2001;28:2289–2296.
7. Jolesz, FA, Talos, IF, Schwartz, RB, et al. Intraoperative magnetic resonance imaging and magnetic resonance imaging-guided therapy for brain tumors. *Neuroimaging Clin N Am* 2002;12:665–683.
8. Jolesz, FA, Bleier, AR, Jakab, P, Ruenzel, PW, Huttl, K, Jako, GJ. MR imaging of laser-tissue interactions. *Radiology* 1988;168:249–253.
9. Zhang, Y, Samulski, TV, Joines, WT, Mattiello, J, Levin, RL, LeBihan, D. On the accuracy of noninvasive thermometry using molecular diffusion magnetic resonance imaging. *Int J Hyperthermia* 1992;8:263–274.
10. Le Bihan D, DJ, Levin RL. Temperature mapping with MR imaging of molecular diffusion: application to hyperthermia. *Radiology* 1989;171:853–857.
11. Parker DL, SV, Sheldon P, Crooks LE, Fussell L. Temperature distribution measurements in two-dimensional NMR imaging. *Med Phys* 1983;10:321–325.
12. Dickinson RJ, HA, Hind AJ, Young IR. Measurement of changes in tissue temperature using MR imaging. *J Comput Assist Tomogr* 1986;10:468–472.
13. Matsumoto R, Mulkern RV, Hushek SG, Jolesz FA. Tissue temperature monitoring for thermal interventional therapy: comparison of T1-weighted MR sequences. *J Magn Reson Imaging* 1994;4:65–70.
14. Bleier, AR, Jolesz, FA, Cohen, MS, et al. Real-time magnetic resonance imaging of laser heat deposition in tissue. *Magn Reson Med* 1991;21:132–137.

15. MacFall, J, Prescott, DM, Fullar, E, Samulski, TV. Temperature dependence of canine brain tissue diffusion coefficient measured in vivo with magnetic resonance echo-planar imaging. *Int J Hyperthermia* 1995;11:73–86.
16. Kuroda K, Abe K, Tsutsumi S, Ishihara Y, Suzuki Y, Sato K. Water proton magnetic resonance spectroscopic imaging. *Biomed Thermol* 1994;13:43–62.
17. Ishihara Y, Calderon A, Watanabe H, Okamoto K, Suzuki Y, Kuroda K. A precise and fast temperature mapping using water proton chemical shift. *Magn Reson Med* 1995;34:814–823.
18. Peters, RD, Hinks, RS, Henkelman, RM. Ex vivo tissue-type independence in proton-resonance frequency shift MR thermometry. *Magn Reson Med* 1998;40:454–459.
19. Kahn, T, Harth, T, Kiwit, JC, Schwarzmaier, HJ, Wald, C, Modder, U. In vivo MRI thermometry using a phase-sensitive sequence: preliminary experience during MRI-guided laser-induced interstitial thermotherapy of brain tumors. *J Magn Reson Imaging* 1998;8:160–164.
20. Vykhodtseva N, Sorrentino V, Jolesz FA, Bronson RT, Hynynen K. MRI detection of the thermal effects of focused ultrasound on the brain. *Ultrasound Med Biol* 2000;26:871–80.
21. McDannold, N, Hynynen, K, Jolesz, F. MRI monitoring of the thermal ablation of tissue: effects of long exposure times. *J Magn Reson Imaging* 2001;13:421–427.
22. Vimeux, FC, De Zwart, JA, Palussiere, J, et al. Real-time control of focused ultrasound heating based on rapid MR thermometry. *Invest Radiol* 1999;34:190–193.
23. Salomir R, Vimeux F, de Zwart JA, Grenier N, Moonen CT. Hyperthermia by MR-guided focused ultrasound: accurate temperature control based on fast MRI and a physical model of local energy deposition and heat conduction. *Magn Reson Med* 2000;43:342–347.
24. Smith NB, Merrilees N, Hynynen K, Dahleh M. Control system for an MRI compatible intracavitary ultrasound array for thermal treatment of prostate disease. *Int J Hyperthermia* 2001;17:271–282.
25. Kahn T, Harth T, Bettag M, et al. Preliminary experience with the application of gadolinium-DTPA before MR imaging-guided laser-induced interstitial thermotherapy of brain tumors. *J Magn Reson Imaging JMRI* 1997;7:226–229.
26. Anzai Y, Lufkin R, Hirschowitz S, Farahani K, Castro DJ. MR imaging-histopathologic correlation of thermal injuries induced with interstitial Nd:YAG laser irradiation in the chronic model. *J Magn Reson Imaging* 1992;2:671–678.
27. Schulze PC, Adams V, Busert C, Bettag M, Kahn T, Schober R. Effects of laser-induced thermotherapy (LITT) on proliferation and apoptosis of glioma cells in rat brain transplantation tumors. *Lasers Surg Med* 2002;30:227–232.
28. Bettag M, Ulrich F, Schober R, Furst G, Langen KJ, Sabel M, Kiwit JC. Stereotactic laser therapy in cerebral gliomas. *Acta Neurochir Suppl (Wien)* 1991;52:81–83.
29. Ascher, PW, Justich, E, Schrottner, O. Interstitial thermotherapy of central brain tumors with the Nd:YAG laser under real-time monitoring by MRI. *J Clin Laser Med Surg* 1991;9:79–83.
30. Kahn T, Bettag M, Ulrich F, et al. MRI-guided laser-induced interstitial thermotherapy of cerebral neoplasms. *J Comput Assist Tomogr* 1994;18:519–532.
31. Kahn T, Bttag M, Harth T, Schwabe B, Schwarzmaier HJ, Modder U. Laser-induced interstitial induced hyperthermia of cerebral tumors with nuclear magnetic resonance tomography control. *Radiologe* 1996;36:713–721.
32. Kettenbach J, Silverman SG, Hata N, et al. Monitoring and visualization techniques for MR-guided laser ablations in an open MR system. *J Magn Reson Imaging* 1998;8:933–943.
33. Hata, N, Morrison, PR, Kettenbach, J, Kikinis, R, Jolesz, FA. Computer-asisted intra-operative MRI monitoring of interstitial laser therapy in the brain: a case report. *J Biomed Optics* 1998;3:304–311.

34. Jolesz, FA and Blumenfeld, SM. Interventional use of magnetic resonance imaging. *Magn Reson Q* 1994;10:85–96.
35. Sakai, T, Fujishima, I, Sugiyama, K, Ryu, H, Uemura, K. Interstitial laserthermia in neurosurgery. *J Clin Laser Med Surg* 1992;10:37–40.
36. Krishnamurthy, S, Powers, SK, Witmer, P, Brown, T. Optimal light dose for interstitial photodynamic therapy in treatment for malignant brain tumors. *Lasers Surg Med* 2000;27:224–234.
37. Reimer, P, Bremer, C, Horch, C, Morgenroth, C, Allkemper, T, Schuierer, G. MR-monitored LITT as a palliative concept in patients with high grade gliomas: preliminary clinical experience. *J Magn Reson Imaging* 1998;8:240–244.
38. Fry WJ, Fry FJ. Fundamental neurological research and human neurosurgery using intense ultrasound. *IRE Trans Med Electron* 1950;ME-7:166–181.
39. Delon-Martin C, Vogt C, Chigner E, Guers C, Chapelon JY, Cathignol D. Venous thrombosis generation by means of high-intensity focused ultrasound. *Ultrasound Med Biol* 1995;21:113–119.
40. Hynynen K, Colucci V, Chung A, Jolesz FA. Noninvasive artery occlusion using MRI guided focused ultrasound. *Ultrasound Med Biol* 1996;22:1071–1077.
41. Hynynen K, McDannold N, Vykhodtseva N, Jolesz FA. Noninvasive MR imaging-guided focal opening of the blood-brain barrier in rabbits. *Radiology* 2001;220:640.
42. Greenleaf WJ, Bolander ME, Sarkar G, Goldring MB, Greenleaf JF. Artificial cavitation nuclei significantly enhance acoustically induced cell transfection. *Ultrasound Med Biol* 1998;24:587–595.
43. Porter TR, Fox R, Kricsfeld A, Xie F. Thrombolytic enhancement with perfluorocarbon exposed sonicated dextrose albumin microbubbles. *Am Heart J* 1996;132:964–968.
44. Guthkelch AN, Carter LP, Cassady JR, et al. Treatment of malignant brain tumors with focused ultrasound hyperthermia and radiation: results of a phase I trial. *J Neurooncol* 1991;10:271–284.
45. Sun J, Hynynen K. Focusing of ultrasound through a human skull: a numerical study. *J Acoust Soc Am* 1998;104:1705–1715.
46. Hynynen K, Jolesz FC. Demonstration of potential noninvasive ultrasound brain therapy through intact skull. *Ultrasound Med Biol* 1998;24:275–283.
47. Clement GT, White J, Hynynen K. Investigation of a large-area phased array for focused ultrasound surgery through the skull. *Phys Med Biol* 2000;45:1071–1083.

13
Gene-Based and Viral-Based Therapies

Manish Aghi, MD, PhD and E. Antonio Chiocca, MD, PhD

INTRODUCTION

Disappointing results in the treatment of aggressive central nervous system (CNS) neoplasms such as glioblastoma multiforme have fueled a search for novel treatment modalities. New drugs and new radiation modalities have and are being tested. Biological materials have also been explored as potential anticancer agents. Such biological materials include immunotoxins, engineered cells that release diffusible anticancer factors, proteins, stem cells, immune- or vaccine-based modalities, and gene-based and virus-based therapies. The latter type of experimental treatment is the subject of this chapter.

Gene-based therapy indicates the process of introducing into a cancer cell a gene that will reverse or destroy its malignant phenotype. Virus-based therapy is a form of gene therapy, the process of infecting cancer cells with a virus that has been genetically altered so as to destroy that cancer cell and spare normal cells selectively. In fact, several historical reports, dating back from the beginning of the last century until the 1980s, described the administration of attenuated viruses to patients afflicted with incurable cancers, yet this approach was never fully tested and/or widely translated, probably because of its relative lack of appeal compared with the emerging modalities of chemotherapy and radiotherapy *(1)*.

The advent of technologies associated with recombinant DNA in the 1970s and 1980s made it possible to engineer viruses genetically. This allowed the generation of (1) replication-defective viruses (designated as vectors), which cannot grow or produce viral proteins in cells and are used to deliver an anticancer gene (gene therapy); and (2) oncolytic viruses that maintain the ability to grow and replicate in infected tumor but not normal cells (oncolytic viral therapy) *(2)*. Considerable scientific and preclinical excitement has surrounded the application of each of these biologic modalities, although recent events related to the death of a patient treated with gene therapy because he was suffering from an inborn error of metabolism have provided a sobering reminder of the highly experimental nature of these endeavors.

Cancer has become the foremost arena in which gene therapy is applied—a recent summary of 600 published gene therapy clinical trials from 1990 to 2001

From: *Minimally Invasive Neurosurgery,* edited by: M.R. Proctor and P.M. Black © Humana Press Inc., Totowa, NJ

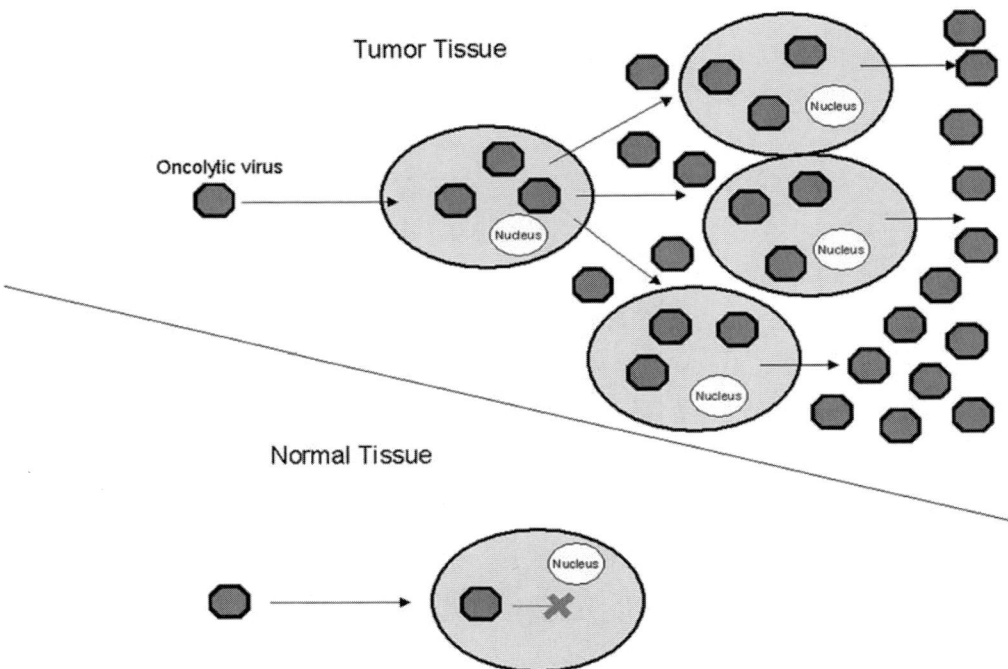

Fig. 1. Selective replication (i.e., growth) and killing of tumor cells by oncolytic virus. An oncolytic virus (hexagon) will infect and grow into multiple progeny viruses within a tumor cell (upper panel). The cell will die and release such progeny into the extracellular milieu. Progeny oncolytic viruses can then go on and infect additional tumor cells, repeating the entire process. Successive waves of infection and replication set up a spreading infection within the tumor that should lead to regression. However, in normal cells, this does not occur, and replication of the initially infecting oncolytic virus will be aborted.

found that 63% of the trials were in the area of cancer, whereas only 13% were for gene replacement in genetic disorders, the purpose of the first gene therapy clinical trial begun in 1989 (3). Cancer gene therapy involves the administration of a vector (most commonly derived from a virus, but also derived from a chemical lipid construct) to deliver a gene that will impede the survival and growth of tumor cells. If the vector is a virus, it will have been gutted of all its endogenous genes, disabling its ability to grow and directly hurt the cell. Therefore, the entire anticancer effect derives from the delivered anticancer cDNA. Oncolytic viruses, instead, directly lyse tumor cells because they retain almost the entire complement of viral genes that allow for production of viral progeny and lysis of the infected cell, but have been modified so as to allow this process to occur selectively in cancer cells and not normal cells (Fig. 1).

As with conventional therapies, there is a therapeutic window for each gene and viral therapy that defines beneficial anticancer vs toxic side effects. Localized administration of vector to the brain tumor can allow for increased selectivity. Other approaches to increase selectivity consist of using tumor-specific

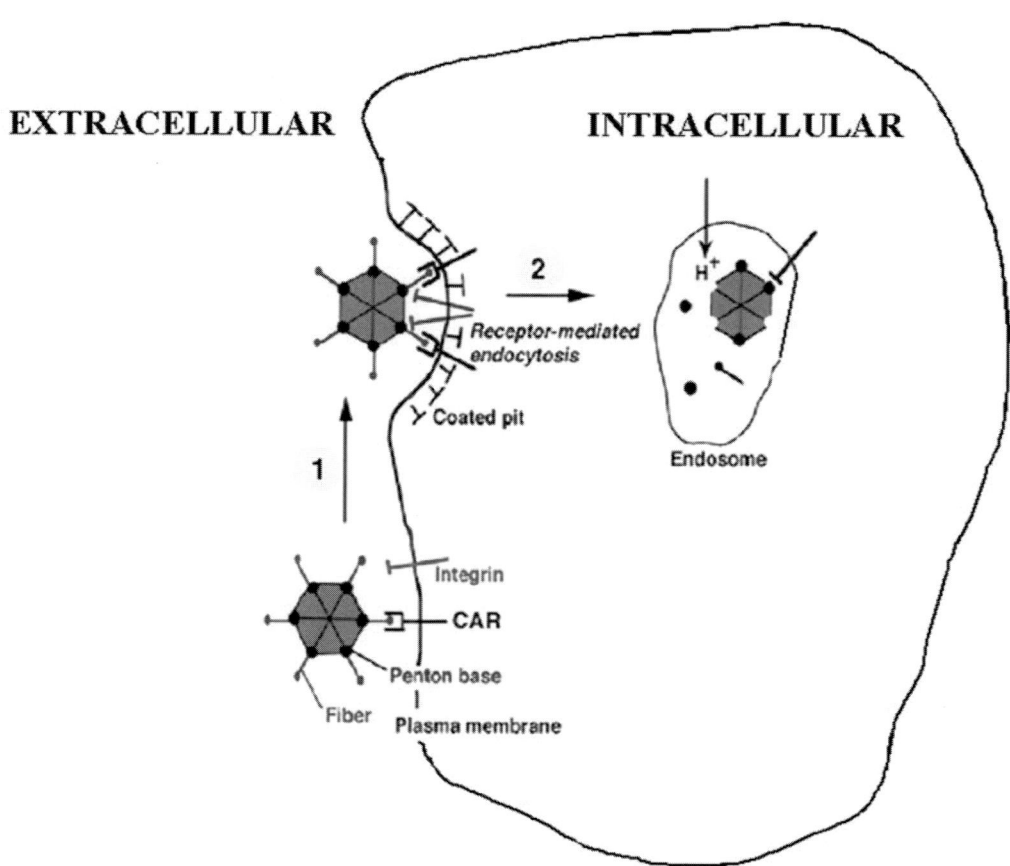

Fig. 2. Entry of adenovirus into cells via specific binding of a viral ligand to a cell surface receptor. Adenovirus serotype 5 (Ad5), the most common serotype employed in gene transfer, enters cells through the following series of steps: 1, specific binding of virion surface fiber molecules (labeled fiber above) to the coxsackie-adenovirus receptor (CAR); 2, adenovirus internalization is then initiated after the interaction of the penton base protein with cell surface integrins $\alpha(v)\beta3$ and $\alpha(v)\beta5$; 3, receptor-mediated endocytosis then occurs; 4, virion particles are disassembled in the acidic environment of the endosome. Once tumor-specific receptors are identified, genetic modification of the virion surface molecules that bind cell surface receptors like CAR could create an engineered virus specifically taken up by tumor cells.

promoters to confer selectivity to the anticancer cDNA or to the replicating oncolytic virus and changing the molecular structure of the surface proteins of the vector or virus in order to target a tumor-specific receptor (Fig. 2).

CNS neoplasms are thought to provide an excellent target for cancer gene therapy because tumor cells are among the few rapidly proliferating cells in the CNS, and most of the gene- or viral-based therapies target cellular division. Proliferation of microglial, endothelial, and glial cells as well as neural stem cells is a much rarer occurrence than that displayed by a glioma cell. Experimentally, viral vectors employed for cancer gene therapy in the brain include those derived from retrovirus, adenovirus, herpes simplex virus-1 (HSV-1), and adeno-associated virus (AAV). Oncolytic viruses employed for brain tumors include HSV-1, adenovirus, reovirus, and poliovirus. Clinically, published gene therapy trials for gliomas have used retroviral and adenoviral vectors to deliver a thymidine kinase cDNA, endowing tumor cells with ganciclovir chemosensitivity. Published oncolytic virus trials for gliomas have used HSV-1 and adenoviral mutants (Table 1).

GENE THERAPY VECTORS FOR GLIOMAS

Retroviruses

Retroviral vectors are RNA viruses converted to DNA by one of the viral enzymes (reverse transcriptase) and then integrated into the host genome at nonspecific sites. With the exception of lentiviruses, retroviruses only integrate into the genomes of rapidly dividing cells, providing an element of tumor selectivity. Most retroviral vectors are derived from the Moloney murine leukemia virus (Mo-MLV), originally developed by Mulligan and Berg in 1981 (4). Retrovirus vectors are generated in vector-producer cells (VPCs), and then they can be harvested from the medium of VPCs at titers of 10^5–10^7 PFU/mL. However, the viral particles themselves are usually too unstable to be injected directly into tumors. Thus, the transfected VPCs must be engrafted into the tumor.

The disadvantages of retroviral vector systems are: *(1)* low titers; *(2)* the need to engraft VPCs, which cannot survive for long periods; *(3)* low transgene capacity—the maximum amount of DNA that can be packaged into a retrovirus allows for only 8 kb of foreign DNA in the vector; and *(4)* risk of insertional mutagenesis if integration disrupts a protooncogene. Possible advantages include: *(1)* integration into dividing cells, allowing long-term gene expression, although long-term gene expression carries with it long term concerns about safety; and *(2)* relatively little toxicity because of replication deficiency with minimal risk of wild-type virus generation and minimal inflammation. Retroviruses have and are being used in 54% of brain tumor gene therapy clinical trials (3).

Adenoviruses

Adenoviruses are nonenveloped DNA viruses causing upper respiratory tract infections. The adenovirus vectors used for gene delivery are derived from subgroup C. Wild-type subgroup C causes a mild upper respiratory infection, which resolves uneventfully in healthy individuals. In an adenoviral vector, the desired transgene is cloned into the E1 gene, thus disrupting it. This gene is essential for adenoviral replication, thus rendering the vector now safe to use because it will grow/replicate in infected cells but will only deliver the transgene.

High titers (up to 10^{12} particles/mL) can be achieved with adenovirus. Limitations include the fact that the viral genome is maintained as an extrachromosomal element that is rapidly lost in dividing cells and the highly immunogenic nature of the vectors. The immunogenic nature of adenovirus may have con-

Table 1
General Biology, Advantages, and Disadvantages of Various Viral Vectors for Cancer Gene Therapy

	HSV-1	Retrovirus	Adenovirus	AAV	Reovirus
General biology					
Genetic material	ds DNA	ds RNA	ds DNA	ss DNA	ds RNA
Lytic?	Yes	No—requires transgene for tumor killing	Yes	Yes	Yes
Integration?	No	Yes—nonspecific integration leading to risk of malignant transformation	No	Yes—site-specific integration	No
Features					
Transgene capacity	30 kb	7.5 kb	10 kb	4.7 kb	Not investigated
Titer	10^{10} PFU/mL	10^6 PFU/mL	10^{12} PFU/mL	10^6 PFU/mL	10^9 PFU/mL
Virion stability	High	Low—need to graft packaging cell line	High	High	High
Specific antiviral agent available	Yes	No	No	No	No
Ease of genetic manipulation	Difficult	Easy	Easy	Easy	Not investigated
Immunogenicity	Moderate	Low	High	Low	Moderate
Wild-type virus infects nonreplicating cells	Yes	No	Yes	Yes	No
Virulence of wild-type virus	Yes	No	Slight	No	No

Abbreviations: HSV-1, herpes simplex virus-1; AAV, adeno-associated virus; ds, double-stranded; ss, single-stranded.

tributed to the death of an 18-yr-old patient after an arterial infusion of a replication-defective adenovirus vector during a gene therapy trial for ornithine transcarbamylase deficiency. This death was attributed to a massive cytokine response to the adenovirus vector, resulting in disseminated intravascular coagulation.

Despite these concerns, adenoviruses are used in a large number of gene therapy trials (3). They are the most commonly used vector in cancer gene therapy trials (32% of these trials), and the second most commonly used vector in brain tumor gene therapy trials (16% of these trials).

Herpesviruses

HSV-1 is an enveloped, double-stranded linear DNA virus whose genome spans 152 kb, encoding more than 80 genes.

HSV-1 has been developed as a vector either by removing some of the essential genes needed for viral replication (recombinant HSV) or by removing the entire viral genome except for a small 300-bp sequence that provides packaging function (amplicon vector). This packaging signal when incorporated into any bacterial plasmid will allow this plasmid to be packaged into an infectious virion.

HSV-1 offers a number of advantages as a vector (Table 1). These advantages include: *(1)* the ease with which high titers (typically 10^{10} infectious particles/mL) can be generated; *(2)* potential for incorporating a large payload of foreign DNA—approx 30 kb of the HSV-1 genome have been estimated to be replaceable by foreign genes with minimal effects on titers or replication; *(3)* neurotropism, rendering gene delivery to the CNS more effective; *(4)* sensitivity to antiherpetic agents like ganciclovir, providing a safety mechanism by which viral replication could be abrogated; and *(5)* the fact that HSV-1 never integrates and persists as an episome even during latency, ensuring that the risk of insertional mutagenesis posed by retroviral vectors is not an issue with HSV-1 vectors. Furthermore, the lack of integration with HSV-1 vectors is not a concern with cancer gene therapy, as immediate tumor killing probably does not require long-term gene expression.

However, there are four challenges that arise when one is working with HSV-1 vectors. First, genetic manipulation of HSV-1 is difficult owing to the large size of the viral DNA. A second potential obstacle when using HSV-1 recombinant vectors is the fact that most humans have preexisting herpes immunity, which could potentially impair gene delivery. Approximately 60–90% of the adult population has been exposed to HSV-1, as determined by the detection of viral DNA and antibodies to HSV-1 in serum (5). Potential neurotoxicity is a third problem inherent to HSV-1 vectors. HSV-1 is a neurotropic human pathogen that can cause a life-threatening encephalitis from primary infection or from reactivation of latent virus. The introduction of HSV-1 vectors could lead to one of two scenarios that could cause a potentially fatal encephalitis: *(1)* recombination with latent wild-type HSV-1 could restore full replicative capacity to the introduced vector; or *(2)* the latent wild-type HSV-1 present in most humans could be reactivated by application of HSV-1 vectors. Finally, the ability of HSV-

1 vectors to infect both dividing and nondividing cells is undesirable for cancer therapy, which requires selective targeting of replicating cells.

Adeno-Associated Virus

Wild-type AAV and AAV vectors depend on the presence of adenovirus for their replication and lytic infection. The vectors can infect quiescent and proliferating cells. Long-term expression can be achieved owing to site-specific integration on human chromosome 19q and transgene amplification. Integration is more efficient in proliferating cells. Aside from the dependence on helper virus, limitations include a small transgene capacity (4.7 kb) and low titers (10^6 infectious particles/mL).

TRANSGENES USED IN CANCER GENE THERAPY

At first, cancer seems to be unsuitable for gene therapy, which originally involved attempts to replace defective genes. Because the vast majority of target cells remain nontransduced after gene therapy, replacement of defective genes would appear to be a suitable approach only for monogenetic disorders, which might benefit from partial restoration of genetic function. Cancer generally arises from a multistep process involving a variety of genetic abnormalities. Cancer gene replacement therapy requires the replacement of multiple genes in every single target cell, since any nontransduced cells would continue rapid replication and quickly pose a threat. As it turns out, cancer gene therapy strategies proved not to be limited to gene replacement. In addition, several of the transgenes employed endow transduced tumor cells with the ability to confer cytotoxicity upon neighboring nontransduced cells—a bystander effect.

The transgenes that have been utilized are divided here into five categories.

Correction of Genetic Defects in Cancer

Some cancer gene therapy approaches have employed the gene replacement approach. In gliomas, early-stage tumor formation is triggered by mutations in the *p53* gene, whereas the later stages of tumor development seen in glioblastoma multiforme are associated with loss of heterozygosity on chromosome 10 and mutation of the epidermal growth factor receptor (EGFR) gene *(16)*.

Introduction of the wild-type *p53* gene into human and rodent glioma cell lines results in growth inhibition in culture *(17)*. Glioma cells transfected with wild-type *p53* display reduced tumorigenicity in nude mice *(18)*. The effects caused by the introduction of wild-type *p53* are independent of whether the parental cell lines expressed mutant or wild-type *p53*.

As of September 2001, 33 clinical protocols employing *p53* gene therapy in adenovirus, retrovirus, or a naked plasmid form have been undertaken, several involving lung cancer and one involving brain tumors. A total of 133 patients have been enrolled. Tumor regressions have been observed in approximately one-third of patients with sufficient information to evaluate responses *(3)*. A group performing one of these trials showed that a slight bystander effect is achieved during *p53* gene therapy *(19)*.

Mutation of the EGFR receptor gene occurs in 40% of all glioblastomas *(20)*. These mutations generate abnormal EGFR receptors that mediate constitutive signaling. The retroviral transfer of a signal-defective mutant EGFR gene to cells overexpressing a constitutively active mutant EGFR caused inactivation of mutated EGFR function in a dominant-negative manner by formation of inactive dimers *(21)*. Although effective at the cellular level, such an approach is unlikely to generate a bystander effect.

Antiangiogenesis

Because tumors depend on angiogenesis for expansion, antiangiogenic therapy has received considerable attention. However, antiangiogenic proteins must be administered in large quantities over long periods to have effects, causing some researchers to consider gene delivery of antiangiogenic factors. In addition to being one of the gene replacement strategies described above, *p53* gene therapy is also an antiangiogenic gene therapy because of the discovery that inducing wild-type *p53* expression in astrocytomas causes release of an angiogenesis inhibitory factor *(22)*.

Angiogenesis is promoted by vascular endothelial growth factor (VEGF), an endothelium-specific mitogen produced by tumors. In one study, a retroviral vector was used to deliver a signaling-defective VEGF receptor that forms inactive dimers with wild-type VEGF receptor *(23)*. Significant inhibition of glioma growth in nude mice was shown when this vector was delivered to endothelial cells near the tumor mass.

Tumors also produce antiangiogenic factors such as angiostatin. An AAV vector expressing angiostatin has been shown to promote long-term survival of mice harboring intracranial gliomas *(24)*.

Immune Response Modifying Genes

Attempts to modify antitumor immune responses have focused on transducing tumor cells with genes that make them more immunogenic. Cytokine genes are the most commonly studied. These studies have been done by infecting tumor cells ex vivo, arresting their growth by irradiation, and then reimplanting them to sustain paracrine secretion of cytokine within the tumor *(25,26)* or by implanting retrovirus producer cell lines intratumorally so that infection occurs *in situ (27,28)*. The former is preferred because it concentrates cytokine production closest to the tumor mass, but it can be difficult to obtain sufficient numbers of tumor cells from patients and to generate large enough numbers of transduced cells.

The cytokines utilized include: (1) interleukin 2 *(25,27)*, an autocrine T-cell growth factor; (2) γ-interferon and interleukin 12 *(26,27,29)*, which promote helper T cells to differentiate into the TH1 subtype important in antitumor responses; and (3) interleukin 4 *(28)* and interferon-β *(30)*, which activate cytotoxic lymphocytes and macrophages. Severe central nervous system toxicity, secondary to brain edema, was documented when interleukin 2 or γ-interferon were secreted by tumor cells intracranially *(27)*.

Gene therapy can be used to generate tumor vaccines. In this model, cells from a tumor are grown in culture, and then infected with a viral vector carrying the gene for granulocyte-macrophage colony-stimulating factor (GM-CSF). This cytokine enhances antigen presentation. After onset of GM-CSF expression, the tumor cells are irradiated to induce growth arrest and then inoculated in the periphery away from the tumor mass. This approach generates a strong immune response against intracranial tumors in animal models (31–34). By infecting ex vivo and vaccinating peripherally, an immune response can be initiated against an intracranial tumor while avoiding the toxicity associated with intracranial cytokine expression.

Eighty-five protocols worldwide have used gene therapy to modify the antitumor immune response. A total of 547 patients have been entered in these ongoing protocols. Major tumor regressions have been observed in 15 of 237 patients with sufficient information to evaluate responses (3). Eight such protocols are under way in brain tumors, with results pending.

Drug Resistance Genes

The transfer of genes into normal cells to augment resistance to chemotherapeutic agents is also under investigation. Bone marrow cells, whose replication rate renders them susceptible to chemotherapy, are the most common targets for this approach. A clinical trial for glioblastoma multiforme involving ex vivo transduction of bone marrow cells with the multiple-drug resistance gene (MDR1) followed by infusion of transduced cells and chemotherapy is under way (3). MDR1 is a cellular efflux pump conferring resistance to hydrophobic drugs such as Taxol, Adriamycin, vincristine, and actinomycin D (35).

Prodrug-Activating Enzymes

Prodrugs are chemicals that are inert over a wide range of doses but are converted into toxic molecules by specific prodrug-activating enzymes. Genes encoding for these enzymes are the most commonly used transgenes in cancer gene therapy because of their prominent bystander effects.

Herpes Simplex Virus Type 1 Thymidine Kinase/Ganciclovir

Ganciclovir (GCV) is an acyclic analog of the natural nucleoside 2'-deoxyguanosine (36). GCV's antiherpetic properties result from its specificity for HSV-thymidine kinase (TK), which is three orders of magnitude more efficient at monophosphorylating GCV than human nucleoside kinase. The resulting GCV-monophosphate is subsequently converted by cellular kinases into toxic GCV-triphosphate. GCV-triphosphate's structural resemblance to 2'-deoxyguanosine triphosphate makes it a substrate for DNA polymerase. GCV binds herpes viral DNA polymerase better than human DNA polymerase. Thus, as an antiviral agent, GCV's specificity for infected cells derives from its preferential affinity for two viral enzymes, thymidine kinase and DNA polymerase. Once bound to herpes DNA polymerase, GCV-triphosphate inhibits the polymerase or is incorporated into DNA, causing DNA chain elongation to terminate (Fig. 3).

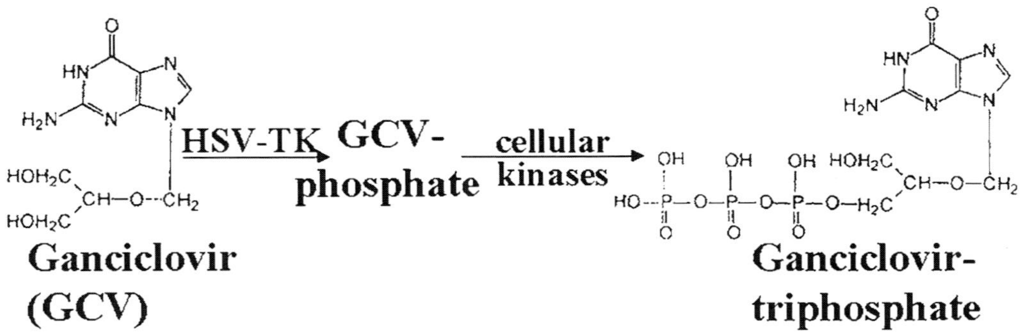

Fig. 3. Metabolism of ganciclovir. Chemical structure of the acyclic nucleoside ganciclovir (GCV), which is monophosphorylated by the enzyme herpes simplex thymidine kinase (HSV-TK). Further phosphorylation by cellular kinases leads to the creation of the toxic metabolite ganciclovir-triphosphate.

Glioma cells transduced and selected to express HSV-TK are 5000-fold more sensitive to GCV than their nontransduced counterparts *(37)*, suggesting that transduction leads to enough HSV-TK expression to phosphorylate enough GCV to inhibit mammalian DNA polymerase. Thus, the poor affinity of mammalian DNA polymerase relative to herpes DNA polymerase for GCV does not impede chemosensitization upon transfection with HSV-TK. Because GCV's effects are limited to DNA, it targets replicating cells, much like the S-phase–specific chemotherapeutic agents.

Efficacy in vivo was demonstrated in a study in which rats harboring intracranial gliosarcoma tumors were treated with intratumoral implantation of a fibroblast packaging cell line secreting HSV-TK-expressing retroviral vectors, followed by intraperitoneal GCV treatment. Treated animals survived more than twice as long as controls *(38)*.

HSV-TK/GCV is commonly used in cancer gene therapy because of its bystander effect. When 10% of murine sarcoma cells express HSV-TK, GCV eradicates the entire mixed population *(39)*. The percentage of cells expressing HSV-TK has to be higher in vivo—subcutaneous tumors have to possess at least 50% HSV-TK–positive cells to be eliminated by GCV treatment *(39)*.

HSV-TK/GCV's bystander effect requires cell-to-cell contact—the HSV-TK bystander effect can be abrogated when HSV-TK-expressing cells are separated from wild-type cells by a filter membrane *(39)*. Whereas HSV-TK cells treated with [^{3}H]GCV contain mostly GCV monophosphate and very little di- and triphosphate, bystander cells contain mostly GCV triphosphate *(40)*. Taken together, these experiments suggest that the bystander effect results from cell-to-cell contact allowing transfer of GCV-triphosphate from HSV-TK$^+$ cells to nontransduced cells—GCV-triphosphate is too polar to cross cell membranes, and thus cell-to-cell contact is required for its transfer. This contact occurs via gap junctions, a hypothesis supported by the fact that the magnitude of the bystander effect correlates with the extent of gap junction-mediated intercellular coupling *(41)*.

There are also two nonspecific explanations for the in vivo HSV-TK bystander effect that are used to explain several in vivo cancer gene therapy bystander effects. First, transduction of dividing endothelial cells may lead to GCV-mediated death of the endothelial cells that comprise the neovasculature of the tumor, causing death of nontansduced and transduced tumor cells *(42)*. Second, the bystander effect may result from an immune response against a nonhuman enzyme like HSV-TK, leading to diffuse cell death affecting neighboring nontransduced cells; or prodrug-mediated death of transduced tumor cells may liberate tumor antigens, generating an immune response that can then target transduced and nontransduced tumor cells *(43,44)*. This hypothesis may explain the observation that eradication of localized tumor deposits in immunocompetent animals sometimes results in the simultaneous immune-mediated regression of anatomically distant metastases, an effect dubbed the distant bystander effect *(45)*. However, whereas the immune system may be an ally in HSV-TK gene therapy, since the bystander effect in vivo is not significantly enhanced relative to that in culture, the role of the immune response in eradicating a single tumor mass may not be substantial, which is noteworthy since brain tumors can cause immunosuppression and many brain tumor patients are treated with dexamethasone.

Although GCV is a prodrug, the doses required for tumor eradication have been slightly toxic in some animal studies. Studies using HSV-TK gene therapy in rodents have found that 150 mg GCV/kg body weight/d was required for complete tumor elimination, and this dose produced some treatment-related mortality *(46)*. Improvements in HSV-TK/GCV gene therapy have been achieved via random sequence mutagenesis of the HSV-TK nucleoside binding site, generating mutant HSV-TK enzymes that display increased phosphorylation of GCV *(47)*.

Tumor cells transduced to express HSV-TK and treated with the antiviral agent acyclovir (ACV) display enhanced sensitivity to radiation in culture and in vivo *(48)*. ACV sensitized cells to radiation regardless of whether its administration preceded or followed radiation. Radiation enhancement when ACV preceded radiation could occur because DNA that has incorporated ACV may be more susceptible to radiation-induced strand breakage; whereas ACV administered following radiation might sensitize cells by inhibiting the polymerase activity required for repair of radiation-induced DNA damage.

Monitoring intratumoral prodrug-activating enzyme expression after gene therapy allows for decisions regarding whether repeated transduction of the tumor is necessary and also helps time prodrug delivery to coincide with maximal transgene expression. The demonstration of noninvasive imaging of HSV-TK gene expression using the substrate [^{131}I]-labeled 2'-fluoro-2'-deoxy-1-β-D-arabinofuranosyl-5-iodo-uracil combined with a clinical gamma camera, single photon emission computed tomography (SPECT), or positron emission tomography *(49)* has led to investigations seeking novel HSV-TK substrates with high imaging sensitivity.

As of September 2001, 62 clinical trials using adenoviruses or retroviruses expressing HSV-TK to treat mesothelioma, ovarian cancer, glioblastoma, breast cancer, melanoma, multiple myeloma, and astrocytoma have been proposed (3). A total of 603 patients have been enrolled, and major tumor regressions have been observed in 13% of patients for whom sufficient information is available.

Cytosine Deaminase/5-Fluorocytosine

5-Fluorocytosine (5-FC), an agent used to treat infections by fungi such as *Candida* and *Cryptococcus neoformans*, is a prodrug converted into the active agent 5-fluorouracil (5FU) by the CD enzyme, which is uniquely expressed in certain fungi and bacteria. Whereas 5-FC is nontoxic to humans because of the lack of cellular CD expression, 5-FU is used to treat colon, pancreatic, and breast cancers. The toxic effects of 5-FU are mediated by three of its intracellular metabolites: 5-fluoro-2'-deoxyuridine-5'-monophosphate (FdUMP), 5-fluoro-2'-deoxyuridine-5'-triphosphate (FdUTP), and 5-fluorouridine-5'-triphosphate (FUTP) (52). FdUMP inhibits the enzyme thymidylate synthetase, which converts deoxyuridylate (dUMP) into thymidylate (dTMP). Because thymidylate synthetase is the only source of *de novo* thymidylate synthesis, a cell treated with 5-FU ultimately becomes deficient in deoxythymidine-5'-triphosphate (dTTP), leading to the incorporation of both uridine triphosphate and FdUTP into DNA. Uracils in DNA are normally removed, but the lack of dTTP leaves them unreplaced and leaves the DNA strand nicked. The nicked DNA cannot be replicated, leading to cell death. 5-FU also targets RNA via incorporation of FUTP into all three types of RNA, where it inhibits mRNA polyadenylation, tRNA methylation, and processing of rRNA precursors. If RNA-directed effects led to toxicity, 5-FU could prove toxic against the 85–95% of the cells in a malignant glioma that are not proliferating at any given time (53), but 5-FU could also prove toxic against permanently arrested cells such as neurons. However, 5-FU's established efficacy in chemotherapy suggests that 5-FU's RNA-directed effects contribute minimally to cytotoxicity in vivo (Fig. 4).

Rodent gliosarcoma cells expressing the *E. coli* cytosine deaminase gene become 77-fold more sensitive to 5-FC in culture (54). In addition, mice whose CD+ tumors were eliminated by 5-FC resist subsequent rechallenge with unmodified wild-type tumor (55). Tumor cells expressing CD may present CD peptides on class I MHC, where they could serve as superantigens, leading to polyclonal activation of T cells (56).

CD/5-FC has a stronger bystander effect than HSV-TK/GCV (57). In culture, a mixture containing 33% CD-expressing cells displayed a dose–response curve identical to cultures containing 100% CD-expressing cells. Some nude mice subcutaneous tumors containing just 4% CD-expressing cells displayed no detectable tumor after 3 wk of 5-FC treatment, and all tumors containing only 2% CD-expressing cells displayed significant tumor regressions after 5-FC treatment. In contrast to HSV-TK/GCV, cell-to-cell contact does not appear to be required for the CD/5-FC bystander effect. Because high-performance liquid chromatography analysis detected 5-FU in the medium of cultured CD-expressing cells after 5-FC treatment, the bystander effect appears to result from 5-FU exiting CD-expressing cells and entering wild-type cells by facilitated diffusion. This mechanism could render the CD/5-FC strategy more effective than

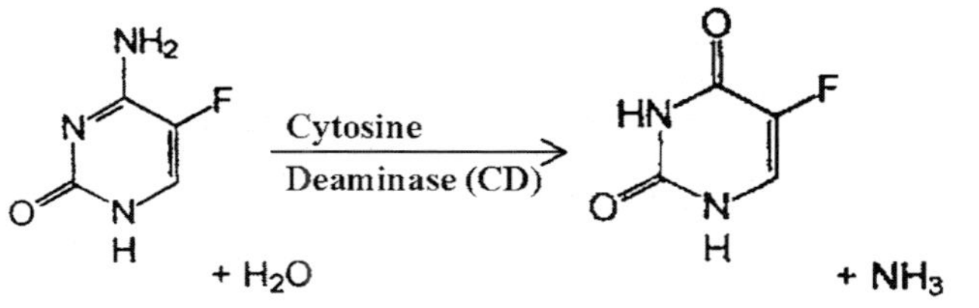

Fig. 4. Metabolism of 5-fluorocytosine. Generation of 5-fluorouracil (5-FU) from 5-fluorocytosine (5-FC) by the *E. coli* cytosine deaminase (CD) enzyme.

HSV-TK/GCV, because the capacity to form gap junctions appears to be lost in most cancer cells *(58)*.

Two studies of CD/5-FC in experimental brain tumors have been performed using adenovirus *(59,60)*. Stereotactic injection of adenovirus expressing CD into established gliomas derived from rat glioma cell lines in syngeneic hosts or human glioma cell lines in immunodeficient mice, followed by systemic administration of 5-FC, resulted in 160% (rat cells) and 137% (human cells) increases in survival time over controls. Treated rodents that died prior to the conclusion of the study showed no histologic signs of viable tumor. In the rat study, large areas of tumor necrosis were surrounded by extensive cerebral edema, suggesting that the strong bystander effect of CD/5-FC gene therapy caused toxicity to surrounding normal tissue and resulted in treatment-related death *(59)*. No such edema was found in the study of human cell lines, a study in which the host rodents were immunodeficient *(60)*.

Four CD/5-FC clinical trials are under way to treat metastatic colon carcinoma of the liver, metastatic breast cancer, prostate cancer, and penile cancer, with no results as of September 2001 *(3)*.

CYTOCHROME P450 2B1/CYCLOPHOSPHAMIDE

Cyclophosphamide (CPA) is one of the most commonly used chemotherapeutic agents. CPA is a prodrug activated by liver-specific enzymes of the cytochrome P450 family. One of these, the rat cytochrome P450 2B1 (CYP2B1), activates CPA with high efficiency *(61)*. This cytochrome hydroxylates CPA, forming 4-hydroxy-cyclophosphamide, an unstable compound that rapidly decomposes into phosphoramide mustard (PM) and acrolein *(61)*. The former is an alkylating agent responsible for the biologic effects of CPA *(61)*. PM-induced DNA alkylation generates intrastrand and interstrand DNA crosslinks. Toxicity occurs because attempting to replicate crosslinked DNA leads to strand breaks. PM alkylates DNA regardless of whether or not a cell is replicating, but toxicity does not occur until replication is attempted, assuming DNA repair has not occurred (Fig. 5).

The efficacy of CPA in treating tumors of the central nervous system has been limited by the fact that, although CPA crosses the blood–brain barrier, its active metabolites can only be generated by liver P450, and these metabolites are

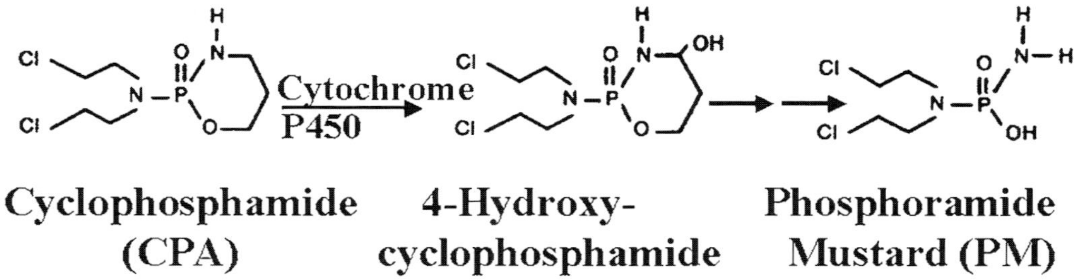

**Cyclophosphamide 4-Hydroxy- Phosphoramide
(CPA) cyclophosphamide Mustard (PM)**

Fig. 5. Metabolism of cyclophosphamide. The mammalian enzyme cytochrome P450 hydroxylates cyclophosphamide (CPA). 4-Hydroxycyclophosphamide then spontaneously decomposes into the toxic metabolite and alkylating agent phosphoramide mustard (PM).

poorly transported across the blood-brain barrier (61). Gene therapy using CYP2B1 to activate CPA was designed primarily for use in brain tumors because other tumor types have ready access to CPA's active metabolites produced by the liver when CPA is administered systemically.

Intratumoral implantation of VPCs releasing retroviral vectors expressing CYP2B1 caused regression of intracerebral rat glioma cells in nude mice after intratumoral or intrathecal CPA administration (62). Development of leptomeningeal tumor infiltration was prevented in most animals, whereas control tumors lacking CYP2B1 exhibited extensive leptomeningeal infiltration. In fact, the regression of parenchymal tumor mass caused by CPA treatment of CYP2B1-transduced cells was not nearly as dramatic as the inhibition of leptomeningeal infiltration observed, suggesting better access of CPA to leptomeningeal infiltrates than to the main tumor mass. Different modes of drug delivery, such as intraarterial administration or intratumoral implantation of polymer-based wafers containing CPA (63), should allow better access of CPA to parenchymal tumors.

When 10% of cultured glioma cells express CYP2B1, CPA causes a 75% decrease in cell proliferation (64). Separating CYP2B1-expressing cells from parental cells by a membrane still allows a bystander effect, and PM appears to be the diffusible metabolite responsible (65).

The P450 system consists of two protein components, the heme-containing P450 and the flavoprotein NADPH-P450 reductase (RED), both embedded in the phospholipid bilayer of the endoplasmic reticulum. RED catalyzes the transfer of electrons required for all microsomal P450-dependent enzyme reactions. Transfecting tumor cells with the RED cDNA enhances CPA sensitivity after infection with recombinant adenovirus expressing CYP2B1 (66). The same group has also used a retroviral vector to deliver various human cytochrome P450 genes to a rat gliosarcoma cell line, with CYP2B6 causing the most dramatic enhancement in CPA sensitivity. These human P450s should prove less immunogenic in human tumor gene therapy.

Three P450/CPA clinical trials are under way, none in brain tumors. Seventeen patients are enrolled as of September 2001, with results pending (3).

ONCOLYTIC VIRUSES

Adenovirus

Adenovirus can be modified to allow for viral growth within tumors in a relatively selective manner. One deletion that confers tumor selectivity is within the E1B region, found in the vector ONYX-015, which restricts viral replication to cells lacking normal p53 function *(13)*. Based on gene mutations alone, this vector could be of use in a majority of human glioblastomas, not only those carrying mutations in the p53 gene *(14)*, but also in those that contain the frequent deletion in CDKN2, whose gene (p14ARF) is required for proper p53 function. Other adenoviral mutants have been constructed so they will grow within tumors that contain mutations/deletions or dysfunctions in the p16/pRB pathway. Another type of mutant will target cells expressing the EGFR or integrins, which are often upregulated in gliomas.

Reovirus

This nonenveloped RNA virus, with little pathogenicity to humans, will replicate/grow and kill selectively only in cells with an activated Ras pathway. This is a common occurrence with gliomas because of either constitutively active EGFR or platelet-derived growth factor receptor (PDGFR). When the virus is administered intravenously to animals bearing subcutaneous tumors, potent antitumor activity occurs in a variety of tumor types *(15)*. Importantly, the virus shows excellent potency and safety profiles in animal models of gliomas. A phase I study is being planned in Canada.

HSV

Since a seminal study from 1991 by Martuza et al. *(2)*, this virus has provided a leading role in applications of oncolytic viruses to cancer therapy. Challenges regarding use of HSV-1 in the treatment of brain tumors have been defined by the fact that the wild-type virus is neurovirulent and infects/replicates/kills both dividing and quiescent cells. Such challenges have been addressed through genetic manipulations with the objective of reducing/eliminating neurovirulence and growth/replication in quiescent normal cells. Viral genes can be deleted through homologous recombination, generating HSV-1 mutants that are less virulent and replication conditional, a term used to describe viruses that replicate selectively in dividing cells. The recombinant HSV-1 viruses that have been studied as anticancer agents fall into three categories: (1) viruses deleted in β-genes involved in nucleic acid metabolism, such as uracil DNA glycosylase or the large subunit of viral ribonucleotide reductase; (2) viruses lacking both copies of the $\gamma 34.5$ gene; and *(3)* viruses with mutations in two or more different genes.

Group 1 vectors share the desirable property of being replication conditional because they only replicate when a dividing cell complements the mutation they carry in an enzyme involved in DNA synthesis. HSV-1 vectors mutated in the large subunit of ribonucleotide reductase, such as hrR3, or in the thymidine kinase gene, such as dlptk, exhibit efficacy in experimental brain tumor models and limited neurotoxicity (6). Despite showing reduced neurovirulence and the ability to infect dividing cells selectively, uracil DNA glycosylase mutants have not been studied as a single mutant in brain tumor therapy, only as part of a double-mutant HSV-1 vector

Group 2 vectors harbor deletions in γ34.5 and include the vectors R3616, R4009, and 1716. These vectors display low neurovirulence. The role of γ34.5 in promoting DNA replication may render a γ34.5 mutant replication conditional because only actively replicating cells express the DNA repair enzymes that perform the same function for the virus as γ34.5 (7). The other reason for possible tumor selectivity resides within the finding that these mutants grow better in cells with an overactive ras pathway, similar to reovirus targeting of this pathway.

The risks of using single mutant HSV-1 vectors (groups 1 and 2) include recombination with latent host virus to restore wild-type phenotype, reactivation of latent virus in the host, and suppressor mutations to restore wild-type phenotype. The risk of recombination with latent host HSV-1 has not yet been investigated. The risk of reactivation was felt to be low based on a study showing that, after adult rats were infected with wild-type HSV-1 and latency was established, intracerebral inoculation of hrR3 failed to cause HSV-1 reactivation (8). There is, however, a risk of viral mutations that restore a wild-type phenotype based on a study showing that, when a strain of HSV-1 with a deletion of the γ34.5 gene is growing, a suppressor mutation in two viral genes can occur, enabling the virus to acquire the wild-type HSV-1 phenotype of sustained late protein synthesis (9).

Concern about these risks led to the design of vectors with dual mutations (group 3). One example of a double mutant HSV-1 vector is 3616UB, generated by introducing a mutation in uracil DNA glycosylase into the γ34.5 mutant R3616 (10). The enhanced safety of the double-mutant 3616UB compared with the single-mutant R3616 was demonstrated in a study in which cultured neurons could still occasionally sustain the replication of R3616, whereas no neurons supported the replication of 3616UB. The most thoroughly studied combination is mutations in hrR3 and γ34.5, a combination found in two vectors, G207 and MGH-1, with the former having completed phase I safety trials. At an multiplicity of infection of 1, cultured rodent gliosarcoma cells are completely killed within 4 d of infection with single mutant hrR3, whereas the double mutants R3616 and MGH-1 result in approx 50% killing (11). Thus, the enhanced safety of double-mutant vectors may compromise their oncolytic potential.

The greater oncolytic effect of a single mutant can be combined with the reduced virulence of a double mutant by deleting ribonucleotide reductase and keeping the γ34.5 gene under transcriptional control of the cell cycle-regulated B-myb promoter, creating a novel oncolytic virus, Myb34.5, that is as oncolytic as a ribonucleotide reductase single mutant and whose safety is currently being investigated (12).

Oncolytic HSV can be further modified by adding anticancer genes, thus combining viral-based with gene-based therapies. One logical selection would be to use ganciclovir, because the HSV oncolytic viruses already express thymidine kinase. However, combining the HSV-TK/GCV strategy with herpes oncolysis can produce complex results because GCV inhibits the propagation of herpes vectors. In gliomas, GCV-mediated oncolysis of tumor cells expressing HSV-TK exceeds GCV-mediated inhibition of hrR3 propagation (50), but in cell lines derived from colorectal carcinomas, GCV's antiviral effect predominates, and GCV promotes the survival of hrR3-infected cells in culture (51). This distinction may be attributable to differences in these tumors' levels of gap junctions. When using HSV-TK-positive herpes vectors, after allowing sufficient time for intratumoral vector spread, GCV could be administered as a safety-ensuring agent that blocks vector spread beyond the tumor. If the tumor happens to express high levels of gap junctions, an additional GCV-mediated oncolysis will occur.

Replacement of the large subunit of HSV-1 ribonucleotide reductase with the CYP2B1 gene has led to the generation of an HSV-1 vector, rRp450, that can kill tumor cells through three modes—viral oncolysis and rendering infected cells sensitive to CPA and GCV. Subcutaneous tumors established from glioma cell lines in immunodeficient mice only regress when treated with rRp450, CPA, and GCV (67).

Oncolytic HSV-1 vectors are being employed in three clinical trials, all designed to treat cancer and two designed to treat brain tumors, as of September 2001 (3).

Poliovirus

This single-stranded RNA virus commonly infects and replicates in anterior horn motoneurons, producing devastating paralytic illnesses in humans. However, deletion of one region of the viral genome and substitution with a sequence from human rhinovirus significantly attenuates this virus, so that it cannot grow in neurons, yet still infects/grows in and kills glioma cells. In another application, poliovirus was disabled so that it would infect tumor cells/grow in them and kill them, but the produced viral progeny was then unable to infect additional cells further.

BRAIN TUMOR GENE THERAPY CLINICAL TRIALS

Three viruses have been studied in completed brain tumor gene therapy clinical trials—retrovirus, adenovirus, and herpesvirus; the former two were genetically modified to express HSV-TK with concurrent GCV administration , and the latter two were used as a replication-conditional oncolytic agent in the absence of GCV administration (*see* Table 2A on p. 287 and 2B on pp. 288-289).

The first study of brain tumor gene therapy in human patients occurred when a retroviral vector carrying HSV-TK was inoculated into recurrent brain tumors in 1992, just 2 yr after the first human gene therapy of any kind was undertaken in a 4-yr-old girl with adenosine deaminase deficiency. The goals of the study were to assess safety, examine the survival of murine VPCs in human tumors, determine the degree of in vivo gene transfer to tumor cells, look for evidence of escape of the genetic vector outside the area of treatment, determine whether intratumoral transplantation of xenogenic cells into human brain tumors elicits an immune response, and detect evidence of local antitumor activity in human tumors. The study involved 15 patients with malignant brain tumors who had failed standard therapy *(68)*. Patients received stereotactic injections of HSV-TK VPCs throughout the MRI gadolinium-enhancing portion of their tumors. Eight patients showed a greater than 25% reduction in gadolinium enhancement on MRI immediately after GCV administration, and four patients showed sustained reduction, but not cure, 4–18 mo after treatment. Quantitative polymerase chain reaction (PCR) and *in situ* hybridization performed on tumors resected 7 d after producer cell implantation revealed a low in vivo transduction efficiency ($\leq 0.17\%$), suggesting that the bystander effect was vital to any observed therapeutic response *(68)*.

These results led to a phase I/II dose-escalating open study running from 1995 to 1996 in France involving 12 patients with recurrent glioblastoma multiforme. The surface of tumor volume remaining had to be 75 cm^2 or less. VPCs were injected at a total dose proportional to tumor surface volume along needle tracks spaced 1 cm apart to a maximum depth of 1.5 cm, followed eventually by GCV treatment. No treatment-related adverse effects occurred. Overall median survival was 206 d, with 25% of the patients surviving longer than 12 mo. One patient was free of recurrence at 2.8 yr after treatment *(69)*.

A similar phase I study was performed in 12 children between ages 2 and 15 treated between 1995 and 1997. These children had recurrent tumors and received 10 mL of VPCs at multiple sites at concentrations of 10^7–10^8 cells/mL, followed eventually by GCV treatment. Disease progression occurred at a median time of 3 mo after treatment, with the three longest times until progression being 5, 10, and 24 mo. No adverse effects were documented *(70)*.

A similar international, multicenter, open-label uncontrolled phase II study occurred between 1997 and 1998. In this study, 48 patients with recurrent GBM underwent optimal tumor resection, at which time a VPC suspension was administered through 0.2-mL (VPC density 10^8 cells/mL) injections spaced 0.5–1 cm apart each time to a depth of 1–2 cm, followed eventually by GCV administration. The VPCs were modified compared with the previous study, with additional unnecessary DNA sequences in the retroviral construct deleted to produce higher retroviral titers and improved transduction rates. The median survival time was 8.6 mo, and the 12-mo survival rate was 27%. Tumor recurrence was absent on MRI in seven patients for at least 6 mo, and for at least 12 mo in two patients. One patient remained recurrence free at 24 mo *(71)*.

To assess further the safety of VPC injections, rate of tumor cell transduction, amplitude of immune response, and degree of antitumor effect, a recent study combined gene marking with a therapeutic trial. In this study, five patients underwent two trials of intratumoral VPC implantation (first, three aliquots of 10^6 VPCs in columns; second, 5 ds later), separated by an intermediate harvest of implanted tumor for neuropathological study, and followed eventually by GCV treatment. Four patients tolerated the procedure well but experienced

Table 2A
Summary of Clinical Trials in Brain Tumor Gene Therapy: *21 Open Trials*[a]

Phase	Country	Investigator	Indication	Gene(s)	Vector	Route	No. of patients
I	Japan	Yoshida	GBM, astrocytoma	IFN-β	none	it	Unknown
III	Multicountry	Maria	GBM	HSV-TK	Retrovirus	it	251
II	Multicountry	Maria	GBM	HSV-TK	Retrovirus	it	13
I/II	Spain	Izquierdo	GBM	HSV-TK	Retrovirus	it	9
I/II	Multicountry	Mulder	GBM	HSV-TK	Retrovirus	it	4
I	Netherlands	Mulder	GBM	IL-2	None	it	3
I	Multicountry	Van Gilder	GBM	HSV-TK	Retrovirus	it	30
I/II	Poland	Kasprzak	GBM, meningioma	IGF-1 triple helix	Plasmid DNA	sc	1
I/II	Switzerland	Seiler	GBM	HSV-TK	Retrovirus	it	Unknown
I	UK	Alberts	GBM, primary or recurrent	None	HSV-1 with γ34.5 deletion	it	9
I	UK	Alberts	GBM, primary or recurrent	None	HSV-1 with γ34.5 deletion	it	Unknown
I	USA	Ilan	GBM	IGF-1 antisense	Lipofection	sc	1
I	USA	Lieberman	GBM	HSV-TK	Adenovirus	it	Unknown
I	USA	Sobol	GBM	IL-2	Retrovirus	sc	1
I	USA	K. Black	GBM	GM-CSF	Plasmid DNA	id	Unknown
I	USA	Eck	GBM	IFN-β	Adenovirus	it	Unknown
I	USA	Hesdorffer	GBM	MDR-1	Retrovirus	bm	5
I	USA	Kun	Recurrent pediatric brain tumors	HSV-TK	Retrovirus	it	2
I	USA	Okada	GBM	IL-4	Retrovirus	id	Unknown
I	USA	Lang	GBM	p53	Adenovirus	it	Unknown
I	USA	Pollack	GBM	IL-4	Retrovirus	sc	Unknown
I	USA	Fetell	Recurrent GBM	HSV-TK	Retrovirus	it	2

[a] *As of September 2001.* Data from open studies were obtained from ref. 3; data from closed studies were obtained from the references given in the table.

Abbreviations: met, metastasis; HSV-TK, herpes simplex virus type 1 thymidine kinase gene; LacZ, *E. coli* β-galactosidase gene; 1716, HSV-1 with mutation in γ34.5 gene; G207, HSV-1 mutated in γ34.5 and large subunit of viral ribonucleotide reductase; it, intratumoral; sc, subcutaneous; id, intradermal; bm, reinfused back into bone marrow after ex vivo gene transfer; No. patients, number of patients enrolled in the trial; VPCs, vector producer cells; VPs, vector particles; retro, retrovirus; adeno, adenovirus; PFU, plaque-forming units; GCV (d), days during which 7 mg/kg twice a day intravenous ganciclovir was given, with day 0 being the day on which tumor resection and viral vector implantation were performed; surv, survival; prog, disease progression as defined by tumor growth or recurrence on MRI; GBM, glioblastoma multiforme; IFN, interferon; IGF, insulin-like growth factor; IL, interleukin; GM-CSF, granulocyte-macrophage colony-stimulating factor; met, metastasis.

Table 2B
Summary of Clinical Trials in Brain Tumor Gene Therapy: *11 Closed Trials*[a]

Phase	Country	Investigator	Indication	Gene(s)	Vector	Route	No. of patients
I	USA	Oldfield	Recurrent GBM or met	HSV-TK	Retrovirus	it	15
I/II	France	Klatzmann	Recurrent GBM	HSV-TK	Retrovirus	it	12
I	USA	Packer	Children with recurrent tumors	HSV-TK	Retrovirus	it	12
I/II	Multicountry	Mariani	GBM	HSV-TK	Retrovirus	it	48
I	USA	Harsh	GBM	HSV-TK	Retrovirus	it	5
III	Multicountry	Rainov	GBM	HSV-TK	Retrovirus	it	248 (124 control, 124 retro)
I	USA	Trask	Recurrent GBM or recurrent	HSV-TK and LacZ	Adenovirus adenovirus	it	13
I/II	Finland	Yla-Herttuala	GBM, primary	HSV-TK	Retrovirus or	it	21 (7 retro; 7 adeno; 7 LacZ)
I	UK	Rampling	Recurrent GBM	No transgene	1716 (HSV-1 mutant)	it	9
I	USA	Markert	Primary or recurrent GBM	No transgene	G207 (HSV-1 mutant)	it	21
I	USA	K. Black	GBM	TGF-B	Plasmid	sc	2
I	USA	Eck	GBM	HSV-TK	Adenovirus	it	13

[a] *See* footnote and abbreviations for Table 2A.

tumor progression. The other developed an abscess after the second operation and died. The abscess was unrelated to the VPS injection and was caused by *Staphylococcus aureus*. Increased HSV-TK enzymatic activity was demonstrated in one tumor specimen. Immunohistochemical confirmation of HSV-TK gene expression was limited only to VPCs, with no detection of activity in tumor cells. Viable tumor cells were seen near HSV-TK–positive VPCs. The lymphocytic immune response was mild *(72)*.

These studies suggested that the HSV-TK gene therapy strategy using retroviral VPCs appeared safe, although potentially limited by poor transduction, with efficacy evaluation only possible by means of an adequately powered, randomized controlled trial. Such a trial occurred by means of a parallel-group phase III trial involving patients recruited between 1996 and 1998 with untreated glioblastoma multiforme randomized into two groups of 124 patients each. The first group received gross resection of tumor on d 0, followed by 50–60 Gy in 2-Gy fractions starting on d 14–21 and continuing for 6 wk. The second group received HSV-TK VPCs (10 mL at a concentration of 10^8 VPC/mL) during craniotomy by means of multiple injections 1 cm in depth, separated by 1 cm *(73)*. Progression-free median survival in the gene therapy group was 180 d compared with 183 d in control subjects. Median survival was 365 vs 354 d,

Treatment period	Virus dose	GCV (d)	Result	Ref.
7/92–12/94	2.5–10 × 10^8 VPCs	8–21	Median surv 8 mo	68
1/95–4/96	6 × 10^7–6 × 10^8 VPCs	8–21	Median surv 7 mo	69
11/95–12/97	10^8–10^9 VPCs	14–27	Median to prog 3 mo	70
1/97–7/98	2 × 10^7 VPCs	14–27	Median surv 9 mo	71
3/98–3/99	10^6 VPCs	14–27	Median surv 8 mo	72
7/96–4/98	10^9 VPCs	14–27	Median surv (d): 365 retro; 354 control	73
12/96–9/98	2 × 10^9–2 × 10^{12} VPs	1–15	Median surv 4 mo	74
1/98–9/99	3×10^8–2 × 10^9 VPCs (retro) 1–6 × 10^{10} VPs (adeno)	5–18 (adeno) 14–27 (retro)	Median surv (mo): 7 (retro); 10 (LacZ); 15 (adeno)	75
11/97–11/99	10^5 PFU	Not given	Median surv 7 mo	76
2/98–5/99	10^6–3 × 10^9 PFU	Not given	Mean to prog 3.5 mo	77
Closed 1997	Not known	Not given	Not known	None
Unknown	Unknown	Unknown	Unknown	None

and 12-mo survival rates were 50 vs 55% in the gene therapy and control groups, respectively. These differences were not statistically significant.

There has been an anecdotal case report of a patient whose malignant glioma responded favorably to treatment with VPC-retrovirus-TK/ganciclovir gene therapy for at least 3 yr. Death from an unrelated cause led to postmortem analysis of the brain. This failed to show evidence of tumor, leading to the assertion of a cure. In spite of this, the results of the phase III trial indicate that significant advances and refinements will be needed to show that this technology can work.

The second vector studied in clinical trials is based on adenovirus. Between 1996 and 1998, 13 patients with recurrent glioblastoma multiforme were treated with a single intratumoral injection in escalating doses that ranged from 2 × 10^9 up to 2 × 10^{12} vector particles (VPs) of a replication-defective adenoviral vector bearing HSV-TK, followed eventually by ganciclovir treatment. Doses of 2 × 10^{11} VPs or less were tolerated, but patients treated with 2 × 10^{12} VPs exhibited CNS toxicity, causing confusion, hyponatremia, and seizures. One patient was reported alive and stable 29.2 mo after treatment, and two patients survived 25 mo before succumbing to tumor progression. Neuropathologic examination of postmortem tissue confirmed intratumoral foci of coagulative necrosis with variable infiltration of residual tumor with macrophages and lymphocytes *(74)*.

Retroviruses were compared with adenoviruses in a phase I/II trial in Finland between 1998 and 1999, in which 21 patients with primary or recurrent glioblastoma multiforme were randomly divided into three groups *(75)*. At the time of surgical resection, the two experimental groups were treated with VPCs producing retroviruses expressing HSV-TK or adenoviruses expressing HSV-TK; the control group received either adenovirus or VPCs expressing *E. coli* β-galactosidase, a marker gene. After subsequent GCV treatment, mean survival times were 7.4 (retrovirus), 8.3 (control), and 15.0 mo (adenovirus). Although the differences between mean survival times of the retrovirus and control groups were not statistically significant, the differences between the adenovirus group and the other two groups were significant ($p < 0.012$). No adverse effects occurred. The explanations offered for the greater efficacy of the adenovirus group were greater titer, a benefit from the inflammatory reaction to adenovirus, and the ability of adenovirus to infect nondividing cells. It is important to remember that the latter two features have also been raised also as safety concerns for adenovirus.

The third virus to undergo clinical trials in brain tumor therapy is HSV-1. Recently, two groups performed phase I dose-escalation safety trials of replication-selective HSVs in the treatment of malignant brain tumors. A Scottish group evaluated the γ34.5 mutant 1716 in nine patients with brain tumors between 1997 and 1999 *(76)*, and a U.S. group evaluated the double γ34.5 and ribonucleotide reductase mutant G207 in 21 patients with brain tumors *(77)*. Patients in the Scottish trial received lower doses of virus (between 10^3 and 10^5 PFU) than patients in the US trial (between 10^6 and 3×10^9 PFU), perhaps because of safety concerns.

In the 1716 trial, three patients each received 10^3, 10^4, and 10^5 PFU of 1716 by a single intratumoral injection *(76)*. No adverse effects, including encephalitis, were seen that could be attributed to the administration of 1716. Five patients died of tumor progression at the conclusion of the 14–24 mo study. The thallium SPECT volumes were smaller in one, stable in two, larger in five, and not assessable in one patient.

In the G207 trial, 21 patients received doses ranging from 10^6 PFU in a single site to 3×10^9 PFU at five sites between 1998 and 1999 *(77)*. Two patients had long-term expression of the β-galactosidase reporter gene found in G207 56 and 157 d after inoculation. No encephalitis was reported or found at autopsy. Four of the 21 patients were alive at the time the results were published. No deaths were attributable to the viral vector. Six of 21 patients had a decrease in the enhancement volume on MRI 1 mo after viral inoculation *(77)*.

Finally, the onoclytic adenovirus ONYX-015 was evaluated in a dose-escalating trial for patients with recurrent malignant glioma between 1999 and 2002 (New Approaches to Brain Tumor Therapy Consortium Trial Number 9701). Injections were performed in brain adjacent to tumor resected at surgery. The treatment was well tolerated by 24 enrolled patients, even at the highest injected dose of 10^{10} PFU.

FUTURE DIRECTIONS

The completed clinical trials in brain tumor gene therapy have offered evidence for the safety of this modality but have suggested that its efficacy will continue to be limited by inefficient transduction, the biggest discrepancy between the experimental rodent studies and the clinical trials. Inefficient transduction will need to be addressed in the laboratory before any larger scale clinical trials are conducted.

The efficiency of transduction could be improved by modifying VPCs or by modifying the means by which they are delivered. Use of migratory VPCs, which have shown the ability to "track" even single tumor cells invading the surrounding normal brain *(78)*, may allow better spatial distribution of VPCs throughout the tumor, particularly in distal areas that become foci of recurrence. The currently used manual injections of VPCs into multiple needle tracks are plagued by the limitations in volume that can be injected at any given time and the reflux that occurs along needle tracks. These problems might be addressed by using 3D neuronavigation techniques and automated slow-speed injection/infusion devices *(79,80)*.

The dependence on the bystander effect and limitations of poor transduction could also be overcome by recruiting the immune response. Hoping that the use of a transgene encoding a secreted protein might overcome the difficulty obtaining extensive HSV-TK transduction, a phase I trial has been launched using a recombinant adenovirus expressing human interferon-β *(81)*.

It could well be that the next step in the development of brain tumor gene therapy will require a multimodal approach combining several of the ideas suggested above. Hopefully, continued gene therapy studies in the laboratory will lead to novel clinical trials capable of improving the outcome for patients diagnosed in the future with malignant gliomas.

REFERENCES

1. Southam CM. Present status of oncolytic virus studies. *NY Acad Sci* 1960;22:656–673.
2. Martuza RL, Malick A, Markert JM, et al. Experimental therapy of human glioma by means of a genetically engineered virus mutant. *Science* 1991;252:854–856.
3. On-line database found at the website for *The Journal of Gene Medicine*. Updated September 2001. http://www.wiley.co.uk/genetherapy/clinical/.
4. Mulligan RC, Berg P. Selection for animal cells that express the Escherichia coli gene coding for xanthineguanine phosphoribosyltransferase. *Proc Natl Acad Sci USA* 1981;78:2072–2076.
5. Boviatsis EJ, Scharf JM, Chase M, et al. Antitumor activity and reporter gene transfer into rat brain neoplasms inoculated with herpes simplex virus vectors defective in thymidine kinase or ribonucleotide reductase. *Gene Therapy* 1994;1:323–331.
6. Boviatsis EJ, Park JS, Sena-Esteves M, Kramm CM, Chase M, Efird JT, et al. Long-term survival of rats harboring brain neoplasms treated with ganciclovir and a herpes simplex virus vector that retains an intact thymidine kinase gene. *Cancer Res* 1994;54:5745–5751.
7. Brown SM, MacLean AR, McKie EA, et al. The herpes simplex virus virulence factor ICP34.5 and the cellular protein MyD116 complex with the proliferating cell

nuclear antigen through the 63-amino-acid domain conserved in ICP34.5, MyD116, and GADD34. *J Virol* 1997;71:9442–9449.
8. Wang Q, Guo J, Jia W. Intracerebral recombinant HSV-1 vector does not reactivate latent HSV-1. *Gene Ther* 1997;4:1300–1304.
9. Mohr I, Gluzman Y. A herpesvirus genetic element which affects translation in the absence of the viral GADD34 function. *EMBO J* 1996;15:4759–4766.
10. Pyles RB, Warnick RE, Chalk CL, et al. A novel multiply-mutated HSV-1 strain for the treatment of human brain tumors. *Hum Gene Ther* 1997;8:533–544.
11. Kramm CM, Chase M, Herrlinger U, et al. Therapeutic efficiency and safety of a second-generation replication-conditional HSV1 vector for brain tumor gene therapy. *Hum Gene Ther* 1997;8:2057–2068.
12. Chung RY, Saeki Y, Chiocca EA. B-myb promoter retargeting of herpes simplex virus γ34.5 gene-mediated virulence toward tumor and cycling cells. *J Virol* 1999; 73:7556–7564.
13. Bischoff JR, Kirn DH, Williams A, et al. An adenovirus mutant that replicates selectively in p53-deficient human tumor cells. *Science* 1996;274:373–376.
14. Hollstein M, Rice K, Greenblatt MS, et al. Database of p53 gene somatic mutations in human tumors and cell lines. *Nucleic Acids Res* 1994;22:3551–3555.
15. Coffey MC, Strong JE, Forsyth PA, Lee PW. Reovirus therapy of tumors with activated ras pathway. *Science* 1998;282:1332–1334.
16. Von Deimling A, Louis DN, Schramm J, Wiestler OD. Astrocytic gliomas: characterization on a molecular genetic basis, in *Molecular Neuro-oncology and Its Impact on the Clinical Management of Brain Tumors* (Wiestler OD, Schlegel U, Schramm J, eds.), Springer-Verlag, Berlin, 1994, pp. 33–42.
17. Mercer WE, Shields MT, Amin M, et al. Negative growth regulation in a glioblastoma tumor cell line that conditionally expresses human wild-type p53. *Proc Natl Acad Sci USA* 1990;87:6166–6170.
18. Asai A, Miyagi Y, Sugiyama A, et al. Negative effects of wild-type p53 and s-Myc on cellular growth and tumorigenecity of glioma cells. *J Neurooncol* 1994;19: 259–268.
19. Roth JA, Nguyen D, Lawrence DD, et al. Retrovirus-mediated wild-type p53 gene transfer to tumors of patients with lung cancer. *Nat Med* 1996;2:985–991.
20. Collins, V.P. Epidermal growth factor receptor gene and its transcripts in glioblastomas, in *Molecular Neuro-oncology and Its Impact on the Clinical Management of Brain Tumors* (Wiestler OD, Schlegel U, Schramm J, eds.), Springer-Verlag, Berlin, 1994, pp. 17–24.
21. Redemann N, Holzmann B, von Ruden T, Wagner EF, Schlessinger J, Ullrich A. Anti-oncogenic activity of signaling-defective epidermal growth receptor mutants. *Mol Cell Biol 1992*;12:491–498.
22. Van Meir EG, Polverini PJ, Chazin VR, Huang HJS, deTribolet N, Cavenee WK. Release of an inhibitor of angiogenesis upon induction of wild type p53 expression in glioblastoma cells. *Nat Genet* 1994;8:171–176.
23. Millauer B, Shawver LK, Plate KH, Risau W, Ulrich A. Glioblastoma growth inhibited *in vivo* by a dominant-negative Flk-1 mutant. *Nature* 1994;367:576–578.
24. Ma H-I, Guo P, Li J, et al. Suppression of intracranial human glioma growth after intramuscular administration of an adeno-associated viral vector expressing angiostatin. *Cancer Res* 2002;62:756–763.
25. Fearon ER, Pardoll DM, Itaya T, et al. Interleukin-2 production by tumor cells bypasses T helper function in the generation of an antitumor response. *Cell* 1990; 60:397–403.

26. Gansbacher B, Bannerji R, Daniels B, Zier K, Cronin K, Gilboa, E. Retroviral vector-mediated gamma-interferon gene transfer into tumor cells generates potent and long lasting antitumor immunity. *Cancer Res* 1990;50:7820–7825.
27. Tjuvajev J, Gansbacher B, Desai R, et al. RG-2 glioma growth attenuation and severe brain edema caused by local production of interleukin-2 and interferon-2. *Cancer Res* 1995;55:1902–1910.
28. Yu JS, Wei MX, Chiocca EA, Martuza RL, Tepper RI. Treatment of glioma by engineered interleukin 4-secreting cells. *Cancer Res* 1993;53:3125–3128.
29. Tahara H, Lotze MT. Antitumor effects of interleukin-12 (IL-12): applications for the immunotherapy and gene therapy of cancer. *Gene Ther* 1994;2:96–106.
30. Qin X-Q, Tao N, Dergay A, et al. Interferon-β gene therapy inhibits tumor formation and causes regression of established tumors in immune-deficient mice. *Proc Natl Acad Sci USA* 1998;95:14411–14416.
31. Herrlinger U, Kramm CM, Johnston KM, et al. Vaccination for experimental gliomas using GM-CSF-transduced glioma cells. *Cancer Gene Ther* 1997;4:345–352.
32. Dranoff GE, Jaffee E, Lazenby A, et al. Vaccination with irradiated tumor cells engineered to secrete murine granulocyte-macrophage colony-stimulating factor stimulates potent, specific, and long-lasting anti-tumor immunity. *Proc Natl Acad Sci U S A* 1993;90:3539–3543.
33. Saito S, Bannerji R, Gansbacher B, et al. Immunotherapy of bladder cancer with cytokine gene-modified tumor vaccines. *Cancer Res* 1994;54:3516–3520.
34. Vieweg J, Rosenthal FM, Banerji R, et al. Imunotherapy of prostate cancer in the Dunning rat model: use of cytokine gene modified tumor vaccines. *Cancer Res* 1994;54:1760–1765.
35. Sorrentino BP, Brandt SJ, Bodine D, et al. Selection of drug-resistant bone marrow cells *in vivo* after retroviral transfer of the human MDR1. *Science* 1992;257:99–103.
36. Faulds D, Heel RC. Ganciclovir: a review of its antiviral activity, pharmacokinetic properties, and therapeutic effciacy in cytomegalovirus infections. *Drugs* 1990;39:597–638.
37. Shewach DS, Zerbe LK, Hughes TL, Roessler BJ, Breakefield XO, Davidson, B.L. Enhanced cytotoxicity of antiviral drugs mediated by adenovirus directed transfer of the herpes simplex virus thymidine kinase gene in rat glioma cells. *Cancer Gene Ther* 1994;1:107–112.
38. Rainov NG, Kramm CM, Aboody-Guterman K, et al. Retrovirus-mediated gene therapy of experimental brain neoplasms using the herpes-simplex virus-thymidine kinase/ganciclovir paradigm. *Cancer Gene Ther* 1996;3:99–106.
39. Freeman SM, Abboud CN, Whartenby KA, et al. The "bystander effect": tumor regression when a fraction of the tumor mass is genetically modified. *Cancer Res* 1993;53:5274–5283.
40. Ishii-Morita H, Agbaria R, Mullen CA, et al. Mechanism of 'bystander effect' killing in the herpes simplex thymidine kinase gene therapy model of cancer treatment. *Gene Therapy* 1997;4:244–251.
41. Fick J, Barker FG, Dazin P, Westphale EM, Beyer EC, Israel MA. The extent of heterocellular communication mediated by gap junctions is predictive of bystander tumor cytotoxicity *in vitro*. *Proc Natl Acad Sci USA* 1995;92:11071–11075.
42. Ram Z, Walbridge S, Shawker T, Culver KW, Blaese RM, Oldfield, E.H. The effect of thymidine kinase transduction and ganciclovir therapy on tumor vasculature and growth of 9L gliomas in rats. *J Neurosurg* 1994;81:256–260.
43. Barba, D., Hardin, J., Sadelain, M., Gage, F.H. Development of anti-tumor immunity following thymidine kinase-mediated killing of experimental brain tumors. *Proc Natl Acad Sci USA* 1994;91:4348–4352.

44. Gagandeep S, Brew R, Green B, et al. Prodrug-activated gene therapy: involvement of an immunological component in the "bystander effect." *Cancer Gene Ther* 1996;3:83–88.
45. Kianmanesh AR, Perrin H, Panis Y, et al. A "distant" bystander effect of suicide gene therapy: regression of nontransduced tumor together with a distant transduced tumor. *Hum Gene Ther* 1997;8:1807–1814.
46. Caruso M, Panis Y, Gagandeep S, Houssin D, Salzmann JL, Klatzmann, D. Regression of established macroscopic liver metastases after *in situ* transduction of a suicide gene. *Proc Natl Acad Sci USA* 1993;90:7024–7028.
47. Black ME, Newcomb TG, Wilson HP, Loeb LA. Creation of drug-specific herpes simplex virus type 1 thymidine kinase mutants for gene therapy. *Proc Natl Acad Sci USA* 1996;93:3525–3529.
48. Kim JH, Kim SH, Kolozsvarky A, Brown SL, Kim OB, Freytag SO. Selective enhancement of radiation response of herpes simplex virus thymidine kinase transduced 9L gliosarcoma cells in vitro and in vivo by antiviral agents. *Int J Radiat Oncol* 1995;33:861–868.
49. Tjuvajev JG, Finn R, Watanabe K, et al. Noninvasive imaging of herpes virus thymidine kinase gene transfer and expression: a potential method for monitoring clinical gene therapy. *Cancer Res* 1996;56:4087–4095.
50. Boviatsis EJ, Park JS, Sena-Esteves M, et al. Long-term survival of rats harboring brain neoplasms treated with ganciclovir and a herpes simplex virus vector that retains an intact thymidine kinase gene. *Cancer Res* 1994;54:5745–5751.
51. Carroll NM, Chase M, Chiocca EA, Tanabe KK. The effect of ganciclovir on herpes simplex virus-mediated oncolysis. *J Surg Res* 1997;69:413–417.
52. Grem JL. 5-fluoropyrimidines, in *Cancer Chemotherapy and Biotherapy: Principles and Practice*, 2nd ed. (Chabner BA, Longo DL, eds.), Lipincott, Philadelphia, 1996, pp. 149–212.
53. Hoshino T, Wilson CB, Rosenblum ML, Barker M. Chemotherapeutic implications of growth fraction and cell cycle time in glioblastomas. *J Neurosurg* 1975;43:127–135.
54. Aghi M, Kramm CM, Chou TC, Breakefield XO Chiocca, E.A. Synergistic anticancer effects of ganciclovir/thymidine kinase and 5-fluorocytosine/cytosine deaminase gene therapies. *J Natl Cancer Inst* 1998;90:370–380.
55. Mullen CA, Coale MM, Lowe RM, Blaese RM. Tumors expressing the cytosine deaminase suicide gene can be eliminated *in vivo* with 5-fluorocytosine and induce protective immunity to wild type tumor. *Cancer Res 1994*;54:1503–1506.
56. Mullen CA, Petropoulous D, Lowe RM. Treatment of microscopic pulmonary metastases with recombinant autologous tumor vaccine expressing interleukin 6 and *Escherichia coli* cytosine deaminase suicide genes. *Cancer Res* 1996;56:1361–1366.
57. Huber BE, Austin EA, Richards CA, Davis ST, Good SS. Metabolism of 5-fluorocytosine to 5-fluorouracil in human colorectal tumor cells transduced with the cytosine deaminase gene: significant antitumor effects when only a small percentage of tumor cells express cytosine deaminase. *Proc Natl Acad Sci USA* 1994;91:8302–8306.
58. Holder JW, Elmore E, Barrett JC. Gap junction function and cancer. *Cancer Res* 1993;53:3475–3485.
59. Dong, Y, Wen, P, Manome, Y, Parr, M, Hirshowitz, Chen, L, et al. *In vivo* replication-deficient adenovirus vector-mediated transduction of the cytosine deaminase gene sensitizes glioma cells to 5-fluorocytosine. *Hum Gene Ther* 1996;7:713–720.
60. Miller CR, Williams CR, Buchsbaum DJ, Gillespie GY. Intratumoral 5-fluorouracil produced by cytosine deaminase/5-fluorocytosine gene therapy is effective for experimental human glioblastomas. *Cancer Res* 2002;62:773–780.

61. Tew KD, Colvin M, Chabner BA. Alkylating agents, in *Cancer Chemotherapy and Biotherapy: Principles and Practice*, 2nd ed. (Chabner BA, Longo DL, eds.), Lippincott, Philadelphia, 1996, pp. 297–332.
62. Wei MX, Tamiya T, Chase M, et al. Experimental tumor therapy in mice using the cyclophosphamide-activating cytochrome P450 2B1 gene. *Hum Gene Ther* 1994;5:969–978.
63. Gopferich A, Alonso MJ, Langer R. Development and characterization of microencapsulated microspheres. *Pharmacol Res* 1994;11:1568–1574.
64. Wei MX, Tamiya T, Rhee RJ, Breakefield XO, Chiocca EA. Diffusible cytotoxic metabolites contribute to the *in vitro* bystander effect associated with the cyclophosphamide/cytochrome P450 2B1 cancer gene therapy paradigm. *Clin Cancer Res* 1995;1:1171–1177.
65. Chen L, Waxman D. Intratumoral activation and enhanced chemotherapeutic effect of oxazaphosphorines following cytochrome P450 gene transfer: development of a combined chemotherapy/cancer gene therapy strategy. *Cancer Res* 1995;55:581–589.
66. Chen L, Yu LJ, Waxman DJ. Potentiation of cytochrome P450/cyclophosphamide-based cancer gene therapy by coexpression of the P450 reductase gene. *Cancer Res* 1997;57:4830–4837.
67. Aghi M, Chou TC, Suling K, et al. Multimodal cancer treatment mediated by a replicating oncolytic virus that delivers the oxazaphosphorine/rat cytochrome P450 2B1 and gancliovir/herpes simplex virus thymidine kinase gene therapies. *Cancer Res* 59:3861–3865; 1999.
68. Ram Z, Culver K, Oshiro E, et al. Summary of results and conclusions of the gene therapy of malignant brain tumors: clinical study. *J Neurosurg* 1995;82:343A.
69. Klatzmann D, Valery CA, Bensimon G, et al. A phase I/II study of herpes simplex virus type 1 thymidine kinase "suicide" gene therapy for recurrent glioblastoma. *Hum Gene Ther* 1998;9:2595–2604.
70. Packer RJ, Raffel C, Villablanca JG, et al. Treatment of progressive or recurrent pediatric malignant supratentorial brain tumors with herpes simplex virus thymidine kinase gene vector-producer cells followed by intravenous ganciclovir administration. *J Neurosurg* 2000;92:249–254.
71. Shand N, Weber F, Mariani L, et al. A phase 1–2 clinical trial of gene therapy for recurrent glioblastoma multiforme by tumor transduction with the herpes simplex thymidine kinase gene followed by ganciclovir. *Hum Gene Ther* 1999;10:2325–2335.
72. Harsh GR, Deisboeck TS, Louis DN, Hilton J, Colvin M, et al. *J Neurosurg* 2000;92:804–811.
73. Rainov NG. A phase III CLinical Evaluation of Herpes Simplex Virus Type 1 Thymidine Kinase and Ganciclovir Gene Therapy as an adjuvant to surgical resection and radiation in adults with previously untreated glioblastoma multiforme. *Hum Gene Ther* 2000;11:2389–2401.
74. Trask TW, Trask RP, Aguilar-Cordova E, et al. Phase I study of adenoviral delivery of the HSV-TK gene and ganciclovir administration in patients with recurrent malignant brain tumors. *Mol Ther* 2000;1:195–203.
75. Sandmair A-M, Loimas S, Puranen P, et al. Thymidine kinase gene therapy for human malignant glioma, using replication-deficient retroviruses or adenoviruses. *Hum Gene Ther* 2000;11:2197–2205.
76. Rampling R, Cruickshank G, Papanastassiou V, et al. Toxicity evaluation of replication-competent herpes simplex virus (ICP 34.5 null mutant 1716) in patients with recurrent malignant glioma. *Gene Ther* 2000;7:859–866.

77. Markert JM, Medlock MD, Rabkin SD, et al. Conditionally replicating herpes simplex virus mutant, G207 for the treatment of malignant glioma: results of a phase I trial. *Gene Ther* 2000;7:867–874.
78. Herrlinger U, Woiciechowski C, Sena-Esteves M, et al. Neural precursor cells for delivery of replication-conditional HSV-1 vectors to intracerebral gliomas. *Mol Ther* 2000;1:347–357.
79. Rutka JT, Taylor M, Mainprize T, et al. Molecular biology and neurosurgery in the third millennium. *Neurosurgery* 2000;46:1034–1051.
80. Lieberman DM, Laske DW, Morrison PF, Bankiewicz KS, Oldfield EH. Convection-enhanced distribution of large molecules in gray matter during interstitial drug infusion. *J Neurosurg* 1995;82:1021–1029.
81. Eck SL, Alavi JB, Judy K, et al. Treatment of recurrent or progressive malignant glioma with a recombinant adenovirus expressing human interferon-beta (H5.010CMVhIFN-β): a phase I trial. *Hum Gene Ther* 2001;12:97–113.

14
Local Delivery Methods Into the CNS

Timothy W. Vogel, MD and Jeffrey N. Bruce, MD

INTRODUCTION

The earliest forms of therapeutic drug delivery to the central nervous system (CNS) were systemically based intravenous and oral preparations. Despite attempts to increase target concentrations with intraarterial delivery or osmotic opening of the blood–brain barrier (BBB), systemic delivery remains hindered by systemic toxicity and the need for extensive drug modification for effective *(80)* BBB penetration. These limitations have provided the impetus for developing strategies of localized treatment for CNS disorders, to circumvent the BBB and increase local drug concentration without systemic toxicity.

A variety of methodologies for local delivery have been developed including direct injection, polymer technology, and convection-enhanced delivery (CED). Although many of these delivery methods are in the early phases of development, they have demonstrated their superiority to systemic methods in experimental models and clinical trials *(8,28)*. By avoiding the systemic circulation, local delivery of therapeutic agents into the CNS allows compounds to reach targeted sites more consistently without undesired tissue binding, protein binding, and enzymatic modification, to promote a more consistent drug uptake *(19)*. The advantage of local delivery for treating CNS disorders is, therefore, the ability to achieve a sufficient concentration of drug at the site of the lesion or defined neuroanatomic region for sufficient duration to produce a therapeutic response *(35)*.

ADVANTAGES OF LOCAL DELIVERY STRATEGIES

Traditional systemic delivery modalities share a common limitation by relying on diffusion across the BBB to distribute a therapeutic agent throughout the CNS *(3)*. Diffusion, especially through solid tissue, is slow and relies on concentration gradients to disperse molecules *(95)*. The increased time needed to establish dispersion reduces the bioavailability of drugs by increasing the potential for drug catabolism and tissue clearance. Methods that rely on diffusion require a high concentration source to establish a sufficient concentration gradient for adequate distribution. The high concentration sources needed to establish sufficient concentration gradients across the BBB can be toxic to both the surrounding cerebral tissue and systemic organ systems *(81)*.

The major advantage of local treatment modalities is that drugs do not have to cross the BBB to reach target destinations *(2)*. Although the BBB has been shown to be disrupted in cerebral tumors and may not be an absolute barrier to therapy, some form of BBB remains either within the tumor or in peritumoral brain *(3,81,83)*. Local treatment avoids this limitation, achieving higher local drug concentrations in the surrounding parenchyma *(5,71,81)*.

An example of the application of local therapy is in the treatment of malignant gliomas, in which tumor dissemination and local recurrence are problematic. Up to 90% of gliomas recur within 2 cm of resection, providing the rationale for local delivery by increasing intratumoral and peritumoral concentrations of therapeutic agent *(1,9,51,28)*. Although this theoretical advantage for decreased tumor recurrence is challenged by some investigators *(28)*, local treatment modalities have been shown to increase significantly patient survival *(53,55,56)*.

Local treatment modalities achieve a higher local drug concentration *(13,51)*, sustain longer target exposure times, and minimize toxicity *(75,77)*. One of the disadvantages of systemic treatment is the brief time a drug is in contact with a targeted area of the CNS. Arterial delivery has been tried in an effort to increase CNS penetration, but its pulsatile nature, its potential for binding tissues outside the CNS, and its increasing tissue clearance before and after reaching the CNS combine to limit the time and dose of exposure. By contrast, local delivery can maintain drug concentration and exposure more uniformly and consistently *(3,5)* through increased drug half-life *(3,75)* by limiting a drug's exposure to tissues, carrier proteins, and cells outside the CNS *(75)*.

Technological advances have produced products engineered to facilitate local delivery strategies. Direct injection with pumps, reservoirs, and catheters offers several advantages when one is attempting to treat patients requiring complex and prolonged delivery schemes with multiple drugs *(20)*. Different rates of drug infusion can be programmed for treatment *(4)*, and refillable pumps and reservoirs avoid the need for multiple injections, surgeries, or invasive procedures. Among the most versatile and effective local delivery strategies is CED, which can treat localized lesions while potentially reaching areas of invaded brain tissue *(71,75,80,83)*. The more uniform concentrations attained with CED achieve a desired therapeutic window for a drug *(75,95)* and provide flexibility for controlling the concentrations over a longer period of treatment time *(81)*. Adjustment of volumes and flow rates allows local concentrations to be altered in a temporal fashion with greater accuracy *(2,80)*. CED also achieves maximal volume of distribution in a shorter time *(75,77,80,95)*. The reduced time translates into less drug catabolism, less nonspecific tissue binding, reduced tissue clearance, and prolonged exposure to the drug *(95)*.

Local delivery modalities provide the advantage of delivering a variety of new classes of therapeutic compounds from neurohormones, trophic factors, neurotransmitters, viruses, immunotherapy, and drugs to a specific site within the CNS *(22)*. This advantage of customizing drug delivery expands the repertoire of drugs that can be used when treating CNS disorders *(11,51)*. The flexibility to apply novel classes of compounds to cellular and molecular targets will help local delivery modalities keep pace with evolving pharmaceutical developments that would otherwise not be feasible with systemic delivery.

EARLY STRATEGIES FOR LOCAL DELIVERY

Direct injection of therapeutic compounds into the CNS is one of the earliest forms of local delivery for CNS lesions. This treatment modality includes intrathecal and intraventricular injections and has been successful in the control of patient pain and in the treatment of leptomeningeal metastases. Direct injection has also been used to facilitate recent advances in gene therapy with viral vectors and immunotherapy with activated lymphocytes. Improved engineering of injection catheters, implantable pumps, and refillable Ommaya reservoirs has expanded the versatility and success of this approach in clinical trials.

Methods of Direct Injection

Injection into the CNS has been studied by targeting different compartments of the CNS. Clinical trials have been conducted using intrathecal, intraventricular, and intracerebral injections. Each route of administration possesses different properties and limitations based on its cellular environment and fluid dynamics. Variables include drug distribution following delivery, time of injection, number of injections, site of infusion, and property of drug or therapy being delivered *(22)*. Clinical trials have utilized reservoirs *(16)*, implantable pumps *(20)*, and catheters *(35)* as delivery devices.

Intrathecal Delivery

The thecal sac and lateral ventricles share many of the same properties of drug distribution and fluid dynamics. Intrathecal injection involves administration of drug into the subarachnoid space, primarily in the lumbar area; intraventricular drug injection refers to infusion into the lateral ventricles. The primary property governing drug distribution within these spaces is bulk flow of cerebrospinal fluid (CSF). CSF flow is directional, with a variable velocity within the CNS that can further affect a drug's distribution *(2)*. Because of CSF flow, the initial concentration of drug is directly proportional to the concentration of the infusate *(2)*. CSF is an ideal medium for drug delivery, allowing therapeutic agents to be delivered unaltered to their targeted site at desired concentrations *(20,22)*. Drug concentration in the CSF is governed by several variables including the number and duration of injections as well as the drug's ability to cross the CSF–brain barrier and distribute further by diffusion *(2,4,22)*.

Intraparenchymal Injection

Drug distribution following local injection into brain parenchyma largely depends on the size and molecular weight of the drug being injected (Fig. 1). Distribution from the point source occurs along a concentration gradient by diffusion, a process that is slow in solid tissue. A larger drug may require repeat injections or a sustained release in order to reach therapeutic levels. An addi-

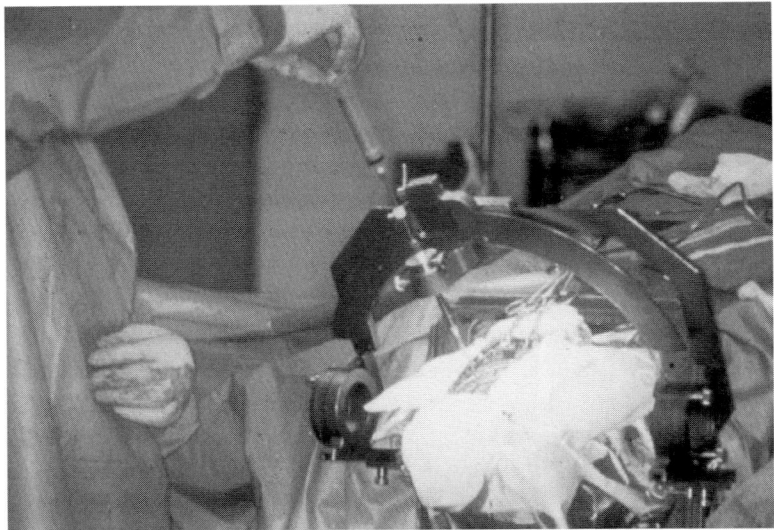

Fig. 1. Direct parenchymal injection under stereotactic guidance has been used in clinical trials to deliver gene therapy to malignant gliomas.

tional factor to consider is the hydrophobicity of the drug being infused, since lipophilic drugs cross into the systemic vasculature and the surrounding CNS more readily, further limiting the volume of distribution. The infusate solution pH and composition should be compatible with the delivery mechanism since corrosive drugs can lead to malfunctioning of delivery devices and treatment failure (22,37). The potential limiting factor for intraparenchymal treatment is neurotoxicity (2,5,34).

Injection Technology

Different mechanical devices have been developed to facilitate intrathecal delivery including the Ommaya reservoir and different implantable pumps. Early efforts to treat intracranial lesions utilized injections through a catheter left outside the cranial vault (5). The Ommaya reservoir was developed for intraventricular therapy (4) and consists of a Silastic catheter connected to a depressible capsule. The capsule is placed subcutaneously under the scalp to prevent infection and the reservoir can be filled by subcutaneous injections. Eventually, pump devices that could be subcutaneously implanted were developed to facilitate drug delivery at a constant rate (5). There are two categories of pumps, vapor pressure and programmable. More recent pumps can electronically control the rate of drug delivery: constant flow, periodic flow, or multiple flow rates (20). Programmable pumps have the advantage of being refillable, so that a sustained treatment regimen can be followed. The pump system has several disadvantages, however; the tubes and materials of the pumps are subject to corrosion (20), and the accumulation of tissue debris, tissue fibrosis, solution residue, and material can block the flow from the pumps. Protein solutions are generally avoided because of the possibility of denaturation within the device. Additional disadvantages include pump failure, infection, and surgical risks associated with improper placement of the catheter *(16)*. A further limitation of the pump system is the limited biodistribution of drug with an exponential drop in concentration from the catheter tip *(4,19,35)*.

Clinical Applications of Direct Injection

Direct injection has a significant history in the treatment of various CNS disorders. The use of catheters *(4,35)*, pumps, and reservoirs continues in conventional patient care. Current pump applications include patient-controlled analgesia (PCA) *(4,20,22)* and treatment of Alzheimer's disease *(4,22)*, spasticity *(22)*, carcinomatous meningitis *(2,4,37)*, leukemia *(4)*, infectious meningitis *(4)*, and malignant gliomas *(2,22)*. Ommaya reservoirs are used in the treatment of meningeal leukemia, meningeal carcinomatosis *(3)*, and infectious meningitis *(4)*. Reservoir technology has been used in experimental immunotheraputic *(27)* protocols to infuse interferon-γ locally into surgical cavities of malignant gliomas. Although no significant improvement in survival occurred, this local treatment was found to be safe and well tolerated in patients *(27)*.

More conventionally, intrathecal delivery via Ommaya reservoirs is used for treatment of leptomeningeal metastases and has resulted in increased survival time and improvement of symptoms. Catheter malposition must be avoided, as it can result in leukencephalopathy in surrounding neurological structures. Other complications include increased intracranial pressure (ICP), infection, and intracranial hemorrhage *(15,16)*. Reservoirs, however, offer significant advantages over multiple lumbar punctures to deliver chemotherapy including improved patient comfort, diminished risk in patients with thrombocytopenia, and a more predictable concentration of drug delivery *(16)*.

Ommaya reservoirs have also been used in the treatment of pediatric tumors, including intralesional chemotherapy of cystic craniopharyngiomas *(17,26)*. Local chemotherapy with bleomycin can avoid systemic side effects, although local toxicity can include hypothalamic dysfunction with hypersomnia, mental change, visual disturbances, thermal dysfunction, and memory impairment. Leakage of bleomycin from the cyst has also been associated with arterial infarcts and subsequent cerebral function *(17)*.

More versatile than reservoirs, implantable pumps have diverse applications in neurosurgery, particularly in the treatment of chronic pain *(5,22)*. Intraspinal morphine, hydromorphone, bupivicane, and analgesic peptides have all been used to control patient pain in inpatient and outpatient settings *(4,22)*. Implantable pumps have also been used for the treatment of spasticity with the intraspinal administration of baclofen *(20,22,37)*. A more recent application of pump technology is in the treatment of Alzheimer's disease. Multicenter double-blind studies in Alzheimer's patients revealed a measurable improvement in behavior and neuropsychological test scores following bethanechol infusion *(20,22)*. Finally, pumps have been used in the treatment of malignant glioma, in which postresection cavities have been targeted. Studies with methotrexate *(19)* achieved higher intratumoral concentrations than could be achieved with systemic administration *(19,22)*. Side effects from intrathecal administration included arachnoiditis; however, intratumoral treatment with methotrexate was well tolerated *(19)*.

Simple direct injection has been used to deliver cells into the CNS. One such study utilized lymphokine-activated killer (LAK) cells engineered with recombinant DNA technology to produce various cytokines *(6)*. LAK cells and cytokines were injected into tumor resection cavities to amplify local tumor immune responses. Clinical efforts have focused on interleukin-2 (IL-2) as a candidate cytokine because of its ability to induce T-cell growth and potentially to amplify T-cell tumoricidal activity *(14,21,23,24,28)*. Side effects of the injection included debilitating fatigue, headaches, and lethargy that were attributed to increased ICP and edema surrounding the injection site. Many side effects were controllable with systemic corticosteroids *(21,23)*. Postmortem biopsy specimens revealed extensive necrosis, gliosis, and infiltration of lymphocytes and macrophages in the area surrounding the injection sites *(23,24)*.

The first gene therapy trial for malignant glioma utilized a direct injection strategy. Patients received stereotactically guided injections of murine fibroblasts that produced retroviruses carrying the herpes simplex virus-thymidine kinase (HSV-tk) gene. The retroviruses would transduce the tumor cells and express the thymidine kinase gene. Patients were then given systemic ganciclovir, which entered transduced tumor cells, where it was phosphorylated by the thymidine kinase gene. The phosphorylated ganciclovir would block DNA replication and be selectively lethal to proliferating cells. The first clinical trial involved 15 patients, 12 with recurrent malignant gliomas, 2 with metastatic melanoma, and 1 with metastatic breast carcinoma. Reduction of the tumor mass occurred in five patients, and survival time improved to more than 11 mo in three patients. Although there were several adverse events (including seizures, meningeal inflammation, headache, and pancytopenia), the study demonstrated the feasibility of intratumoral injection of retrovirus-producing cells for patients with malignant gliomas. Interestingly, no replication-competent retroviruses were found in the systemic circulation of the patients treated with direct injection *(48,49)*. Similar phase I and II studies have verified the usefulness of the HSV-tk strategy for the treatment of malignant gliomas *(42,45,46,48)*.

CNS disorders other than malignant gliomas may be treated with direct injection, as suggested by recent research in Parkinson's disease *(44)*. Injection of dopaminergic neuroprotection and regeneration chemicals and studies with neurotophic factors in clinical trials *(88)* are under way. Although therapeutic efficacy has yet to be shown, these studies do not suggest an increased risk of toxicity with intracerebral injections.

IMPLANTABLE POLYMERS

The use of biodegradable wafers and microspheres combined with a variety of chemotherapeutic and immunotherapeutic agents has established this local treatment modality as a versatile investigative approach for interstitial treatment of CNS lesions. The investigation culminated with US Food and Drug

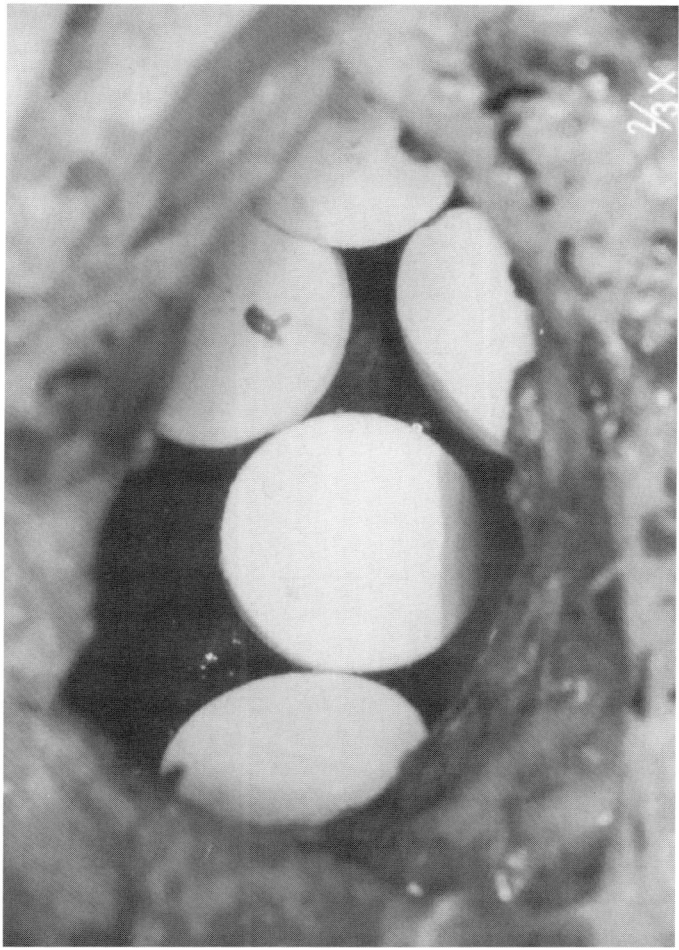

Fig. 2. Gliadel wafers placed into a tumor cavity following resection of a recurrent malignant glioma.

Administration (FDA) approval of wafers (Gliadel) impregnated with 1,3-*bis* (2,chloroethyl)-1-nitrosurea (BCNU; also called carmustine) in 1996 for use in the treatment of malignant gliomas (Fig. 2) *(38)*. The clinical results validate efforts to utilize local delivery as a feasible strategy for treating gliomas; however, its impact on survival has not lived up to expectations.

Principles of Interstitial Polymer Therapy

Polymer technology was introduced with development of a polymer that would release drug at a timed rate from the intact polymer matrix. This led to the design of a polymer matrix that would degrade within the interstitium of the CNS, releasing its impregnated drug into the brain's parenchyma *(4)*. These approaches depend on diffusion for distribution within the brain *(2)*.

The prototype polymer developed using an intact matrix was the ethylene-vinyl acetate copolymer (EVAc). This matrix is capable of releasing a host of drugs ranging from high- to low-molecular-weight compounds *(4)*. The release rate of drug is largely governed by the properties of the matrix, its permeability, its reactivity to the surrounding interstitium, and its interaction with the loaded drug. The EVAc matrix has been subsequently used in clinical treatment for glaucoma with pilocarpine, vaginal contraception with progesterone, and intratumoral glioma therapy with BCNU *(5)*. Silicone rubber, a long-lasting matrix, has also been used with 5-fluoruracil (5-FU) in clinical efforts *(4,12)*.

The degradable poly-[bis(*p*-carboxyphenoxy)propane]-sebacic acid copolymer (PCPP-SA) was used for glioma therapy in clinical trials. PCPP-SA and its metabolites have been shown to be nonmutagenic, noncytotoxic, and non-teratogenic *(4)* and to elicit only a minimal inflammatory reaction (gliosis) in vivo *(5,8)*. This matrix is degraded by alteration of the polyanhydride bonds that constitute the matrix. The release of drugs from the biodegradable polymer system depends on diffusion of the drug from the polymer and degradation properties of the matrix *(4)*. A variety of drugs can be incorporated into the matrix provided they do not chemically modify or interact with the backbone PCPP-SA *(5)*.

PCPP-SA is primarily designed for hydrophobic agents, such as BCNU, but its use with hydrophilic agents has been complicated by degradation of the impregnated drug *(5)*. An additional matrix fatty acid dimer-sebacic acid (FAD-SC) was approved for clinical trials for the delivery of hydrophilic agents. The FAD-SC polymer prevents degradation of the loaded drug and allows for its delivery to a lesion *(5)*. An additional polymer matrix has been developed using a poly(lactide-co-glyoclide) polymer *(5,29,67)*, which enables the polymer to form microspheres *(29)*. Microspheres can be introduced into a lesion with stereotactic placement or during surgical resection *(5,57)*. Animal and clinical studies with microspheres loaded with 5-FU or various cytokines have shown promise in the treatment of malignant gliomas and the development of tumor vaccines *(29,30,68)*.

The volume of distribution of drug and its sustained delivery are largely dependent on concentration gradients established by drug diffusion *(7,28)*. These properties are determined primarily by the drug loaded into the polymer matrix *(51)*. This mechanism is ultimately responsible for the limited volume of distribution that can be achieved since diffusion is exceedingly slow in solid tissues. A transient increase in interstitial fluid may promote a limited degree of convection that may occur as a result of increased ICP at the site of polymer insertion *(7,61)*. Diffusion remains the primary mechanism by which drugs are delivered with polymer implants and can be verified with experiments that show an exponential decrease in drug concentration as distance from the polymer implant is increased *(2,12)*. This is the likely explanation for the limited efficacy in clinical trials.

Experiments to optimize the therapeutic delivery and volume of distribution with polymers have focused on two facets. The first is altering the matrix and its structure. The second is changing the concentration of the drug loaded into the polymer *(8,10,28,51,56)*. Subsequent studies revealed that changing to 50% PCPP and 50% SA offered no improvement in survival, but when the BCNU was increased to 20%, an increase in survival was possible while maintaining limited toxicity *(8)*.

Although most studies report a mild gliosis to the polymer at autopsy, there may be more significant adverse effects. Severe brain edema unresponsive to corticosteroid therapy, perioperative seizures, wound infections, CSF leaks, sepsis, wound dehiscence, and cyst formation have all been reported *(3,8,28)*. Intracranial air collection and fragments of a degradable polymer are a concern, as they may migrate through the parenchyma and penetrate the ventricular system, contributing to the observed CSF leaks and chemical meningitis *(28)*. Wound dehiscence is thought to be caused by inhibition of epidermal cell growth by BCNU leaking from the wafer. Gliosis in response to the polymer may, however, be advantageous, as it may help to recruit components of the inflammatory response, further suppressing tumor growth *(28,58)*.

A further limiting factor is that the polymers, unlike pumps, CED, and reservoirs, cannot be refilled with the therapeutic agent of choice. This translates into subsequent surgeries for placement of additional drug wafers if the therapeutic response is suboptimal. Finally, the possibility of developing tumor resistance to a single therapeutic agent when it is released from a polymer has been explored *(5)*.

Clinical Applications of Polymer Technology

Research investigations with polymer technology have included its use in the treatment of malignant gliomas, cerebral infections *(51)*, Parkinson's disease *(57,60)*, Huntington's disease *(59)*, cerebral edema with dexamethasone release *(57)*, and models of tumor metastasis with breast cancer. The diversity is a reflection of the unique versatility of polymer technology to address a wide range of CNS disorders.

The initial studies completed with polymer wafers centered on the treatment of malignant gliomas. Initial animal studies *(13,51)* and phase I/II clinical studies *(10)* focused on establishing the safety, efficacy, and combination of drug and polymer that would be optimal. These initial studies were responsible for the FDA's approval of Gliadel wafers, 3.85% BCNU impregnated in a 20% PPCA, and 80% SA polymer *(10)*. Early results from phase I/II clinical trials revealed that the wafers could be used safely in a population of patients with histologically graded III and IV astrocytomas. This study helped to establish the aforementioned BCNU dose of 3.85% and helped elucidate that increased dose did not necessarily result in improved clinical outcome. Patients did experience cerebral edema; however, no significant adverse events were found to be attributable to the wafers.

A subsequent prospective clinical study randomized placebo-controlled patients and 222 patients with malignant gliomas from 27 centers in the United States and Canadal *(56)*. Patients with glioblastoma multiforme (GBM) had the most significant improvement with the drug-loaded wafers, although overall results showed minimal improvement in survival. As with the previous study,

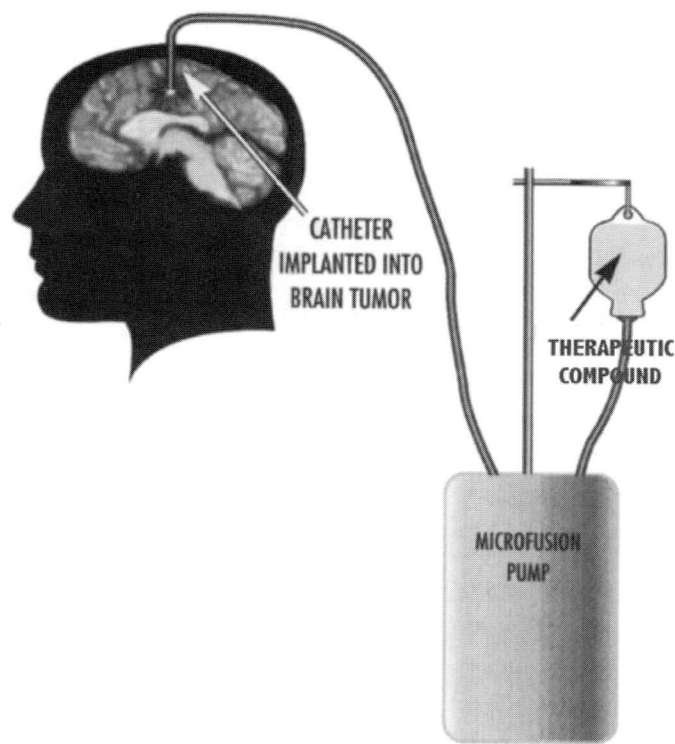

Fig. 3. Diagram demonstrating convection-enhanced delivery. Therapeutic compounds are slowly pumped into a catheter implanted in brain tissue. A pressure gradient is established that distributes the compound through the interstitial space by bulk flow.

cerebral edema occurred and was treated with corticosteroids *(28,56)*. Subsequent studies helped to establish Gliadel wafers as acceptable treatments for patients undergoing their initial surgery for GBM *(28)*. Further studies, repeated in 1997 *(53)*and 1999 *(28)*, revealed that a significant complication rate is associated with polymer treatment using Gliadel wafers.

These studies elucidated the pharmacokinetics of the Gliadel system, demonstrating that BCNU was released in vivo over a period of three weeks with 50% of the drug being released within the first 24 h and 95% of the BCNU being released in 120 h *(3,61)*. Wafers were found to degrade within 6–8 wk. Further characterization of the pharmacokinetics revealed that the depth of BCNU was predicted to be limited to 5mm at 100 h, owing to a high transvascular permeability and rapid reabsorption into the systemic circulation *(28)*. Measurable penetration of BCNU may be limited to 1 to 2 cm from the site of implantation *(28)*, but effective therapeutic concentrations are even more limited, with a millimeter range that limits its effect on invaded brain tissue.

Additional clinical research with BCNU wafers has explored its use in a model of breast cancer metastasis to the brain *(43)* and in combination with radiation *(9)*. Initial results have shown promise in combining radiation therapy with polymer technology including the use of halogenated pyrimidines as potent radiosensitizers for human gliomas *(63)*. Studies using IUdR impregnated in a PCPP-SA polymer coupled with radiation to treat malignant gliomas are currently under way *(63)*. Additional chemotherapeutic agents being investigated include mitoxanthrone, doxetaxel, and platinum base *(3)*.

As polymer technology moves into the future, its versatility as a treatment modality may make it suitable for targeting specific molecular proteins and signal transduction cascades. One such example is the use of O^6-benzylguanine to potentiate the antitumor effect of BCNU polymers *(55)*. Recent studies coupling immunotherapy and polymer technology have utilized IL-2 coupled with BCNU or carboplatin wafers *(58,60)*. This combined approach to treatment may be helpful when one is trying to avoid tumor cell resistance.

CONVECTION ENHANCED DELIVERY

Mathematical modeling, physiological studies, and increasing numbers of animal and clinical studies have helped to establish CED as one of the most promising of future strategies for the treatment of CNS disorders. The perpetual efforts to improve on local delivery techniques have helped move this method to the forefront, as it has distinct advantages over other local treatment modalities. CED has been described in the scientific literature by different names, including convection-enhanced intracerebral infusion, high-flow microinfusion, high-flow interstitial infusion, direct intraparenchymal controlled-rate infusion, intracerebral clysis, and direct convective delivery (Fig. 3) *(95)*. The term CED has emerged as the current accepted nomenclature.

Principles

Within the extracellular environment of the CNS, fluid can move either through diffusion along concentration gradients or by bulk flow along pressure gradients. Whereas diffusion has a limited capacity to deliver high-molecular-weight solutes, bulk flow is largely independent of size and molecular weight *(75)*. Bulk flow can, therefore, achieve homogenous solution concentrations that are less dependent on molecular size. In the CNS, volumes of distribution achievable with bulk flow strategies such as CED are orders of magnitude greater than those achievable with diffusion strategies including direct injection, polymers, or systemic delivery.

CED involves infusion of a solution into the brain interstitium through a microcannula, thereby establishing a positive pressure gradient for flow *(83)*. The delivered infusate moves radially outward from the cannula to penetrate the surrounding parenchyma *(75)*. The interstitial velocities achieved exceed those present endogenously, and drug is allowed to follow fiber tracts present in white and gray matter *(80)*. An additional feature of CED is precise placement of the cannula through stereotactic technology, allowing delivery to specific and eloquent areas of the brain *(97)*. Lesions of rat brainstem and spinal cord and of primate globus pallida have been successfully targeted, suggesting that CED can address varying CNS disorders in a site-specific manner *(85–87,97)*

The volume of distribution achievable by the infusion is determined by several variables including the rate of infusion, tissue architecture, the size of the cannula, the volume of infusion, and the rate of efflux. A possible dependence on dose has also been suggested *(84)*. Rate of infusion is shown to be an essential determinant in the success of CED *(74)*. Rates of infusion for CED are in the range of several microliters per minute and are optimal for establishing the high-flow microinfusion pressures required for effective drug delivery *(78)*. If, however, these rates are exceeded, there can be leak-back through the cannula tract and subsequent loss of infusion pressure *(77)*. To avoid an artificially low resistance pathway created by the cannula placement, a small cannula is preferred to a large one *(74)*.

The architecture of the tissue being infused also helps determine the volume of distribution achieved in CED *(75)*. Placement of the cannula into white or gray matter exploits the inherent fluid dynamic differences between these two microenvironments. The high-flow microinfusion utilized by CED is dependent on channels that develop in the brain's parenchyma and allow passage of solutions and molecules *(71)*. Convective gradients normally exist within white matter as a result of anisotropic pathways along the parallel myelinated fibers *(83,84)*. The parallel arrangement of these oriented fiber tracks creates a state with low resistance to interstitial infusion *(81,83)*. CED infusion into white matter tracks therefore attains a greater volume of distribution along these low-resistance pathways *(71,78)*. The gray matter, in contrast, is more uniform, and a more spherical volume of distribution can be obtained *(2)*. This is significant when considering both the type of lesion treated and the placement of the cannula into the brain. Appropriate targeting can obtain desired volumes of distribution and allow for the specific targeting of local lesions.

The volume of infusion determines the volume of distribution through a linear relationship *(75,77,87)*. Through this linear relationship, equilibrium is eventually reached at the edge of the drug delivery sphere radiating from the cannula after a certain volume has been infused. At the periphery of the sphere, the rate of infusion is equal to the rate of efflux. At the periphery, diffusion works to carry drug further into the parenchyma, and the property of exponential decline in drug concentration away from the equilibrium point is applicable *(2,81)*. Excessive tissue binding, leak-back through the cannula tract, large infusion rates, and differing flow patterns between white and gray matter can affect the linear ratio between infusion volume and volume of distribution.

When applying CED in practice, the properties of the infusate, including the efflux and clearance of these same molecules, must be taken into consideration, as they determine the volume of distribution. Clearance of the infusate is ultimately by catabolism, efflux through the BBB to the systemic vasculature, and dilution in the CSF *(75,95)*. Efflux may also be influenced by P-glycoprotein, an ATP-dependent efflux pump with broad substrate specificity *(66,89,98,94)*. The process of efflux associated with CED is counterintuitive. Increased vascular permeability actually acts to increase drug efflux and lowers the subsequent volume of distribution with CED *(2)*. It becomes hypothetically desirable, therefore, to use drugs that are more hydrophilic in order to reduce crossing of the

BBB *(69)*. Longer half-lives, larger local concentrations, and larger volume of distribution achieved with CED help to promote the efflux of infusate following infusion.

Several methods have been used to measure the volume of distribution with CED including autoradiography with radioactive isotopes *(74,75,77,81)* and histological sections after dye injection. The various dyes used to visualize the extent of spread of the infusate include fluorescein isothiocyanante *(87,95)* and Evans Blue *(78)*. The effects of treatment can be easily measured with these techniques and coupled with magnetic resonance imaging technology to monitor the progression of various CNS lesions *(84,95)*.

Neurotoxic events are the limiting factors in treatment and dictate the dose and rate of infusion *(2,81)*. The toxicity can be divided into two components: mass effect related to increased volume of infusion and neurotoxicity from direct effects of drug on neurons and glial cells *(81)*. The mild increase in ICP during infusion *(77,80,84)* is thought to be minimal *(95)* and has not been shown to alter local tissue structure significantly. Although remodeling of the parenchyma with dilation of channels in the interstitium can occur, it has not been associated with neuronal dysfunction *(78,81)*. CED has also been documented to cause a mild gliosis that results either from the infusate or the infusion process. This inflammation is associated with increased glialfibrillary acidic protein immunoreactivity in the CNS local environment surrounding the cannula *(78)*. This is a sensitive marker for astrocytic responses to neuronal trauma *(75)* and possibly represents a reversible phenomenon that results from changes in the interstitium *(78)* without significant changes to neuronal functioning. Each particular infusate will have its own toxicity profile associated with CED. These complications should be addressed when one is considering clinical trials and further research efforts. Indeed, the pH, the osmolarity, and the ionic composition of the infusate solution should be considered as well *(2)*. The various cells of the CNS have different tolerances to different drugs, and further work needs to clarify these potential side effects of treatment with CED.

A final limitation to CED revolves around its inherent dependence on the directional bulk flow in the treatment of gliomas. If a tumor is removed, edema that had been present quickly resolves. The associated convection of fluid is now directed into the resection cavity and effectively reverses the direction of the pressure gradient *(3)*. CED may potentially be limited to a role as a pretreatment method or as an alternative treatment for recurring lesions *(3)*.

Clinical Applications

A more uniform and predictable distribution of drug, a larger volume of distribution, and the potential for treating eloquent areas of the brainstem and spinal cord have helped support CED as a leading treatment modality for CNS disorders. To capitalize on these advantages, researchers have sought to couple this method with the latest treatment modalities made available in oncology, virology, and immunology. Researchers have targeted gliomas and discussed treating other CNS disorders such as Parkinson's disease and Huntington's disease with CED *(97)*. Progress has primarily come in the realm of establishing

CED as a safe and efficacious method with animal models that has been effectively translated into human clinical trials *(96,97)*.

Studies thus far have used models to apply CED to a variety of therapeutic agents to treat gliomas and other biochemical imbalances in the CNS. The various agents utilized include those involving chemotherapy *(75,77,78,90,91)*, immunotherapy *(92)*, and genetic targeting *(71)*. The ideal therapeutic agent for CED takes advantage of its potential to deliver therapy to a larger volume of distribution more quickly with greater control of local concentrations *(69)*. Drugs chosen for treatment with CED, however, are held to the same standards used for systemic treatment, namely, specificity for the lesion, lack of local toxicity, pharmacodynamic stability, and some lipophilicity to promote entry into the cell.

Capitalizing on the wealth of knowledge surrounding the genetic and protein signal transduction cascades involved in tumorigenesis, researchers are now using CED to target specific enzymes *(82)* involved in aberrant DNA replication. One such family of nuclear enzymes is the topoisomerase group that the cell uses to coordinate unwinding of the DNA strands to replication and DNA repair. This enzyme is a prime candidate for CED treatment, given its essential role in regulation of DNA turnover *(69)*. Drugs such as the family of campothecins, which specifically target topoisomerase I, have been shown to be effective in the clinical treatment of gliomas. CED was shown to improve long-term survival, local concentration, and volume of distribution in animal glioma models *(69)*. Clinical trials with chemotherapeutic agents such as topotecan and paclitaxel are currently underway in glioma patients *(76)*. If successful, a new horizon for chemotherapeutic approaches to human gliomas may be opened for future research efforts.

Further studies have sought to establish the efficacy of using CED with novel treatment approaches such as antisense oligonucleotides *(71)*, cytokines *(72,92)*, and immunotoxins. The strategy that is furthest developed in clinical trials involves immunotoxins, which are molecules composed of a ligand such as transferrin or Il-4 that will bind with high specificity to rapidly dividing glioma cells, coupled with a toxin that will inhibit cell proliferation or induce apoptosis, such as diphtheria toxin or *Pseudomonas* toxin. The diphtheria–transferrin toxin was used with CED to treat patients with recurrent gliomas since systemic delivery would not be feasible with such a complex macromolecule. By bypassing the systemic circulation, the large molecular weight (140-kDa) protein product could be delivered unaltered at high concentrations to tumors in the CNS. The advantage of using the transferrin receptor as a target is that it is up-regulated on rapidly dividing cells, including gliomas, conferring a high level of glioma specificity while avoiding local toxicity to surrounding neurons. Once inside the cells, diphtheria toxin can function to inhibit cell signaling and induce apoptosis within the tumor. In a phase I trial, tumor regression occurred in 60% of patients (9/15) treated, with complete remission in two patients. More importantly, delivery of this immunotoxin was well tolerated, and toxicity was minimal at lower doses *(70)*. Seizures and focal brain injury were the primary complications in this study and occurred only at higher doses. This study offers the first promising result of using CED in conjunction with immunotherapy to treat human gliomas.

Success with the transferrin–diphtheria immunotoxin led to the development of other toxin conjugates for high-grade gliomas, including a formulation coupling IL-4 with *Pseudomonas* toxin. As with transferrin, IL-4 receptors are overexpressed in malignant glioma cells but not on other cells in the CNS, allowing the IL-4–pseudomonas organism conjugate to achieve a high degree of specificity. The *Pseudomonas* toxin is toxic to malignant glioma cells and induces apoptosis within tumors by ADP ribosylation of elongation factor 2, which is used in translation to form cellular proteins. In the initial clinical study, 6/9 patients had a responding tumor that underwent necrosis, while the neurotoxicity was minimal. Increased ICP was associated with pretreatment edema but was also associated with necrotic tumor-induced edema. Both factors are believed to have contributed to some level of toxicity seen in the few patients who experienced altered neurological function. The need for further studies on CED-induced toxicity is evident; however, the results of coupling CED with novel antitumor compounds show promise for a significant contribution to glioma therapy in the future (72).

Although most CED investigations have involved the treatment of gliomas, this strategy may prove to be more applicable to other CNS disease states, particularly those with more limited anatomic targets. Research on treating diseases such as Parkinson's and Huntington's with CED offers new hope for applying animal studies to human disease states (97). Additional work with CED to address spinal cord injury offers yet another avenue for exploring the applications of this treatment modality (85–87). The ultimate test for CED is to demonstrate its efficacy in clinical trials and to provide information for the development of future therapeutic modalities. Future studies will also be needed to investigate infusion parameters to optimize volumes of distribution. The development of appropriate contrast agents and imaging methods will lead to safer and more effective clinical uses of CED and more individualized therapy.

CONCLUSIONS

Local delivery strategies have proved to be safe and effective in providing new treatment alternatives for various CNS lesions and diseases. Gliomas are the most established area of research with local delivery. These aggressive lesions have remained resistant to conventional treatment methods and require new treatment options. Local delivery strategies have evolved from local injection to polymer technology to CED, to meet these demands. As neurosurgeons move forward, they will need to address the growing need for new technology, and CED may offer the most promise. CED will allow versatility for incorporating new chemotherapeutic and immunotherapeutic agents into clinical studies, as it has already been validated as a safe treatment strategy in clinical trials. Ongoing and future clinical trials will further elucidate the safety and efficacy of CED and the other local delivery strategies with previously untested agents in the hope of improving the treatment of CNS diseases.

REFERENCES

1. Buahin K, Brem H, et al. Interstitial chemotherapy of experimental brain tumors: comparison of intratumoral injection versus polymeric controlled release. *J Neurooncol* 1995;26:103–110.
2. Groothius DR. The blood-brain and blood-tumor barriers: a review of strategies for increasing drug delivery. *Neurooncology* 2000;2:45–59.
3. Giese A, Westphal M. Treatment of malignant glioma: a problem beyond the margins of resection. *J Cancer Res Clin Oncol* 2001;127:217–225.
4. Tamargo RJ, Brem H. Drug delivery to the central nervous system: a review. *Neurosurg Q* 1992;2:259–279.
5. Walter KA, Tamargo RJ, et al. Intratumoral chemotherapy. *Neurosurgery* 1995;37:1129–1145.
6. Tashiro T, Yoshida J, et al. Reinforced cytotoxicity of lymphokine-activated killer cells toward glioma cells by transfection with the tumor necrosis factor-alpha gene. *J Neurosurg* 1993;78:252–256.
7. Fung LK, Ewend MG, et al. Pharmacokinetics of interstitial delivery of carmustine, 4-hydroperoxycyclophosphamide, and paclitaxel from a biodegradable polymer implant in the monkey brain. *Cancer Res* 1998;58:672–684.
8. Sipos EP, Tyler B, et al. optimizing interstitial delivery of BCNU from controlled release polymers for the treatment of brain tumors. *Cancer Chemother Pharmacology* 1997;39:383–389.
9. Ewend MG, Williams JA, et al. local delivery of chemotherapy and concurrent external beam radiotherapy prolongs survival in metastatic brain tumor models. *Cancer Res* 1996;56:5217–5223.
10. Brem H, Mahaley MS, et al. Interstitial chemotherapy with drug polymer implants for the treatment of recurrent gliomas. *J Neurosurg* 1991;74:441–446.
11. Brem H, Tamargo RJ, et al. biodegradable polymers for controlled delivery of chemotherapy with and without radiation therapy in the monkey brain. *J Neurosurg* 1994;80:283–290.
12. Tomita T. Interstitial chemotherapy for brain tumors: review. *J Neurooncol* 1991;10:57–74.
13. Grossman SA, Reinhard C, et al. The intracerebral distribution of BCNU delivered by surgically implanted biodegradable polymers. *J Neurosurg* 1992;76:640–647.
14. Merchant RE, McVicar DW, et al. Treatment of recurrent malignant glioma by repeated intracerebral injections of human recombinant interleukin-2 alone or in combination with systemic interferon-alpha. results of a phase I clinical trial. *J Neurooncol* 1992;12:75–83.
15. Chamberlain MC, Kormanik PA, et al. complications associated with intraventricular chemotherapy in patients with leptomeningeal metastases. *J Neurosurg* 1997;87:694–699.
16. Sanberg DI, Bilsky MH, et al. ommaya reservoirs for the treatment of leptomeningeal metastases. *Neurosurgery* 2000;47:49–55.
17. Park DY, Park JY, et al. Outcome of postoperative intratumoral bleomycin injection for cystic craniopharygioma. *J Korean Med Sci* 2002;17:254–259.
18. Nirenberg D, Harbaugh R, et al. Continuous intratumoral infusion of methotrexate for recurrent glioblastoma: a pilot study. *Neurosurgery* 1991;28:752–761.
20. Madrid Y, Feigenbaum L, et al. New directions in the delivery of drugs and other substances to the central nervous system. *Adv Pharmacol* 1991;22:299–321.
21. Merchant RE, Merchant LH, et al. Intralesional infusion of lymphokine-activated killer (lak) cells and recombinant interleukin-2 (rIL-2) for the treatment of patients with malignant brain tumor. *Neurosurgery* 1988;23:725–732.

22. Harbaugh RE, Saunders RL, et al. Use of implantable pumps for central nervous system drug infusions to treat neurological disease. *Neurosurgery* 1988;23: 693–697.
23. Atkinson LL, Merchant RE, et al. sterile abscesses in glioma patients treated by intraparenchymal injection of lymphokine-activated killer cells and recombinant interleukin-2: case reports. *Neurosurgery* 1989;25:805–809.
24. Merchant RE, Ellison MD, et al. Immunotherapy for malignant glioma using human recombinant interleukin-2 and activated autologous lymphocytes. *J Neurooncol* 1990;8:173–188.
25. Morantz RA, Kimler BF, et al. Bleomycin and brain tumors. *J Neurooncol* 1983;1: 249–255.
26. Takahashi H, Nakazawa N, et al. Evaluation of postoperative intratumoral injection of bleomycin for craniopharyngioma in children. *J Neurosurg* 1985;62:120–127.
27. Farkklia M, Jaaskelainen J, et al. Randomised, controlled study of intratumoral recombinant gamma-interferon treatment in newly diagnosed glioblastoma. *Br J Cancer* 1994;70:138–141.
28. Jacobs SK, Wilson DJ, et al. Interleukin-2 or autologous lymphokine-activated killer cell treatment of malignant glioma: phase I trial. *J Cancer Res* 1986;40: 2101–2104
29. Menei P, Venier MC, et al. Local and sustained delivery of 5-fluoruracil from biodegradable microspheres for the radiosensitization of glioblastoma. *Cancer* 1999;86:325–330.
30. Menei P, Boisdron-Celle M, et al. Effect of stereotactic implantation of biodegradable 5-fluorouracil-loaded microspheres in healthy and C6 glioma-bearing rats. *Neurosurgery* 1996;39:117–123.
31. Emerich DF, Tracy MA, et al. Biocompatibility of poly(DL-lactide-*co*-glycolide) microspheres implanted into the brain. *Cell Transplant* 1999;8:47–58.
32. Kimler BF, Liu C, et al. Intracerebral chemotherapy in the 9L rat brain tumor model. *J Neurooncol* 1992;14:191–200.
33. Lum JT, Nguyen T, et al. Drug distribution in solid tissue of the brain following chronic local perfusion utilizing implanted osmotic minipumps. *J Pharm Methods* 1984;12:141–147.
34. Bouvier G, Penn RD, et al. Direct delivery of medication into a brain tumor through multiple chronically implanted catheters. *Neurosurgery* 1987;20:286–291.
35. Laske DW, Morrison PF, et al. chronic interstitial infusion of protein to primate brain: determination of drug distribution and clearance with single-photon emission computerized tomography imaging. *J Neurosurg* 1997;87:586–594.
36. Yoshida TK, Shimizu K, et al. Intrathecal chemotherapy with ACNU in a meningeal gliomatosis rat model. *J Neurosurg* 1992;77:778–782.
37. Penn RD, York MM, et al. Catheter Systems for Intrathecal Drug Delivery. *J Neurosurg* 1995;83:215–217.
38. Engelhard HH. The role of interstitial BCNU chemotherapy in the treatment of malignant glioma. *Surg Neurol* 2000;53:458–464.
39. Hlavaty J, Hlubinova K, et al. Treatment of rat gliomas with recombinant retrovirus harboring herpes simplex virus thymidine kinase suicide gene. *Neoplasma* 1997;44:342–347.
40. Chen SH, Shine HD, et al. Gene therapy for brain tumors: regression of experimental gliomas by adenovirus-mediated gene transfer. *Proc Natl Acad Sci USA* 1994;91:3054–3057.
41. Vincent AJPE, Vogels R, et al. Herpes simplex virus thymidine kinase gene therapy for rat malignant brain tumors. *Hum Gene Ther* 1996;7:197–205.

42. Shand N, Weber F, et al. A phase 1–2 clinical trial of gene therapy for recurrent glioblastoma multiforme by tumor transduction with the herpes simplex thymidine kinase gene follow by ganciclovir. *Hum Gene Ther* 1999;10:2325–2335.
43. Ewend MG, Sampath P, et al. Local delivery of chemotherapy prolongs survival in experimental brain metastases from breast carcinoma. *Neurosurgery* 1998;43:1185–1193.
44. Horellou P, Sabate O, et al. Adenovirus-mediated gene transfer to the central nervous system for parkinson's disease. *Exp Neurol* 1997;144:131–138.
45. Floeth FW, Aulich A, et al. MR imaging and single-photon emission CT findings after gene therapy for human glioblastoma. *AJNR* 2001;22:1517–1527.
46. Long Z, Li LP, et al. Biosafety monitoring of patients receiving intracerebral injections of murine retroviral vector producer cells. *Hum Gene Ther* 1998;9:1165–1172.
47. Ram Z, Culver KW, et al. Therapy of malignant brain tumors by intratumoral implantation of retroviral vector-producing cells. *Nat Med* 1997;3:1354–1361.
48. Alemany R, Gomez-Manzano C, et al. Gene therapy for gliomas: molecular targets, adenoviral vectors, and oncolytic adenoviruses. *Experimental Cell Res* 1999;252:1–12.
49. Ram Z, Culver KW, et al. Therapy of malignant brain tumors by intratumoral implantation of retroviral vector-producing cells. *Nat Med* 1997;3:1354–1361.
50. Laske DW, Morrison PF, et al. Chronic interstitial infusion of protein to primate brain: determination of drug distribution and clearance with single photon emission computerized tomography imaging. *J Neurosurg* 1997;87:586–594.
51. Tamargo RJ, Myseros JS, et al. Interstitial chemotherapy of the 9L gliosarcoma: controlled release polymers for drug delivery in the brain. *Cancer Res* 1993;53:329–333.
52. Brem H, Ewend MG, et al. the safety of interstitial chemotherapy with bcnu-loaded polymer followed by radiation therapy in the treatment of newly diagnosed malignant gliomas: phase I trial. *J Neurooncol* 1995;26:111–123.
53. Valtonen S, Timonen U, et al. Interstitial chemotherapy with carmustine-loaded polymers for high-grade gliomas: a randomized double-blind study. *Neurosurgery* 1997;41:44–49.
54. Rhines, LD, Sampath P, et al. O^6-Benzylguanine potentiates the antitumor effect of locally delivered carmustine against an intracranial rat glioma. *Cancer Res* 2000;60:6307–6310.
55. Quinn JA, Pluda J, et al. Phase II trial of carmustine plus O (6)-benzylguanine for patients with nitrosurea-resistant recurrent or progressive malignant glioma. *J Clinical Oncology* 2002;20:2277–2283.
56. Brem H, Plantadosi S, et al. Placebo-controlled trial of safety and efficacy of intraoperative controlled delivery by biodegradable polymers of chemotherapy for recurrent gliomas. *Lancet* 1995;345:1008–1012.
57. Madrid Y, Langer LF, et al. New directions in the delivery of drugs and other substances to the central nervous system. *Adv Pharmacol* 1991;22:299–324.
58. Sampath P, Hanes J, et al. Paracrine immunotherapy with interleukin-2 and local chemotherapy is synergistic in the treatment of experimental brain tumors. *Cancer Res* 1999;59:2107–2114.
59. Emerich DF, Bruhn S, et al. Cellular delivery of CFTF but not NT-4/5 prevents degeneration of striatal neurons in a rodent model of Huntington's disease. *Cell Transplant* 1998;7:213–225.
60. Linder MD, Emerich DF, et al. Therapeutic potential of a polymer-encapsulated L-DOPA and dopamine-producing cell line in rodent and primate models of Parkinson's disease. *Cell Transplant* 1998;7:165–174.
61. Fleming AB, Saltzman WM, et al. Pharmacokinetics of the carmustine implant. *Clin Pharmacokinet* 2002;41:403–419.

62. Yuan X, Tabassi K, et al. Implantable polymers for tirapazamine treatments of experimental intracranial malignant glioma. *Radiat Oncol Invest* 1999;7:218–230.
63. Yuan X, Dillehay LE, et al. IUdR polymers for combined continuous low-dose rate and high-dose rate sensitization of experimental human malignant glioma. *Int J Cancer* 2001;96:118–125.
64. Bouvier G, Penn RD, et al. Direct delivery of medication into a brain tumor through multiple chronically implanted catheters. *Neurosurgery* 1987;20:286–291.
65. Lum, JT, Nguyen T, et al. drug distribution in solid tissue of the brain following chronic perfusion utilizing implanted osmotic minipumps. *J Pharmacol Methods* 1984;12:141–147.
66. Hendriske NH, Schinkel AH, et al. Complete *in vivo* reversal of P-glycoprotein pump function in the blood-brain barrier visualized with positron emission tomography. *Br J Pharmacology* 1998;124:1413–1418.
67. Emerich DF, Tracy MA, et al. Biocompatibility of poly(DL-lactide-*co*-glycolide) microspheres implanted into the brain. *Cell Transplant* 1999;8:47–58.
68. Golumbek PT, Azhari R, et al. controlled release, biodegradable cytokine depots: a new approach in cancer vaccine design. *Cancer Res* 1993;53:5841–5844.
69. Kaiser MG, Parsa AT, Fine RL, et al. Tissue distribution and antitumor activity of topotecan delivered by intracerebral clysis in a rat glioma model. *Neurosurgery* 2000;47:1391–1399.
70. Laske DW, et al. Tumor regression with regional distribution of the targeted toxin TF-CRM107 I patients with malignant brain tumors. *Nat Med* 1997;3:1362–1367.
71. Broaddus WC, Prabhu SS, et al. Distribution and stability of antisense phosphorothioate oligonucleotides in rodent brain following direct intraparenchmyal controlled-rate infusion. *J Neurosurg* 1998;88:734–742.
72. Rand RW, Kreitman RJ, et al. Intratumoral administration of recombinant circularly permutated interleukin-4–*pseudomonas* exotoxin in patients with high-grade glioma. *Clin Cancer Res* 2000;6:2157–2165.
73. Heimberger AB, Archer GE, et al. Temozolmide delivered by intracerebral microinfusion is safe and efficacious against malignant gliomas in rats. *Clin Cancer Res* 2001;6:4148–4153.
74. Chen MY, Lonser RR, et al. variables affecting convection enhanced delivery to the striatum: a systemic examination of rate of infusion, cannula size, InfU S ate concentration, and tissue-cannula sealing time. *J Neurosurg* 1999;90:315–320.
75. Lieberman DM, Laske DW, et al. Convection enhanced distribution of large molecules in gray matter during interstitial drug infusion. *J Neurosurg* 1995;82:1021–1029.
76. Mardor Y, Roth Y, et al. Monitoring response to convection enhanced taxol delivery in brain tumor patients using diffusions-weighted magnetic resonance imaging. *Cancer Res* 2001;1:4971–4973.
77. Bobo RH, Laske DW, et al. Convection-enhanced delivery of macromolecules in the brain. *Proc Natl Acad Sci USA* 1994;91:2076–2080.
78. Prabhu SS, Broaddus WC, et al. Distribution of macromolecular dyes in brain using positive pressure infusion: a model for direct controlled delivery of therapeutic agents. *Surg Neurol* 1998;50:367–375.
79. Nirenberg D, Harbaugh R, et al. Continuous infusion of methotrexate for recurrent glioblastoma: a pilot study. *Neurosurgery* 1991;28:752–761.
80. Morrison, PF, Laske DW, et al. High-flow microinfusion: tissue penetration and pharmacodynamics. *Am J of Physiology* 1994;266:R292-R305.
81. Groothuis DR, Ward S, et al. Comparison of ^{14}C-sucrose delivery to the brain by intravenous, intraventricular, and convection-enhanced intracerebral infusion. *J Neurosurg* 1999;90:321–331.

82. Viola JJ, Agbaria R, et al. *In situ* cyclopentenyl cytosine infusion for the treatment of experimental brain tumors. *Cancer Res* 1995;55:1306–1309.
83. Geer CP, Grossman SA. Interstitial fluid flow along white matter tracts: a potentially important mechanism for the dissemination of primary brain tumors. *J Neurooncol* 1997;32:193–201.
84. Kroll RA, Pagel MA, et al. Increasing volume of distribution to the brain with interstitial infusion: dose, rather than convection, might be the most important factor. *Neurosurgery* 1996;38:746–753.
85. Wood JD, Lonser RR, et al. Convective delivery of macromolecules into the naïve and traumatized spinal cords of rats. *J Neurosurg (Spine I)* 1999;90:115–120.
86. Lonser RR, Gogate N, et al. Direct convective delivery of macromolecules to the spinal cord. *J Neurosurg* 1998;89:616–622.
87. Sandberg DI, Edgar MA, et al. Convection-enhanced delivery into the rat brainstem. *J Neurosurg* 2002;96:885–891.
88. Nutt JG. Burchiel KJ., et al. Randomized, double-blind trial of glial cell line-derived neurotrophic factor (GDNF) in PD. *Neurology* 2003;60:69–73.
89. de Lange ECM, de Boer BAG, et al. Microdialysis for pharmacokinetic analysis of drug transport to the brain. *Adv Drug Dev Rev* 1999;36:211–227.
90. Engelhard HH, Duncan HA, et al. Therapeutic effects of sodium butyrate on glioma cells in vitro and in the rat C6 glioma model. *Neurosurgery* 2001;48:616–625.
91. Kimler BF, Liu C, et al. Intracerebral chemotherapy in the 9L rat brain tumor model. *J Neurooncol* 1992;14:191–200.
92. Kikuchi T, Akasaki Y., et al. Antitumor activity of interleukin-18 on mouse glioma cells. *J Immunother* 2000;23:184–189.
93. Miller CR, Williams CR, et al. Intratumoral 5-fluorouracil produced by cytosine deaminase/5-fluorocytosine gene therapy is effective for experimental human glioblastomas. *Cancer Res* 2002;62:773–780.
94. Schinkel AH. P-glycoprotein, a gatekeeper in the blood-brain barrier. *Adv Drug Deliv Rev* 1999;36:179–194.
95. Bruce JN, Falavigna A, et al. Intracerebral clysis in a rat glioma model. *Neurosurgery* 2000;46:683–691.
96. Ram Z, Culver KW, et al. *In situ* retroviral-mediated gene transfer for the treatment of brain tumors in rats. *Cancer Res* 1997;53:83–88.
97. Lieberman DM, Corthesy ME, et al. Reversal of experimental parkinsonism by using selective chemical ablation of the medial globus pallidus. *J Neurosurg* 1999;90:928–934.
98. Tamai I, Tsuji A. Drug delivery through the blood-brain barrier. *Adv Drug Deliv Rev* 1996;19:401–424.

Part II

Specialties

15
Minimally Invasive Pediatric Neurosurgery

Michael Weaver, MD and Mark R. Proctor, MD

INTRODUCTION

Pediatric neurosurgery, which by its nature overlaps multiple neurosurgical subspecialties, has benefited greatly from the advances in minimally invasive neurosurgical techniques. Not only can it take advantage of the progress in the areas of vascular, spine, trauma, and tumor neurosurgery, but as a subspecialty it has significantly advanced the minimally invasive treatment of hydrocephalus and intraventricular lesions.

There have been substantial technological advances in the treatment of hydrocephalus in the past half century. Ventricular shunts, our current mainstay of treatment, can be considered a minimally invasive alternative to the techniques that preceded them for the treatment of hydrocephalus. However, neuroendoscopy is now the leading edge technology in the treatment of this condition and has become an important part of the armamentarium of all pediatric neurosurgeons. The current goal in hydrocephalus is to treat the patient without a shunt, or at least to simplify shunt systems as much as possible by fenestration of loculated fluid spaces. In this chapter we review how pediatric neurosurgeons employ minimally invasive techniques in their practice for the treatment of hydrocephalus, cysts, tumors, and vascular and congenital abnormalities of the brain and spine.

HYDROCEPHALUS

Endoscopy

Hydrocephalus is a common entity in pediatric neurosurgery, and treatment often encompasses a large percentage of the neurosurgical volume in a pediatric institution. Whether the condition has been caused by congenital etiologies, intraventricular hemorrhage, infection, or tumors, minimally invasive techniques are becoming the standard in its treatment. Minimally invasive techniques using the endoscope and image guidance have led to improved shunt placement, simplification of shunt systems, and shunt independence in select patients.

From: *Minimally Invasive Neurosurgery*, edited by: M.R. Proctor and P.M. Black © Humana Press Inc., Totowa, NJ

A significant development in pediatric neurosurgery during the past decade has been the evolution of neuroendoscopy and its application to the management of childhood hydrocephalus. The first endoscopic neurosurgical procedure was performed by Lespinasse, a urologist, in 1910. He used a cystoscope to fulgurate the choroid plexus in two children (1). Walter Dandy used a "ventriculoscope" (a rigid cystoscope) to treat hydrocephalus via choroid plexus fulguration or third ventriculostomy (2), but this fell out of favor with the development of cerebrol spinal fluid (CSF) diversion catheters. However, the cerebral ventricles, when pathologically dilated, are ideally suited to neurosurgical endoscopy. This fact, along with technological advances in optics and imaging, have brought on a resurgence in endoscopy for the treatment of pediatric hydrocephalus.

Armed with the endoscope as both a diagnostic and therapeutic surgical adjunct, the neurosurgeon can now fenestrate cysts and obstructing membranes. This permits the conversion of complicated shunts into more easily managed systems, and in many instances diversion of CSF can be accomplished without valve-regulated shunt systems. Advance planning of the endoscopic procedure with high-resolution neuroimaging helps to minimize potential confusion when the neurosurgeon encounters variable anatomy within the ventricular system. This can also be combined with stereotactic techniques for more precise localization when anatomy is altered by pathology.

Therapeutic procedures aimed at treating hydrocephalus with the endoscope can be divided into shunt catheter placement, membrane fenestration, and, in limited conditions, tumor resection aimed at relieving ventricular obstruction.

Many studies indicate that ventricular catheter blockage is the most common site of the shunt obstruction. Although no study has demonstrated improved shunt patency with catheter tip position (3,4), it is suggested by the fact that the most commonly found materials causing ventricular catheter obstruction are connective, glial, and granulomatous tissue. Concerning the optimal placement of the ventricular portion of a shunt system, endoscopy serves as an adjunct in that it provides an intraoperative confirmation of optimal catheter placement. This may be particularly useful in cases of multiple ventricular septations or small ventricles. Image guidance, especially employing intraoperative ultrasound, has also been responsible for improved catheter placement in ventricular shunting procedures. In very difficult cases, stereotactic image guidance or intraoperative planar imaging can also be useful. Although optimizing catheter tip position in the frontal horn may not be necessary for shunt longevity, confirmation of placement within the ventricle as opposed to a CSF cistern using these techniques has certainly prevented many reoperations.

Neonatal germinal matrix hemorrhage, as well as meningitis, usually produces a multiloculated hydrocephalus. This condition can lead to complex shunt systems and numerous shunt revisions in patients unfortunate enough to have loculated hydrocephalus. A variety of therapeutic options are available to treat multiloculated hydrocephalus, including placement of multiple shunt catheters, stereotactic aspiration, craniotomy with lysis of septations, and endoscopic fenestrations. Unfortunately, none is entirely effective in all cases, and the treatment of these children often involves combining two or more of these techniques. Cystic membranes often collapse and scar around shunt catheters, necessitating frequent revisions or placement of additional shunt catheters, thus creating complex shunts. Stereotactic aspiration effectively decompresses the cyst, but the wall is neither devascularized nor widely fenestrated, increasing the probability for future recurrence. Craniotomy for cyst fenestration can effectively reduce the rate of shunt revisions or repeat craniotomies, although access to all loculations is not always feasible, and the procedure can be quite complex. Endoscopic cyst fenestration has been reported to provide a safe and less invasive, yet effective, therapeutic alternative without the higher rate of failure (5). The endoscope can be used through a burr hole or as an adjunct to loculated spaces during an open craniotomy. Although shunt independence is not always possible, reducing the number of shunt catheters can reduce the risk of infection and greatly simplify operative revisions at the time of a shunt malfunction.

Third Ventriculostomy

Third ventriculostomy was first performed by Dandy in 1922, and soon thereafter Mixter reported the first endoscopic third ventriculostomy (6). The introduction of shunting procedures by Holter and colleagues in the early 1950s brought about a dramatic improvement in the treatment of hydrocephalus, and thereafter third ventriculostomy and ablation of the choroid plexus fell out of vogue. Renewed interest in the technique resurfaced with improved endoscopic technology and the realization that shunt-dependent hydrocephalus has a significant long-term morbidity including infection, need for operative revision, and increased risk of death. In 1978, Vries (7) reported the utility of the endoscopic third ventriculostomy with the use of modern instrumentation, and a second wave of interest has emerged.

The effectiveness of third ventriculostomy is highly dependent on patient selection. The ideal candidate is a patient with adolescent- or adult-onset aqueductal stenosis, with a predicted response rate of 80–90% (8,9), Because most hydrocephalus patients do not fit this category, the decision must be made on a patient-by-patient basis. Inherent in this decision is the consideration of what constitutes a success, which in turn is dependent on the initial indications for the procedure. In newly diagnosed hydrocephalus, the desired effect of treatment is the abatement or reversal of symptoms caused by increased intracranial pressure and reduction in ventriculomegaly. However, for third ventriculostomy it is interesting that symptoms may resolve without a significant change in ventricular size (10). Whereas this may seem counterintuitive, as normalization of ventricular size often seems a sign of successful treatment in a shunted patient, there are definite advantages in maintaining enlarged ventricles in a patient with chronic ventriculomegaly. For instance, the physiological drainage offered by third ventriculostomy seems to reduce the rate of subdural formation seen when these same patients with chronic ventriculomegaly are shunted.

A second group of patients who benefit from third ventriculostomy are those who are already shunted but have had shunt-related complications, such as frequent obstructions, difficulty in achieving the proper intracranial pressure dynamics, and shunt infections. The goal in this population may be to make them less shunt-dependent, or to minimize the malfunction rate, or to free them from shunts altogether. Patients with noncommunicating hydrocephalus, who are known to decline rapidly with life-threatening symptoms when their shunt fails, may be aided by third ventriculostomy even if they remain shunt dependent. Conversion of noncommunicating to communicating hydrocephalus gives a much larger CSF reserve and can thereby make shunt failures in these same individuals a less urgent surgical imperative, with less chance of a morbid outcome.

Beyond selection of appropriate patients based on underlying disease and age considerations, other practical issues should be addressed. The preoperative image of choice is the magnetic resonance imaging (MRI). This modality allows for a more accurate assessment of third ventricular anatomy (i.e., width of the floor, attenuated floor, and bulging down into the interpeduncular cistern). Several contraindications to third ventriculostomy exist. Owing to the possibility of intraoperative bleeding, patients who have received prior brain radiation therapy may be at greater risk from endoscopy. Patients with fungal basal meningitis are poor candidates secondary to thickening of the floor and obliteration of the interpeduncular cisterns. The preoperative MRI may identify vascular abnormalities involving the basilar apex, thereby obviating endoscopic exploration. Patients with grossly abnormal anatomy, such as severely involved Chiari II syndromes, may be at an increased risk because of the inability to identify anatomical landmarks *(11)*.

The complication rate of third ventriculostomy has not been clearly defined, although it is considered to be low in experienced hands. Jones et al. *(12)* attempted 103 third ventriculostomies and had a 6% complication rate, with no mortalities reported. Numerous isolated complications have been reported following endoscopic third ventriculostomy, including scalp abscesses, ataxia, drowsiness, hypothalamic damage (i.e., SIADH, DI, aberrant temperature regulation), cardiac arrest, injury to the basilar artery (i.e., catastrophic hemorrhage, pseudoaneurysm formation, and stroke), and visual impairment.

Implanted Shunts

Some recent advances in shunt technology have led to more minimally invasive approaches to hydrocephalus in select patients. Adjustable valves serve as a good example. Although they do not seem to have affected shunt failure rates *(13)*, there are two definite patient populations in whom these valves have allowed for fewer surgical procedures. The first includes those with severe ventriculomegaly, who generally need a higher pressure valve early on to prevent overdrainage and subdural formation, but a lower pressure later on as the ventricles decrease in size to allow for adequate drainage. The second involves those with slit ventricle syndrome, in whom gradually turning the valve pressure up has allowed for progressive dilation of the ventricles over time.

Since most shunt failures are proximal blockages of the ventricular catheter, percutaneous clearance of the ventricular catheter has recently been employed as a method of avoiding shunt surgery at the time of a failure. Two methods, one involving endoscopic exploration of the catheter itself combined with coagulation to clear the blockage, and the other being ultrasonic disruption of the blockage, are both currently under investigation *(14,15)*, In both cases the catheter is entered percutaneously, without a skin incision. Success rates have been reported comparable to those for open surgical exchange of the catheter.

Laparoscopic assisted placement of the distal shunt, into either the pleura or the peritoneum, is another way in which minimally invasive techniques are aiding in the treatment of hydrocephalus *(16)*.

INTRACRANIAL CYSTS

The treatment of intra- and extraventricular cysts has also become significantly less invasive over time. Craniotomy is often effective because wide fenestration of septations is possible. However, this is obviously a maximally invasive technique. Others have advocated shunting of cysts *(17)*. This can be associated with failures secondary to scarring and collapse of the cyst around the catheter, requiring surgical revision. Stereotactic aspiration is appealing owing to the minimally invasive nature of the procedure, but cyst recurrence is likely, secondary to closure of the small fenestration. Endoscopy coupled with an image guidance system allows for an accurate, safe approach and wide fenestration of the cysts. It combines the success of open fenestration techniques with the minimally invasive advantages offered by the improved optics of an endoscope. It is especially useful for suprasellar arachnoid cysts extending up to the third ventricle and causing hydrocephalus, where through and through fenestration is often successful at treating both the cyst and the hydrocephalus without need for craniotomy or shunting (Fig. 1; *see* Color Plate 6 following p. 112).

TUMOR BIOPSY/RESECTION

Tumor surgery has greatly benefited from minimally invasive techniques including limited corridors of entry, preoperative embolization, brachytherapy, image guidance, and endocopic assistance. Many of these techniques are discussed in other chapters, but the use of the endoscope in pediatric tumor surgery is worth discussing here. The endoscope can be employed to biopsy and/or resect intraventricular tumors safely. Midline lesions that abut the ventricular system pose an increased surgical risk with stereotactic methods owing to the proximity of critical neurovascular structures, and they also require a large craniotomy to attain the necessary exposure. Ventricular endoscopy may allow safe biopsy in such cases, again touting the advantage of directly visualizing the tumor and the ability to select a less vascular portion of the lesion. In general, endoscopic biopsy is contraindicated in highly vascular lesions as it is hard to control bleeding with the endoscope. The risk of intraventricular seeding of the tumor must be considered, although endoscopy may be advantageous compared with craniotomy because immediate whole craniospinal radiotherapy can be initiated following the minimally invasive endoscopic surgery. Endoscopic biopsy of germinoma in the posterior third ventricle is an

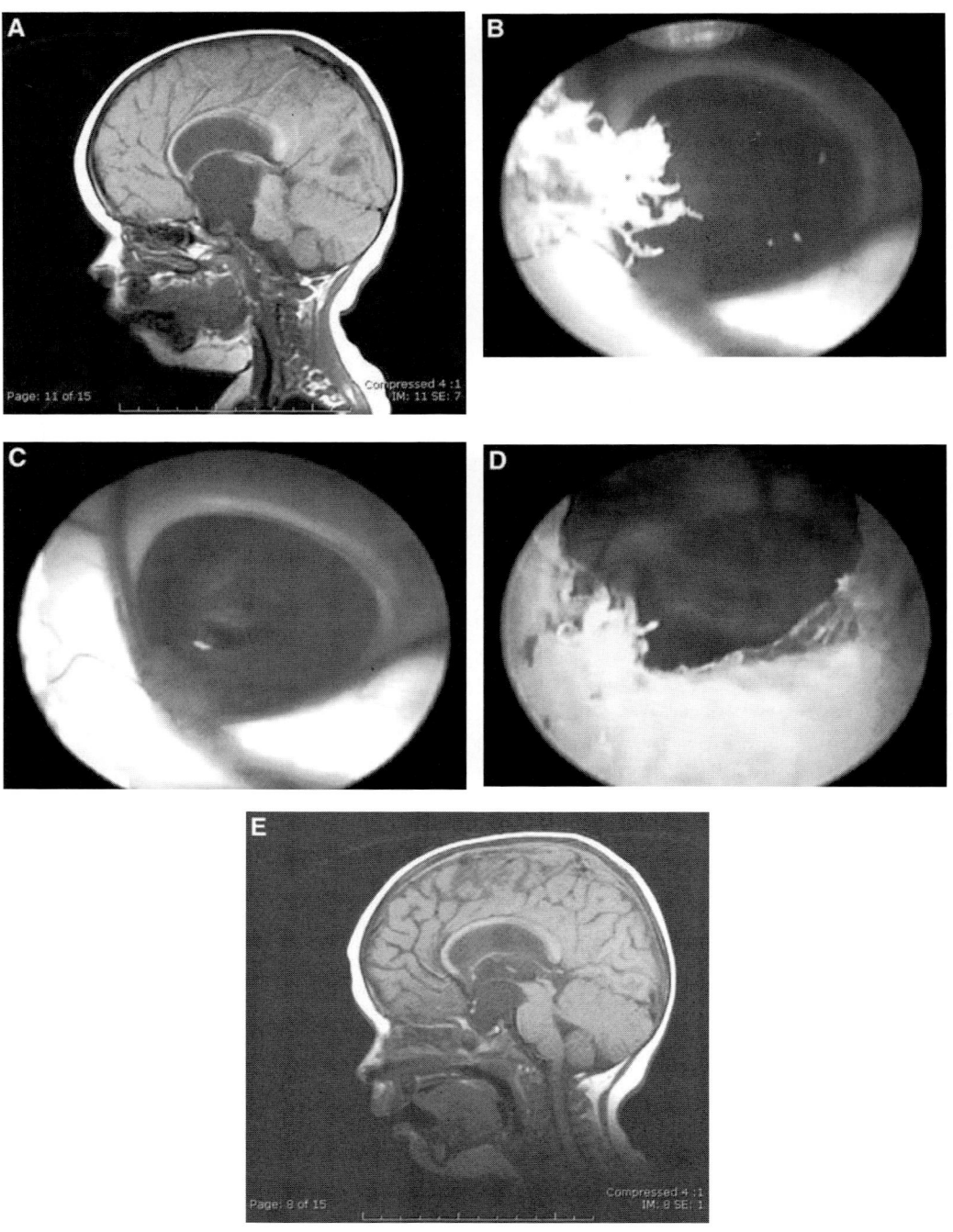

Fig. 1. (A) Preoperative sagittal MRI image of large suprasellar cyst causing obstructive hydrocephalus. **(B)** Endoscopic view at the foramen of Monroe prior to cyst fenestration. **(C)** View after initial puncture through the cyst wall. **(D)** Endoscopic image after wide fenestration of the cyst with the pituitary gland and infundibulum visible through the cyst wall. **(E)** Postoperative sagittal MRI revealing decreased cyst size and reestablishment of normal third ventricle anatomy. (Figure courtesy of Dr. Liliana Goumnerova. *See* Color Plate 6 following p. 112.)

excellent example of this. For cases presenting with hydrocephalus, the tumor can be biopsied with either associated third ventriculostomy or immediate postoperative irradiation to treat the hydrocephalus. There is an existing literature on use of the endoscope to resect colloid cysts of the third ventricle (18) with a low complication and recurrence rate; as comfort levels and technology grow, the use of endoscopy will only grow.

CRANIOSYNOSTOSIS

Premature closure of skull sutures is associated with compensatory cranial and facial deformational changes that often require major reconstructive procedures. In the early years of synostosis surgery, releases at an early age were felt to be the standard of care for treating these patients. Strip craniectomy, a technique first reported in the late 1800s (19) that involves the removal of the fused suture, was for many years the preferred treatment for craniosynostosis, However, over time it was felt that the cosmetic results were often disappointing, and the surgeries required large incisions and frequent need for blood transfusion since extensive scalp mobilization was required for adequate exposure. In a child less than 2 mo of age, skull exposure alone can lead to significant blood loss. Furthermore, the failure to correct the skull shape adequately in a significant percentage of patients led to the evolution of cranial vault remodeling as the preferred technique for synostosis repair. Obviously, these procedures continue to use large bicoronal skin incisions and have an even greater likelihood of blood tranfusion.

The significant invasiveness of current procedures, combined with the advent of newer technologies, has recently brought about innovative approaches in craniosynostosis repair that combine the old and the new. Multiple authors, following the lead of Jimenez and Barone (20,21), have described combined techniques using small incisions, endocopic strip craniectomies, and postoperative orthotic cranial banding to correct synostosis. This allows for a minimally invasive, low blood loss way of doing strip craniectomies, with the orthosis leading to improved cosmetic outcomes compared with the stand-alone strip craniectomies. Endoscopic strip craniectomy is now commonly being used in children less than 2 mo of age to treat sagittal synostosis, with more recent use of the technique for coronal and metopic synostosis as well. The endoscope has minimized the scalp incision, decreased the blood loss, and shortened the operative and recovery time; the authors believe the clinical result is acceptable. The endoscopic technique does have the disadvantage of requiring the patient to wear a molding helmet postoperatively both to help reshape the cranium and to maintain head shapes in the long term. Jimenez advocates the use of the helmet until the child is 1 yr of age. Many consider this a significant drawback to the technique and would rather pursue a more aggressive surgical approach without the need for postoperative orthosis.

Some authors have combined open techniques with more minimally invasive techniques to try and take advantage of each. These newer procedures tend to involve multiple strategically located smaller incisions, along with use of the endoscope, to achieve results similar to those of open procedures in a minimally invasive fashion, involving less blood loss. Although the newer procedures in craniofacial surgery seem to involve lower transfusion rates and shorter operative times than more conventional procedures, the ultimate outcome measures of function and appearance are harder to compare. Although the cephalic index data appear favorable in the correction of sagittal synostosis *(21)*, there are fewer well-accepted objective measurements for the comparison of coronal and metopic synostosis repairs.

VASCULAR ABNORMALITIES

Endovascular treatment of vascular malformations is becoming safer and more effective in obliterating lesions that were traditionally treated with large craniotomies and brain surgeries. Combining endovascular therapy with radiation has permitted "bloodless" surgery for many of the smaller vascular lesions located in eloquent areas of the brain. Much of this is covered in other chapters and is not reviewed here; however, one disease process deserves special attention.

Vein of Galen malformation is a disease process specific to pediatric neurosurgery. These lesions, which comprise a fistulous connection of the arterial circulation to the vein of Galen or nearby venous structures with resultant dilation of the vein of Galen, can have significant effects on newborns. In some less fortunate cases, the circulatory steal is so severe that children are born with severe hypoxic–ischemic encephalopathy and often do not survive. However, others are born with more benign symptoms such as high-output cardiac failure or hydrocephalus. Although some lesions can thrombose without treatment *(22)*, the majority require obliteration. Endovascular obliteration of the fistula, either from the arterial or venous side, has become the treatment of choice, and open surgery is now really just of historical interest for the treatment of vein of Galen malformations. The results are often remarkable, with instantaneous resolution of the heart failure and the children often going on to live normal lives *(23)*.

SPINAL ABNORMALITIES

As with vascular lesions, many minimally invasive spine procedures mimic those in the adult population and do not need special attention in this chapter. However, some spine pathologies are specific to children. Intrauterine myelomeningocele closures are changing the face of traditional spinal surgery and perhaps blurring the boundaries of disease as we have the opportunity to intervene so early that the sequelae of disease do not even develop. In many respects this would be minimally invasive, but the hypothesis remains to be proved. In addition, it introduces ethical issues, as what may be less invasive for the baby is clearly maximally invasive for the mother.

In the authors' personal experience, tethered cord release is becoming significantly less invasive. Procedures for filar lipomas, done previously with large incisions and laminectomies, are now done microscopically with small incisions and operating between adjacent lamina. It remains to be seen whether endoscopic techniques might be applicable to this surgery in the future.

In general, smaller incisions and exposure seem to be significantly aiding pediatric spine procedures. This is especially true because the bone healing in children is so robust that simply exposing additional levels or facets can lead to unwanted autofusion of the spinal column. Pediatric neurosurgeons often take advantage of this robust fusion in other ways by performing laminoplasty in place of laminectomy, as it is likely that the child's bone will fuse and reestablish normal anatomy.

PAIN/SPASTICITY

Pediatric neurosurgery has witnessed significant minimally invasive advances in the treatment of spasticity. Although it is still being performed, selective dorsal rhizotomy has seen a marked falloff in favor of the insertion of baclofen pumps. In these procedures, a lumbar puncture or lumbar drain is performed to allow for a test dose of intrathecal baclofen. If this is successful, the definitive implanted pump can then be inserted by implanting a lumbar catheter, which is then tunneled subcutaneously and attached to a small, refillable pump placed in the subcutaneous space in the abdominal wall. Depending on the level of spasticity, the cathether tip can be placed all the way up to the cervical region from the lumbar space (24). Intrathecal baclofen pump implantation has improved quality of life and helped to reduce the need for the multiple orthopedic procedures that are often performed to release contracted tendons and "locked" joints in the patients with severe spasticity.

EPILEPSY

The neurosurgeon's role in treating epilepsy has ranged from small craniotomies and resection of focal lesions to hemispherectomy. Large brain resection for intractable seizures has fallen out of vogue primarily because of more effective anticonvulsant medications and better electrophysiological monitoring, permitting a more precise localization of epileptiform focus. In the last decade, a relatively minimally invasive technique has gained acceptance as a viable alternative in treating epilepsy. In patients for whom monitoring cannot accurately localize a seizure focus or who have bilateral foci, with poor seizure control despite administration of multiple oral anticonvulsants, vagal nerve stimulation provides a safe and effective option. At many centers, this technique has replaced corpus collosotomy as the treatment of choice for poorly localized secondarily generalizing epilepsy. It is a safe, well-tolerated procedure that can improve the seizure frequency and severity in many patients (25).

CONCLUSIONS

Pediatric neurosurgery as a specialty has benefited perhaps more than any other neurosurgical subspecialty from minimally invasive techniques. It has revolutionized the treatment of hydrocephalus for many patients, leaving them free of shunts or with fewer shunt catheters. Craniosynostosis repair is at a crossroads where a whole new method of correction can be offered as an option to some patients. Treatment of tumors, vascular lesions, spine pathology, epilepsy, and spasticity in children are all being revolutionized. The possibilities are many, and new technologies will continue to be integrated on a regular basis.

REFERENCES

1. Guazzo EP. Recent advances in pediatric neurosurgery. *Arch Dis Child* 1993;69: 335–337.
2. Harris LW. Endoscopic techniques in neurosurgery. *Microsurgery* 1994;15:541–546.
3. Villavicencio AT, Leveque JC, et al. Comparison of revision rates following endoscopically versus nonendoscopically placed ventricular shunt catheters. *Surg Neurol* 2003;59:375–379; discussion 379–380.
4. Bierbrauer KS, Storrs BB, et al. A prospective, randomized study of shunt function and infections as a function of shunt placement. *Pediatr Neurosurg* 1990;16: 287–291.
5. Gangemi, M, Maiuri F, et al. Endoscopic treatment of para- and intraventricular cerebrospinal fluid cysts. *Minim Invasive Neurosurg* 2000;43:153–158.
6. Jimenez DF. Third ventriculostomy, in *Intracranial Endoscopic Neurosurgery* (Jimenez DF, ed.), *American Association of Neurological Surgeons*, Park Ridge, IL, 1998, p. 108.
7. Vries J. An endoscopic technique for third ventriculostomy. *Surg Neurol* 1978;9: 165–168.
8. Choi JU, Kim DS, et al. Endoscopic surgery for obstructive hydrocephalus. *Yonsei Med J* 1999;40:600–607.
9. Feng, H, Huang G, et al. Endoscopic third ventriculostomy in the management of obstructive hydrocephalus: an outcome analysis. *J Neurosurg* 2004;100:626–633.
10. Kulkarni AV, Drake JM, et al. Imaging correlates of successful endoscopic third ventriculostomy. *J Neurosurg* 2000;92:915–919.
11. Cartmill, M, Jaspan T, et al. Neuroendoscopic third ventriculostomy in dysmorphic brains. *Childs Nerv Syst* 2001;17:391–394.
12. Jones RF, Kwok BC, et al. Neuroendoscopic third ventriculostomy. A practical alternative to extracranial shunts in non-communicating hydrocephalus. *Acta Neurochir Suppl (Wien)* 1994;61:79–83.
13. Zemack, G, Romner B. Seven years of clinical experience with the programmable Codman Hakim valve: a retrospective study of 583 patients. *J Neurosurg* 2000;92: 941–948.
14. Pattisapu JV, Trumble ER, et al. Percutaneous endoscopic recanalization of the catheter: a new technique of proximal shunt revision. *Neurosurgery* 1999;45:1361–6; discussion 1366–1367.
15. Ginsberg HJ, Sum A, Drake JM, Cobbold RS. Ventriculoperitoneal shunt flow dependency on the number of patent holes in a ventricular catheter. *Pediatr Neurosurg* 2000;33:7–11.
16. Fanelli RD, Mellinger DN, et al. Laparoscopic ventriculoperitoneal shunt placement: a single-trocar technique. *Surg Endosc* 2000;14:641–643.
17. Ciricillo SF, Cogen PH, et al. Intracranial arachnoid cysts in children. A comparison of the effects of fenestration and shunting. *J Neurosurg* 1991;74:230–235.
18. King WA, Ullman JS, Frazee JG, Post KD, Bergsneider M. Endoscopic resection of colloid cysts: surgical considerations using the rigid endoscope. *Neurosurgery* 1999;44:1103–1109; discussion 1109–1111.

19. Shillito JJ, Matson DD: Craniosynostosis: A review of 519 surgical patients. *Pediatrics* 1968;41:829–853.
20. Barone, CM, Jimenez DF. Endoscopic craniectomy for early correction of craniosynostosis. *Plast Reconstr Surg* 1999;104:1965–1973; discussion 1974–1975.
21. Jimenez DF, Barone CM, et al. Early management of craniosynostosis using endoscopic-assisted strip craniectomies and cranial orthotic molding therapy. *Pediatrics* 2000;110:97–104.
22. Nikas DC, Proctor MR, et al. Spontaneous thrombosis of vein of Galen aneurysmal malformation. *Pediatr Neurosurg* 1999;31:33–39.
23. Mitchell PJ, Rosenfeld JV, et al. Endovascular management of vein of Galen aneurysmal malformations presenting in the neonatal period. *AJNR Am J Neuroradiol* 2001;22:1403–1409.
24. Burns, AS, Meythaler JM. Intrathecal baclofen in tetraplegia of spinal origin: efficacy for upper extremity hypertonia. *Spinal Cord* 2001;39:413–419.
25. FineSmith RB, Zampella E, et al. Vagal nerve stimulator: a new approach to medically refractory epilepsy. *N Engl J Med* 1999;96:37–40.

16
Minimally Invasive Techniques in Vascular Neurosurgery

Prithvi Narayan, MD and Daniel L. Barrow, MD

INTRODUCTION

A number of options exist to minimize the invasiveness of surgical intervention for neurovascular disorders. These include techniques such as endovascular therapy and stereotactic radiosurgery, which eliminate or reduce the need for traditional surgical approaches, and surgical adjuncts such as image guidance and microsurgical techniques, which reduce the invasiveness of those traditional surgical approaches.

Endovascular management of cerebrovascular disorders was first developed by Serbinenko and introduced to the Western world by Debrun *(1,2)*. Initially used to treat carotid cavernous fistulae, endovascular techniques have advanced rapidly with the development of modern catheters and devices and currently provide therapeutic options for the management of a large number of cerebrovascular disorders. For selected cerebrovascular disorders, such as cavernous malformations, there is currently no endovascular option. Endovascular therapy may serve as an adjunct to the surgical treatment of selected conditions such as arteriovenous malformations (AVMs) to reduce the morbidity of the definitive vascular procedure or, as is the case with intracranial aneurysms, may provide a therapeutic alternative to open surgery.

Image guidance is of less value in vascular neurosurgery than in other areas of the specialty. This technique can be of great assistance in localizing vascular malformations such as AVMs or cavernous malformations that are below the surface of the brain, minimizing retraction and dissection, and more accurately placing a craniotomy. A role for image guidance in the treatment of intracranial aneurysms and any benefit of reduction in the size of the craniotomy for addressing intracranial aneurysms remain speculative.

Stereotactic radiosurgery is a minimally invasive neurosurgical option for selected neurovascular disorders. The greatest experience has been in the treatment of AVMs of the brain, for which stereotactic radiosurgery has been successful in obliterating well-selected lesions. In many instances, it is an alternative to open neurosurgical resection. The efficacy of stereotactic radiosurgery in the treatment of cavernous malformations is unproven and more controversial.

The most valuable minimally invasive technique in vascular neurosurgery remains microsurgery. Despite remarkable advances in endovascular therapy, it should be pointed out that the field of microsurgery is not static, and advances in this discipline continue. Use of the operating microscope, combined with appropriate microsurgical instruments and a knowledge of microneurosurgical anatomy, allows one to utilize cisternal anatomy to obtain brain relaxation and exposure of the vascular lesion with minimal or no retraction. Furthermore, sulcal approaches to selected vascular lesions are one of the most important minimally invasive techniques in vascular neurosurgery. Skull base techniques are used to remove bone, minimize brain retraction, open surgical corridors, and bring the surgeon closer to the pathology.

The potential usefulness of each of these minimally invasive techniques varies significantly with the specific neurovascular pathology. This chapter discusses the pathological entities most commonly encountered in a neurovascular practice and the role of minimally invasive procedures in the management of these disorders.

ANEURYSMS

Microsurgery

Surgical treatment of intracranial aneurysms originated in the 1930s, prior to which the treatment of choice was hunterian ligation of the parent vessel. The morbidity and mortality were quite high before the advent of the operating microscope. Refinement of microscopic technology and development of microsurgical techniques have established clip ligation as a time-honored, durable, and standard treatment for intracranial aneurysms. A thorough knowledge of the cisternal and vascular anatomy and microsurgical navigation through the cisterns, with egress of cerebrospinal fluid (CSF) affording brain relaxation, has established surgical clip ligation as a minimally invasive, low-risk, and efficacious treatment option for these lesions. The pterional approach, described by Yasargil and Fox (3), is the most widely used approach compared with bifrontal and frontolateral craniotomies for access to the anterior circulation. A criticism of this approach has been the limited resection of the gyrus rectus necessary for exposure and control of the anterior communicating (ACOM) artery complex despite the lack of evidence of adverse neurological sequelae. Also, the cosmetic results from a standard pterional approach can be disturbing owing to temporalis muscle atrophy. This has given impetus to the development of minimally invasive surgical techniques (4–6).

The goal of microsurgical techniques developed during the last few decades has been to reduce iatrogenic trauma and improve postoperative outcomes. This has been enhanced by the increased sophistication of microscopes, neuronavigation systems, stereotactic techniques, and intraoperative endoscopes. Concomitantly, there has been an evolution of diagnostic and preoperative imaging techniques allowing precise localization of lesions and providing exquisite anatomic details for operative planning. These developments have led to the keyhole concept of microneurosurgery.

A transorbital keyhole approach to ACOM artery aneurysms has recently been described (7). The rationale behind this technique is to render the dissection of the ACOM complex completely extracerebral, obviating the need for or minimizing the gyrus rectus resection. Also, temporalis muscle dissection is minimized. The eyebrow keyhole approach is another attempt at reducing the invasiveness of standard microsurgery (8). The skin incision is made in the lateral two-thirds of the eyebrow, followed by a small supraorbital craniotomy. This is especially useful cosmetically in people with receding hairlines. Paladino et al. (8) used this approach with an endoscope to visualize the neck better to treat 37 patients with 40 intracranial aneurysms with no mortality and excellent cosmetic results.

The disadvantages of the keyhole approach are the narrow viewing angles, limited space for manipulating microinstruments, and reduced operating field light intensity. One method of improving the light intensity with keyhole craniotomies is the use of endoscopes. The first endoscopic neurosurgical procedure was performed in 1910 to cauterize the choroid plexus in hydrocephalic infants (9). Since then, endoscopic technology has undergone major advances (10,11). The introduction of the rigid rod lens scope has revived interest in neuroendoscopy. There are a growing number of applications for treating lesions in the intraventricular and subarachnoid spaces. Recently, Kalavakonda et al. (12) described the use of an endoscope in assisting microsurgery for aneurysms in 55 patients with 79 aneurysms. The endoscope reportedly provides additional views not available with a standard microscope. In 26 aneurysms, the authors reported that endoscopic assistance provided a better view than would have been possible with the microscope alone. However, in more than half the cases, the endoscope did not seem to provide useful information.

The use of navigation systems in aneurysm surgery is limited. 3D subtraction angiography and 3D computed tomographic angiography (CTA) are emerging technologies that may be useful for preoperative planning in patients with intracranial aneurysms (13,14). However, their use in determining the size and placement of craniotomies is limited. In our experience, these advances have been more useful in determining the viability of endovascular options and more often in revealing anatomic details that suggest surgical clip ligation may be better suited for a particular aneurysm.

It has been suggested that keyhole microneurosurgery may contribute to improved postoperative results through shorter hospitalization times by reducing complications such as bleeding, infection, CSF leak, and neurological deterioration with brain retraction (8). Although it certainly is a useful addition to the armamentarium for microsurgery, its routine use is not recommended. Simplicity and cosmetic results are important in craniotomies, but it should not be at the expense of safety and efficacy.

Endovascular Treatment

Endovascular treatment of intracranial aneurysms began in the 1960s and 1970s. Serbinenko (1), with the creation of a latex detachable balloon for endovascular obliteration, is arguably the father of endovascular therapy. In 1981, Debrun et al. *(2)* used detachable balloons for parent vessel occlusion in patients with giant aneurysms and began the North American experience. Subsequently balloon occlusion of aneurysms was replaced by coil embolization. Guido Guglielmi invented detachable coils, which revolutionized the endovascular treatment of aneurysms through the development of Guglielmi detachable coils (GDCs; Boston Scientific/Target Therapeutics, Fremont, CA) *(15)*. The major advantage of this system is the softness and compliance of the coil, allowing packing of the aneurysm dome. Other benefits include controlled delivery and retrievability. However, the GDC technique has some limitations. Large and giant aneurysms, as well as wide-necked and complex aneurysms, are difficult to pack densely with this technique. This led to the development of adjuncts to coiling, such as balloon remodeling *(16)* and stenting *(17–20)*. In the remodeling technique, the balloon not only functions as an external barrier and prevents coils from escaping into the parent artery, but also allows for tighter packing of the dome with coils. The development of new flexible, intravascular stents has further improved the density of packing. Stents function as scaffolds, preventing the coils from escaping into the parent vessel. (Fig. 1) The safety and efficacy of this technique have been reported recently *(17–21)*. Recently, the Neuroform microdelivery stent system (SMART Therapeutics, San Leandro, CA) has been approved for use with embolic coils specifically for the treatment of wide-necked saccular aneurysms. Its efficacy remains to be established.

Endovascular therapy has generated not only great enthusiasm but also great controversy because of its potential therapeutic benefits vs lack of long-term data to establish its durability. The International Subarachnoid Aneurysm Trial Collaborative Group (ISAT) reported the results of its randomized trial of coiling vs clipping of intracranial aneurysms *(22)*. In this study, 9559 patients with subarachnoid hemorrhage (SAH) were seen in multiple centers. Of these, 7416 patients were excluded form the study and 2143 were randomized. At the end of 1 yr, 190 of 801 patients (23.7%) allocated to endovascular treatment were dependent or dead compared with 243 of 793 (30.6%) allocated to surgery. The relative risk reduction was 22.6%, with an absolute risk reduction of 6.9%. The conclusions reached from the trial's data were that endovascular coiling is significantly more likely to result in survival free of disability 1 yr after SAH than neurosurgical treatment. Longer term follow-up, however, is vital to answer the question of durability of benefit *(22)*.

This study has come under criticism for a number of reasons, including selection bias, the large number of patients who were not randomized, short follow-up, and subjective outcome assessment. The overwhelming majority of patients randomized had small aneurysms *(93%)* on the anterior circulation (97.3%) and were good grade *(88%) (22)*. Outcomes after aneurysm treatment should be determined by the rate of periprocedural complications and the success in the reduction of rebleeding. One of the great drawbacks of endovascular therapy with the current technology is the incomplete obliteration of the dome of the aneurysm which can directly result in increased rebleeding rates. Therefore, a

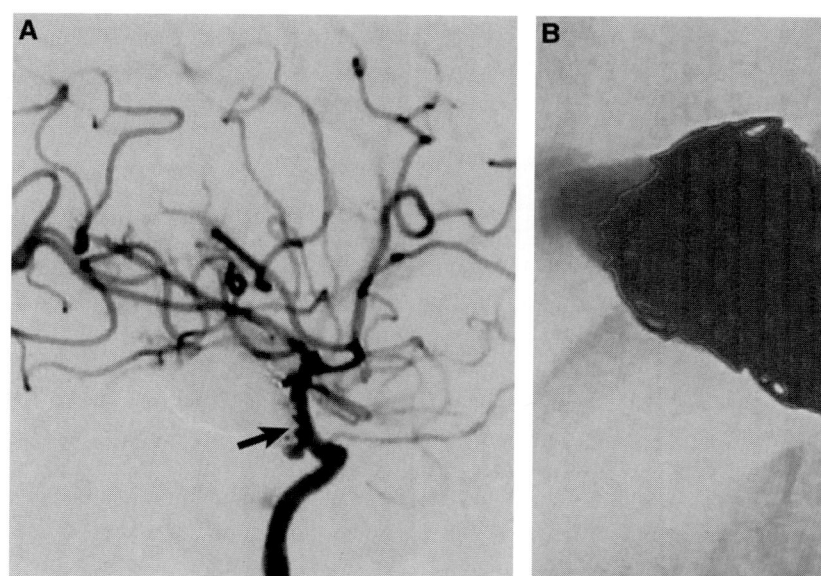

Fig. 1. Stent coiling of intracranial aneurysm. **(A)** Right internal carotid angiogram after endovascular coiling of large aneurysm involving the entire lateral wall of the carotid. Note the irregular interface between the coil mass and the lumen of the parent artery (arrow). **(B)** Anteroposterior film demonstrates endovascular stent (arrow) within the lumen of the carotid bolstering the coil mass within the wide-necked aneurysm.

1-yr follow-up is insufficient to establish the durability of coiling compared with clipping. There has also been a tendency to apply the ISAT data to all patients harboring intracranial aneurysms. This is dangerous since endovascular coiling of all aneurysms irrespective of the width of the neck, dome-to-neck ratio, and complexity of the vascular anatomy could result in higher complications. Another striking aspect of the ISAT trial is the poor surgical outcome. This highly selective patient population had a higher rate (almost 10%) of poor outcome compared with similar patient populations in large prospective surgical series. Despite these criticisms, it should be acknowledged that endovascular therapy is a viable alternative treatment for intracranial aneurysms in carefully selected patients. The angiographic and long-term follow-up data from the ISAT trial may shed some light on the rebleeding rates and patient outcomes. Until there is clear evidence of improved outcomes with endovascular therapy, surgical clip ligation should be considered the first line of therapy, especially in good-grade patients harboring aneurysms.

ARTERIOVENOUS MALFORMATIONS

Microsurgery

Surgery for the treatment of AVMs yielded dismal results until the introduction of angiography and microsurgical techniques in the 1940s and the 1960s, respectively. The goal of surgical treatment for most AVMs is to cure the malformation and eliminate the risk of hemorrhage. An important advantage of surgery over other treatment options such as radiosurgery and endovascular techniques is the immediate protection from hemorrhage. Despite the various advances in endovascular technology and radiosurgery, microsurgical resection remains the treatment of choice for most parenchymal AVMs *(23–25)*.

Various surgical treatment concepts have evolved depending on the size and natural history of the lesions. These include staged resections or combination with preoperative embolization or radiosurgery *(26–28)*. The tenet of microsurgery for AVMs is the resection of the nidus with minimal hemorrhage and brain retraction. There is no place for minimally invasive, small craniotomy flaps in AVM resection. A wide exposure is important to accommodate brain swelling, identify the surface and vascular anatomy, and allow for safe resection of the AVM in the event of catastrophic bleeding.

Stereotactically guided resection of AVMs was one of the first applications of this modality *(29)*. Although its value for the volumetric resection of tumors is widely accepted, its use in AVM resection has been slow to take off. AVMs, similar to tumors, can be defined by volumes in stereotactic space based on imaging. It seems logical that image guidance can be used to identify the margins of the nidus and the major feeding arteries. Recently, a novel method using image guidance for the resection of AVMs in 22 patients was described *(30)*. Preoperative helical CTA with 3D reconstruction was obtained, and intraoperative neuronavigation was used. Temporary clips were placed on all identifiable feeding arteries greater than 3 mm in diameter to decompress the nidus. The dissection was then performed along the main draining veins based on image guidance. The morbidity and mortality rates were 14 and 0%, respectively. The 4-mo follow-up was too short to make any meaningful conclusions compared with the literature. Larger published series with longer follow-ups are needed to determine whether surgical outcomes can be improved with these evolving techniques.

Endovascular Treatment

The endovascular treatment of AVMs has made significant progress since the obliteration of a carotid-cavernous fistula (CCF) with a muscle embolus reported by Barney Brooks in 1931 *(31)*. This led to the search for an ideal embolic agent in the following years, including silastic spheres, spheres with silk sutures to increase thrombogenicity, porcelain beads, Gelfoam, steel balls, and Teflon-coated spheres *(32–34)*. The major drawback of these early attempts was the lack of microcatheters and control over the emboli, which resulted in unacceptable morbidity and neurological deficits. Advances in imaging techniques and delivery catheters and development of a solidifying liquid embolic agent *(35)* have revolutionized modern-day embolization (Fig. 2). Roadmapping techniques allow the interventionalist to advance the catheter safely in tortuous arteries using a negative map of the vascular tree with a superimposed image of the catheter tip. Despite these major advances, endovascular treatment of AVMs remains primarily an adjunct to microsurgery or radio-

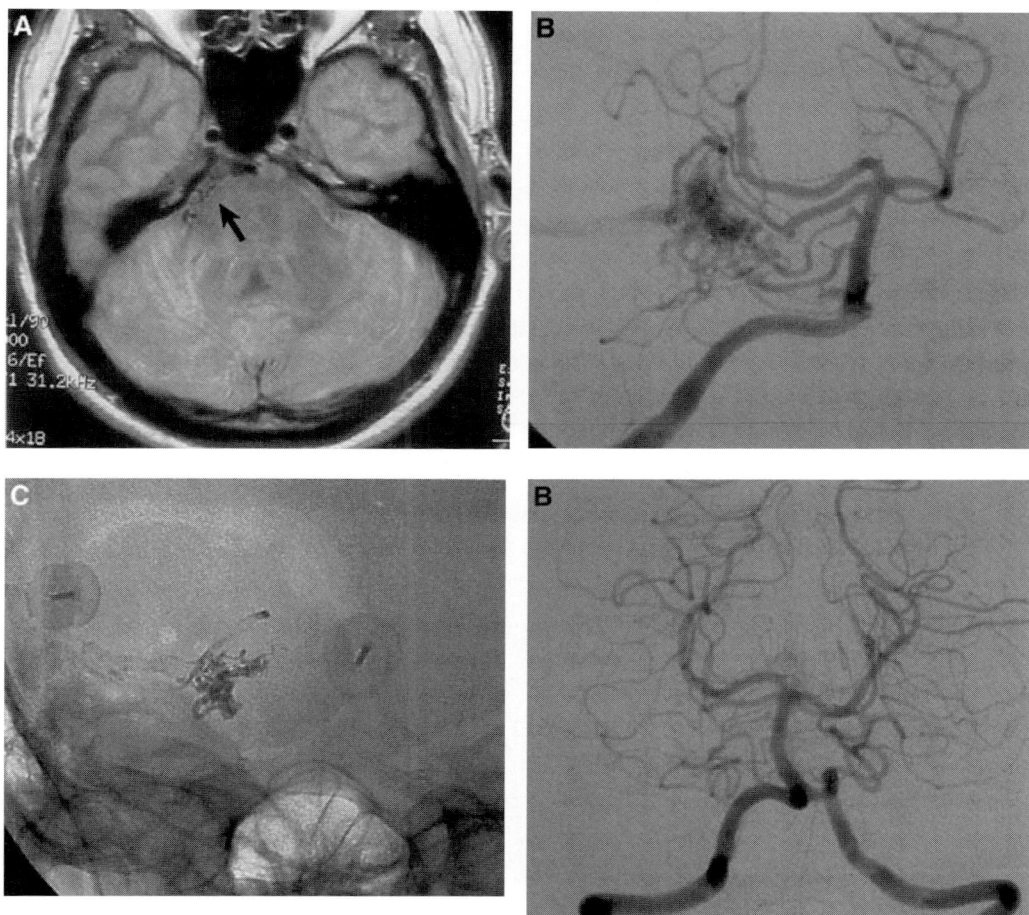

Fig. 2. Embolization of pial arteriovenous malformation. **(A)** Axial MRI shows small AVM on lateral edge of brainstem (arrow). **(B)** AP vertebral angiogram reveals the AVM fed by a single branch of the anterior inferior cerebellar artery. **(C)** AP film shows "glue" in nidus of AVM after embolization. **(D)** AP vertebral angiogram after embolization documents complete obliteration of AVM.

surgery. Complete obliteration of AVMs is possible only in rare cases, and the morbidity associated with it is not insignificant.

Radiosurgery

Radiosurgery is a viable minimally invasive treatment alternative for AVMs that are not suitable for surgical resection. Radiosurgery appears to induce a pathological process in the nidus that leads to gradual thickening of the vessels, leading to thrombosis *(36,37)*. Obliteration rates from 70 to 98% have been reported, depending on the nidus volume and the dose delivered *(38)*. Larger AVMs pose a greater problem with lower obliteration rates owing to the difficulty of defining the complete nidus volume and using reduced doses for safety. Incomplete obliteration fails to reduce the risk of hemorrhage, thereby requiring other treatment modalities such as surgery, embolization, or alternate strategies of radiosurgery. Repetitive radiosurgery is an evolving concept. A 2-yr obliteration rate of 62% (62 of 101 patients) was reported by Karlson et al. *(39)* after repetitive radiosurgery to treat AVMs. Fourteen patients developed radiation-induced deficits and six experienced additional hemorrhage. This concept will continue to evolve as more AVMs in critical areas continue to be treated with this modality. Another strategy for large AVMs is prospectively staged radiosurgery, in which two adjacent volumes of the AVM nidus are treated at intervals of 3–6 mo. This allows for the delivery of a larger total dose and minimizes radiation to adjacent normal tissue *(40)*.

DURAL ARTERIOVENOUS MALFORMATIONS

Advances in endovascular therapy have established this modality as the primary treatment option for a majority of dural arteriovenous malformations (DAVMs). Transvenous embolization is the preferred route (Fig. 3). For those lesions that are not amenable to endovascular therapy, surgical interruption of the venous drainage provides immediate elimination of the lesion.

The treatment of DAVMs with radiosurgery is highly controversial. Link et al. *(41)* have recently reported on the use of stereotactic radiosurgery for the treatment of DAVMs as the primary treatment modality. The protocol involved radiosurgery followed by transarterial embolization 48 h after the radiation. The authors reported good results in their short-term follow-up (1 yr) of the 105 patients with various DAVMs. Although knowledge of the natural history of DAVMs is incomplete, it is well known that those lesions associated with leptomeningeal venous drainage have a very aggressive clinical course compared to those draining into a dural sinus *(42,43)*. The former are associated with rates of intracranial hemorrhage, nonhemorrhagic neurological deficit, and mortality of 14.2, 10.9, and 19.3% per lesion per year, respectively *(43)*. In these cases, the use of stereotactic radiosurgery, with its long interval to therapeutic benefit, exposes the patient to unnecessary risks, especially when the fistulae can be immediately obliterated by endovascular or surgical interruption of the venous drainage. In addition, partial treatment of these lesions may turn them into more aggressive ones by altering the venous drainage pattern. Although radiosurgery is a less invasive treatment modality, its efficacy in the treatment of DAVMs has not been established.

CAVERNOUS MALFORMATIONS

Cavernous malformations are angiographically occult; therefore, endovascular techniques have no role in the treatment of these lesions. Although the natural history of these lesions is incompletely understood and variable, it is significantly more benign than the natural course of AVMs. Nonoperative therapy is probably the best course for most incidentally discovered cavernous malformations. Symptomatic lesions are best treated with standard microsurgical

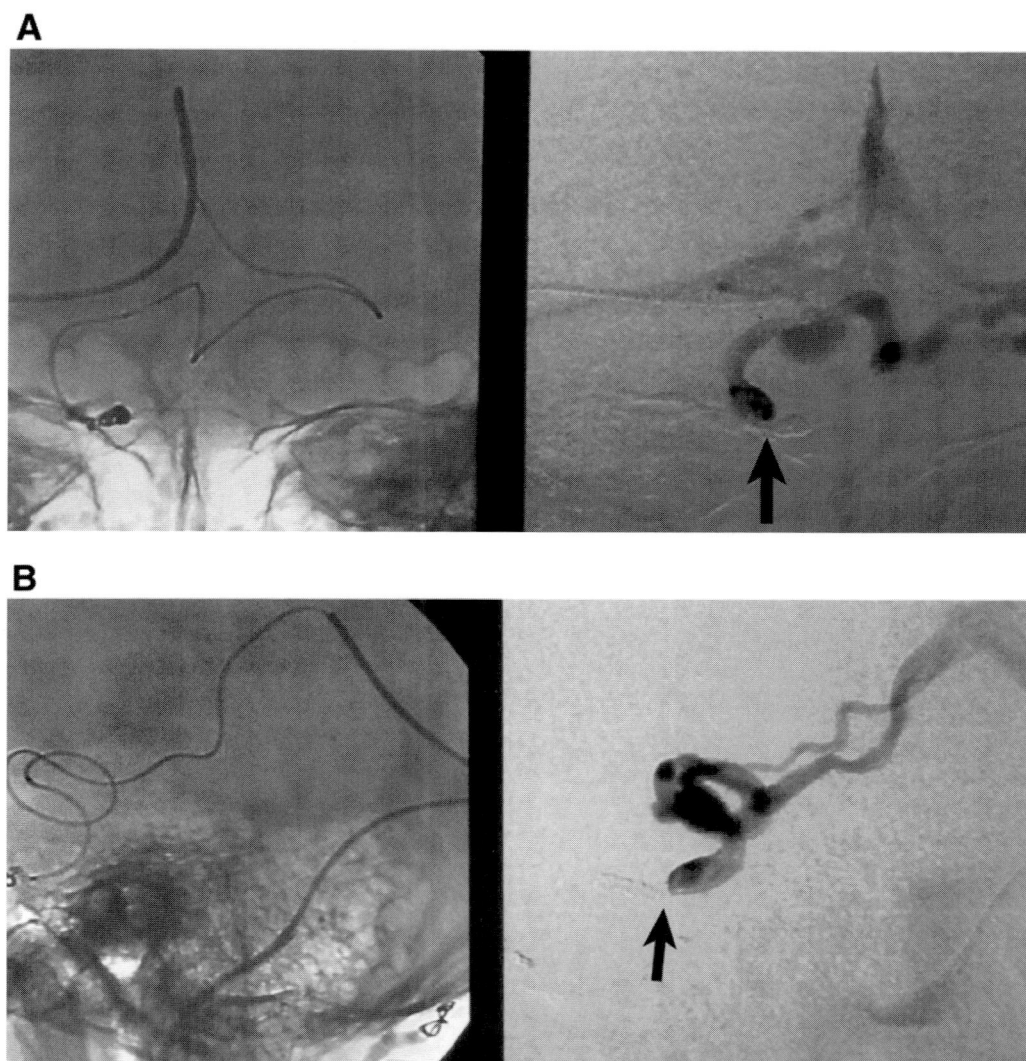

Fig. 3. Transvenous embolization of dural arteriovenous fistula. **(A)** AP and **(B)** lateral venograms through a microcatheter placed at the precise site of the fistula. Arrows point to endovascular coils deposited at the site of the fistula to obliterate the lesion.

techniques. A useful addition to the surgical armamentarium is the availability of intraoperative stereotactic localization. A number of frameless stereotactic systems are now available with acceptable accuracy that are extremely useful for planning small craniotomies, locating deep-seated lesions, minimizing brain retraction, and limiting the corticectomy. (Fig. 4)

Radiosurgery has been attempted for the treatment of deep-seated cavernous malformations *(14)*. There is a higher incidence of complications compared with similar series of patients with AVMs. This is probably owing to the deleterious

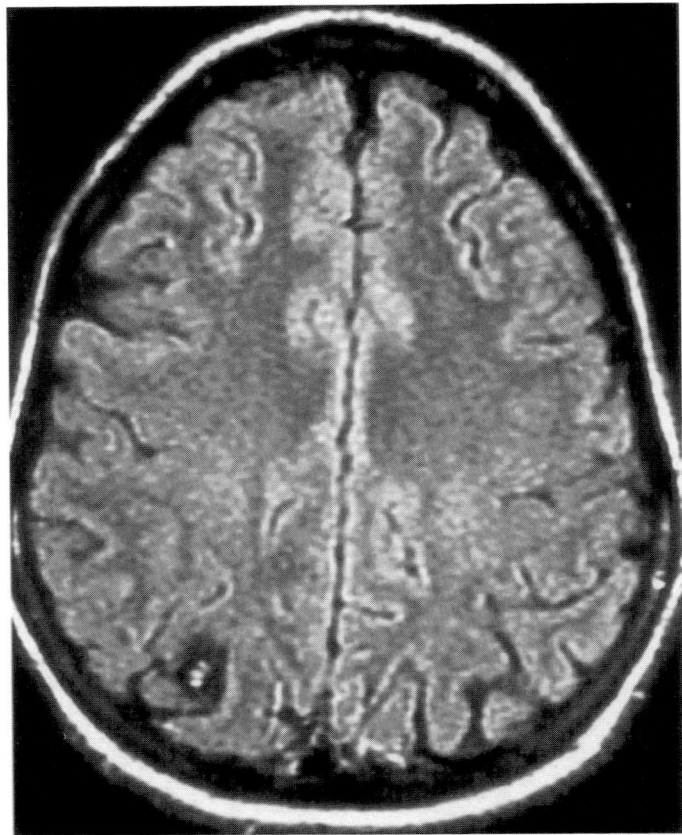

Fig. 4. Frameless stereotactic localization of cavernous malformation. Axial MRI shows small cavernous malformation below the surface of the brain that was readily located and removed utilizing frameless stereotactic guidance.

effects of radiation injury. It is also well known that cavernous malformations undergo spontaneous reduction in size after a hemorrhage. Although it has been suggested that radiosurgery may reduce the subsequent risk of hemorrhage, this remains to be proved, and evidence of disappearance of cavernous malformations following radiosurgery is lacking. Because of these factors, radiosurgery is not recommended as a treatment option for these lesions except experimentally, utilizing carefully selected criteria. An exception to this is extracerebral cavernous malformations of the middle fossae. Surgical extirpation of these lesions can be formidable because of their propensity to cause life-threatening intraoperative hemorrhages. Initial biopsy followed by radiosurgery and surgical resection provides the best results *(44)*.

CAROTID CAVERNOUS FISTULAE (CCF)

Endovascular technology has advanced to the point that it has monopolized the treatment of CCF. The creation of microcatheters and a variety of embolic agents has established this modality as the treatment of choice for CCFs. The goal of therapy is to obliterate the fistula and preserve the parent artery. In rare cases, the cavernous carotid artery may have to be sacrificed to preserve visual function. CCFs are classified into two types: direct and indirect, with indirect fistula further classified on the basis of arterial supply *(45)*. The direct, or type A, fistula is generally posttraumatic in nature and involves a direct connection between the internal carotid artery (ICA) and cavernous sinus. These may also result from rupture of an intracavernous aneurysm. The indirect type is an arteriovenous fistula located within the dura surrounding the cavernous sinus and is characterized by multiple arteries from the dura supplying the fistule. Type B CCFs are supplied by small branches of the cavernous segment of the ICA and is exceedingly rare. Type C CCFs are supplied by dural branches of the external carotid artery. Type D CCFs are supplied by branches from both the internal and external carotid arteries *(45)*.

The transarterial approach is preferred for most direct CCFs. Alternatively, the transvenous approach can be used when the transarterial route is impossible. The cavernous sinus can be accessed either through the inferior petrosal sinus or the superior ophthalmic vein *(46,47)*. In complex cases, a combination of the two may be necessary. Surgical exposure of the sinus may be necessary when the endovascular routes are impermeable or embolic materials result in venous outflow obstruction leading to clinical deterioration *(48)*. More recently, we have utilized an approach to selected cases through transorbital puncture of the cavernous sinus through the superior orbital fissure *(49)*. The transvenous route carries the lowest risk but also the lowest success rate owing to difficulty in negotiating the multicompartmental sinuses *(50)*.

The treatment of indirect CCFs is through the tranvenous route. The multiple arterial feeders supplying these lesions make transarterial embolization less successful. Continued advances in catheter technology and embolic agents may improve the obliteration rates, with minimal complications.

FUTURE TRENDS

The trend toward making microneurosurgery less invasive continues with advances in neuronavigation, and neuroendoscopy and refinement of skull base techniques and surgical approaches to minimize brain retraction. Robotics in microneurosurgery seems to be the next wave of technological innovation to minimize the invasiveness of standard techniques. Certainly, they cannot replace surgeons. Their primary use in neurosurgery would be dexterity enhancement with dampening of physiologic tremor. This may then allow one to operate through narrow corridors safely with the use of endoscopes. Surgery using robotic systems has already been applied in many surgical fields such as the Robodoc System (Integrated Surgical Systems, Davis, CA) for hip joint replacement surgery *(51)*, and the da Vinci System (Intuitive Surgical, Sunnyvale, CA) for coronary artery bypass surgery *(52)*. The Neu-Robot telecontrolled micromanipulator system currently under development and in preliminary testing seems to be promising in terms of improving accuracy while minimizing invasiveness. This system has been tested on cadavers to open the sylvian fissure and the floor of the third ventricle through a single burr hole working through multiple working channels (53). Whether these technological advances will make a difference in terms of patient outcome remains to be seen.

Despite the controversies surrounding the use of endovascular therapy in neurosurgery, the use of this modality is increasing exponentially. Several centers throughout the world have adopted this modality as the treatment of choice for intracranial aneurysms. The general thinking is that the current concepts and technology are in evolution, and with improvements in coils, embolic materials, microcatheters, and stents, this modality will become the definitive therapy for many neurovascular disorders. Similarly, rapid developments in neuroimaging, stereotactic techniques, and robotic technology are contributing to the improvement of results and expanding the indications for stereotactic radiosurgery.

The future is exciting, with unlimited scope for these new technological advances to enhance patient care. It is important that with such dramatic advances, patient care and outcome be the sole determinant of the treatment paradigm rather than technology.

REFERENCE

1. Serbinenko FA. Balloon catheterization and occlusion of major cerebral vessels. *J Neurosurg* 1974;41:125–145.
2. Debrun G, Fox A, Drake C, Peerless S, Girvin J, Ferguson G. Giant unclippable aneurysms: treatment with balloons. *AJNR* 1981;2:167–173.
3. Yasargil MG, Fox JL. The microsurgical approach to intracranial aneurysms. *Surg Neurol* 1975;3:7–14.
4. Brock M, Dietz H. The small frontolateral approach for the microsurgical treatment of intracranial aneurysms. *Neurochirurgia* 1978;21:185–191.
5. Fukushima T, Miyazaki S, Takusagawa Y, Reichman M. Unilateral interhemispheric keyhole approach for anterior cerebral artery aneurysms. *Acta Neurochir Suppl* 1991;53:42–47.
6. Yeh H, Tew JM Jr. Anterior interhemispheric approach to aneurysms of the anterior communicating artery. *Surg Neurol* 1985;23:98–100.
7. Steiger HJ, Schmid-Elsaesser R, Stummer W, Uhl E. Transorbital keyhole approach to anterior communicating artery aneurysms. *Neurosurgery* 2001;48:347–352.
8. Paladino J, Pirker N, Stimac D, Stern-Padovan R. Eyebrow keyhole approach in vascular neurosurgery. *Minim Invas Neurosurg* 1998;41:200–203.
9. Cohen AR. Endoscopic neurosurgery, in *Neurosurgery*, vol. 1. (Wilkins RH, Rengachary SS, eds.), McGraw Hill, New York, 1996, pp. 539–546.
10. Gieger M, Cohen AR. The history of neuroendoscopy, in *Minimally Invasive Techniques in Neurosurgery* (Cohen AR, Haines SJ, eds.), Williams & Wilkins, Baltimore, 1995, pp. 1–5.
11. Hopf NJ, Perneczky A. Endoscopic neurosurgery and endoscope-assisted microneurosurgery for the treatment of intracranial cysts. *Neurosurgery* 1998;43:1330–1337.
12. Kalavakonda C, Sekhar LN, Ramachandran P, Hechl P. Endoscope-assisted microsurgery for intracranial aneurysms. *Neurosurgery* 2002;51:1119–1127.

13. Anxionnat R, Bracard S, Ducrocq X, et al. Intracranial aneurysms: clinical value of 3D digital subtraction angiography in the therapeutic decision and endovascular treatment. *Radiology* 2001;218:799–808.
14. Kondziolka D, Lunsford LD, Coffey RJ. Stereotactic radiosurgery of angiographically occult vascular malformations: indications and preliminary experience. *Neurosurgery* 1990;27:892–900.
15. Guglielmi G, Vinuela F, Duckwiler G, et al. Endovascular treatment of posterior circulation aneurysms by electrothrombosis using electrically detachable coils. *J Neurosurg* 1992;77:515–524.
16. Moret J, Cognard C, Weill A, Castaings L, Rey A. Reconstruction technic in the treatment of wide-neck intracranial aneurysms. *J Neuroradiol* 1997;24:30–44.
17. Bracard S, Anxionnat R, Da Costa E, Lebedinsky A, Scomazzoni F, Picard L. Combined endovascular stenting and endosaccular coiling for the treatment of a wide-necked intracranial vertebral aneurysm. *Intervent Neuroradiol* 1999;5:245–249.
18. Higashida RT, Smith W, Gress D, et al. Intravascular stent and endovascular coil placement for a ruptured fusiform aneurysm of the basilar artery. *J Neurosurg* 1997;87:944–949.
19. Lanzino G, Wakhloo AK, Fessler RD, Hartney ML, Guterman LR, Hopkins LN. Efficacy and current limitations of intravascular stents for intracranial internal carotid, vertebral, and basilar artery aneurysms. *J Neurosurg* 1999;91:538–546.
20. Wakhloo AK, Lanzino G, Lieber BB, Hopkins LN. Stents for intracranial aneurysms. *Neurosurgery* 1998;43:377–379.
21. Sekhon LH, Morgan MK, Sorby W, Grinnell V. Combined endovascular stent implantation and endosaccular coil placement for the treatment of a wide-necked vertebral artery aneurysm. *Neurosurgery* 1998;43:380–384.
22. Molyneux A, Kerr R, Stratton I, et al. International Subarachnoid Aneurysm Trial (ISAT) of neurosurgical clipping versus endovascular coiling in 2143 patients with ruptured intracranial aneurysms: a randomised trial. *Lancet* 2002;360:1267–74.
23. Pikus HJ, Beach ML, Harbaugh RE. Microsurgical treatment of arteriovenous malformations: analysis and comparison with stereotactic radiosurgery. *J Neurosurg* 1998;88:641–646.
24. Pollock BE, Lunsford LD, Kondziolka D, Maitz A, Flickinger JC. Patient outcomes after stereotactic radiosurgery for "operable" arteriovenous malformations. *Neurosurgery* 1994;35:1–8.
25. Sisti MB, Kader A, Stein BM. Microsurgery for 67 intracranial arteriovenous malformations less than 3 cm in diameter. *J Neurosurg* 1990;79:653–660.
26. Andrews BT, Wilson CB: Staged treatment of arteriovenous malformations of the brain. *Neurosurgery* 1987;21:314–323.
27. Bonnal J, Born JD, Hans P. One-stage excision of high-flow arteriovenous malformation. *J Neurosurg* 1985;62:128–131.
28. Spetzler RF, Martin NA, Carter P, Flom R, Raudzens PA, Wilkinson E. Surgical management of large AVMs by staged embolization and operative excision. *J Neurosurg* 1987;67:17–28.
29. Guiot G, Rougerie J, Sachs M, Herzog E, Molina P. Repérage stéréotaxique des malformations vasculaires profondes intracérébrales. *Semin Hop* 1960;36:1134–1143.
30. Muacevic A, Hans-Jakob S. Computer-assisted resection of cerebral arteriovenous malformations. *Neurosurgery* 1999;45:1164–1175.
31. Brooks B. Discussion of paper by Noland L, Taylor AS. *Trans South Surg Assoc* 1931;43:176–177.
32. Luessenhop AJ, Spence WT. Artificial embolization of cerebral arteries. *JAMA* 1960;172:1153–1155.

33. Luessenhop AJ, Kachmann R, Shevlin W, Ferrero AA. Clinical evaluation of artificial embolization in the management of large cerebral arteriovenous malformations. *J Neurosurg* 195;23:400–417.
34. Boulos R, Kricheff II, Chase NE. Value of cerebral angiography in the embolization treatment of cerebral arteriovenous malformations. *Radiology* 1970;97:65–70.
35. Kerber C. Balloon catheter with a calibrated leak. *Radiology* 1976;120:547–550.
36. Ogilvy CS. Radiation therapy for arteriovenous malformations: a review. *Neurosurgery* 1990;26:725–735.
37. Yamamoto M, Jimbo M, Kobayashi M. Long term results of radiosurgery for arteriovenous malformation: neurodiagnostic imaging and histological studies of angiographically confirmed nidus obliteration. *Surg Neurol* 1992;37:219–230.
38. Lunsford LD, Kondziolka D, Flickinger JC, et al. Stereotactic radiosurgery for arteriovenous malformations of the brain. *J Neurosurg* 1991;75:512–524.
39. Karlsson B, Kihlstrom L, Lindquist C. Gamma knife radiosurgery for previously irradiated arteriovenous malformations. *Neurosurgery* 1998;42:1–6.
40. Niranjan A, Lunsford LD. Radiosurgery: Where we were, are, and may be in the third millenium. *Neurosurgery* 2000;46:531–543.
41. Link MJ, Pollock BE, Nichols DA, et al. Stereotactic radiosurgery for dural arteriovenous ristulae, in *Contemporary Stereotactic Radiosurgery: Technique and Evaluation* (Pollock BE, ed.), Futura Publishing Company, Armonk, NY, 2002, pp. 109–137.
42. Davies MA, Saleh J, terBrugge K, Willinsky R, Wallace MC. The natural history and management of intracranial dural arteriovenous fistula. Part 1: Benign lesions. *Intervent Neuroradiol* 1997;3:295–302.
43. Davies MA, terBrugge K, Willinsky R, Wallace MC. The natural history and management of intracranial dural arteriovenous fistulae. Part 2: Aggressive lesions. *Intervent Neuroradiol* 1997;3:303–311.
44. Rigamonti D, Pappas CTE, Spetzler RF, et al. Extracerebral cavernous angiomas of the middle fossa. *Neurosurgery* 1990;27:306–310.
45. Barrow DL, Spector R, Braun I, et al. Classification and treatment of spontaneous carotid-cavernous sinus fistulas. *J Neurosurg* 1985;62:248–256.
46. Berenstein A, Manelfe C. Transjugular approach to carotid cavernous fistulas. *Mt Sinai J Med* 1981;48:255–258.
47. Uflacker R, Lima S, Ribas G, et al. Carotid-cavernous fistulas: embolization through the superior ophthalmic vein approach. *Radiology* 1986;159:175–179.
48. Parkinson D. A surgical approach to the cavernous portion of the carotid artery. *J Neurosurg* 1965;23:474–483.
49. Workman MJ, Dion JE, Tong FC, Cloft HG. Treatment of trapped CCF by direct puncture of the cavernous sinus by intraocular trans—SOF approach. Case report and anatomical basis. *Intervent Neuroradiol* 2002;8:299–304.
50. Jensen ME, Dion JE. Carotid Cavernous Sinus Fistulae, in *The Practice of Neurosurgery*, vol. 2. (Tindall GT, Cooper PR, Barrow DL, eds.), Williams & Wilkins Baltimore, 1996, pp. 2243–2260.
51. Bargar WL, Bauer A, Borner M. Primary and revision total hip replacement using the Robodoc system. *Clin Orthop* 1998;354:8291.
52. Autschbach R, Onnasch JF, Falk V, et al. The Leipzig experience with robotic valve surgery. *J Card Surg* 2000;15:82–87.
53. Hongo K, Kobayashi S, Kakizawa Y, et al. NeuRobot: telecontrolled micromanipulator system for minimally invasive microneurosurgery—preliminary results. *Neurosurgery* 2002;51:985–988.

17
Minimally Invasive Treatment for Brain Tumors

Dennis S. Oh, MD and Peter M. Black, MD, PhD

INTRODUCTION

Minimally invasive techniques have significantly changed our ability to do expert and safe surgery for brain tumors. These techniques include neuroendoscopy, image-guided surgery in the traditional operating room, intraoperative imaging, radiosurgery, laser hypothermia, and focused ultrasound. With these, the contemporary neurosurgical oncologist has a powerful armamentarium to help in the management of brain and spinal cord tumors.

MINIMALLY INVASIVE NEUROSURGERY AS MINIMALLY DISRUPTIVE NEUROSURGERY

Minimally invasive neurosurgery is typically thought to be surgery through small openings. However, there is another interpretation. This interpretation suggests that minimally invasive neurosurgery is surgery minimally disruptive to the patient. Although it may not have a small opening in the scalp or the bone, it has as a goal the least possible effect on brain tissue around the abnormality being dealt with.

This concept of minimally disruptive neurosurgery is extremely important as a general principle for neurosurgical oncology in the last decade. Such techniques as brain mapping, functional magnetic resonance (MR), magnetoencephalography, and other systems that establish safe trajectories are valuable in achieving this goal.

Carrying out surgical procedures under intravenous sedation anesthesia has allowed the surgeon to operate in areas of vision, primary motor, or sensory cortex and in speech areas with significantly greater resection and lessening of morbidity *(1,2)*. These techniques for low-grade gliomas, for example, allow resection of a tumor that may often act as an extraaxial mass, displacing tissue rather than destroying it. For larger malignant tumors, similar resection can be done with accuracy and safety *(3,4)*.

Carrying out surgery under intravenous sedation allows direct mapping of the brain. However, a number of preoperative technologies that have also been used for achieving this kind of minimal invasiveness with minimal disruption. These include magnetoencephalography, functional MR, and diffusion tensor

From: *Minimally Invasive Neurosurgery*, edited by: M.R. Proctor and P.M. Black © Humana Press Inc., Totowa, NJ

imaging. Magnetoencephalography (5–9) uses the magnetic field of the brain to evaluate the region where a particular function is represented and is particularly useful for motor cortex analysis. It requires very sophisticated equipment and staff.

Functional MR appears to assess the change in blood flow on the surface of the cortex that accompanies a particular activity such as arm or hand movement or speech (10–12). Again, it requires sophisticated paradigms both for testing and analysis of data, (13–15), but is an extremely useful technology. Diffusion tensor imaging allows analysis of the fiber tracts leading from the cortex to the brainstem (16–18) It can be extremely helpful in defining motor and sensory tracts noninvasively (19,20).

Taken together, these techniques, which emphasize minimal disruption and therefore minimal invasiveness in the patient's life, have made neurosurgical oncology a newly revitalized specialty. For glioblastoma multiforme, they allow resection of discrete tumor, which markedly improves the morbidity after surgery and seems to increase survival (21–23). For low-grade gliomas, they have similarly revolutionized our ability to resect tumors. For metastatic tumors, it is now possible to combine them with localization techniques to be able to remove tumors even from eloquent areas (24).

NEUROENDOSCOPY IN TUMOR SURGERY

Endoscopy has not had the same revolutionary impact in brain tumor surgery as it has in general and gastrointestinal surgery or in thoracic oncology. This may be because the brain does not have abundant open channels that can be readily used as navigational pathways. The use of endoscopy has been limited primarily to the ventricular system, to pituitary surgery, and to some extent to verification of resection in some sites such as the internal auditory meatus.

Intraventricular Tumors

As has been discussed elsewhere, neuroendoscopy has been suggested for a variety of uses including both biopsy and resection of tumors and cysts of the brain and ventricular system (25–28). Clearly, its most important application is for intraventricular tumors (29). Pineal region tumors can be biopsied and partially resected (30,31), and colloid cysts of the third ventricle may also be removed.

These tumors account for fewer than 5% of adult neurosurgical oncology cases, although they may be slightly more common in pediatric practice. The morbidity of endoscopy is primarily bleeding and is approx 2–3%. Its ability to biopsy tumors is great, but the capacity to remove tumors with endoscopic techniques is extremely limited. Tumors that are cystic may be removed.

Pituitary Tumors

Perhaps the most successful recent application of endoscopy has been in resecting pituitary adenomas (32–34). The endoscope in this case allows the use of a small opening at the back of the nostril and thereby avoids having to elevate a large flap. In experienced hands, it will permit very satisfactory resection of an adenoma. Usually both nostrils are used, one for visualization and the other for manipulation. In this application the major problem is bleeding, which can be significant and can obscure the surgical field, making it difficult to identify the structure being manipulated. For large, bloody adenomas, this could be a major problem. The reason for considering endoscopic surgery is that the morbidity of nose manipulation (35,36), including the need for nasal packs for more than a day, is lessened and patients may go home within a day or two of their procedure. Despite these advantages, this technique has not become the norm for most pituitary surgeons. The endoscope can, however, be very helpful in confirming that there is removal of tumor laterally and also superiorly when there may be some question of suprasellar residual tumor (37).

Other Endoscopic Applications

Some surgeons have suggested that the internal auditory meatus can be inspected with a small endoscope, for residual tumor in vestibular schwannoma surgery (38–40), or in skull base surgery potential components can be inspected, including what may be behind residual tumor.

Summary

Although neuroendoscopy has been suggested as being useful for a number of applications in tumor surgery, its use remains the preview of a few surgeons and has not been generalized for all neurosurgical applications.

SMALL INCISIONS FOR TRADITIONAL PROCEDURES

In the late 1990s, some microneurosurgeons made a strong case for small openings to manage traditional neurosurgical procedures such as aneurysm clipping. This was equated with silver dollar openings in such procedures as vascular repositioning and anterior circulation aneurysm surgery. Often these claims were associated with claims of virtuoso capability in neurosurgery, and it became difficult to separate the advantages of minimal invasive management from self-promotion. However, it is clear that microsurgical approaches lessened morbidity enough at sites such as the cerebellar pontine angle or the circle of Willis for us neurosurgeons to think of more parsimonious openings and approaches. This in turn led to the general concept of small, discrete operative approaches rather than the more traditional exploratory flap.

The influence of this on neurosurgical practice is very important. With small openings, healing is quicker, incisions are more attractive, and, in general, the impact on the body is sufficiently less that such incisions dramatically change a patient's response to the surgery. This is particularly true in the posterior fossa.

IMAGE-GUIDED SURGERY IN THE TRADITIONAL OPERATING ROOM

The most influential technology for minimally invasive brain tumor surgery has been image-guided surgery using navigational devices in the traditional operating room. These have allowed accurate localization of tumors and resection from areas previously thought impossible. They have further allowed smaller incisions, especially over the cortex, with such precision that they produce the concept of earlier management of some benign tumors as well as definitive surgical management of malignant tumors, such as metastatic lesions.

The concept behind these devices is fairly straightforward. They use reconstruction of a MR scan to create the image of a mass and then the registration through fiducials or surface registration to superimpose that image on the patient's actual physiognomy. When this is done, the surgeon can use the image created preoperatively to guide him or her.

Many systems available with a number of different advantages. They include the Stealth System (Medtronic), the InstaTrak System (General Electric), the ISG Viewing Wand (ISG Technologies), and others. They all have common features: (1) preoperative acquisition of MR or computed tomography scans by specific protocols, (2) reconstruction capacities with differing sophistication of segmentation of tumor in other areas, (3) a registration system that might include scalp fuducials or surface-to-surface registration, and (4) a navigational system, which links the computer with the actual image. There may be substantial variations in any of these. The Instatrak system from General Electric, for example, uses an electromagnetic system rather than a visual system. This allows the surgeon to avoid blockage of navigation by blind sight obstruction. These techniques have truly changed tumor surgery. For glioma surgery, they allow identification of the sites and margins of low-grade gliomas. Dr. Patrick Kelly *(41,42)* in the early days and, more recently, Drs. Mitchell Berger, Peter Black, and others have reported on this capacity. For malignant gliomas, including glioblastoma, they have also demonstrated the capacity to localize the margins; taken in conjunction with the intravenous sedation and other systems discussed previously, they have also increased our ability to do aggressive surgery. This has lessened morbidity and increased survival for patients *(21–23,43,44)*. The most striking applications, however, may be in metastatic tumors. The new techniques allow identification of small tumors or tumors that are in eloquent areas with great precision *(45,46)*. The issue of brain shift, discussed later, is not as much of a problem.

These techniques have made a difference not only for metastatic tumors but also for convexity meningiomas. They allow accurate localization of a mass. This means that tumors that once required large craniotomy flaps can now be resected with a small linear incision and essentially cured in patients who have many years before them. This can be an extremely helpful solution for the problem of continued monitoring and uncertainty about seizures and other manifestations of tumor.

INTRAOPERATIVE IMAGING

Further development in the capacity to do image-guided surgery is the recent creation of intraoperative imaging for immediate confirmation of surgical manipulation. Over the last decade a number of solutions to the problem of immediate verification of surgical effect have been offered *(47)*.

One of the earliest was the GE Signa System, which has an open MR design allowing navigation in real time within the magnet and immediate update of resection *(48)*. This technology allows surgery to be done in the magnet. The patient is managed in precisely the same way he or she would be in a traditional operating room. All the instruments and anesthesia equipment are nonmagnetic. The result is an operating system in which the surgeon has MRI vision with the capacity to confirm his or her surgical effect immediately.

Using this device, which is situated at the Brigham and Women's Hospital in Boston, our group has done over 700 craniotomies for brain tumor. These have primarily been resections for low-grade or recurrent tumors, although anaplastic gliomas and glioblastomas have also been removed in this device. Our complication rate has been the same as in the traditional operating room. In terms of infection and other surgical problems, the instance of immediate neurologic deficit is lower than in the traditional operating room because of the ability to see residual tumor. With transsphenoidal procedures, the leakage of spinal fluid is slightly more prevalent because more aggressive surgery is suggested.

A similar solution to the problem of intraoperative verification of removal is the concept of moving the patient into and out of the MR scanner. This has been particularly useful in the Siemens Magnetom System, in which the operating table is moved in and out of the scanning device. Fahlbusch et al. have used this concept, first for the 0.2-T scanner and then for the 1.5-T scanner, with very good intraoperative pictures *(49,50)*. (*See* Chapter 6.)

A third solution has been to bring the scanner to the patient. An elaborate example of this is the IMRIS System, in which the 1.5-T intraoperative MR scanner is brought from a shielded cage into the region of the patient to obtain high-quality images and verify removal of tissue *(51)*. One advantage of this system is that the room can be used for traditional surgery when it is not being used for intraoperative imaging. Such devices have been described in detail, and the applications they bring to tumor surgery are significant, with markedly improved resections. They have also demonstrated their usefulness for low-grade gliomas, pituitary adenomas, and malignant gliomas.

A variant that is increasing in popularity is the Odin PoleStar System, which gives a limited view of the brain, and has modest navigational capacities but can be used within the traditional operating room *(52,53)*. This is a very low-field (0.1-T) magnet, but it may be useful for some applications.

These developments in image-guided surgery have made it possible to consider very different approaches to be certain that the desired result is achieved in planning surgery. They are extremely important as new advances in minimally invasive neurosurgery.

These techniques may also be combined with other minimally invasive techniques so that endoscopy, for example, can be combined with image-guided frameless systems or the intraoperative MR to think about new ways of guiding endoscopes *(54–56)*.

LOCAL APPLICATIONS AND CHEMOTHERAPY

One of the most interesting and potentially important minimally invasive therapies for brain tumors is the future potential for local applications of gene therapy and chemotherapy (also discussed in Chapters 13 and 14). Infusion technology with catheters in tumor or ventricles for convection-enhanced delivery is one example; another is the application of cells or slow-release polymers to the tumor bed (57–59). It may be possible for the patient then to benefit from minimally invasive techniques for direct and local chemotherapy (60,61) and gene therapy (62,63).

FUTURE MINIMALLY INVASIVE SYSTEMS

Following the concept of minimal invasion, several technologies are now being developed that may further change our capacity to deal with specific tumors. One of these is laser hypothermia, in which a laser fiber is introduced to the center of a lesion (64). The changes that occur with heating can be followed nicely, and the patient can have complete destruction of the lesion. Examples of this use include a hypothalamic hamartoma or low-grade glioma of the hypothalamus.

A second future potential therapy is focused ultrasound (65–67). With the capacity to calculate differential absorption of energy through the skull, it is possible to develop the technology of multiple source high-energy ultrasound that can destroy a target noninvasively. This is still in the development phase but may be an important addition as well. (*See* Chapter 12.)

SUMMARY AND CONCLUSION

Neurosurgical oncology has been transformed by the capacity to do minimally invasive neurosurgery. If minimal disruptiois included, the world of brain tumor surgery is markedly different today than it was even a decade ago. Image-guided neurosurgery whether in the traditional operating room or with intraoperative imaging has made a substantial difference. The ability to do brain mapping and use intravenous sedation anesthesia techniques has further limited the potential problems of this surgery.

REFERENCES

1. Jaaskelainen J, Randell T. Awake craniotomy in glioma surgery. *Acta Neurochir-Supp* 2003;88:31–35.
2. Danks R, Aglio L, Black P. Craniotomy under local anesthesia and monitored conscious sedation for the resection of tumors involving eloquent cortex. *J Neuroncol* 2000;49:131–139.
3. Signorelli F, Guyotat J, Isnard J, Schneider F, Mohammedi R, Bret P. The value of cortical stimulation applied to the surgery of malignant gliomas in language areas. *Neurol Sci* 2001;22:3–10.
4. Meyer F, Bates L, Goerss S, Friedman J, Windschitl W, Duffy J, et al. Awake craniotomy for aggressive resection of primary gliomas located in eloquent brain. *Mayo Clin Proc* 2001;76:677–687.

5. Papanicolaou A, Simos P, Breier J, et al. Magnetoencephalographic mapping of the language-specific cortex. *J Neurosurg* 1999;90:85–93.
6. Schiffbauer H, Berger M, Ferrari P, Freudenstein D, Rowley H, Roberts T. Preoperative magnetic source imaging for brain tumor surgery: a quantitative comparison with intraoperative sensory and motor mapping. *J Neurosurg* 2002;97:1333–1342.
7. Castillo E, Simos P, Wheless J, et al. Integrating sensory and motor mapping in a comprehensive MEG protocol: clinical validity and replicability. *Neuroimage* 2004;21:973–983.
8. Taniguchi M, Kato A, Ninomiya H, Hirata M, Cheyne D, Robinson S, et al. Cerebral motor control in patients with gliomas around the central sulcus studied with spatially filtered magnetoencephalography. *J Neurol Neurosurg Psychiatry* 2004;75:466–471.
9. Kamada K, Houkin K, Takeuchi F, et al. Visualization of the eloquent motor system by integration of MEG, functional, and anisotropic diffusion-weighted MRI in functional neuronavigation. *Surg Neurol* 2003;59:352–361.
10. Wilkinson I, Romanowski C, Jellinek D, Morris J, Griffiths P. Motor functional MRI for preoperative and intraoperative neurosurgical guidance. *Br J Radiol* 2003;76:98–103.
11. Roux F, Boulanouar K, Lotterie J, Mejdoubi M, LeSage J, Berry I. Language functional magnetic resonance imaging in preoperative assessment of language areas: correlation with direct cortical stimulation. *Neurosurgery* 2003;52:1335–1345.
12. Baciu M, Le Bas J, Segebarth C, Benabid A. Presurgical fMRI evaluation of cerebral reorganization and motor deficit in patients with tumors and vascular malformations. *Eur J Radiol* 2003;46:139–146.
13. Moritz C, Haughton V. Functional MR imaging: paradigms for clinical preoperative mapping. *Magn Reson Imaging Clin N Am* 2003;11:529–542.
14. Kamba M, Sung Y, Ogawa S. A dynamic system model-based technique for functional MRI data analysis. *Neuroimage* 2004;22:179–187.
15. Yoo S, Talos I, Golby A, Black P, Panych L. Evaluating requirements for spatial resolution of fMRI for neurosurgical planning. *Hum Brain Mapp* 2004;21:34–43.
16. Clark C, Barrick T, Murphy M, Bell B. White matter fiber tracking in patients with space-occupying lesions of the brain: a new technique for neurosurgical planning. *Neuroimage* 2003;20:1601–1608.
17. Barboriak D. Imaging of brain tumors with diffusion-weighted and diffusion tensor MR imaging. *Magn Reson Imaging Clin N Am* 2003;11:379–401.
18. Yamada K, Kizu O, Mori S, et al. Brain fiber tracking with clinically feasible diffusion-tensor MR imaging: initial experience. *Radiology* 2003;227:295–301.
19. Wakana S, Jiang H, Nagae-Poetscher L, van Zijl P, Mori S. Fiber tract-based atlas of human white matter anatomy. *Radiology* 2004;230:77–87.
20. Price S, Burnet N, Donovan T, et al. Diffusion tensor imaging of brain tumors at 3T: a potential too for assessing white matter tract invasion? *Clin Radiol* 2003;58:455–462.
21. Keles G, Anderson B, Berger M. The effect of extent of resection on time to tumor progression and survival in patients with glioblastoma multiforme of the cerebral hemisphere. *Surg Neurol* 1999;52:371–379.
22. Hentschel S, Sawaya R. Optimizing outcomes with maximal surgical resection of malignant gliomas. *Cancer Control* 2003;10:109–114.
23. Laws E, Parney I, Huang W, et alg. Survival following surgery and prognostic factors for recently diagnosed malignant glioma: data from the Glioma Outcomes Project. *J Neurosurg* 2003;99:467–473.

24. Weinberg J, Lang F, Sawaya R. Surgical management of brain metastases. *Curr Oncol Rep* 2001;3:476–483.
25. Fries G, Perneczky A. Intracranial endoscopy. *Adv Tech Stand Neurosurg* 1999;25: 21–60.
26. Macarthur D, Buxton N, Punt J, Vloeberghs M, Robertson I. The role of neuroendoscopy in the management of brain tumours. *Br J Neurosurg* 2002;16:465–470.
27. Buxton N, Vloeberghs M, Punt J. Flexible neuroendoscopic treatment of suprasellar arachnoid cysts. *Br J Neurosurg* 1999;13:316–318.
28. Kirollos R, Javadpour M, May P, Mallucci C. Endoscopic treatment of suprasellar and third ventricle-related arachnoid cysts. *Childs Nerv Sys* 2001;17:713–718.
29. Yurtseven T, Ersahin Y, Demirtas E, Mutluer S. Neuroendoscopic biopsy for intraventricular tumors. *Minim Invas Neurosurg* 2003;46:293–299.
30. Ferrer E, Santamarta D, Garcia-Fructuoso G, Caral L, Rumia J. Neuroendoscopic management of pineal region tumours. *Acta Neurochirur* 1997;139:12–20.
31. Robinson S, Cohen A. The role of neuroendoscopy in the treatment of pineal region tumors. *Surg Neurol* 1997;48:360–365.
32. Jho H, Carrau R, Ko Y. Endoscopic pituitary surgery, in *Neurosurgical Operative Atlas*, vol. 5 (Rengachary S, Wilkins R, eds.), American Association of Neurological Surgeons, Park Ridge, IL, 1996, pp. 1–12.
33. Jho H, Carrau R. Endoscopic endonasal transphenoidal surgery: experience with 50 patients. *J Neurosurg* 1997;87:44–51.
34. Cusimano M, Fenton R. A technique for endoscopic pituitary tumor removal. *Neurosurg Focus* 1996;1.
35. Yaniv E, Rappaport Z. Endoscopic transseptal transsphenoidal surgery for pituitary tumors. *Neurosurgery* 1997;40:944–946.
36. Koren I, Hadar T, Rappaport Z, Yaniv E. Endoscopic transnasal transsphenoidal microsurgery versus the sublabial approach for the treatment of pituitary tumors: endonasal complications. *Laryngoscope* 1999;109:1838–1840.
37. Jarrahy R, Berci G, Shahinian H. Assessment of the efficacy of endoscopy in pituitary adenoma resection. *Arch Otolaryngol Head Neck Surg* 2000;126:1487–1490.
38. Tatagiba M, Matthies C, Samii M. Microendoscopy of the internal auditory canal in vestibular schwannoma surgery. *Neurosurgery* 1996;38:737–740.
39. McKennan K. Endoscopy of the internal auditory canal during hearing conservation acoustic tumor surgery. *Am J Otol* 1993;14:259–262.
40. Low W. Enhancing hearing preservation in endoscopic-assisted excision of acoustic neuroma via the retrosigmoid approach. *J Laryngol Otol* 1999;113:973–977.
41. Kelly P. Computer-assisted stereotaxis: new approaches for management of intracranial intraaxial tumors. *Neurology* 1986;36:535–541.
42. Kelly P. Volumetric stereotactic surgical resection of intra-axial brain mass lesions. *Mayo Clin Proc* 1988;63:1186–1198.
43. Johannesen T, Langmark F, Lote K. Progress in long-term survival in adult patients with supratentorial low-grade gliomas: a population-based study of 993 patients in whom tumors were diagnosed between 1970 and 1993. *J Neurosurg* 2003;99:854–862.
44. Berger M, Rostomily R. Low grade gliomas: functional mapping resection strategies, extent of resection, and outcome. *J Neurooncol* 1997;34:85–101.
45. Tan T, Black P. Image-guided craniotomy for cerebral metastases: techniques and outcomes. *Neurosurgery* 2003;53:82–89.
46. Kelly P, Kall B, Goerss S. Results of computed tomography-based computer-assisted stereotactic resection of metastatic intracranial tumors. *Neurosurgery* 1988; 22:7–17.

47. Lipson A, Gargollo P, Black P. Intraoperative magnetic resonance imaging: considerations for the operating room of the future. *J Clin Neurosci* 2001;8:305–310.
48. Black P, Alexander E 3rd, Martin C, et al. Craniotomy for tumor treatment in an intraoperative magnetic resonance imaging unit. *Neurosurgery* 1999;45:423–431.
49. Nimsky C, Ganslandt O, von Keller B, Fahlbusch R. Preliminary experience in glioma surgery with intraoperative high-field MRI. *Acta Neurochir Suppl* 2003;88:21–29.
50. Fahlbusch R, Ganslandt O, Nimsky C. Intraoperative imaging with open magnetic resonance imaging and neuronavigation. *Childs Nerv Syst* 2000;16:829–831.
51. Sutherland G, Kaibara T, Louw D, Hoult D, Tomanek B, Saunders J. A mobile high-field magnetic resonance system for neurosurgery. *J Neurosurg* 1999;91:804–813.
52. Kanner A, Vogelbaum M, Mayberg M, Weisenberger J, Barnett G. Intracranial navigation by using low-field intraoperative magnetic resonance imaging: preliminary experience. *J Neurosurg* 2002;97:1115–1124.
53. Hadani M, Katznelson E, Zuk Y, Sinai R. A novel real-time intraoperative MR imaging system for conventional neurosurgical operating rooms. Presented at the *American Association of Neurological Surgeons Annual Meeting*, San Francisco, CA, 2000.
54. Schroeder H, Wagner W, Tschiltschke W, Gaab M. Frameless neuronavigation in intracranial endoscopic neurosurgery. *J Neurosurg* 2001;94:72–79.
55. Gumprecht H, Trost H, Lumenta C. Neuroendoscopy combined with frameless neuronavigation. *Br J Neurosurg* 2000;14:129–131.
56. Burtscher J, Dessl A, Maurer H, Seiwald M, Felber S. Virtual neuroendoscopy, a comparative magnetic resonance and anatomical study. *Minim Invas Neurosurg* 1999;42:113–117.
57. Haroun R, Brem H. Local drug delivery. *Curr Opin Oncol* 2000;12:187–93.
58. Broaddus W, Gillies G, Kucharczyk J. Minimally invasive procedures: advances in image-guided delivery of drug and cell therapies into the central nervous system. *Neuroimaging Clin N Am* 2001;11:727–735.
59. Read T, Thorsen F, Bjerkvig R. Localised delivery of therapeutic agents to CNS malignancies: old and new approaches. *Curr Pharm Biotechnol* 2002;3:257–273.
60. Sampson J, Akabani G, Archer G, et al. Progress report of a phase 1 study of the intracerebral microinfusion of a recombinant chimeric protein composed of transforming growth factor (TGF)-alpha and a mutated form of the Pseudomonas exotoxin termed PE-38 (TP-38) for the treatment of malignant brain tumors. *J Neurooncol* 2003;65:27–35.
61. Kunwar S. Convection enhanced delivery of IL13-PE38QQR for treatment of recurrent malignant glioma: presentation of interim findings from ongoing phase 1 studies. *Acta Neurochir Suppl* 2003;88:105–111.
62. Ren H, Boulikas T, Lundstrom K, Soling A, Warnke P, Rainov N. Immunogene therapy of recurrent glioblastoma multiforme with a liposomally encapsulated replication-incompetent Semliki forest virus vector carrying the human interleukin-12 gene—a phase I/II clinical protocol. *J Neurooncol* 2003;64:147–154. Erratum in: *J Neurooncol* 2003;65:191.
63. Rainov N, Kramm C. Vector delivery methods and targeting strategies for gene therapy of brain tumors. *Curr Gene Ther* 2001;1:367–383.
64. Kettenbach J, Silverman S, Hata N, et al. Monitoring and visualization techniques for MR-guided laser ablations in an open MR system. *J Magn Reson Imaging* 1998;8:933–943.

65. Jaaskelainen J. Non-invasive transcranial high intensity focused ultrasound (HIFUS) under MRI thermometry and guidance in the treatment of brain lesions. *Acta Neurochir Suppl* 2003;88:57–60.
66. Vykhodtseva N, Sorrentino V, Jolesz F, Bronson R, Hynynen K. MRI detection of thermal effects of focused ultrasound on the brain. *Ultrasound Med Biol* 2000;26: 871–880.
67. Hynynen K, Vykhodtseva N, Chung A, Sorrentino V, Colucci V, Jolesz F. Thermal effects of focused ultrasound on the brain: determination with MR imaging. *Radiology* 1997;204:247–253.

18
New Directions in Spinal Surgery

Ian F. Dunn, MD and Marc E. Eichler, MD

INTRODUCTION

Evolving technological sophistication has resulted in ongoing modifications of traditional surgical approaches to correct disorders of the spinal axis. Advances in instrumentation and pre- and intraoperative imaging have fueled a move toward minimally invasive, minimal access spine surgery *(1)*, by which the same surgical goals of conventional open techniques are met through a smaller access corridor. An early and now well-accepted example is the surgical approach to a herniated paracentral lumbar disc, originally performed via complete laminectomy and now performed by microsurgical discectomy thorough a 15–25-mm incision and hemilaminectomy.

This chapter reviews current concepts in minimal access spinal surgery. We first focus on modifications of traditional posterior and anterior approaches and then evaluate the increasing role of completely novel approaches, such as kyphoplasty for the treatment of vertebral compression fractures or the use of intraoperative magnetic resonance imaging (MRI) to define surgical anatomy better. Lastly, we discuss advances in biologic instrumentation such as bone morphogenetic proteins and bioabsorbable polymers.

POSTERIOR APPROACHES AND THEIR MODIFICATIONS
Discectomy

The complete laminectomy and transdural approach to herniated lumbar discs, first propounded by Mixter and Barr, was long ago replaced by strategies to reduce blood loss, incision length, and intraoperative morbidity. Currently, a microsurgical discectomy through a 15–25-mm incision is the standard treatment for lumbar disc herniation, with success rates between 88 and 98% *(2–8)*. The widespread acceptance of microsurgical discectomy as a successful and low-risk alternative to the conventional approach of a wide laminectomy, fueled the search for even less invasive approaches. For example, chemonucleolysis, percutaneous nucleotomy, and laser discectomy, are all attempts to refine microdiscectomy further for the treatment of lumbar disc disease *(9–13)*.

Recent strategies to refine minimally invasive approaches have focused on endoscopically assisted discectomy. Initial reports involved the use of endoscopy

From: *Minimally Invasive Neurosurgery*, edited by: M.R. Proctor and P.M. Black © Humana Press Inc., Totowa, NJ

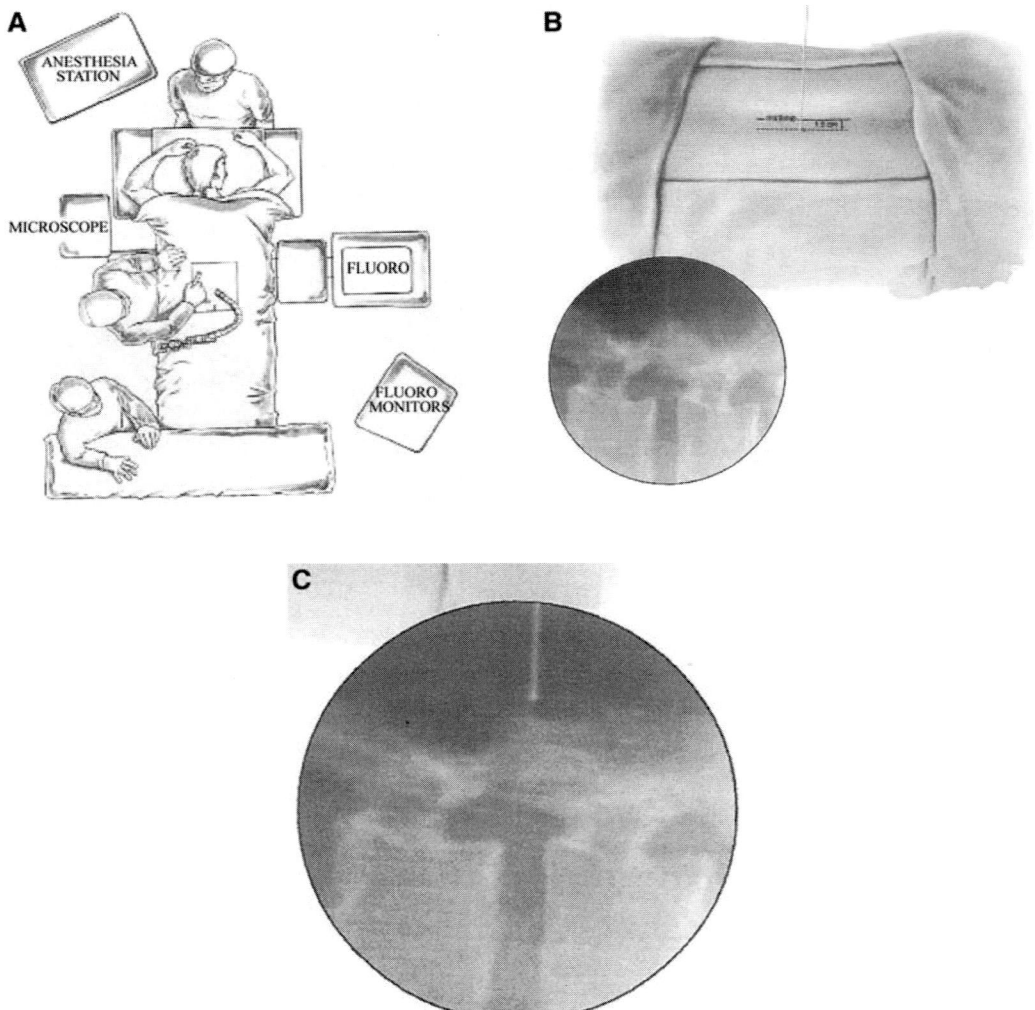

Fig. 1. (A) Typical operating room setup for a left-sided disc herniation. The location of the microscope should be determined prior to the case by the neurosurgeon. **(B)** A 20-gage spinal needle is inserted into the paraspinous musculature one fingerbreadth (1–1.5 cm) off the midline at the appropriate disc level. Location is confirmed using lateral C-arm fluoroscopy. The spinal needle is removed, and a vertical incision through the fascia is made at the puncture site. **(C)** A guidewire has been placed through the incision and directed toward the inferior aspect of the superior lamina. **(D)** A cannulated soft tissue dilator is inserted over the guide wire using a twisting motion. **(E)** Second and third dilators are sequentially placed over the initial dilator down to the lamina, and the endoscope is attached.

to facilitate percutaneous nucleotomy *(11)*. The approach is comprised of a biportal system with instruments in one port and the endoscope in the other. Mayer and Brock have described their percutaneous endoscopic lumbar discectomy (PELD) technique *(13)*. They employed straight, angled, and flexible rigid

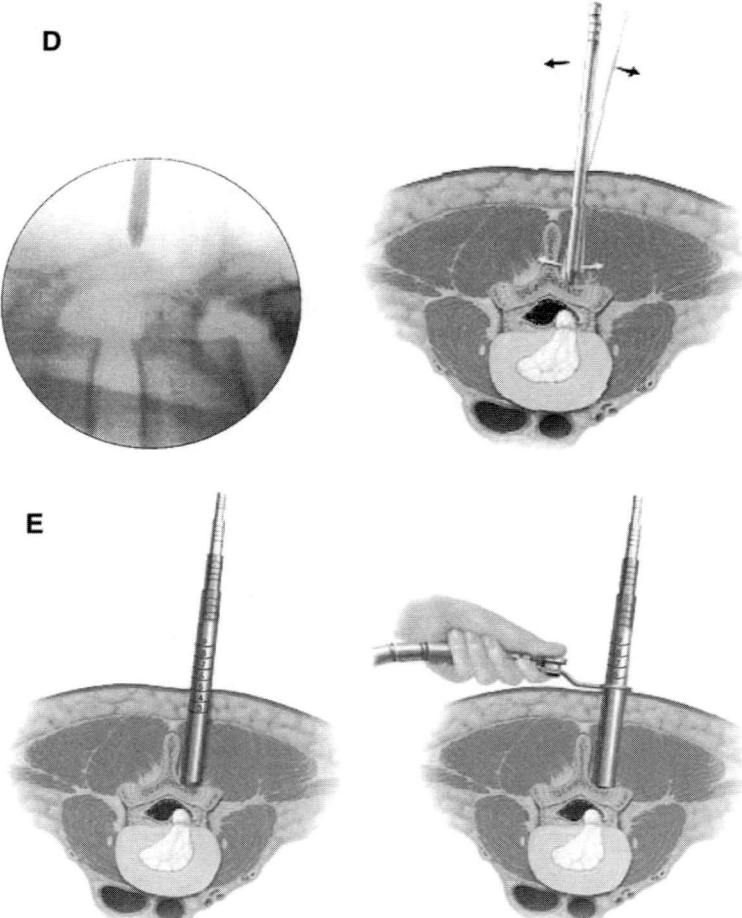

Fig. 1. *(continued)*

forceps, an automated high-power suction shaver/cutter system, and monitoring with a 70°-angled endoscope for contained or small noncontained disc fragments. They reported results comparable to those of open microdiscectomy *(14,15)*. It should be noted that this technique does not permit bony decompression and employs only intermittent endoscopy through one cannula. Other authors have since presented notably improved endoscopic approaches, including transforaminal or foraminoscopic techniques *(16,17)*. Such techniques expand endosurgical indications to include free fragments along with small noncontained and contained disc herniations by utilizing smaller and more flexible endoscopes. These smaller endoscopes are able to pass into the spinal canal to allow better visualization of disc and nerve roots.

The latest innovation of the endoscopic discectomy is a hybrid between PELD and the open microsurgical discetomy called microendoscopic discectomy (MED). First described by Smith and Foley in 1998 *(18)*, this procedure employs a K-wire followed by sequential, as well as continuous, endoscopy to provide a portal through which a hemilaminectomy and discectomy may be performed. The endoscopically guided surgery begins with level confirmation by fluoroscopy followed by a 15-mm vertical incision just off midline and placement of a K-wire onto the inferior aspect of the superior lamina under fluoroscopic guidance (Fig. 1). A series of dilators of progressively increasing diameter are placed over the K-wire and aid in sweeping the paraspinal musculature off the lamina. The working channel is then placed over the final dilator and the endoscope attached (Fig. 2). A standard microdiscectomy with hemilaminectomy and (rarely) medial facetectomy is then performed, followed by identification and protection of the nerve root. This sequential dilator system, the METRx-MED system (Medtronic Sofamor Danek), has also been designed so that an operating microscope may be used rather than an endoscope. Complications are similar to those associated with open microdiscectomy. The particular strengths of the METRx-MED system over other minimally invasive endoscopic techniques for herniated discs is that it allows the surgeon to address not only contained lumbar disc herniations but also free-fragment disc pathology and symptomatic lateral recess stenosis secondary to bony hypertrophy. Initial results have been promising, with more than 85% of patients reporting excellent results and a mean hospital stay of 9.5 h *(18)*; data from longer term follow-up have corroborated these initial encouraging results *(19)*. Cost–benefit analyses will assist in determining whether the added expense of the dilator system is outweighed by faster recovery and decreased hospital stay.

Fusion: Posterior Lumbar Interbody Fusion (PLIF) and Transforaminal Lumbar Interbody Fusion (TLIF)

PLIF

Much has changed since Mercer's contention in 1936 *(20)* that although "the ideal operation for fusing the spine would be an interbody fusion . . . the surgical difficulties encountered in performing such a feat would make the operation technically impossible" *(21)*. Cloward popularized the technique and described the earliest large case series a few years later, reporting an 85% rate of satisfactory outcomes among 331 patients. His published indications were "the treatment of low back pain with or without sciatica due to lumbar disc disease" *(21)*, with the goals of surgery including decompression of the entrapped neural elements, enlargement of the intervertebral foramina through disc space elevation, disc removal, and stabilization of the motion segment.

Cloward's original technique for interbody fusion has since been modified. Traditionally, graft choice was morcellized or structural autologous corticocancellous iliac crest bone. Present alternatives now include allograft cancellous blocks, calcium carbonate, and, more recently, hybrid spacers such as metallic or carbon fiber ramps and circular cages filled with osteoconductive and osteoinductive materials *(22–25)* (Fig. 3). Cage implants and spacers have understandably gained in popularity owing to the availability of a wide range

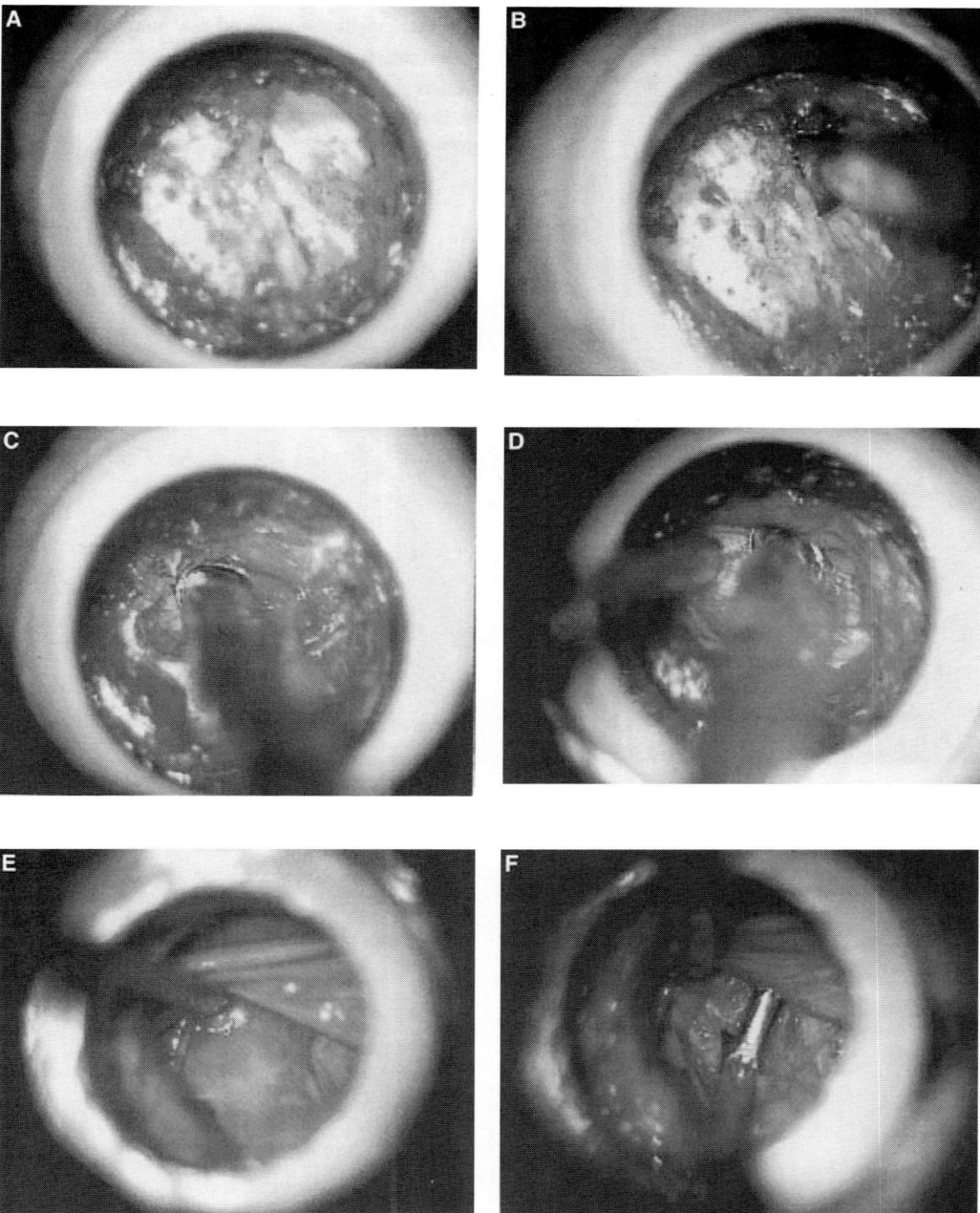

Fig. 2. (A) Electrocautery is used to help with soft tissue dissection and hemostasis. **(B)** The laminar edge is identified, and the ligamentum flavum is detached from the undersurface of the lamina with a small angled curet. **(C)** A hemilaminotomy is accomplished with a Kerrison punch or high-speed drill. **(D)** The ligamentum flavum is then penetrated with a curet and removed with a Kerrison punch. **(E)** The thecal sac and nerve root are identified and retracted medially using a Penfield dissector. **(F)** An annulotomy can then be performed if necessary and the herniated disc is then removed with a pituitary rongeur.

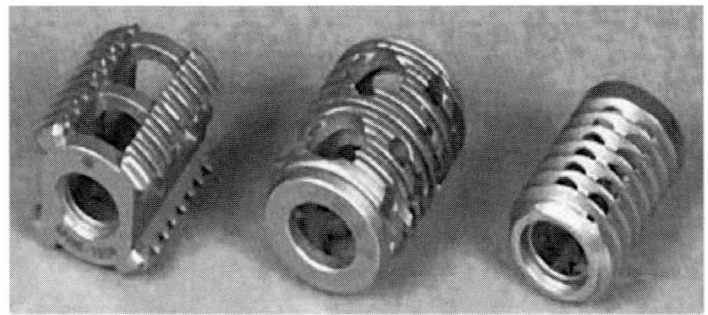

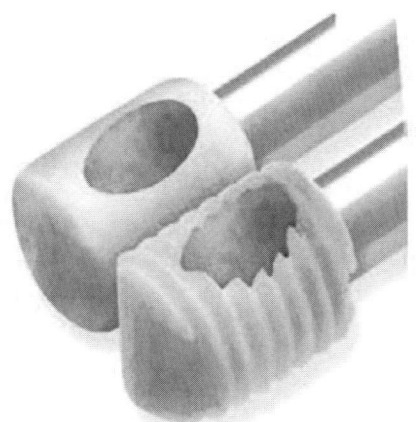 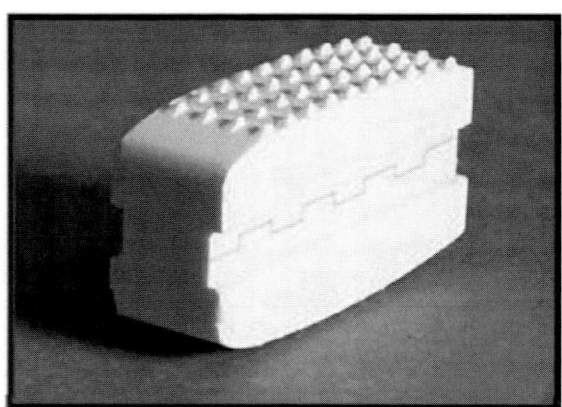

Fig. 3. Various titanium cages, allograft bone dowels, and allograft cancellous blocks are just some of the implements used as interbody spaces.

of shapes and sizes and to the equal or greater stiffness of metallic cage designs compared with allograft bone graft in biomechanical studies (26–30). Current choices for cage implants are cylindrical devices with openings that allow bone ingrowth, promoting fusion. Examples include the Ray TFC Threaded Fusion Cage (Surgical Dynamics, Norwalk, CT), the BAK cage (Spine Tech, Minneapolis, MN), the cylindrical threaded interbody fusion device (Sofamor-Danek, Memphis, TN), and the Brantigan I/F cage (Depuy AcroMed, Raynham, MA).

The introduction of adjunctive segmental instrumentation for improved spinal manipulation and stability (31,32) has been as significant as the evolution in graft choices. Adjunctive segmental instrumental involves the use of pedicle screws and plate distraction to elevate the disc space and allow for ease of interbody graft placement, restoring normal disc space height and enlarging the neural foramina. These technical developments have aided in expanding the indications for posterior interbody fusion to include spondylolisthesis, recurrent disc herniation, failed back surgery syndrome, bilateral or massive midline disc herniation, segmental instability, and degenerative disc disease with mechanical back pain.

Minimally Invasive PLIF

The technical obstacles first voiced by Mercer in performing posterior interbody fusion have been overcome, and authors have since reported excellent outcomes in 85% of patients with fusion rates of more than 90% *(33,34)* using instrumented PLIF. Significant emphasis is now being placed on ways to reduce iatrogenic injury to the dorsal musculoligamentous complex during open PLIF with a view toward more rapid patient recovery and shorter hospital stays. Khoo et al. *(35)* were the first to report their experience with the minimally invasive percutaneous PLIF (MIP-PLIF) in a cadaveric and patient series. Building on earlier work describing percutaneously placed pedicle screws, they used a combination of the METRx-MED endoscopic/microscopic tubular dilator system (Medtronic Sofamor-Danek), Tangent (Medtronic) interbody instruments, and Sextant percutaneous pedicle screw system *(36,37)*. Each of the three patients presented with mechanical back pain, L4 or L5 radiculopathies, and grade I L4–5 spondylolistheses.

Patients were positioned prone on the Wilson frame and Jackson table, and the appropriate laminofacet junction was targeted by fluoroscopy. A stab incision was made 1–1.5 inches off midline to permit fluoroscopically guided docking of the Steinman pin on the appropriate facet. The incision was then extended to a total length of 2 cm to permit introduction of the METRx sequential dilator and tubular retractor system to dilate the lumbar musculature in a manner similar to that described above for the microendoscopic discectomy. A standard PLIF decompressive hemilaminotomy and discecotomy was performed through the METRx portal under microscopic guidance, after which interbody distractors were placed to a final distraction between 10 and 12 mm, depending on the patient's initial lateral radiographs. The contralateral hemilaminotomy and discectomy were then performed in similar fashion and the distractor placed. Both endplates were prepared under endoscopic guidance with the round shaver and cutting chisel to remove any remaining cartilage, disc material, or soft tissue and to prepare graft troughs for the Tangent allograft.

For bone graft, the authors employed a combination of morcellized autograft from the hemilaminotomies and iliac crest, as well as two Tangent allografts of between 10 and 12 mm in height and 22 mm in length placed with a long inserter handle. Placement was confirmed by fluoroscopy. The METRx/MD tubular retractor device was then removed for percutaneous pedicle screw placement, which began with positioning a #11 Jamshidi needle on the appropriate lumbar pedicle under fluoroscopic guidance. The initial trajectory of the pedicle screws was then established by K-wire guidance followed by sequential dilation of the tract with METRx/MD dilators, and finally a preparatory tap passed over the K-wire. Sextant pedicle screws were then placed under fluoroscopic guidance, each attached to a screw extender (Fig. 4).

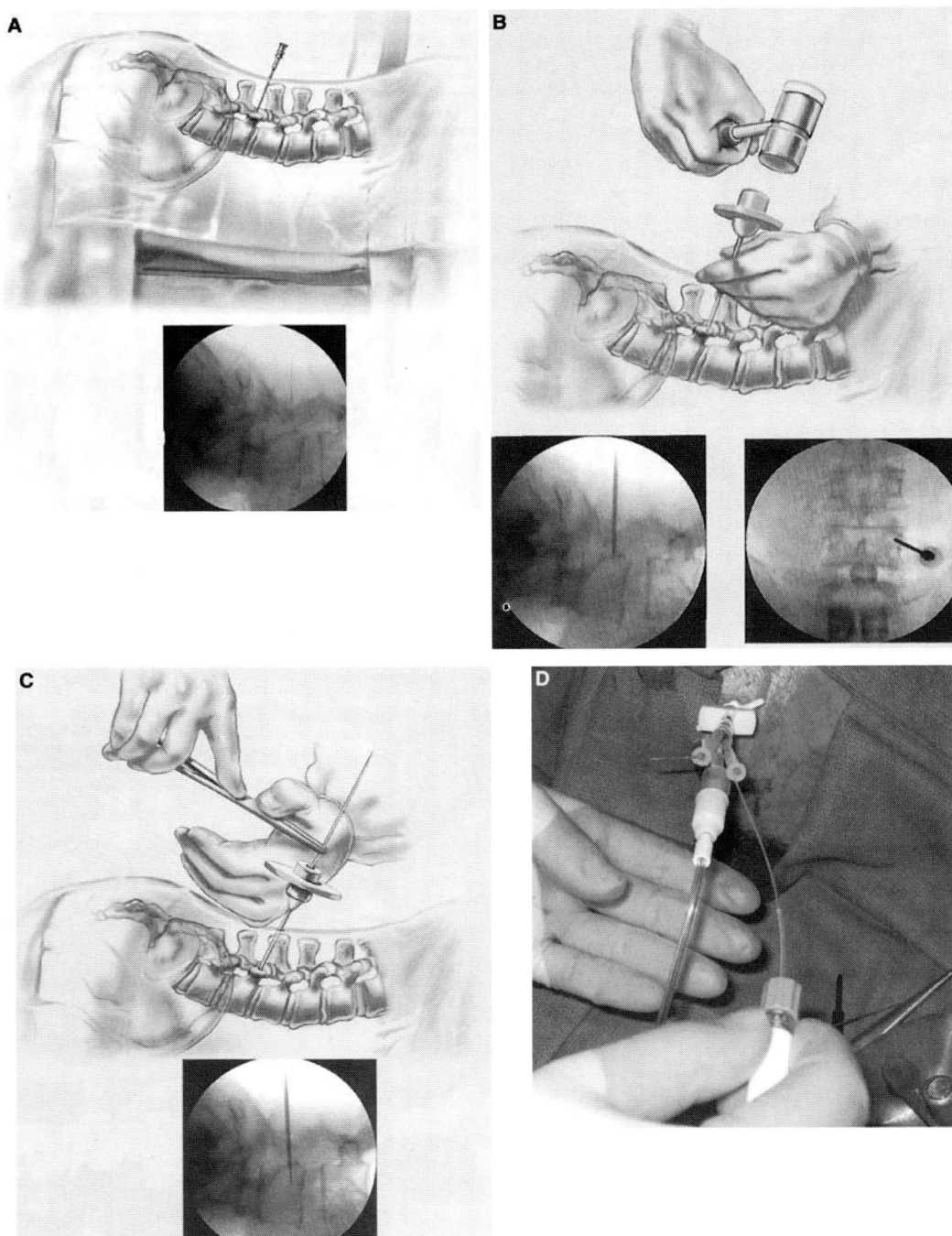

Fig. 4. (A) A 22-gage spinal needle is placed on the appropriate lumbar pedicle under fluoroscopic guidance at the intersection of the facet and transverse process. **(B)** An 11-gage bone biopsy needle is then used to gain access to the pedicle. Utilizing AP and lateral fluoroscopy, the needle is advanced partially through the pedicle. **(C)** The inner trocar of the needle is removed, and a guidewire is then inserted through the needle into the pedicle. The needle is then removed. **(D)** A cannulated awl is then placed over the guidewire and advanced through the pedicle.

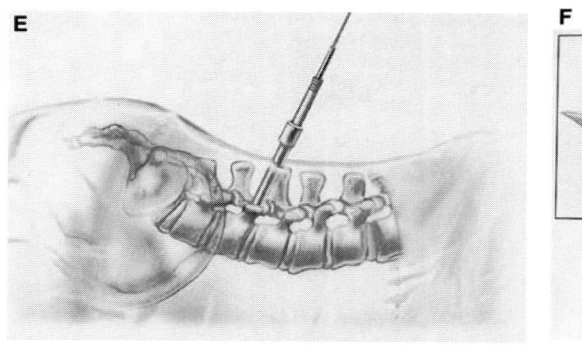
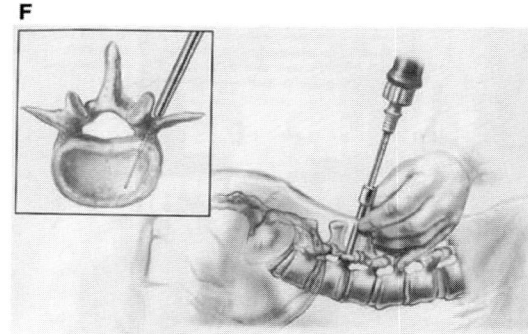
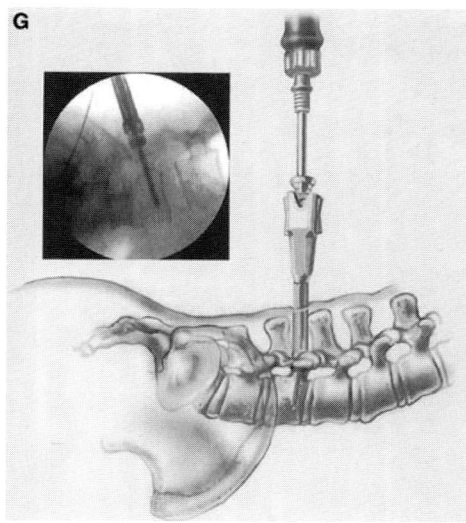

Fig. 4. (E) Dilators are then utilized to dilate the fascia and muscle to allow eventual screw placement. **(F)** The pedicle is prepared for screw placement by placing a tap over the guidewire and tapping the pedicle. **(G)** Pedicle screws are then placed using a screw extender assembly.

Rod attachment with the Sextant system depends on precise alignment of the screw heads by connecting the screw extenders outside the skin. The rod is precontoured in increments of either 5 mm for 1 level cases or 1 cm for 2 level cases. The rod inserter is an arc-shaped device that attaches to the screw extenders. This ensures the precise geometrical arrangement permitting the rod inserter attached to the rod to swing through a small stab incision through subcutaneous tissue and fascia along a path subtended by the screw heads. Rod positioning in the screw heads was confirmed fluoroscopically. Then a hex driver is passed through the extender sleeve, engaging the locking bolts to lock the screw to the rod while simultaneously releasing the screws from their extension sleeves by a torque-limiting break-off force. The rod inserter is then swung out of the stab wound (Fig. 5).

Fessler's group reported decreased length of stay (mean 2.8 d), decreased need for intravenous narcotic pain medication, and solid fusion by anteropos-

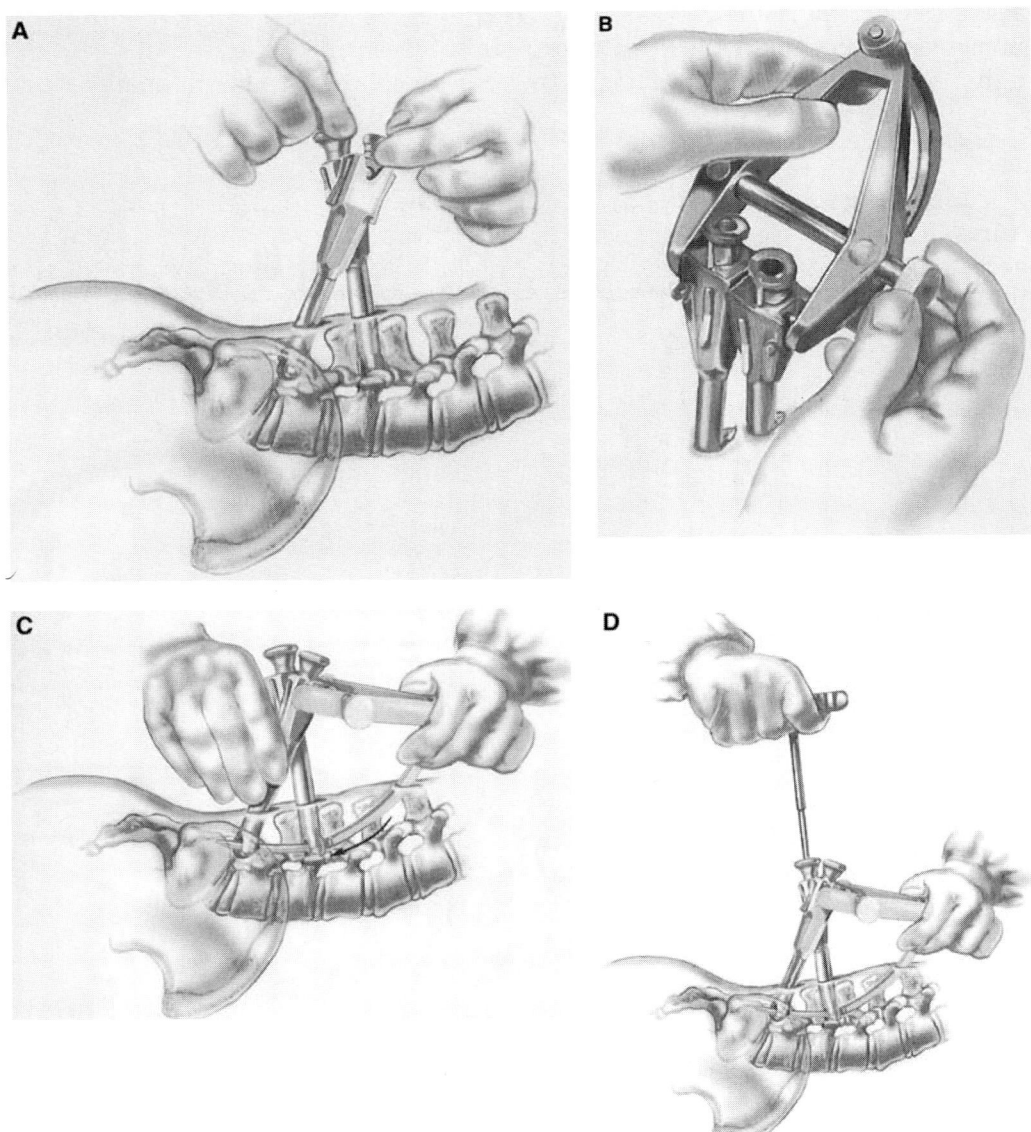

Fig. 5. (A) After placement of two pedicle screws into, the extenders are rotated so there is no gap between them. **(B)** A rod inserter is attached to the screw/extender assembly. **(C)** Appropriate rod length is then determined using templates, and a small skin incision is utilized to insert the rod through the screw heads. **(D)** After verifying with AP and lateral views that the rod is seated in the heads of both screws, the set screws are then tightened.

terior (AP)/lateral plain radiographs *(35)*. Initial results with the MIP-PLIF technique—although only with three patients—are promising enough to merit larger scale comparisons of this technique with the conventional instrumented PLIF. Combining this technique with the use of synthetic cage implants could also represent a viable modification. However, as with most new minimally invasive procedures, widespread adoption of this procedure is contingent not only on larger scale efficacy studies but also on solid cost–benefit analyses that take into account the expense of all required equipment.

TLIF

The transforaminal lumbar interbody fusion (TLIF) is a relatively new procedure. It is a modification of the PLIF procedure but offers the advantage of access to the spinal canal and disc unilaterally through the foramen, thereby minimizing retraction on the nerve roots and dural sac. This approach reduces the risk of neurologic injury and spares the posterior tension band. Additionally, the TLIF achieves a single-stage circumferential fusion through a posterior approach alone and as such may be considered a minimally invasive alternative to a combined anterior/posterior approach or instrumented PLIF.

First developed in 1982 *(38)*, the TLIF has been performed in patients with mechanical back pain and radiculopathy with or without spondylolisthesis and especially in patients who have had previous surgery *(39,40)*. The patient is placed in the prone position and a midline incision is made and transverse processes exposed after subperiosteal dissection of the paraspinous muscles. If the patient has a radiculopathy, the laminectomy and inferior facetectomy are performed on the side of the radicular pain; otherwise, the side of bony decompression is chosen arbitrarily. The contralateral interspinous ligament and ligamentum flavum are left intact. The nerve root is identified and protected. Thereafter, pedicle screws are placed in standard fashion; however, some authors perform this step before unilateral bony exposure *(40)*. A discectomy is then performed from the side of the laminectomy, the endplates are prepared for graft placement by removing the posterior lip of the endplate and exposing bleeding cancellous bone, and the interspace is distracted for maximum disc height. Cancellous bone is packed anterolaterally and two cages are placed, the first contralaterally and the second on the ipsilateral side. All interbody material is placed through the unilateral approach. Disc space distraction is released and the rod–screw system tightened, after which cancellous bone graft is laid over the decorticated transverse processes to complete the circumferential fusion *(39–41)*.

Initial results in small retrospective case series have been encouraging, with fusion rates and patient satisfaction between 85–90% and 75–85%, respectively *(39–42)*. Complications included transient L5 injury and cerebrospinal fluid (CSF) leak. Although surgically demanding, the TLIF is a viable alternative to conventional approaches to circumferential fusion in degenerative lumbar spine disease, offering maximal stability through minimal posterior column disruption. Furthermore, it is an attractive choice in patients with scarring from prior operations.

MINIMALLY INVASIVE ANTERIOR APPROACHES: THORACOSCOPY AND ANTERIOR LUMBAR INTERBODY FUSION (ALIF)

Thoracoscopy

Thoracoscopic surgery is a standard tool in thoracic surgery for a variety of indications *(43,44)* owing to the lower rates of morbidity compared with open thoracotomy. In the early 1950s, spinal indications for thoracoscopy were limited to accessing the spine in cases of Potts disease *(45)*. However, improvements in thoracoscopy have permitted improved access to the disc space, vertebral bodies, spinal cord, nerve roots, and sympathetic chain, allowing neurosurgeons to utilize endoscopic approaches to the thoracic spine with increasing frequency and for varied indications.

Unique features of this rapidly evolving technology include the type of anesthesia employed and the equipment used. In most cases, patients undergoing thoracoscopic surgery are ventilated by single-lung ventilation to allow manipulation of the other lung for access to the spine. Patients need thorough preoperative evaluations to ascertain whether their cardiorespiratory systems can handle a potentially lengthy operation under single-lung ventilation. The equipment used in thoracoscopy is also radically different from the standard operative set. The components of a thorascopic imaging system include a telescope, light source, video camera, and projection system. Standard telescopes for endoscopic procedures are 5–10 mm rigid scopes that transmit an image to a video camera on the opposite end. The camera contains one to three charge-coupled devices (CCDs), which convert photons to electrical signals that are then processed into a video image. Endoscopes may also be angled so that the angle of view varies from a perpendicular axis; both the 0- and 30-degree scopes are commonly employed in spine surgery. Trocars are key elements of the endoscopy set and are the access devices to the thoracic cavity through which the endoscope and surgical instruments are introduced. Unlike in laparoscopy, the thoracic cavity does not require carbon dioxide insufflation; thus trocars need not be "closed" to retain the insufflated gas. Lastly, a wide range of surgical instruments designed specifically for endoscopic use are available, including fan retractors, suction-irrigators, clip appliers, needle holders, electrocautery, and standard tools for bony decompression engineered for use through a trocar.

Sympathectomy

Exposure and ligation of the sympathetic chain is exceedingly amenable to thoracoscopic intervention. The most common clinical indication for the procedure is palmar hyperhidrosis but can also include axillary sweating, facial sweating (blushing), and upper extremity pain syndromes *(46–51)*. Although the lateral decubitus position is favored for a unilateral sympathectomy, some have advocated a supine approach if bilateral sympathectomies are contemplated *(46)*. A biportal approach is most commonly used with trocars introduced in the third and fifth intercostal spaces as the ipsilateral lung is collapsed by the anesthesiologist. The lung is carefully retracted, and the pleura overlying the vertebra is divided to expose the T2 and T3 ganglia, which supply the sympathetic innervation to the lower trunk of the brachial plexus and ipsilateral upper extremity. Great care is taken to avoid the stellate ganglion and azygos vein located just cephalad to the second rib. Once exposed, the T2 ganglion, as well as its eponymous ventral ramus—the nerve of Kuntz—and the T3 ganglion are cauterized. Once hemostasis is achieved, an

18- or 20-Fr chest tube is placed through one of the portals, and trocars are removed. The lung can then be reinflated and a Valsalva maneuver applied during incisional closure to prevent pneumothorax. Chest tubes are removed either the same or the following day. Reported rates of symptomatic alleviation are nearing 100% with minimal lengths of stay and infrequent complications, which have included Horner's syndrome, intercostal neuralgia, and compensatory hyperhidrosis (46,47,52–58).

Discectomy

Anterior approaches to the thoracic spinal column are recommended for ventral disc herniations, with thoracotomy remaining the standard open procedure that provides optimal exposure to the anterior spinal canal. Although costotransversectomy and transpedicular techniques avoid opening the chest, direct visualization of the ventral spinal cord is compromised, making midline calcified discs particularly difficult to address owing to poor ventral visualization. The thoracoscopic discectomy is an alternative to open surgical approaches in the treatment of thoracic disc herniation. Thoracoscopic discectomy allows adequate ventral exposure and is advantageous over the open techniques because of decreased postoperative pain, less shoulder girdle dysfunction, reduced blood loss and morbidity, and decreased hospital stays (59–61).

For thorascopic discectomy, patients are placed in the left or right lateral decubitus position depending on the laterality of the disc extrusion. Bilateral herniations are usually approached from the right to avoid the ascending thoracic aorta (62–64). The appropriate level is scouted with C-arm fluoroscopy, and up to four portals are placed in the anterior and posterior axillary lines after the lung is deflated. The ipsilateral lung is mobilized off the anterior surface of the spine, and the level is definitively determined by counting ribs, beginning caudally. The pleura overlying the associated rib and disc space is mobilized, and costotransvese and costovertebral ligaments are detached to facilitate removal of the proximal 2–3 cm of rib and superior pedicle. This allows visualization of the anterolateral aspect of the dura, to expose the disc space. At this point, further decompression requires the creation of a trough in the dorsal aspect of the disc space and vertebral bodies above and below the disc space to facilitate maximal removal of disc material. Disc material is then removed in standard fashion with a pituitary rongeur and angled curets (Fig. 6). Chest tubes are placed through existing portals before closing and are usually left in for no longer than 24 h, depending on output. Indications include myelopathy and thoracic radicular pain. Results from thoracoscopic discectomy are encouraging, with symptomatic improvement in 70–89% of patients and more than 85% of patients reporting satisfaction with the procedure. Operative time was shorter in a series comparing thoracoscopy with thoracotomy; reported complications included durotomy, hemothorax, pleural effusion, misidentified level, and retained disc fragment. Practitioners have emphasized the technically demanding nature of thoracoscopic discectomy (59–67).

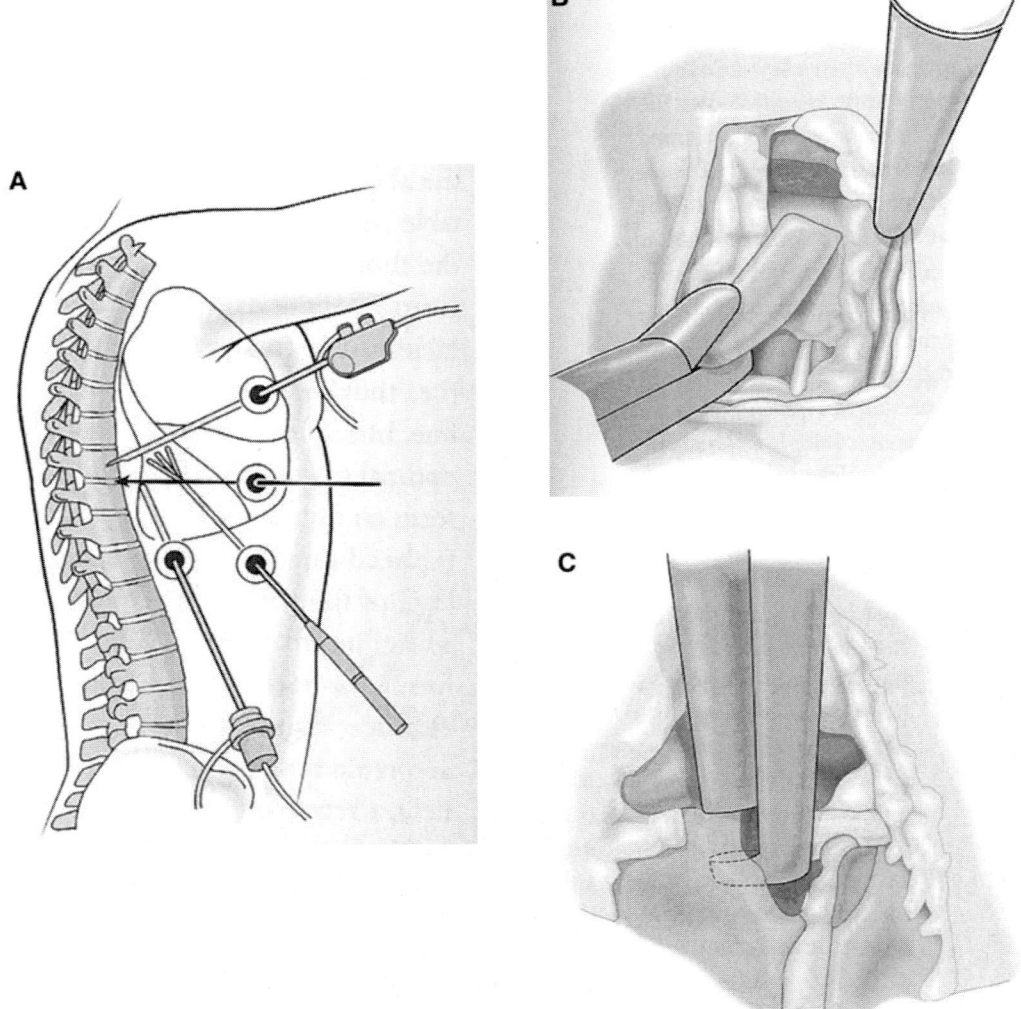

Fig. 6. (A) Four portals are placed in the anterior and posterior axillary lines of a patient in the lateral decubitus position after the lung is deflated. **(B)** The ipsilateral lung is mobilized off the anterior surface of the spine, fluoroscopy is utilized to confirm the appropriate level, and the pleura overlying the associated rib and disc space is mobilized to facilitate removal of the proximal 2–3 cm of rib and superior pedicle. **(C)** The superior portion of the pedicle is removed using a diamond burr and a Kerrison rongeur. The dura can then be visualized.

Corpectomy/Vertebrectomy and Fusion

Operative techniques in thoracoscopic spine surgery have broadened as technical aspects of the procedure have advanced. Present indications include not only discectomy and sympathectomy but also corpectomy, vertebrectomy, anterior instrumentation, and corrective procedures for adult and pediatric scoliosis. Vertebrectomy and corpectomy have been performed with identical indications as open surgery including myelopathy or radiculopathy from infection, tumor, vertebral body fractures, and large transdural heavily calcified discs *(68–70)*. Port placement and patient positioning are similar to discectomy. The proximal 3 cm of rib head above and below the involved vertebral body are resected to expose the pedicles, and dura and disc spaces above and below the level(s) of pathology are prepared. This is followed by the fashioning of a large cavity in the vertebral body with a combination of an osteotome, drill, curet, and rongeur. The posterior longitudinal ligament (PLL) is taken, and the endplates of the vertebral bodies above and below are decorticated in preparation for graft placement. Candidate grafts have included autologous iliac crest, allograft humerus, distractible titanium mesh cages, and methylmethacrylate introduced through Silastic tubing telescoped into the superior and inferior endplates spanning the vertebrectomy *(68–71)*. Grafts are brought through the portal end and positioned in standard fashion with a combination of Babcocks, impactors, and tamps. Anterior plate stabilization after grafting to prevent excessive movement of the spine and graft displacement may be accomplished with the Z-plate (Sofamor-Danek) or with the more recently described MACS-TL plate (Aesculap, Tuttlingen, Germany) *(71)*.

Proponents of the techniques cite less blood loss, less chest tube drainage, less pain medication usage, and shorter intensive care unit and hospital stays compared with the patients who undergo thoracotomy as reasons to favor the thoracoscopy *(48,68–71)*. Furthermore, anterior and anterolateral reconstruction with grafting and plate stabilization offers the biomechanical advantage of anterior and middle column restoration. However, disadvantages include poor exposure of the posterior elements and potential complications including pneumothorax, hemothorax, chylothorax, atelectasis, pneumonia, injury to any thoracic or mediastinal vascular and visceral structures, spinal instability, cardiac arrhythmias, and spinal cord injury.

ALIF/Laparoscopic ALIF

Minimally invasive posterior approaches to the lumbar spine have previously been discussed. Anterior lumbar interbody fusion (ALIF) has emerged as an alternative approach to the surgical treatment of degenerative disc disease and spondylolisthesis (reviewed in refs. 72 and 73). ALIF results in decreased operative time, reduced blood loss, and decreased postoperative pain and hospital stays compared with conventional posterior fusion techniques *(73–75)*. Additionally, ALIF proponents maintain that anterior column reconstruction is biomechanically superior to posterior column reconstruction and avoids paraspinal muscle trauma and denervation compared with posterior techniques.

There are currently two minimally invasive ALIF techniques that have improved on the traditional open laparotomy: the mini-open ALIF and the laparoscopic ALIF. The mini-open technique, first described by Mayer in 1997, reduces postoperative morbidity by using a smaller incision combined with a muscle-splitting exposure *(76,77)*. Access to the lumbar interspaces is obtained by making a 4-cm transverse paramedian incision in the supine or left lateral

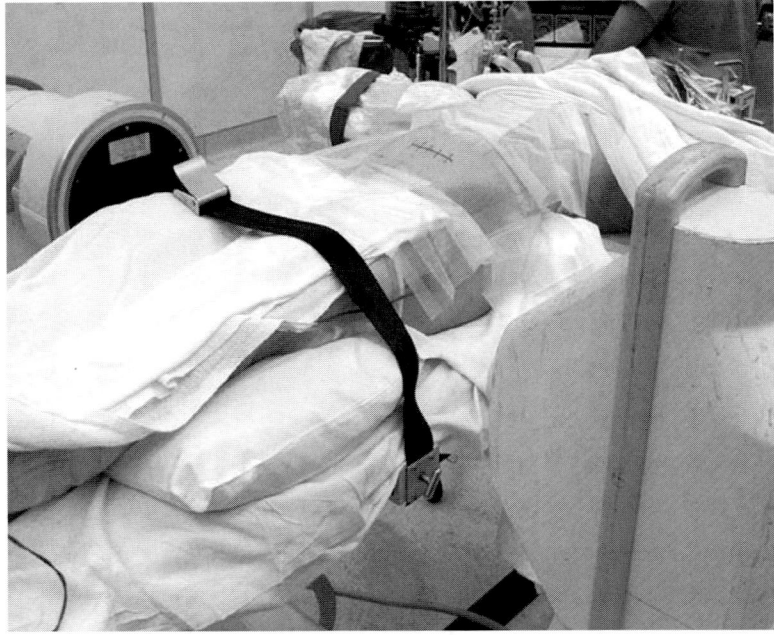

Fig. 7. Positioning and incisions for a mini-open ALIF at the L4–5 level.

decubitus patient at the appropriate level (Fig. 7). This is followed by a muscle-splitting dissection through external obliques, internal obliques, transverse abdominus, and traversalis fascia to the retroperitoneal space. For the psoas muscle, genitofemoral nerve, iliac vessel bifurcation, and lumbar interspace, any of a number of retractor systems (we use the Syn retractor from Synthes) may be introduced to retract the peritoneal contents to enlarge the surgical corridor. At the L4–5 level, care must be taken to avoid avulsing the iliolumbar vein. The iliac vessels should also be handled carefully; often only the right iliacs require mobilization. Complete disc space exposure at L5–S1 requires mobilization of the hypogastric nerve plexus, which if injured may lead to retrograde ejaculation in men. As such, dissecting tools like the Kittner should be used instead of electrocautery once the disc space is visualized. Once the disc space and neighboring endplates are appropriately exposed, an annulotomy and discectomy are performed followed by preparation of the neighboring endplates by removal of the remaining cartilaginous attachments. Candidate grafts include autograft, femoral ring allograft, titanium cages, and carbon fiber cages. The particular interbody graft employed often depends on the surgeon's predilections. Fusion rates at 6 mo are approx 90–95%, and reported complications include visceral injury, vascular injury, retrograde ejaculation, and, more commonly, postoperative ileus *(73–76,78,79)*.

The overall safety and efficacy of the laparoscopic ALIF, first described by Obenchian and Zucherman *(80,81)*, has been reported *(82–86)*. However, a growing list of comparative studies indicates that the laparoscopic approach does not confer any particular advantage to the surgeon performing a mini-

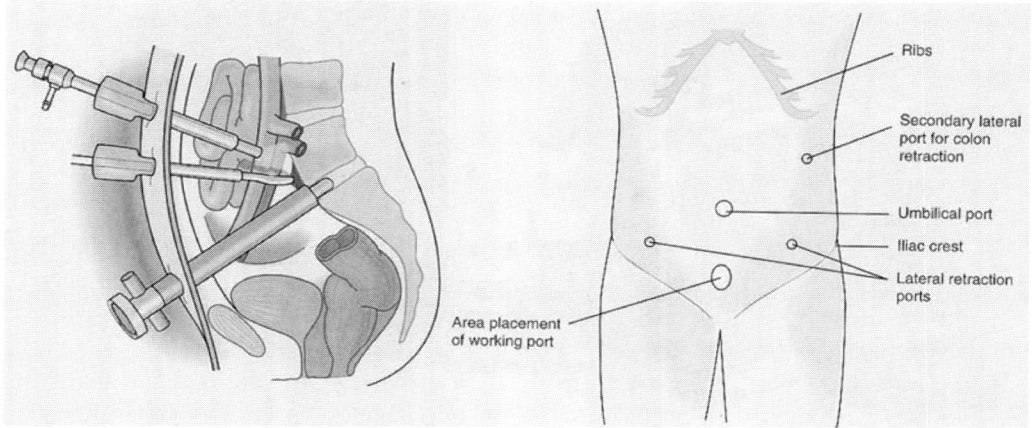

Fig. 8. AP and lateral diagrams showing a laparoscopic L5–S1 ALIF.

open ALIF *(74,78,79)*. A report by Zdeblick and David on mini-open vs laparoscopic ALIF at the L4–5 level noted a statistically significant increase in complications in the laparoscopic group compared with the open group (20% vs 4%) and overall found no convincing reasons to support a laparoscopic ALIF at the L4–5 level (Fig. 8). More recently, Kaiser et al. *(78)* performed a retrospective analysis on their experiences using the mini-open ALIF and the laparoscopic ALIF. They reported an increase in mean operative time for the laparoscopic ALIF at the L5–S1 level and also a striking increase in the incidence of retrograde ejaculation in patients undergoing the laparoscopic approach compared with the mini-open procedure (45% vs 6%). They theorized that mobilization of the hypograstric plexus with laparoscopic tools was somehow more traumatic than sweeping the plexus off the disc space with cottonoids under direct visualization. Other authors have also reported increased complication rates in patients undergoing laparoscopic ALIF instead of mini-open ALIF. The authors noted not only an increased number of complications during the laparoscopic approach but also a 20–35% necessity to convert the laparoscopic approach to an open one to enhance exposure *(74,87)*. Interbody graft choice is also limited by the laparoscopic approach. Moreover, length of hospital stay, blood loss, and postoperative discomfort—parameters that make minimally invasive procedures more attractive than conventional open approaches—are similar between the two approaches.

KYPHOPLASTY: PERCUTANEOUS AND OPEN

Percutaneous Kyphoplasty

Percutaneous techniques of stabilizing thoracic and lumbar compression fractures were first developed in France by Deramond in the late 1980s to treat pain from aggressive vertebral hemangiomas *(88)*. Current techniques for these fractures now include vertebroplasty and kyphoplasty. Vertebroplasty is the minimally invasive internal fixation of a vertebral compression fracture (VCF) by the percutaneous injection of polymethylmethacrylate (PMMA) under high pressures into the involved vertebral body. However, this approach does not restore vertebral height. Kyphoplasty, developed more recently, addresses not only the fracture but also the resultant kyphotic spinal deformity. This technique employs a minimally invasive inflatable bone tamp to restore body height, leaving a cavity that is filled with PMMA, which is injected at lower pressures. Both kyphoplasty and vertebroplasty were developed specifically for pain reduction in patients with VCFs. This section reviews the techniques and expanding indications for the minimally invasive internal fixation and reduction of VCFs, focusing particularly on kyphoplasty.

Kyphoplasty procedures are commonly performed under local anesthesia but can also be performed under general anesthesia. In the lumbar spine, a transpedicular route is favored; an extrapedicular route is used in the thoracic spine. During kyphoplasty, the patient is positioned prone, and an 11-gage trocar with a cannula is introduced through the pedicle into the posterior aspect of the vertebral body using biplanar fluoroscopic guidance. In an attempt to restore the collapsed vertebra to a normal position, an inflatable balloon tamp is introduced through the cannula and inflated under controlled pressure. The balloon is typically inflated to a maximum of 250 psi with 1.5–6 mL of saline, creating a space within the vertebral body for the injection of PMMA cement. The balloon is then withdrawn, and PMMA mixed with barium is injected into the vertebral body under fluoroscopic control to ensure that the cement remains within the vertebral body *(89–91)* (Fig 9).

Osteoporosis

Vertebroplasty and kyphoplasty have been studied most extensively in the treatment of painful osteporotic VCFs and are now viable alternatives to conservative bracing or open surgical reduction and fixation. Patients with osteoporotic VCFs have progressive kyphosis, chronic pain, and impaired ambulatory capacity, which can also lead to depression, malnutrition, and diminished pulmonary function *(92)*. Osteoporotic VCFs are now the most common etiology of vertebral body fractures, with nearly 700,000 new VCFs sustained each year *(93)*. Patients with these fractures rarely present with neurologic deficits, making percutaenous intervention feasible, provided the posterior elements and posterior cortical wall of the vertebral body are intact and no radiographic retropulsed bone in the spinal canal is evident.

One goal of these techniques is to reduce pain by stabilizing the fracture. Data from veretebroplasty have been encouraging, with more than 60% of patients reporting a significant improvement in pain and more than 50% of patients reporting improved ambulation *(94–96)*. However, the relatively high rate of PMMA extravasation reported during vertebroplasty for a variety of indications is concerning. Epidural and foraminal extravasation of PMMA has been reported to occur in 26–70% of treated levels, whereas a recent study reported only a 2.7% incidence of such extravasation in kyphoplasty *(89,97–99)*. The reduction of PMMA extravasation in kyphoplasty is probably related to

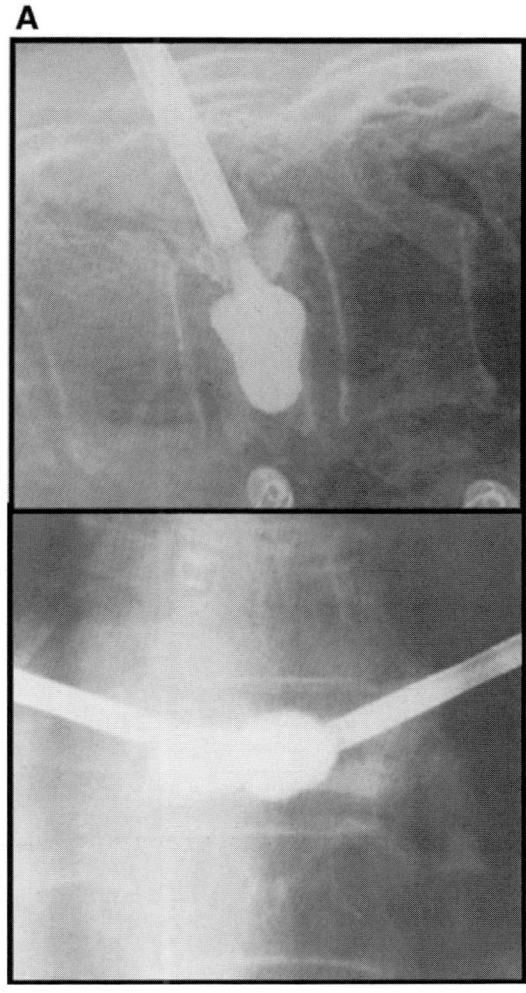
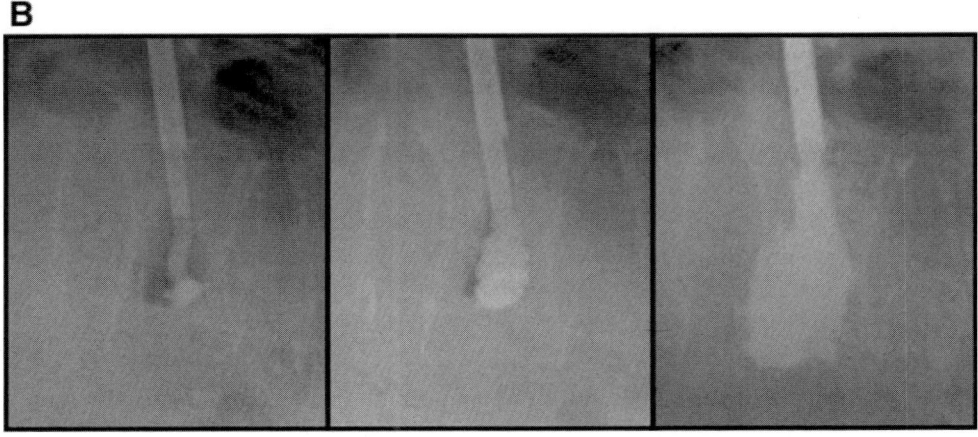

Fig. 9. **(A)** Fluoroscopy reveals an inflated kyphoplasty balloon under controlled pressure in a previously collapsed thoracic osteoporotic compression fracture. **(B)** PMMA is injected into the space in the vertebral body created by the balloon tamp.

injection of cement at the lower pressures permitted by the creation of a bone cavity.

In kyphoplasty, goals of therapy include restoration of body height and sagittal spinal alignment as well as fracture stabilization and pain relief. Initial studies with short-term follow up reported that more than 90% of patients had improvement in symptoms following kyphoplasty with an average body height restoration of 35–40%, and longer term studies also noted substantial symptomatic improvements *(89,90,95)*.

Osteolytic Metastatic Disease

Nonsurgical treatment options for malignant spinal disease now include percutaneous fracture stabilization techniques along with traditional options like analgesia, radiotherapy, hormone therapy, bisphosphonates, cytotoxic drugs, embolization, and bracing. Multiple myeloma has received particular attention because 70–100% of cases have bony involvement in the form of painful compression fractures at multiple levels throughout the vertebral column. Although the disease remains incurable, advances in chemotherapeutic options have focused attention on reducing the attendant morbidity. Data on kyphoplasty for osteolytic metastatic disease from myeloma and other types of cancer have been encouraging, with authors reporting alleviation of pain and body height restoration of an average 35–45% *(91,100)*.

Future Directions

Kyphoplasty is rapidly becoming an important therapeutic option for neurosurgeons treating vertebral compression fractures from osteoporosis and metastatic disease. Kyphoplasty's effectiveness for reducing pain, restoring vertebral body height, and on the improving functional outcome in patients warrant its practice by neurosurgeons. Future refinements will undoubtedly include clarification of the ideal time to perform kyphoplasty after a fracture, as well as the use of select bone substitutes rather than PMMA. Furthermore, biomechanical studies will help us to understand the effects of kyphoplasty on surrounding structures and could complement our existing knowledge of vertebroplasty mechanics. Lastly, we await data on the long-term efficacy of percutaneously fixed and restored vertebral bodies.

Open Kyphoplasty

Kyphoplasty may also be performed during open surgery, offering a new adjunct to surgical treatment of those compression fractures that involve posterior cortical compromise and/or retropulsion of bone into the spinal canal with or without neurologic deficits. Currently, these fractures are contraindications to percutaneous kyphoplasty owing to the potential for causing or exacerbating neurologic injury and increased risk of epidural PMMA extravasation. Boszczyk et al. *(101)* reported good pain relief and kyphosis correction in 17 of 23 patients who underwent a microsurgical interlaminary kyphoplasty or vertebroplasty. Their approach lies between percutaneous augmentation and conventional open reconstruction on the treatment continuum *(101)*. Boszczyk's results complement earlier work by Wenger and Markwalder, who are advocates of the benefits of open kyphoplasty, which helps with better visualization of vertebral body anatomy and the spinal canal during vertebral body stabilization by kyphoplasty *(102)*.

ADVANCES IN BIOLOGIC INSTRUMENTATION: BONE MORPHOGENETIC PROTEINS AND BIOABSORBABLE POLYMERS

Bone Morphogenetic Proteins

Evolving technological sophistication has allowed the development of minimal access surgery. Equally exciting is the ongoing research into biologically based techniques for spinal fusion and their nascent clinical applications. Receiving particular attention from spine surgeons are the bone morphogenetic proteins (BMPs). In 1965 the existence of BMPs, a class of low-molecular-weight glycoproteins, was first proposed, and BMPs are now recognized as playing vital roles in inducing bone formation *(103–105)*. They appear to play critical roles in the formation and maturation of skeletal tissues, with isoforms BMP-2 and BMP-7 receiving particular attention.

Naturally, the osteoinductive ability of BMPs, leading to *de novo* bone formation, has led to considerable interest in using these proteins to enhance spinal arthrodesis, either in concert with auto- or allograft or as stand-alone fusion inducers. Early clinical trials with recombinant human BMP-2 (rhBMP-2) have been encouraging. Boden et al. *(106)* compared lumbar interbody arthrodesis using autograft iliac crest vs a tapered cylindrical threaded fusion cage filled with rhBMP-2 and collagen carrier protein. The study included 14 patients with single-level lumbar degenerative disc disease refractory to nonoperative management who were randomly placed into either the rhBMP-2 group or the control autograft group. After 6 mo, radiographic arthrodesis had occurred more reliably in the rhBMP-2 group with superior outcomes measures *(106)*. Other studies have shown successful laparoscopic ALIF fusions using rhBMP-2-soaked collagen sponges placed within tapered titanium cages *(107)*. In addition, other authors have shown superior rates of lumbar fusion using tapered titanium fusion cages "packed" with rhBMP-2 compared with laparoscopic ALIF utilizing autologous iliac crest bone graft *(108)*.

The demonstrated efficacy of BMP-2 for inducing bony fusion—and the absence of associated serious side effects—has led to Food and Drug Administration approval of rhBMP-2 for lumbar interbody fusion with titanium cages. Continued research will focus both on appropriate carrier matrices through which to deliver and release recombinant BMPs and the potential for rhBMP-2 delivery by gene therapy *(109)*.

Bioabsorbable Polymers

New techniques for stabilizing adjacent spinal segments while waiting for bony fusion are also emerging. Although conventional metallic spinal implants are effective in maintaining spinal alignment and preventing graft migration, they have disadvantages such as degraded imaging, occasional failure and migration, and fusion stress shielding. Thus, interest in bioabsorbable implants has emerged. Bioabsorbable polymers have several advantages: they are radi-

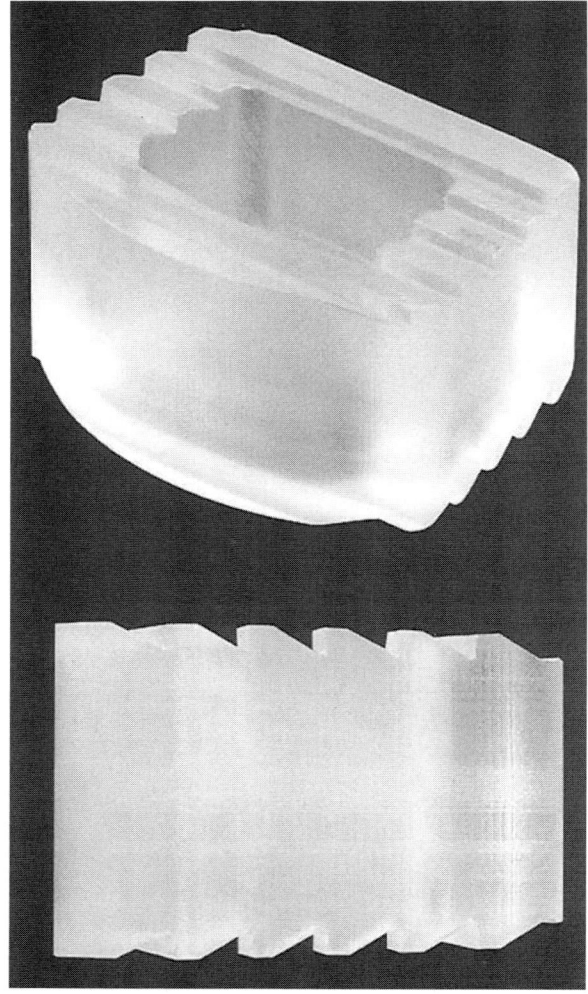

Fig. 10. A radiolucent resorbable implant (Cornerstone HSR).

olucent, lack of metallic implant migration, have no of radiographic artifact, and have the ability to transfer axial loads from implant to bone as the implant degrades over time *(110,111)* (Fig 10). The polymers utilized most often for spinal applications are poly-lactic acid (PLA) and poly-glycolic acid (PGA).

The utility of bioabsorbable plates in anterior cervical discectomy has been demonstrated in a small number of patients. The bioabsorbable implants showed enough structural strength to maintain disc space height during the fusion process but appeared to prevent stress shielding, thereby enhancing bony fusion *(112)*. More recent work demonstrated successful fusion in one- and two-level anterior cervical discectomies using the Macropore bioabsorbable plate and screw system (Macropore, San Diego, CA). This plate has the added benefit that the PLA construct is translucent, thereby allowing visualization of the endplates and disc space during plate application *(113)*. In posterior applications, 3-yr follow-up using PLA cages in lumbar interbody fusion in animal models has shown adequate fusion and maintenance of cage height at 6 mo, as well as 50% cage reabsorption at 36 mo *(114)*. Subach et al. *(115)* reported on a series of 15 patients with spondylosis or spondylolisthesis in whom bioabsorbable cages were placed bilaterally with posterior instrumentation; 6-mo follow-up showed maintenance of disc height and foraminal diameter.

The clear advantages of a bioabsorbable system include the stability of adjacent segments during bony fusion, the eventual transfer of axial load from implant to bone as the implant degrades over time, and the avoidance of metal-related complications such as migration and imaging artifact. Larger scale studies will determine efficacy and feasibility on a statistically significant scale.

NOVEL IMAGE-GUIDANCE TECHNIQUES: INTRAOPERATIVE MRI

The development of the intraoperative MRI (iMRI) system by the Brigham and Women's Hospital and General Electric Medical Systems represented a significant advance in surgical navigation. The iMRI system allows neurosurgeons to obtain real-time dynamic imaging during surgery as opposed to relying on preoperative imaging registered with a patient's anatomy *(116)*. The current 0.5-T iMRI (SIGNA SP, Boston, MA) has a vertical gap within its magnet, allowing space for surgeons on either side of the operating table, which is enclosed within the magnet. The iMRI images may be acquired during the surgery and may be obtained in conjunction with optical tracking of surgical instruments. The images are viewed on monitors within the magnet gap. The images are constantly updated to help eliminate errors that can arise during frame-based or frameless navigation systems. Use of the iMRI in cranial surgery has been well described, and it is particularly useful in defining tumor margins during resection and accounting for brain shift, which may occur during tumor debulking.

The first spinal procedure using iMRI guidance was performed in 1996 for the evacuation of an extraaxial cervical cyst, followed shortly thereafter by cervical decompression for myelopathy *(116)*. Since then, other spinal procedures performed in the iMRI have included lumbar discectomies, anterior cervical discectomies with all graft fusion, cervical vertebrectomies with allograft fusion, cervical foraminotomies, and decompressive cervical laminectomy *(117)*. The iMRI was able to provide fast and precise localization in all the listed cases and allowed determination of the degree of neural decompression in more than 80% of cases. Future applications of the iMRI for spine surgery will undoubtedly include its use in the resection of spine and spinal cord tumors and the refinement of trajectory planning for spinal endoscopy or screw fixation.

CONCLUSIONS

This chapter has reviewed the application of new minimal access techniques to the conventional surgical approaches for the treatment of spine disease. The common theme behind the derivation of these newer technical approaches is that "less is more," that is, a minimally invasive approach is *a priori* superior to the same procedure performed in a conventional "open" fashion. Although procedures such as the thorascopic sympathectomy support this contention compared with open thoracotomy, other minimally invasive approaches, like the laparoscopic ALIF, have shown fewer advantages compared with more conventional open techniques. The best approach is the one that yields the superior outcome. Cases in which minimally invasive techniques are proving to be as effective as conventional open approaches bear consideration, especially when procedural costs, decreased hospital stays, and decreased postoperative discomfort can be obtained while still achieving similar outcomes. The application of advancing technologies to age-old problems in spinal surgery has certainly provided neurosurgeons with numerous innovative ways to treat patients; however, sound clinical decision making is still the foundation required to apply these new techniques.

REFERENCES

1. Fessler RG. Minimally invasive spine surgery. *Neurosurgery* 2002;51(5 suppl): iii–iv.
2. Mixter WJ, Barr JS. Rupture of intervertebral disc with involvement of the spinal canal. *N Engl J Med* 1934;211:210–215.
3. Wilson DH, Kenning J. Microsurgical lumbar discectomy. *Neurosurgery* 1979;4: 137–140.
4. Andrews DW, Lavyne MH. Retrospective analysis of microsurgical and standard lumbar discectomy. *Spine* 1990;15:329–335.
5. Silvers HR. Microsurgical versus standard lumbar discectomy. *Neurosurgery* 1988;22:837–841.
6. Maroon JC, Abla A. The microlumbar discectomy. *Clin Neurosurg* 1986;33: 407–417.
7. Ebeling U, Reichenberg W, Reulen HJ. Results of microsurgical lumbar discectomy. *Acta Neurochir (Wien)* 1986;81:45–52.
8. Caspar W, Campbell B, Barbier DD, Kretschummer R, Gotfried Y. The Caspar microsurgical discectomy and comparison with a conventional standard lumbar disc procedure. *Neurosurgery* 1991;28:78–87.
9. Javid MJ, Nordby EJ: Current status of chymopapain for herniated nucleus pulposus. *Neurosurg Q* 1994;4:92–101.
10. Choy DSJ, Case RB, Fielding W, Hughes J, Liebler W, Ascher P: Percutaneous laser nucleolysis of lumbar disc. *N Engl J Med* 1987;317:771–772.
11. Friedman WA. Percutaneous discectomy:. Neurosurgery. 13:542–547, 1983.
12. Schreiber A, Leu H. Percutaneous nucleotomy. *Orthopedics* 1991;14:439–444.
13. Mayer HM, Brock M. Percutaneous endoscopic discectomy. *J Neurosurg* 1993;78: 216–225.
14. Mayer HM, Brock M. Percutaneous endoscopic lumbar discectomy (PELD). *Neurosurg Rev* 1993;16:115–20.
15. Mayer HM, Brock M, Berlien HP, Weber B. Percutaneous endoscopic laser discectomy (PELD). A new surgical technique for non-sequestrated lumbar discs. *Acta Neurochir Suppl (Wien)* 1992;54:53–58.
16. Ditsworth DA. Endoscopic transforaminal lumbar discectomy and reconfiguration: a postero-lateral approach into the spinal canal. *Surg Neurol* 1998;49:588–597.
17. Mathews HH. Transforaminal endoscopic microdiscectomy. *Neurosurg Clin N Am* 1996;7:59–63.

18. Smith MW, Foley KT. MED: The first 100 cases. Presented at the *Annual Meeting of the Congress of Neurological Surgeons*, Seattle, WA, October, 1998
19. Brayda-Bruno M, Cinnella P: Posterior endoscopic discectomy (and other procedures. *Eur Spine J* 2000;9(suppl):S24-S29.
20. Mercer W. Spondylolisthesis with a description of a new method of operative treatment and notes of ten cases. *Ed Med J Neurosurg* 1936;43:545.
21. Cloward RB. The treatment of ruptured intervertebral discs by vertebral body fusion:. *J Neurosurg* 1953;10:154–168.
22. Brodke DS, Dick JC, Kunz DN, McCabe R, Zdeblick TA. Posterior lumbar interbody fusion:. *Spine* 1997;22:26–31.
23. Lin PM. Technique and complications of posterior lumbar interbody fusion, in *Lumbar Interbody Fusion* (Lin PM, Gill K, eds.), Aspen Publishers, Rockville, 1989, pp. 171–199.
24. Onesti ST, Ashkenazi E. The Ray threaded fusion cage for posterior lumbar interbody fusion. *Neurosurgery* 1998;42:200–205.
25. Brislin B, Vaccaro AR. Advances in posterior lumbar interbody fusion. *Orthop Clin North Am* 2002;33:367–374.
26. Brodke DS, Dick JC, Kunz DN, et al. Posterior lumbar interbody fusion: a biomechanical comparison, including a new threaded cage. *Spin* 1997;22:26–31.
27. Lund T, Oxland R, Jost B, et al. Interbody cage stabilization in the lumbar spine: biomechanical evaluation of cage design, posterior instrumentation, and bone density. *J Bone Joint Surg B* 1998;80:351–359.
28. Brantigan JW, Steffee AD. A carbon fiber implant to aid interbody lumbar fusion: two-year clinical results in the first 26 patients. *Spin* 1993;18:2106–2107.
29. Brantigan JW, Steffee AD, Geiger JM. A carbon fiber implant to aid interbody lumbar fusion: mechanical testing. *Spin* 1991;16(6S):S277-s282.
30. Rapoff AJ, Ghanayem AJ, Zdeblick TA. Biomechanical comparison of posterior lumbar interbody fusion cages. *Spin* 1997;22:2375–2379.
31. Enker P, Steffee AD. Interbody fusion and instrumentation. *Clin Ortho* 1994;300: 90–101.
32. Steffee AD, Sitkowski J. Posterior lumbar interbody fusion and plates. *Clin Ortho* 1988;227:99–102.
33. Lanzino G, Shaffrey CI, Ray CD. Posterior lumbar interbody fusion, *Spine Surgery: Techniques, Complication Avoidance, and Management* in (Benzel EC, ed.), Churchill Livingstone, Philadelphia, 1999, pp. 311–331.
34. Gill K, Blumenthal SL. Posterior lumbar interbody fusion. *Acta Orthop Scand* 1993;64(suppl 251):108–110.
35. Khoo LT, Palmer S, Laich DT, Fessler RG Minimally invasive percutaneous posterior lumbar interbody fusion. *Neurosurgery* 2002;51(5 suppl):166–161.
36. Foley KT, Gupta SK. Percutaneous pedicle screw fixation of the lumbar spine: preliminary clinical results. *J Neurosurg* 2002;97(1 suppl):7–12.
37. Foley KT, Gupta SK, Justis JR, Sherman MC. Percutaneous pedicle screw fixation of the lumbar spine. *Neurosurg Focus* 2001;10:Article 10.
38. Harms J, Rolinger H. A one-stage procedure in operative treatment of spondylolistheses. *Z Orthop Ihre Grenzgeb* 1982;120:343347.
39. Rosenberg WS, Mummaneni PV. Transforaminal lumbar interbody fusion: technique, complications, and early results. *Neurosurgery* 2001;48:569–574;
40. Salehi SA, Tawk R, Ganju A, LaMarca F, Liu JC, Ondra SL. Transforaminal lumbar interbody fusion: surgical technique and results in 24 patients. *Neurosurgery* 2004;54:368–374.

41. Whitecloud TS, Roesch WW, Ricciardi JE. Transforaminal interbody fusion versus anterior-posterior interbody fusion of the lumbar spine. *J Spinal Disord* 2001;14:100–103.
42. Lowe TG, Tahernia AD, O'Brien MF, Smith DA. Unilateral transforaminal posterior lumbar interbody fusion (TLIF): indications, technique, and 2-year results. *J Spinal Disord Tech* 2002;15:31–38.
43. Mack MJ, Aronoff RJ, Acuff TE, Douthit MB, Bowman RT, Ryan WH: Present role of thoracoscopy in the diagnosis and treatment of diseases of the chest. *Ann Thorac Surg* 1992; 54:403–409.
44. Kaiser LR: Video-assisted thoracic surgery. *Ann Surg* 1994;220:720–734.
45. Kux E. The endoscopic approach to the vegetative nervous system and its therapeutic possibilities. *Dis Chest* 1951;20:139–147.
46. Johnson JP, Patel NP. Uniportal and biportal endoscopic thoracic sympathectomy. *Neurosurgery* 2002;51(5 suppl):79–83.
47. Han PP, Gottfried ON, Kenny KJ, Dickman CA. Biportal thoracoscopic sympathectomy: surgical techniques and clinical results for the treatment of hyperhidrosis.. *Neurosurgery* 2002;50:306–312.
48. Han PP, Kenny K, Dickman CA. Thoracoscopic approaches to the thoracic spine: experience with 241 surgical procedures. *Neurosurgery* 2002;51(5 suppl):88–95.
49. Cloward RB. Hyperhidrosis. *J Neurosurg* 1969;30:545–551.
50. Byrne J, Walsh TN, Hederman WP. Endoscopic transthoracic electrocautery of the sympathetic chain for palmar and axillary hyperhidrosis. *Br J Surg* 1990;77:1046–1049.
51. Horgan K, O'Flanagan S, Duignan PJ, Hederman W. Palmar and axillary hyperhidrosis treated with sympathectomy by transthoracic endoscopic electrocoagulation. *Br J Surg* 1984;71:1002.
52. Edmonson RA, Banerjee AK, Rennie JA. Endoscopic transthoracic sympathectomy in the treatment of hyperhidrosis. *Ann Surg* 1992;215:289–293.
53. Friedel G, Linder A, Toomes H. Selective video-assisted thoracoscopic sympathectomy. *Thorac Cardiovasc Surg* 1993;41:245–248.
54. Lin CC. A new method of thoracoscopic transthoracic in hyperhidrosis palmaris. *Surg Endosc* 1990;4:224–226.
55. Banerjee AK, Edmondson R, Rennie JA. Endoscopic transthoracic electrocautery of the sympathetic chain for palmar and axillary hyperhidrosis. *Br J Surg* 1990;77:1435–1436.
56. Claes G, Gothberg G. Endoscopic transthoracic electrocautery of the sympathetic chain for palmar and axillary hyperhidrosis. *Br J Surg* 1991;78:760.
57. Robertson DP, Simpson RK, Rose JE, Garza JS. Video-assisted endoscopic thoracic ganglionectomy. *J Neurosurg* 1993;79:238–240.
58. Drott C, Gothberg G, Claes G. Endoscopic procedures of the upper thoracic sympathetic chain:. *Arch Surg* 1993;128:237–241.
59. Regan JJ, McAfee PC, Mack MJ: Thoracoscopic disc surgery, in *Atlas of Endoscopic Spine Surgery* (Regan JJ, McAfee PC, Mack MJ, eds.), Quality Medical Publishing, St. Louis, 1995, pp. 12–17.
60. Rosenthal D, Rosenthal R, de Simone A. Removal of a protruded thoracic disc using microsurgical endoscopy. *Spine* 1994;19:10871091.
61. Rosenthal D, Dickman CA. Thoracoscopic microsurgical excision of herniated thoracic discs. *J Neurosurg* 1998;9:224–235.
62. Dickman CA, Karahalios DG. Thoracoscopic spinal surgery. *Clin Neurosurg* 1996;43:392–422.
63. Dickman CA, Rosenthal D, Regan JJ. Reoperation for herniated thoracic discs. *J Neurosurg* 1999;91(suppl 2):157–162.

64. Dickman CA, Rosenthal DJ, Perin NI: Thoracoscopic microsurgical discectomy, in *Thoracoscopic Spine Surgery* (Dickman CA, Rosenthal DJ, Perin NI, eds.), Thieme, New York, 1999, pp. 221–244.
65. Johnson JP, Filler AG, McBride DC: Endoscopic thoracic discectomy. *Neurosurg Focus* 2000;9:Article 11.
66. Oskouian RJ Jr, Johnson JP, Regan JJ. Thoracoscopic microdiscectomy. *Neurosurgery* 2002;50:103–109.
67. Anand N, Regan JJ. Video-assisted thoracoscopic surgery for thoracic disc disease: classification and outcome study of 100 consecutive cases with a 2-year minimum follow-up period. *Spine* 2002;27:871–879.
68. McAfee PC, Regan JR, Fedder IL, Mack MJ, Geis WP. Anterior thoracic corpectomy for spinal cord decompression performed endoscopically. *Surg Laparosc Endosc* 1995;5:339–348.
69. Visocchi M, Masferrer R, Sonntag VK, Dickman CA. Thoracoscopic approaches to the thoracic spine. *Acta Neurochir (Wien)* 1998;140:737–43.
70. McAfee PC. Thoracoscopic corpectomy and fusion, in *Atlas of Endoscopic Spine Surgery* (Regan JJ, McAfee PC, Mack MJ, eds.), Quality Medical Publishing, St. Louis, 1995, pp. 189–99.
71. Khoo LT, Beisse R, Potulski M. Thoracoscopic-assisted treatment of thoracic and lumbar fractures: a series of 371 consecutive cases. *Neurosurgery* 2002;51(5 suppl): 104–117.
72. Kozak JA, Heilman AE, O'Brien JP. Anterior lumbar fusion options. *Clin Orthop* 1994;300:45–51.
73. Zdeblick TA, Warden KE, Zou D, McAfee PC, Abitbol JJ. Anterior spinal fixators. *Spine* 1993;18:513–517.
74. Zdeblick T, David S. A prospective comparison of surgical approach for anterior L4L5 fusion. *Spine* 2000;25:2682–2687.
75. Regan J, Yuan H, McAfee P. Laparoscopic fusion of the lumbar spine:. *Spine* 1999;24:402–411.
76. Mayer HM. A new microsurgical technique for minimally invasive anterior lumbar interbody fusion. *Spine* 1997;22:691–700.
77. Dezawa A, Yamane T, Mikami H, Miki H. Retroperitoneal laparoscopic lateral approach to the lumbar spine. *J Spinal Disord* 2000;13:138–143.
78. Kaiser MG, Haid RW Jr, Subach BR, Miller JS, Smith CD, Rodts GE Jr. Comparison of the mini-open versus laparoscopic approach for anterior lumbar interbody fusion: a retrospective review. *Neurosurgery* 2002;51:97–103.
79. Chung SK, Lee SH, Lim SR, Kim DY, Jang JS, Nam KS, Lee HY. Comparative study of laparoscopic L5-S1 fusion versus open mini-ALIF, with a minimum 2-year follow-up. *Eur Spine J* 2003;12:613–617.
80. Obenchain TG. Laparoscopic lumbar discectomy. *J Laparoendosc Surg* 1991;1: 145–149.
81. Zucherman JF, Zdeblick TA, Bailey SA, Mahvi D, Hsu KY, Kohrs D. Instrumented laparoscopic spinal fusion. *Spine* 1995;2:2029–2035.
82. McLaughlin M, Haid R, Rodts GE, Miller J. Current role of anterior lumbar interbody fusion in lumbar spine disorders. *Semin Neurosurg* 2000;11:221–229.
83. McLaughlin M, Zhang J, Subach B, Haid R, Rodts GE. Laparoscopic anterior lumbar interbody fusion. *Neurosurg Focus* 1999;7:16.
84. McLaughlin M, Comey C, Haid R. Laparoscopic anterior lumbar interbody fusion. *Contemp Neurosur* 1998;20.
85. Mahvi DM, Zdeblick TA. A prospective study of laparoscopic spinal fusion. *Ann Surg* 1996;224:85–90.

86. Mathews HH, Evans MT, Molligan HJ, Long BH. Laparoscopic discectomy with anterior lumbar interbody fusion. *Spine* 1995;20:1797–1802.
87. Liu JC, Ondra SL, Angelos P, Ganju A, Landers ML. *Is laparoscopic anterior lumbar interbody fusion a useful minimally invasive procedure? Neurosurgery* 2002;51(5 suppl): 155–1558.
88. Galibert P, Deramond H, Rosat P, Le Gars D. Preliminary note on the treatment of vertebral angioma by percutaneous acrylic vertebroplasty. *Neurochirurgie* 1987;33: 166–168.
89. Coumans JV, Reinhardt MK, Lieberman IH. Kyphoplasty for vertebral compression fractures: 1-year clinical outcomes from a prospective study. *J Neurosurg* 2003;99(1 suppl):44–50.
90. Lieberman IH, Dudeney S, Reinhardt MK, Bell G. Initial outcome and efficacy of "kyphoplasty" in the treatment of painful osteoporotic vertebral compression fractures. *Spine* 2001;26:1631–1638.
91. Dudeney S, Lieberman IH, Reinhardt MK, Hussein M. Kyphoplasty in the treatment of osteolytic vertebral compression fractures as a result of multiple myeloma. *J Clin Oncol* 2002;20:2382–2387.
92. Silverman SL. The clinical consequences of vertebral compression fracture. *Bone* 1992;13 suppl 2:S27-s31.
93. Riggs BL, Melton LJ 3rd. The worldwide problem of osteoporosis: insights afforded by epidemiology. *Bone* 1995;17(5 suppl):505S-511S.
94. Barr JD, Barr MS, Lemley TJ, McCann RM. Percutaneous vertebroplasty for pain relief and spinal stabilization. *Spine* 2000;25:923–928.
95. Garfin SR, Yuan HA, Reiley MA. New technologies in spine: kyphoplasty and vertebroplasty for the treatment of painful osteoporotic compression fractures. *Spine* 2001;26:1511–1155.
96. Amar AP, Larsen DW, Esnaashari N, Albuquerque FC, Lavine SD, Teitelbaum GP Percutaneous transpedicular polymethylmethacrylate vertebroplasty for the treatment of spinal compression fractures. *Neurosurgery* 2001;49:1105–1114; discussion 1114–1145.
97. Ryu KS, Park CK, Kim MC, Kang JK. Dose-dependent epidural leakage of polymethylmethacrylate after percutaneous vertebroplasty in patients with osteoporotic vertebral compression fractures. *J Neurosurg* 2002;96(1 suppl):56–61.
98. Jensen ME, Evans AJ, Mathis JM, Kallmes DF, Cloft HJ, Dion JE. Percutaneous polymethylmethacrylate vertebroplasty in the treatment of osteoporotic vertebral body compression fractures: technical aspects. *AJNR Am J Neuroradiol* 1997;18: 1897–1904.
99. Cotten A, Dewatre F, Cortet B, et al. Percutaneous vertebroplasty for osteolytic metastases and myeloma: effects of the percentage of lesion filling and the leakage of methyl methacrylate at clinical follow-up. *Radiology* 1996;200:525–530.
100. Fourney DR, Schomer DF, Nader R, et al. Percutaneous vertebroplasty and kyphoplasty for painful vertebral body fractures in cancer patients. *J Neurosurg* 2003;98(1 suppl):21–30.
101. Boszczyk BM, Bierschneider M, Schmid K, Grillhosl A, Robert B, Jaksche H. Microsurgical interlaminary vertebro- and kyphoplasty for severe osteoporotic fractures. *J Neurosurg* 2004;100(1 suppl):32–37.
102. Wenger M, Markwalder TM. Surgically controlled, transpedicular methyl methacrylate vertebroplasty with fluoroscopic guidance. *Acta Neurochir (Wien)* 1999;141:625–631.
103. Urist MR. Bone: formation by autoinduction. *Scienc* 1965;150:893–899.
104. Khan SN, Sandhu HS, Lane JM, Cammisa FP Jr, Girardi FP. Bone morphogenetic proteins: relevance in spine surgery. *Orthop Clin North Am* 2002;33:447–463, ix.

105. Sandhu HS, Khan SN. Recombinant human bone morphogenetic protein-2: use in spinal fusion applications. *J Bone Joint Surg Am* 2003;85A(suppl 3):89–95.
106. Boden SD, Zdeblick TA, Sandhu HS, Heim SE. The use of rhBMP-2 in interbody fusion cages. Definitive evidence of osteoinduction in humans: a preliminary report. *Spine* 2000;25:376–381.
107. Kleeman TJ, Ahn UM, Talbot-Kleeman A. Laparoscopic anterior lumbar interbody fusion with rhBMP-2: a prospective study of clinical and radiographic outcomes. *Spine* 2001;26:2751–2756.
108. Burkus JK, Gornet MF, Dickman CA, Zdeblick TA. Anterior lumbar interbody fusion using rhBMP-2 with tapered interbody cages. *J Spinal Disord Tech* 2002;15:337–349.
109. Yoon ST, Boden SD. Spine fusion by gene therapy. *Gene Ther* 2004;11:360–367.
110. Vaccaro AR, Madkgan L. Spinal applications of bioabsorbable implants. *J Neurosurg* 2002;97(4 suppl):407–412.
111. Ciccone WJ, Motz C, Bentley C, et al. Bioabsorbable implants in orthopaedics: new developments and clinical applications. *J Am Acad Orthod Sur* 2001;9:280–288.
112. Taylor WR. Anterior cervical buttress plate using bioabsorbable implant in routine anterior cervical discectomy. What's new session, oral presentation, *AANs/CNS Section on Disorders of the Spine and Peripheral Nerves*, Phoenix, AZ February 14–17, 2001.
113. Park MS, Aryan HE, Ozgur BM, Jandial R, Taylor WR. Stabilization of anterior cervical spine with bioabsorbable polymer in one- and two-level fusions. *Neurosurgery* 2004;54:631–635.
114. van Dijk M, Smit TH, Burger EH, Wuisman PI. Bioabsorbable poly-L-lactic acid cages for lumbar interbody fusion: three-year follow-up radiographic, histologic, and histomorphometric analysis in goats. *Spine* 2002;27:2706–2714.
115. Subach BR, Haid RW, Rodts GE, et al. Posterior lumbar interbody fusion (PLIF) using an impacted, bioabsorbable device. *AANS, Joint Section on Spineal Disorders and Peripher Nerves*. Orlando, FL, February 28–March 2, 2001.
116. Black PM, Moriarty T, Alexander E 3rd, et al. Development and implementation of intraoperative magnetic resonance imaging and its neurosurgical applications. *Neurosurgery* 1997;41:831–842.
117. Woodard EJ, Leon SP, Moriarty TM, Quinones A, Zamani AA, Jolesz FA. Initial experience with intraoperative magnetic resonance imaging in spine surgery. *Spine* 2001;26:410–417.

19
Endoscopic Techniques in the Management of Carpal Tunnel Syndrome

David F. Jimenez, MD, FACS

INTRODUCTION

Carpal tunnel syndrome (CTS) represents the most common form of peripheral nerve entrapment. Although idiopathic and systemic etiologies are not uncommon, repetitive and stressful wrist motion activities represent a large majority of the cases. Its clinical presentation is classic, and diagnosis can easily be corroborated with electrodiagnostic studies. As a single clinical entity, CTS was not recognized until 1854, when it was first described by Paget [1]. His description included a patient who sustained traumatic compressive injury of the median nerve at the distal radius. Subsequently, in 1880, Putnam [2] reported on a series of patients who presented with symptoms consistent with CTS. The first report of surgical release of a compressed median nerve following a traumatic injury was by Learmonth in 1933 [3]. In 1946, Cannon and Love [4] first reported the first surgical release of a nontraumatic entrapped median nerve at the wrist. However, beginning in 1950, and during the subsequent two decades, Phalen [5–10] reported on a large number of patients with idiopathic spontaneous CTS, treated by surgical transection of the transverse carpal ligament. He is acknowledged as single-handedly popularizing the surgical treatment of CTS.

In all surgical procedures, the basic principle in the treatment of CTS is the sectioning of the transverse carpal ligament, thereby increasing the carpal tunnel's capacity. The main variation between the open surgical releases centers around the location and length of the incisions. Some advocate small (<2 cm) palmar incisions, whereas others are proponents of long incisions extending from midpalm across the distal wrist crease and into the forearm. In all these procedures, normal structures (dermis, subcutaneous fat, palmar fat pad, palmar aponeurosis, and palmar brevis muscle) are sectioned and dissected to gain access to the transverse carpal ligament. In the process, dissection of these richly innervated structures can lead to longer and more painful recovery periods. As with many other minimally invasive techniques introduced into neurosurgery, the goals of endoscopic carpal tunnel release include less postoperative pain, less tissue disruption, earlier return to work, increased patient satisfaction, and

From: *Minimally Invasive Neurosurgery,* edited by: M.R. Proctor and P.M. Black © Humana Press Inc., Totowa, NJ

comparable or better outcomes to proven open surgical techniques. This chapter describes the different types of endoscopic carpal tunnel releases and the author's preferred method for sectioning the transverse carpal ligament.

ENDOSCOPIC TECHNIQUES

The first report of an endoscopic technique for the release of an entrapped median nerve in the carpal tunnel was by the Japanese orthopedist Okutsu in 1987 *(11)*. An accomplished arthroscopist, Okutsu presented a single-portal (one incision) approach using a rigid arthroscope. In his introduction of the technique, he described a single transverse incision proximal to the distal wrist crease. Dissection through the antebrachial fascia allowed placement of a clear tubular plastic sheath for the introduction of a 30-degree rigid arthroscope. By rotating the arthroscope 90 degrees counterclockwise or clockwise, he achieved visualization of the carpal tunnel contents. A hook shaped cutting blade was inserted along side of the sheath, and under direct visualization, the transverse carpal ligament was cut in its entirety. He reported a 99.4% success rate in 750 procedures *(12,13)*. His instrumentation was never marketed or approved in North America, and the only experiences available are those reported by him. Nonetheless, his report led others to refine endoscopic techniques further and present large series of patients in subsequent years.

Endoscopic approaches to the carpal tunnel are divided into two groups depending on the number of incisions made to accomplish the procedure. Single-portal techniques have been reported by Okutsu *(11)*, Menon *(14)*, et al. Agee *(15–17)*, and Worseg et al. *(18)*. In all of these procedures, a single incision is made in the distal volar forearm, and access to the carpal tunnel in gained proximally. A variety of endoscopic systems have been designed that allow the surgeon to cut the transverse carpal ligament in its entirety and under direct visualization. Some of the systems had flaws and had to be redesigned after a number of serious complications occurred *(17)*. Biportal techniques refer to a group of procedures that utilize two small incisions to gain access and visualization to the carpal tunnel. Originally described by Chow *(19)* in 1989, the first biportal technique consisted of a small transverse incision in the distal forearm and a small stab incision in the midpalm. Chow first described a transbursal approach with dissection of the ulnar neurovascular bundle. A high number of ulnar postoperative paresthesias led to modification of the technique to a subligamentous approach by Resnik and Miller *(20)*. Using similar landmarks and with smaller, more ergonomic instruments, Brown et al. *(21,22)* introduced a biportal technique that has proved to be safe, reliable, and effective. The Brown biportal technique is the author's preferred method for releasing the carpal tunnel and is described in detail in this chapter.

SURGICAL ANATOMY

The median nerve originates from nerve roots that comprise the lateral and medial cords of the brachial plexus. As the nerve enters the arm, it does not branch until it passes below the elbow ultimately to innervate the numerous wrist and digital flexors. As it enters the hand, the median nerve innervates the LOAF muscles, which include the first and second lumbricales, the opponens pollicis, the abductor pollicis brevis, and the flexor pollicis brevis. The recurrent motor branch, which may arise in the carpal tunnel, can reach the thenar muscles either by looping around the distal end of the transverse carpal ligament (most common type) or through the ligament anywhere along its length. The motor branch innervates the abductor pollicis brevis, the opponens pollicis, and the superficial head of the flexor pollicis brevis. The palmar cutaneous branch of the median nerve exits the median nerve prior to its entry into the carpal tunnel and then travels superficially alongside the median nerve into the palm, where it divides into a medial and lateral branch supplying the skin over the median eminence and extending medially to the fourth metacarpal bone. The branch most commonly originates about 2 cm proximal to the proximal border of the flexor retinaculum but may have a variable origin and course. The sensory supply of the median nerve extends to the radial $3^1/_2$ digits of the hand via the common palmar digital branches. The rest of the sensory innervation of the hand is supplied by the sensory branch of the ulnar nerve as it branches from the main trunk in the distal forearm and immediately radial to the tendon of the flexor carpi ulnaris.

The floor of the carpal tunnel is comprised of the carpal bones, the ligamentous extensions between the carpal bones, and the overlying radiocarpal ligament. The roof of the tunnel is formed by the transverse carpal ligament as it extends radially from the tuberosity of the scaphoid and the crest of the trapezius to its ulnar attachments at the hook of the hamate and the pisiform bone. Proximally, the transverse carpal ligament blends with the fibers of the antebrachial fascia at the distal wrist crease. The ligament extends distally into the palmar approx 3.0 ± 0.25 cm to end near Kaplan's cardinal line. Kaplan's cardinal line is a line defined to be parallel to the distal palmar crease; it runs along the base of the fully extended thumb. In relation to an endoscopic approach to the carpal tunnel, several key anatomical features need to be highlighted.

Access to the tunnel is made ulnar to the palmaris longus, whereas the median nerve is located radial to the palmaris longus, thereby keeping it well away from the endoscopic instrumentation. Although the recurrent motor branch of the median nerve has a variety of branching patterns, the most common is the extraligamentous and recurrent type extending radially to the thenar musculature. Again, this anatomical arrangement keeps the motor branch away from the endoscopic approach. By placing the proximal incision immediately ulnar to the palmaris longus, the surgeon stays away from both the main ulnar nerve and its cutaneous sensory branch. By aiming the distal incision to the third web space, entrance into Guyon's canal is avoided as well as any ulnar neurovascular injuries. By placing the distal incision immediately distal (≤ 1cm) to the distal end of the transverse carpal ligament, the vascular palmar arch is easily avoided. Therefore, an anatomically safe corridor exists between the proximal and distal incisions located immediately radial to the hook of the hamate, where the transverse carpal ligament can be safely and completely sectioned to release the compromised carpal tunnel (Fig. 1).

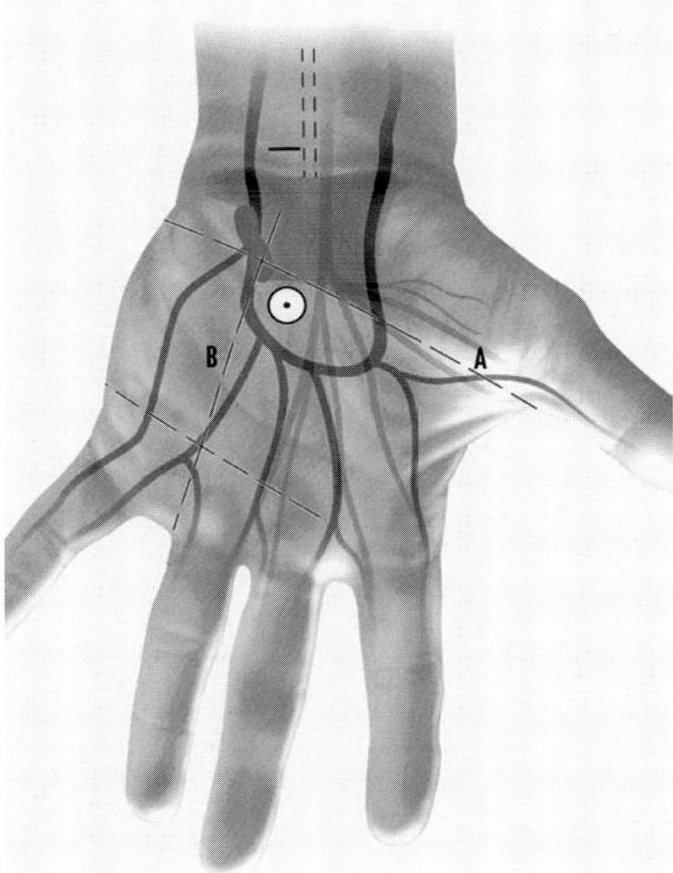

Fig. 1. Diagram demonstrates key anatomical landmarks. A proximal incision is made 1–2 cm proximal to the distal wrist crease on the ulnar side of the palmaris longus tendon. A distal wound is made within a 1-cm-radius circle with an epicenter at 4 cm distal to the wrist crease along the third web space. Line A depicts Kaplan's cardinal line. The intersection of line B with line A points to the location of the hook of the hamate. Median nerve is located on the radial side of the palmaris longus tendon.

SURGICAL PROCEDURE

After careful assessment of the different types of endoscopic approaches to the carpal tunnel, it is the author's preference to use the biportal technique described by Brown. This section depicts that procedure in detail. As with any open technique, the type of anesthesia used is the surgeon's choice. Local, regional (Bier block), or general nonendotracheal anesthesia can be used. Insertion of the endoscopic instrumentation can cause discomfort and pain to the patient, making local anesthesia less desirable. Regional anesthesia via Bier block can be used in most patients safely and rapidly with little discomfort. This type of anesthesia is particularly useful in patients with higher American Society of Anesthesiologiest (ASA) grades, in those with a history of esophageal

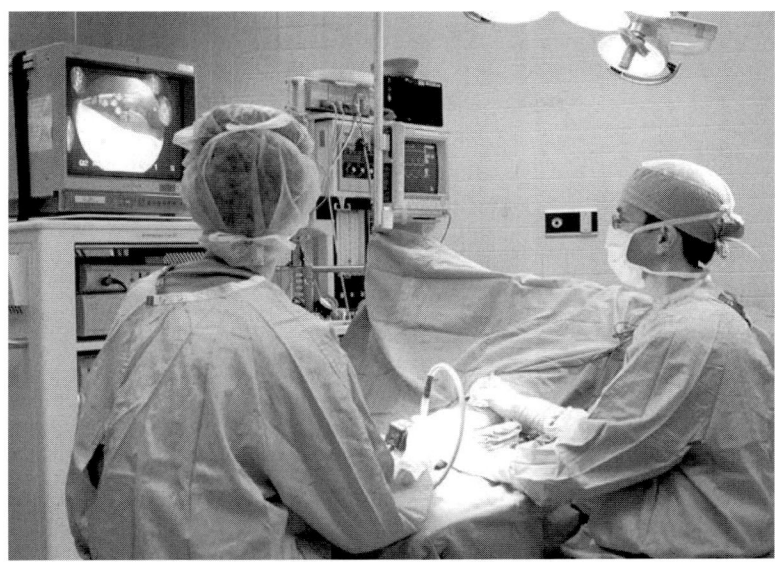

Fig. 2. Operating room configuration shows the surgeon with his dominant hand closest to the patient, sitting directly across from the TV monitor. Assistant sits at the end of the table and helps with management of the endoscope and other equipment.

reflux, and in those for whom general anesthesia in contraindicated. In healthy, otherwise well individuals, general anesthesia with a laryngeal mask airway and intravenous sedation can also be safely used. Induction is achieved with a bolus of propofol followed by a maintenance dose during a very short procedure time. At the end of the procedure, the patients awaken quickly and can be discharged home within 1–2 hr.

As with any endoscopic surgery, the video equipment is connected and checked for proper functioning prior to anesthetic induction. It is imperative that the appropriate orientation be obtained so that the TV monitor image correlates with the appropriate spatial orientation of the patient. The operating room set-up is somewhat different than the standard carpal tunnel surgery. The surgeon should sit with his/her dominant hand toward the patient. The TV monitor is then placed directly across from the surgeon, and the scrub nurse/assistant sits at the end of the patient's extended arm. The scrub nurse is situated between the surgeon and the first assistant if one is available for the procedure (Fig. 2).

The skin marks must be properly localized and marked at this point. The distal wrist crease is the most important landmark because all others are based on its location. Location of the palmaris longus tendon is corroborated by asking the patient to flex the wrist and oppose the thumb and fifth digit. The proximal incision is made in an area located between 1 and 2 cm proximal to the distal wrist crease and immediately ulnar to palmaris longus tendon (Fig. 3). The length of this incision should be 1 cm or less. The distal incision is made along a line perpendicular to the distal wrist crease and running towards the third

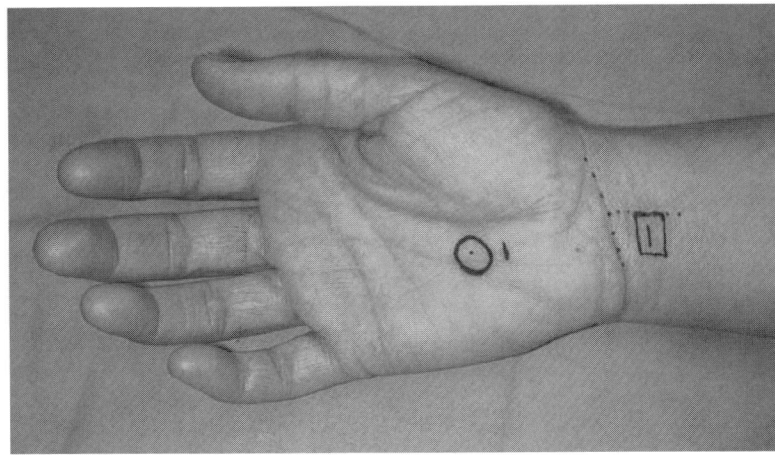

Fig. 3. Intraoperative photograph shows the location of the two skin portals. A proximal incision is made 1–2 cm proximal to the distal wrist crease ulnar to the palmaris longus. A second portal is made within a 1-cm circle located 4 cm distal to the distal wrist crease along the third web space.

web space. Along that line, a point is marked 3 cm distal to the distal wrist crease. In most patients, this will mark the end of the transverse carpal ligament ±0.5 cm. On the same line, another dot is marked at 4 cm distal to the wrist crease. and a .5-cm circle is drawn circumferentially around the 4-cm mark. This circle encompasses the safe area where the second distal portal can be made. One should note that the corridor between the proximal and distal portals encompasses an area where only the transverse carpal tunnel is present and where it is safe to section it.

Following the induction of anesthesia, the arm is elevated, and a rubber Esmarch bandage is applied to exsanguinate the extremities. A tourniquet is applied and inflated to pressures above systolic, and the Esmarch bandage is removed. The hand is then freely held and placed in a slight extension on a pair of rolled-up towels. The proximal incision is made, taking care not to extend it more than 1 cm in the ulnar direction. Tenotomy scissors are then used to spread the subcutaneous tissue apart and allow visualization of the antebrachial fascial fibers. These are easily identified by visualizing white glistening fibers running in multiple directions. Following exposure of the antebrachial fascia, the fibers are spread apart bluntly with the tips of the scissors. Care should be taken not to cut the fascial fibers, as this may inadvertently lead to sectioning of a tendon. Following blunt dissection of the antebrachial fascia, the longitudinally running fibers of the tendons can be easily visualized. No attempt is made to visualize the median nerve. A pair of Adson forceps is used to grasp and elevate the distal edge of the divided antebrachial fascia. A synovial elevator is then gently inserted under the fascial fibers and advanced distally at an acute angle of approx 60° (Fig. 4).

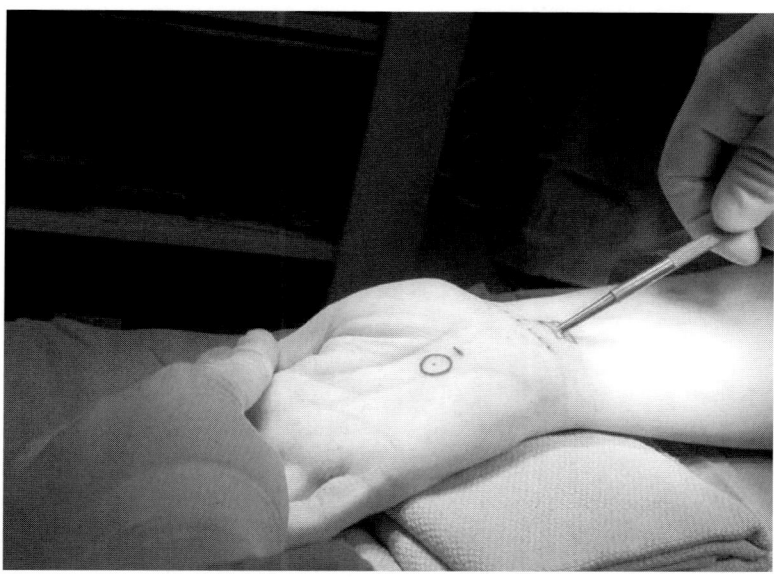

Fig. 4. The synovial elevator is placed through the dissected fibers of the antebrachial fascia and into the carpal tunnel. Note that the original angle of insertion is between 45 and 60°.

Once inside the carpal tunnel, the tip of the synovial elevator is directed superficially in order to strip the synovium from the undersurface of the transversely running fibers of the transverse carpal ligament (TCL). This anatomical arrangement will produce a "washboard"-type sensation as the tip of the elevator moves across these transversely oriented fibers. By palpating this washboard sensation, the surgeon corroborates that the synovial elevator is inside the carpal tunnel. As the tip of the elevator is advanced distally past the distal edge of the TCL, the washboard feeling will disappear, thereby indicating the location of the distal end of the TCL.

Once these internal landmarks are palpated and prior to removal of the synovial elevator, the antebrachial fascial edge should be grasped in order to maintain an open tract into the carpal tunnel. Next, an obturator–canula assembly is inserted into this tract beneath the TCL (Fig. 5). As the tip of the obturator is passed distally into the carpal tunnel, the patient's hand and wrist should be maintained in a neutral position. The obturator should be gently pressed radially against the hook of the hamate. This maneuver will ensure that Guyon's canal is not entered. Once the obturator tip is passed beyond the hook of the hamate, the wrist is extended to approx 30°. As the tip of the obturator approaches the previously drawn circle, the surgeon's nondominant hand is used to apply pressure over the obturator (Fig. 6). The tip of the obturator is easily felt under the skin and at this point, only the skin should lie between the surgeon's thumb and the obturator's tip. A #15 blade is used to create a small stab wound over the tip of the obturator, which is then gently pushed through this skin incision (Fig. 7).

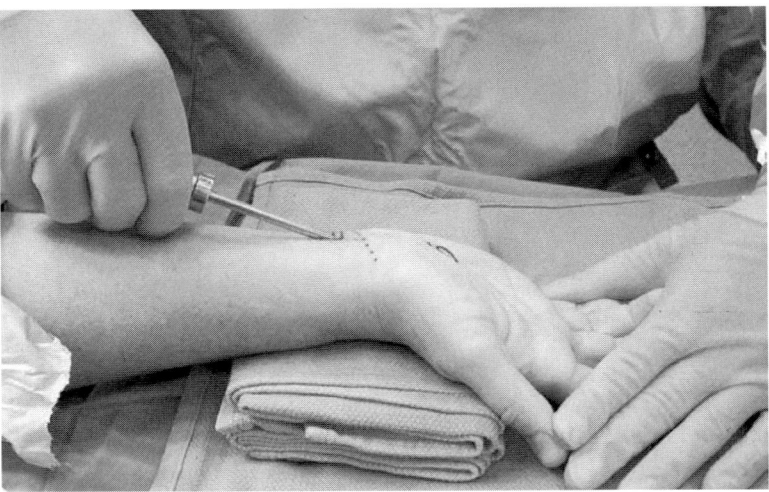

Fig. 5. The obturator–cannula assembly is inserted into the same compartment as the synovial elevator. Using the tip of the assembly, the "washboard" sensation can be felt, ensuring that the assembly is inside the carpal tunnel.

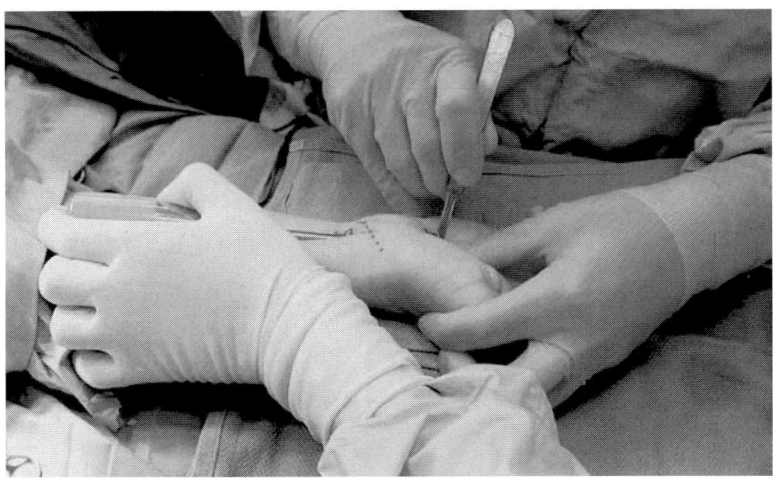

Fig. 6. The surgeon's nondominant hand presses tightly against the skin over the obturator tip. As the assistant pushes the obturator handle, a scalpel is used to make a stab incision over the tip of the obturator.

Once the obturator is removed and the canula is left inside the carpal tunnel, it is then gently rotated approx 10–15° ulnarward (Fig. 8). The endoscope is then inserted at the distal end of the canula (Fig. 9) and advanced proximally to allow full visualization of the undersurface of the TCL. The wide glistening fibers of the TCL should be easily visualized. If there are remnants of synovium, these can be gently removed with a hooked instrument or with a rasper. The distal end of the TCL will be easily visualized as the yellow fat pad will easily

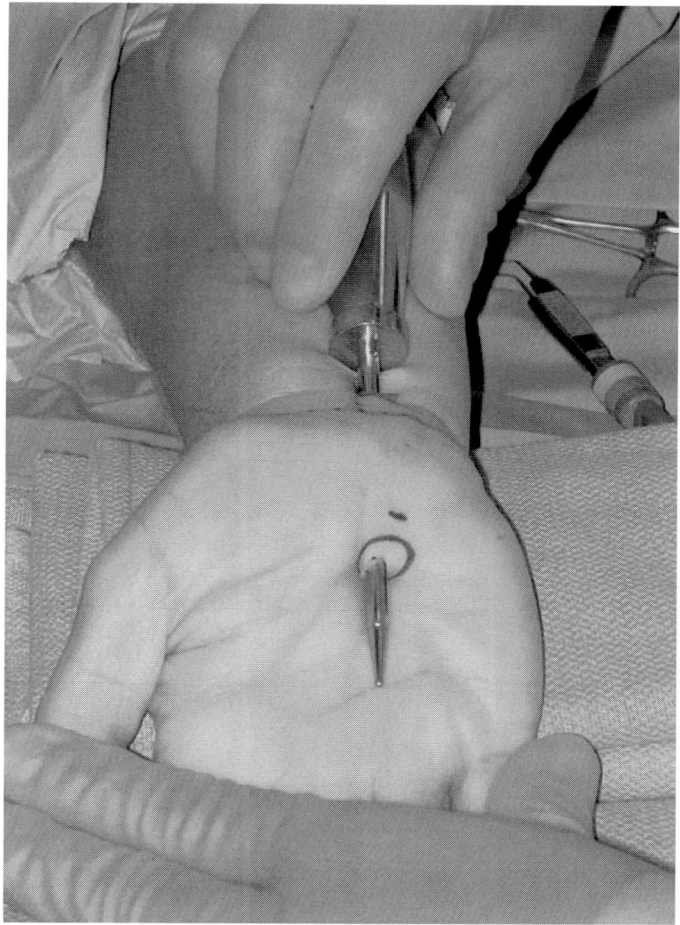

Fig. 7. The obturator–cannula assembly inside the carpal tunnel. Note its entrance through the proximal portal and its exit within the circle located 4 cm distal to the distal wrist crease.

drape over the edge of the ligament. A hooked blade is then inserted using the surgeon's dominant hand through the proximal opening in the canula (Fig. 10). As the endoscope is advanced proximally and the blade is advanced distally, these two instruments should come to rest close to each other. Following this, the blade and the endoscope are moved in unison with the separation of 0.5–1 cm. Before sectioning the TCL, care must be taken to note whether there are any longitudinally running fibers in the field of vision. If this is the case, one must suspect that a tendon is trapped above the slotted cannula. Care must be taken not to section any fiber that is running longitudinally, as this may be either a tendon or a nerve.

Once the entirety of the undersurface of the TCL is well visualized, the blade is then hooked onto the distal end of the TCL and steadily moved proximally to section the ligament under direct visualization (Fig. 11). Depending on the

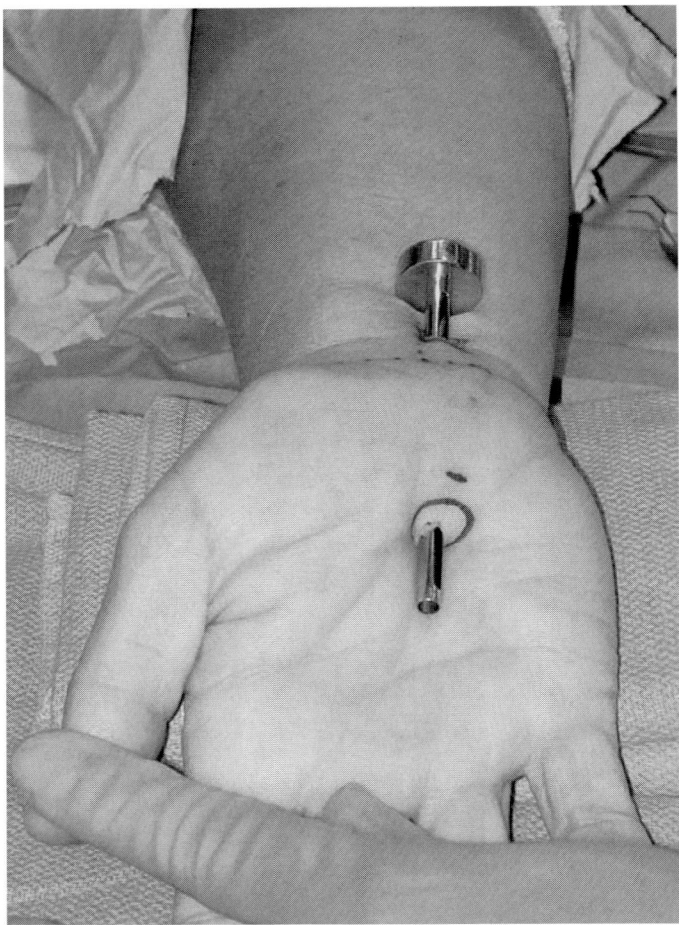

Fig. 8. The obturator has been removed, leaving the open cannula in place. Note that the cannula has been rotated approx 15° ulnarward, thereby directing the dissecting knife away from the median nerve.

severity of the syndrome, multiple passes may be needed to section the TCL in its entirety. Once the ligament is sectioned, the fat pad will fall into endoscopic view and obscure visualization. As this occurs, one can be assured that the ligament has been completely sectioned. At this point, the slotted cannula is removed, and, if a Tinel's sign has been found preoperatively proximal to the distal wrist crease, a proximal volar fasciotomy can be performed using a pair of tenotomy scissors under direct visualization (Fig. 12). The tourniquet is taken down, pressure is applied, and hemostasis obtained as necessary. Several single nonabsorbable sutures are used to close the skin edges. To prevent hyperflexion of the wrist at the early stages, a short-volar splint is used, leaving the fingers free to be used. Sutures are removed within 1 wk, and the patient may return to full use of the hand after suture removal.

Endoscopy in Carpal Tunnel Syndrome

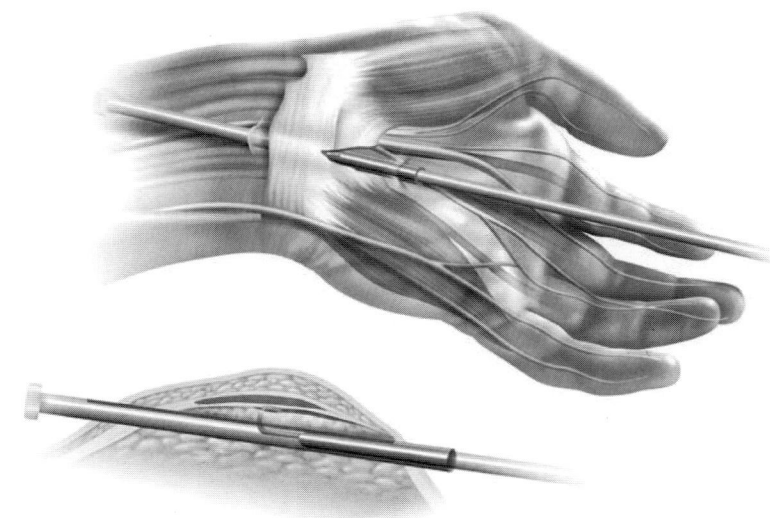

Fig. 9. Drawings depict the transverse carpal ligament being sectioned midway. The wrist is slightly hyperextended as the ligament is sectioned. Lower diagram shows that only the ligament cut and the superficial structures are left intact.

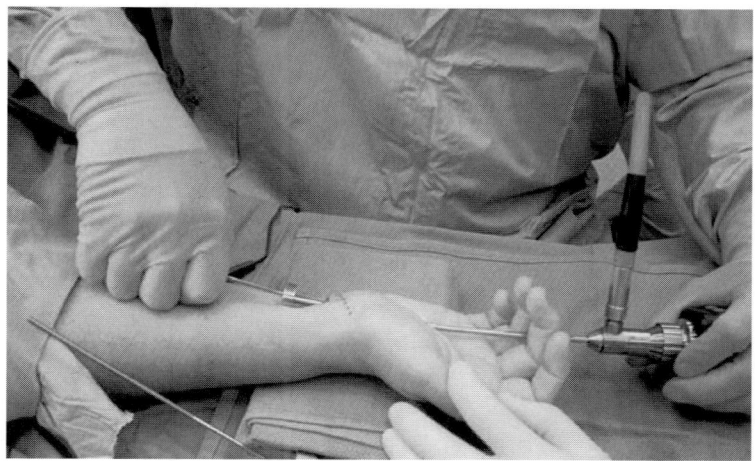

Fig. 10. As the endoscope is guided with the nondominant hand, the hooked knife is controlled with the dominant hand and used to section the transverse carpal ligament under direct visualization.

RESULTS

As previously reported by the author *(23)* in an extensive review of the literature, a total of 8068 endoscopic carpal tunnel release procedures have been reported (Table 1). These reports were classified according to the technique used and the type of study conducted. The success rate varied between 78 and 100%, although the definition of success was not uniform from paper to paper.

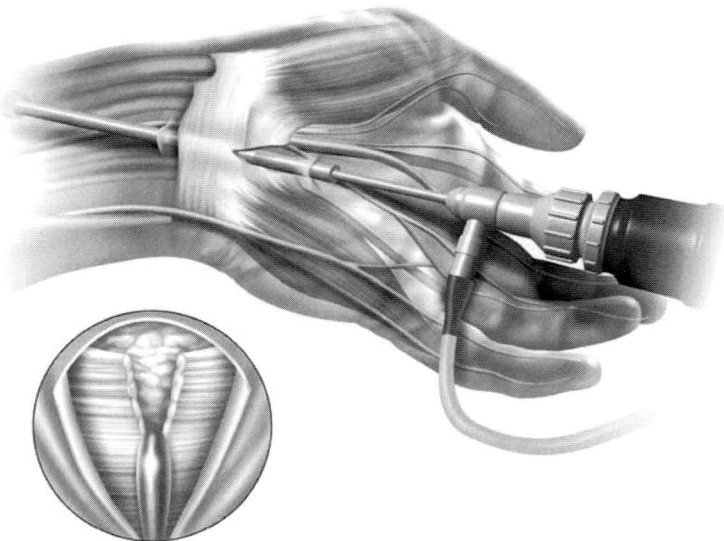

Fig. 11. Diagram demonstrates the insertion of the endoscope through the distal incision. As the endoscope is advanced proximally, the cutting blade is advanced distally until they meet. Both instruments are then moved in unison. Insert shows endoscopic view of transverse carpal ligament being sectioned.

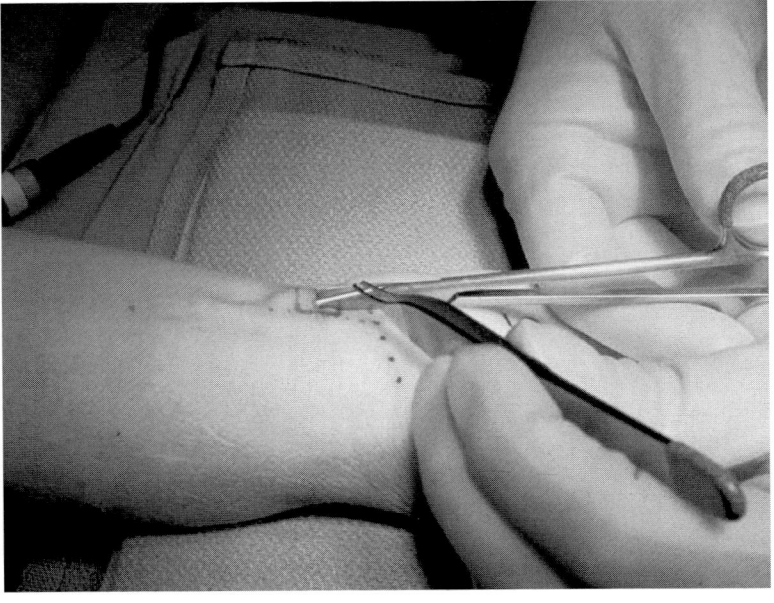

Fig. 12. A proximal volar fasciotomy can be easily performed with tenotomy scissors if there are clinical signs of nerve compression proximal to the distal wrist crease.

Table 1
Summary of Reported Cases According to Type of Endoscopic Technique Performed

Method	No. of patients	No. of procedures	Avg. patient age (yr)	Success rate (%)	Complication rate (%)	Failure rate (%)
Chow	3505	4112	46.05	98.3	1.87	1.44
Brown	1464	1472	57	96.01	1.41	1.78
Agee	1463	1570	47.2	96.2	1.83	1.44
Okutsu	508	750	54.07	99.63	0.4	0.3
Menon	87	100	48.3	94	9	0.6
Worseg	64	64	58	95	1.56	4.7
Total	7091	8068	51.77	96.52	2.67	2.61

Return to work times averaged 21.75 d, ranging between 4 and 39.8 d. Patients not receiving Workers' Compensation had a mean return to work time of 17.8 days, ranging between 10.8 and 22.3 d.

Nine articles have been published describing results obtained using Agee's monoportal technique in a total of 1463 patients undergoing 1570 procedures *(15–17,24–28)*. The combined success rate reported in these articles was 96.2%, with a complication rate of 1.83% and a failure rate of 1.44%. The complications associated with this technique include reflex sympathetic dystrophy, ulnar neuropraxias, palmar sensory loss, infection, pillar pain, weak grip, scar tenderness, flexor digitorum sublimis laceration, and hematoma. Three articles were published describing results obtained using the original singe-portal Okutsu technique in a total of 508 patients undergoing 750 procedures *(13,29,30)*. Okutsu reported a success rate of 99.63%, with a complication rate of 0.4% and a failure rate of 0.3%. The only reported complication was a subcutaneous hematoma. The articles published by Menon *(14,31)* on his technique reported a total of 87 patients undergoing 100 procedures. He reported a success rate of 94% and the highest complication rate of all articles, at 9%, and a recurrence rate of 0.6%. Complications reported included pillar pain, neuropraxia, and ulnar nerve communicating branch injury. Only one article *(18)* dealt with Worseg's technique, and it was included for completeness. He reported on 64 procedures in 64 patients. The success rate was 95%, with a complication rate of 1.56% and the highest failure rate of 4.7%. Complications reported included postoperative pain and transient neuropraxia of the third common digital nerve.

The most widely performed and reported procedure was Chow's dual-portal technique. There were 20 articles describing 3505 patients undergoing 4112 procedures *(3,19,20,27,28,32–46)*. The average success rate reported in these publications was 98.3%, with a complication rate of 1.87% and a failure rate of 1.44% Complications included ulnar nerve neuropraxia and paresthesias, which were most common when ulnar nerve retraction was used during the earlier transbursal method. The incidence of ulnar nerve neuropraxia decreased with the advent of the extrabursal method. Other complications included reflex sympathetic dystrophy, superficial palmar arch injury, interdigital lesion,

Guyon's canal release, and scarring *(47)*. A total of 1464 patients underwent surgery via Brown's dual-portal technique *(21,22)*. A total of 1472 procedures were performed with a reported success rate of 96%, a complication rate of 1.41%, and a failure rate of 1.78%. Transient paresthesias, reflex sympathetic dystrophy, and injury to the superficial palmar arch were reported complications with this procedure. Five papers dealt strictly with complications of endoscopic techniques *(48–52)*. Complications reported included transection of the motor branch of the ulnar nerve, laceration of the ulnar nerve at Guyon's canal, pseudoaneurysm of the superficial palmar arch, median nerve transection, and laceration of the flexor digitorum superficialis four and five.

CONCLUSIONS

The introduction of endoscopic techniques to the management of CTS has greatly improved patient satisfaction while achieving results similar to those of the open technique. Proper training is paramount to successful outcomes. For those surgeons not familiar with endoscopy, the learning curve can be somewhat steep. Nevertheless, by following simple anatomical and surgical principles, this procedure can be safely and successfully done. Careful patient selection is also important for good results. Contraindications include patients with previous carpal tunnel surgery, history of wrist fractures, or anatomical anomalies (ganglion cysts, tumors) or patients with tenosynovitis. In properly selected patients, endoscopic carpal tunnel release provides an excellent surgical option with superior results.

REFERENCES

1. Paget J. *Lectures on Surgical Pathology: Delivered at the Royal College of Surgeons of England*. Lindsay & Blakiston, Philadelphia, 1854, p. 42.
2. Putnam JJ. A series of cases of paraesthesia, mainly of the hands, of periodical occurrence, and possibly of vaso-motor origin. *Arch Med* 1880;4:147–162.
3. Learmonth JR. The principle of decompression in the treatment of certain diseases of peripheral nerves. *Surg Clin North Am* 1933;13:905–913.
4. Cannon BW, Love JG. Tardy median palsy; median neuritis; median thenar neuritis amenable to surgery. *Surgery* 1946;20:210–216.
5. Phalen GS. The carpal tunnel syndrome. Clinical evaluation of 598 hands. *Clin Orthop* 1972;83:29–40.
6. Phalen GS. The carpal tunnel syndrome. Seventeen years' experience in diagnosis and treatment of six hundred fifty-four hands. *J Bone Joint Surg (Am)* 1966;48:211–228.
7. Phalen GS. Reflections on 21 years' experience with the carpal-tunnel syndrome. *JAMA* 1970;212:1365–1367.
8. Phalen GS. Spontaneous compression of the median nerve at the wrist. *JAMA* 1951;145:1128–1133.
9. Phalen GS, Gardner WJ, La Londe AA. Neuropathy of the median nerve due to compression beneath the transverse carpal ligament. *J Bone Joint Surg (Am)* 1950;32:109–112.
10. Phalen GS, Kendrick JI. Compression neuropathy of the median nerve in the carpal tunnel. *JAMA* 1957;164:524–530.

11. Okutsu I, Ninomiya S, Natsuyama M et al. Subcutaneous operation and examination under universal endoscope. *J Jpn Orthop Assoc* 1987;61:491–498. (Jpn)
12. Okutsu I, Hamanaka I, Ninomiya S, et al. Results of endoscopic management of carpal-tunnel syndrome in long-term haemodialysis versus idiopathic patients. *Nephrol Dial Transplant* 1993;8:1110–1114.
13. Okutsu I, Ninomiya S, Takatori Y. Results of endoscopic management of carpal tunnel syndrome. *Orthop Rev* 1993;22:81–87.
14. Menon J. Endoscopic carpal tunnel release, a single portal technique. *Contemp Orthop* 1993;26:109–116.
15. Agee JM, McCarroll HR, Tortosa RD, et al. Endoscopic release of the carpal tunnel: a randomized prospective multicenter study. *J Hand Surg (Am)* 1992;17:987–995.
16. Agee JM, McCarroll HR, North ER. Endoscopic carpal tunnel release using the single proximal incision technique. *Hand Clin* 1994;10:647–659.
17. Agee JM, Peimer CA, Pyrek JD, et al. Endoscopic carpal tunnel release: a prospective study of complications and surgical experience. *J Hand Surg (Am)* 1995;20:165–171.
18. Worseg AP, Kuzbari R, Korak K, et al. Endoscopic carpal tunnel release using a single-portal system. *Br J Plast Surg* 1996;49:1–10.
19. Chow JC. Endoscopic release of the carpal ligament: a new technique for carpal tunnel syndrome. *Arthroscopy* 1989;5:19–24.
20. Resnick CT, Miller BW. Endoscopic carpal tunnel release using the subligamentous two-portal technique. *Contemp Surg* 1991;22:269–277.
21. Brown MG, Keyser B, Rothenberg ES. Endoscopic carpal tunnel release. *J Hand Surg (Am)* 1992;17:1009–1011.
22. Brown MG, Rothenberg ES, Keyser B, et al. Results of 1236 endoscopic carpal tunnel release procedures using the Brown technique. *Contemp Orthop* 1993;27:251–258.
23. Jimenez DF, Gibbs SR, Clapper AT. Endoscopic treatment of carpal tunnel syndrome: a critical review. *Neurosurg Focus* 1997;3(1):Article 6.
24. Brown RA, Gelberman RH, Seiler JG III, et al. Carpal tunnel release. A prospective, randomized assessment of open and endoscopic methods. *J Bone Joint Surg (Am)* 1993;75:1265–1275.
25. Elmaraghy MW, Hurst LN. Single-portal endoscopic carpal tunnel release: Agee carpal tunnel release system. *Ann Plast Surg* 1996;36:286–291.
26. Feinstein PA. Endoscopic carpal tunnel release in a community-based series. *J Hand Surg (Am)* 1993;18:451–454.
27. McDonough JW, Gruenloh TJ. A comparison of endoscopic and open carpal tunnel release. *Wis Med J* 1993;92:675–677.
28. Palmer DH, Paulson JC, Lane-Larsen CL, et al. Endoscopic carpal tunnel release: a comparison of two techniques with open release. *Arthroscopy* 1993;9:498–508.
29. Okutsu I, Ninomiya S, Hamanaka I, et al. Measurement of pressure in the carpal canal before and after endoscopic management of carpal tunnel syndrome. *J Bone Joint Surg (Am)* 1989;71:679–683.
30. Okutsu I, Ninomiya S, Takatori Y, et al. Endoscopic management of carpal tunnel syndrome. *Arthroscopy* 1989;5:11–18.
31. Menon J. Endoscopic carpal tunnel release: preliminary report. *Arthroscopy* 1994;10:31–38.
32. Arner M, Hagberg L, Rosen B. Sensory disturbances after two-portal endoscopic carpal tunnel release: a preliminary report. *J Hand Surg (Am)* 1994;19:548–551.

33. Chow JC. The Chow technique of endoscopic release of the carpal ligament for carpal tunnel syndrome: four years of clinical results. *Arthroscopy* 1993;9:301–314.
34. Chow JC. Endoscopic carpal tunnel release. Two-portal technique. *Hand Clin* 1994;10:637–646.
35. Chow JC. Endoscopic release of the carpal ligament for carpal tunnel syndrome: 22-month clinical result. *Arthroscopy* 1990;6:288–296.
36. Erdmann MW. Endoscopic carpal tunnel decompression. *J Hand Surg (Br)* 1994; 19:5–13.
37. Friol JP, Chaise F, Gaisne E. Endoscopic decompression from the median nerve to the carpal canal. *Ann Chir Main Memb Suppl* 1994;13:162–171. (Fr)
38. Hallock GG, Lutz DA. Prospective comparison of minimal incision "open" and two-portal endoscopic carpal tunnel release. *Plast Reconstr Surg* 1995;96:941–947.
39. Jacobsen MB, Rahme H. A prospective, randomized study with an independent observer comparing open carpal tunnel release with endoscopic carpal tunnel release. *J Hand Surg (Br)* 1996;21:202–204.
40. Kelly CP, Pulisetti D, Jamieson AM. Early experience with endoscopic carpal tunnel release. *J Hand Surg (Br)* 1994;19:18–21.
41. Lewicky RT. Endoscopic carpal tunnel release: the guide tube technique. *Arthroscopy* 1994;10:39–49.
42. Nagle DJ, Fischer TJ, Harris GD, et al. A multicenter prospective review of 640 endoscopic carpal tunnel releases using the transbursal and extrabursal Chow techniques. *Arthroscopy* 1996;12:139–143.
43. Roth JH, Richards RS, MacLeod MD. Endoscopic carpal tunnel release. *Can J Surg* 1994;37:189–193.
44. Skoff HD, Sklar R. Endoscopic median nerve decompression: early experience. *Plast Reconstr Surg* 1994;94:691–694.
45. Slattery PG. Endoscopic carpal tunnel release. Use of the modified Chow technique in 215 cases. *Med J Aust* 1994;160:104–107.
46. Viegas SF, Pollard A, Kaminski K. Carpal arch alteration and related clinical status after endoscopic carpal tunnel release. *J Hand Surg (Am)* 1992;17:1012–1016.
47. Luallin SR, Toby EB. Incidental Guyon's canal release during attempted endoscopic carpal tunnel release: an anatomical study and report of two cases. *Arthroscopy* 1993;9:382–386.
48. Cobb TK, Carmichael SW, Cooney WP. The ulnar neurovascular bundle at the wrist. A technical note on endoscopic carpal tunnel release. *J Hand Surg (Br)* 1994; 19:24–26.
49. De Smet L, Fabry G. Transection of the motor branch of the ulnar nerve as a complication of two-portal endoscopic carpal tunnel release: a case report. *J Hand Surg (Am)* 1995;20:18–19.
50. Murphy RX Jr, Jennings JF, Wukich DK. Major neurovascular complications of endoscopic carpal tunnel release. *J Hand Surg (Am)* 1994;19:114–118.
51. Nath RK, Mackinnon SE, Weeks PM. Ulnar nerve transection as a complication of two-portal endoscopic carpal tunnel release: a case report. *J Hand Surg (Am)* 1993; 18:896–898.
52. Scoggin JF, Whipple TL. A potential complication of endoscopic carpal tunnel release. *Arthroscopy* 1992;8:363–365.

20
Minimally Invasive Procedures in Traumatic Brain Injury

Edward Ahn, MD, William C. Chiu, MD, Max Wintermark, MD, Bizhan Aarabi, MD, and Howard Eisenberg, MD

INTRODUCTION

Minimally invasive procedures (either diagnostic or therapeutic, neurosurgical or multidisciplinary) play a major role in the management of patients with traumatic brain injury (TBI). Minimalism is the backbone of multimodality monitoring, which plays such an important role in preventing secondary cerebral insults and neurological decline *(1–5)*. Such surgical techniques are also used in respiratory and nutritional management of patients with severe head injury who need long-term rehabilitation *(6)*.

Multimodality monitoring measures used in neurotrauma intensive care units include SpO_2, End-Tidal pCO_2, intracranial pressure (ICP), cerebral perfusion pressure (CPP), $SjVO_2$, $PbrO_2$ and perhaps in the future microdialysis *(7–11)*. Minimally invasive surgical techniques are used in percutaneous drainage of subdural hematomas, percutaneous tracheostomy, and gastrojejunostomies *(6,12,13)*.

Prior to sectional imaging, treatment of TBI was primarily based on anecdotal expert opinion and not evidence based. Studies of Quickenstd *(14)* indicated increased intracranial pressure in TBI; however, Lundberg and Langfitt for the first time showed us how important it was to monitor intracranial pressure *(14–16)*. In the 1970s, with the introduction of the Glasgow Coma Scale GCS and computed tomography (CT) scan, clinicians attempted a more aggressive approach in managing severe head injury *(17)*. The importance of ICP in outcome was clearly defined by Miller et al. *(18)*. Experimental and clinical studies indicated low cerebral blood flow very early after major head trauma, setting the stage for the introduction of monitoring CPP and the state of brain tissue oxygenation by jugular bulb oxygen saturation and brain tissue oxygenation *(19–22)*. Whether microdialysis and continuous monitoring of cerebral blood flow (CBF) will become a part of our daily monitoring of brain metabolism remains to be seen *(23)*.

From: *Minimally Invasive Neurosurgery*, edited by: M.R. Proctor and P.M. Black © Humana Press Inc., Totowa, NJ

ICP MONITORING

Parenchymal Devices

ICP monitors can be placed early in the care of severe TBI with relatively low risk. Generally, the upper threshold for treatment of intracranial hypertension is 20–25 mmHg. Pressure transducers are commercially available in sterile packages and can be inserted to determine ICP rapidly.

With the patient supine, the head is raised to approx 30° The preferred insertion site is the right frontal cortex at Kocher's point: 1–2 cm anterior to the coronal suture, which can be palpated, and 2–3 cm off the midline (24). However, the surgeon may choose to insert on the left side or in a slightly removed site in effort to avoid areas of contusion or craniotomy flaps. The hair is shaved, and the site of insertion is marked. The skin is cleaned with a combination of alcohol and povidone–iodine. The area is draped with sterile towels and drape. After the injection of local anesthesia, a stab incision is made with a #11 scalpel. In the Camino monitoring kit (Integra NeuroSciences), a drill bit is provided that has an adjustable safety stop. A hex wrench is used to set the safety stop approx 5 mm clear from the thread on the bit. The drill bit is then fastened to a twist drill and a hole is made carefully through the skull and across the inner table (Fig. 1A). After drilling, the Camino bolt is screwed completely into the hole (Fig. 1B). A stylet is then inserted into the bolt for the purpose of piercing the dura. After this step, cerebrospinal fluid (CSF) may exit through the bolt opening (Fig. 1C).

To zero the monitor, the transducer connecter is attached to the monitor's preamp connector. Either the surgeon or the assistant, while preserving sterile boundaries, then calibrates the monitor using the provided screwdriver so that atmospheric pressure registers as zero. The pressure transducer is then inserted into the bolt to approx the 5-cm mark (Fig. 1D), which allows the tip to be 5 mm beyond the end of the bolt in the subarachnoid space. A waveform should be confirmed on the monitor with an ICP value. The transducer is then secured in place by tightening the compression cap on top of the bolt. A strain relief sheath slides down over the transducer catheter and is secured on the compression cap (Fig. 1E). Dressing for the bolt is gauze wrapped around the area of insertion and soaked with povidone–iodine solution.

External Ventricular Drainage

In the treatment of severe TBI, an intraventricular catheter (IVC) or external ventriculostomy is a treatment modality for intracranial hypertension. The advantage to this device is that it can transduce ICP readings while therapeutically lowering ICP with the external drainage of CSF. Additional risks include ventriculostomy-related CSF infection and intraparenchymal hemorrhage (25).

The standard insertion site is Kocher's point in the right frontal lobe, which is 1–2 cm anterior to the coronal suture and 2–3 cm off the midline, or the mid-pupillary line. However, the ventriculostomy can be made on the left side depending on the presence of underlying subarachnoid hemorrhage, intraparenchymal hemorrhage, or intraventricular hemorrhage or depending on the

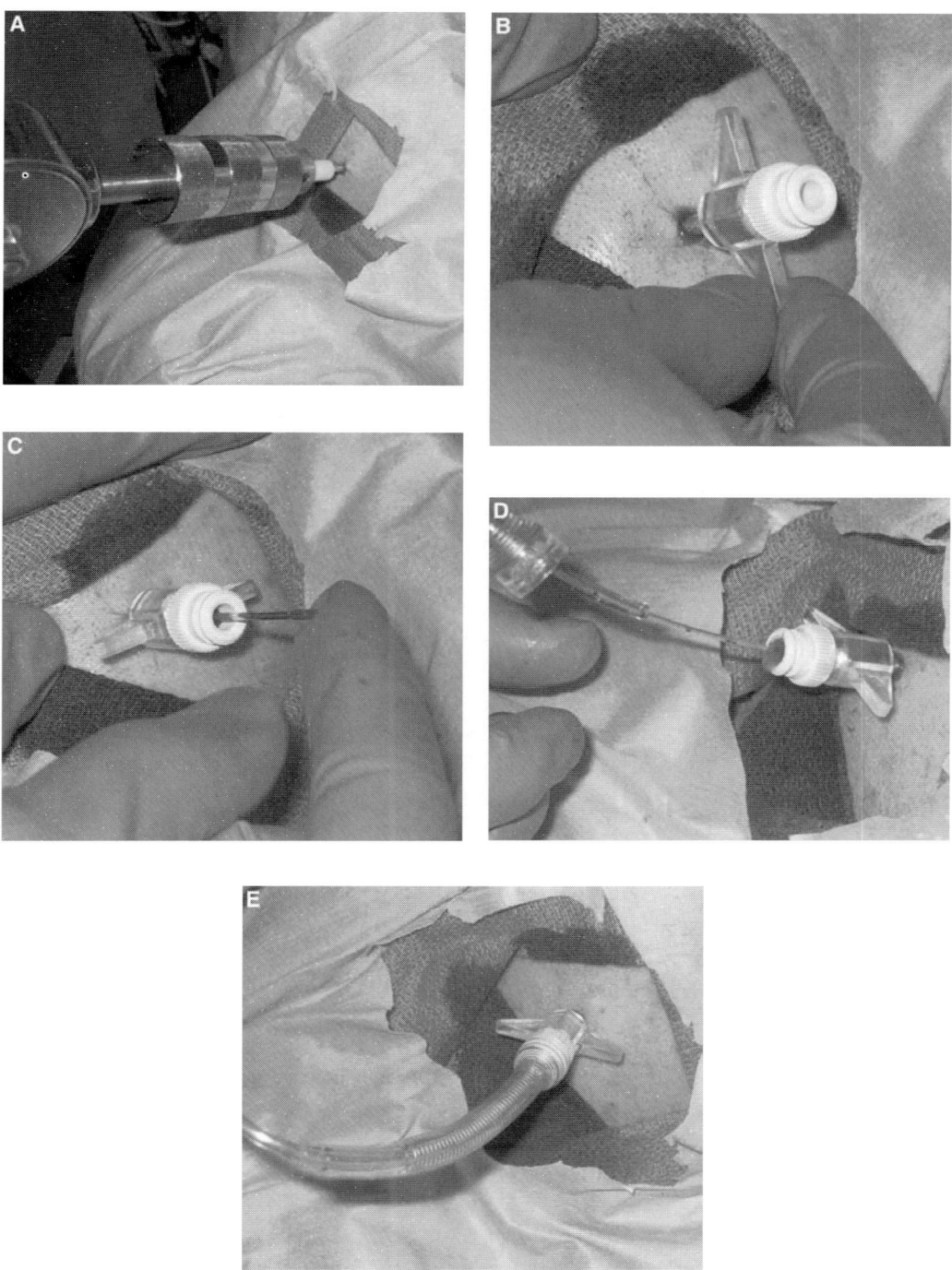

Fig. 1. Insertion of the Camino (Integra NeuroSciences) ICP monitor. The drill bit safety stop is adjusted and fitted to a twist drill. **(A)** A hole is carefully made through the skull. **(B)** The bolt is screwed into the hole. **(C)** The stylet is advanced to the first marking to pierce the dura. **(D)** The transducer is inserted to the 5-cm mark. **(E)** After screwing the compression cap, the sheath slides over the catheter and is secured.

characteristics of the lateral ventricle on imaging studies. Often severe TBI results in slit ventricles from edema, which may be more severe on one side than the other.

With the patient supine, the hair is shaved, and the site of insertion is marked. The skin is cleaned with a combination of alcohol and povidone–iodine. The area is draped in sterile fashion. After the injection of local anesthetic, a 3-cm linear incision is made over the planned site of insertion. After self-retaining retraction, the periosteum is cleared with an elevator. The coronal suture should then be visible. With a twist drill, a hole is made through the skull 1–2 cm anterior to the suture (Fig. 2A). Bone at the inner table can be cleared with a curet.

The dura is then incised with a cruciate incision. The intraventricular catheter, along with the inner stylet, is inserted through this hole in a direction that is orthogonal to the plane of the skull (Fig. 2B). This angle can be approximated by aiming toward the ipsilateral medial canthus in the coronal plane and toward the ipsilateral tragus of the ear in the sagittal plane. The Ghajar guide was developed to direct the catheter in the orthogonal plane if this angle cannot be determined visually *(26,27)*. Both CT-guided *(28)* and ultrasound-guided *(29)* techniques have been proposed to assist in tapping the ventricular system.

The target for the catheter tip is in the frontal horn of the lateral ventricle above the intraventricular foramen of Monroe. The catheter with a stylet should be inserted from 4 to 5 cm in an adult. A change in resistance should be felt when the catheter tip enters the ventricle. When CSF rises through the column of the catheter, the stylet is removed. The surgeon may advance the catheter an additional centimeter while ensuring the continual flow of CSF. A trocar is attached to the end of the catheter, and it is tunneled in the subgaleal space to an exit point about 3–5 cm away from the incision. With the trocar still under the skin, a tunnel stitch may be passed around the trocar using a curved needle (Fig. 2C). Once the trocar is pulled out of the scalp, this stitch can be tied to reduce the risk of CSF leak around the subgaleal catheter. The catheter can then be secured to the skin at the exit site using a pursestring stitch.

The catheter is connected to a three-way stopcock. One port is connected to a drainage bag, and the other is connected a pressure transducer (Fig. 2D). Either the tubing to the transducer is filled with sterile preservative-free saline, or the column is allowed to fill with CSF. Once the transducer is attached to a pressure monitor, a waveform and ICP value can be confirmed. The skin is closed and sterile dressing is applied. The stopcock can be turned so that the transducer directly reads the ICP from the catheter. If the stopcock is turned so that all three ports are open, there is continuous drainage into the bag, which is raised to a set level relative to the patient's ear. Note that an accurate ICP reading is reflected only while the stopcock is turned off to the drainage bag.

Epidural, Subarachnoid, and Subdural Devices

Intracranial pressure can also be monitored by implanting devices in the epidural space (Ladd monitor), the subdural space, or the subarachnoid region

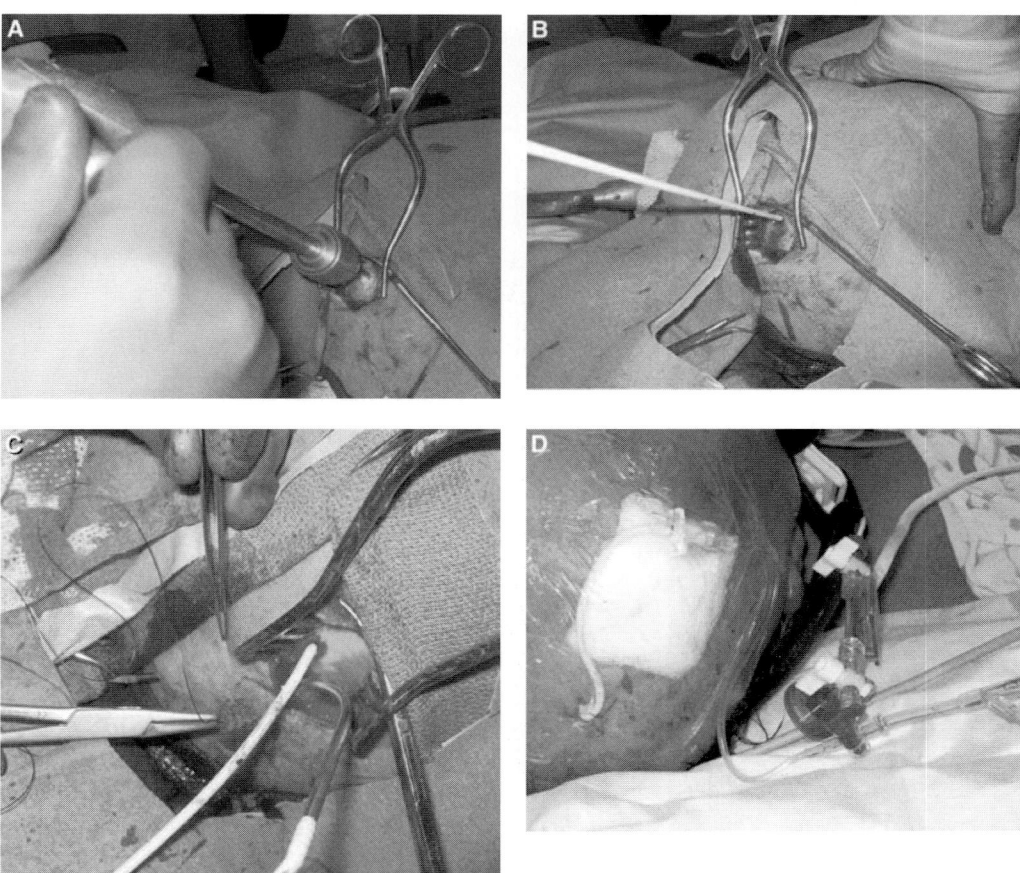

Fig. 2. Insertion of an intraventricular catheter (IVC). **(A)** A twist drill is used to make a burr hole. **(B)** While feeling for facial landmarks with one hand, the surgeon uses the other hand to pass the catheter in a direction that is orthogonal to the plane of the skull at the burr hole. **(C)** While the catheter trocar still lies in the subgaleal space, a suture is passed around it. This suture is then tied around the catheter to reduce the risk of CSF leakage. **(D)** A three-way stopcock connects the IVC (left), drainage bag (right), and fluid-filled pressure transducer (above).

(Richmond screw). The main advantage of these devices is that they are less invasive and are less likely to cause postoperative infection. Epidural drains are especially worthwhile in patients with coagulopathies. These devices tend to overexpress the intracranial pressure and may drift frequently. To place the Ladd monitor one places a burr hole near the coronal suture and 3–5 cm off the midline, dissects the dura, and places the pneumatic device in the epidural space. To place the Richmond screw, a twist drill is placed in that region, the dura is opened, and the screw is fixed in the skull, producing a fluid column connecting to the subarachnoid space. This fluid column is connected to a pressure sensor followed by calibration (Fig. 3).

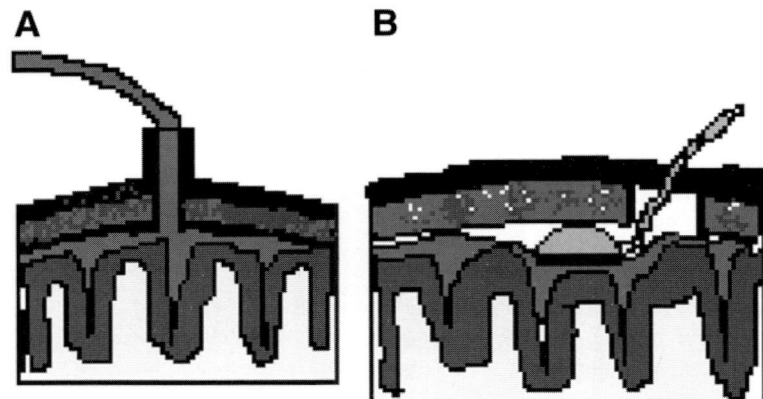

Fig. 3. (A) Richmond bolt fixed into the skull with opened dura in order to monitor intracranial pressure through a fluid filled tube connected to a strain gauge sensor. **(B)** Epidural sensor (pneumatic) placed over the dura and connected a box for calibration of a pneumatic device such as Ladd Monitor.

BRAIN TISSUE OXYGEN MONITORING

Licox Device

Investigators have proposed the prognostic value of monitoring brain tissue oxygenation ($p_{bt}O_2$) in the setting of TBI *(21,29a)*. The goal of monitoring $p_{bt}O_2$ is to provide additional information about the local cerebral perfusion of injured cerebral tissue.

The patient is prepared in a similar fashion as in the insertion of the ICP monitor described above. The standard insertion site at Kocher's point may be used, or the surgeon may choose to aim the probe toward a specific tissue in question. $p_{bt}O_2$ monitors such as the Licox (Integra NeuroSciences) are commercially available. To begin, the drill stop on the drill bit is adjusted to penetrate the skull. A small incision is made, and a burr hole is made with the twist drill. The dura is then incised with a #11 scalpel. The bolt is twisted into the hole (Fig. 4A). Subsequent insertion of the stylet through the bolt ensures an adequate dural opening.

An introducer with three ports (ICP, oxygen, and temperature) is inserted through the bolt, and the compression screw is loosely fastened around it (Fig. 4B). The ICP transducer, or Camino, is calibrated as described above and inserted through the appropriate port of the introducer in lieu of its obturator. The ICP tracing can be visualized on the monitor to ensure placement in the subarachnoid space or parenchymal surface. The depth of the Camino catheter is adjusted by pulling the white plastic sleeve until the black ring is visible (Fig. 4C). The catheter is then secured by tightening the adjacent compressor cap. The oxygen and temperature probes are then inserted in the remaining ports and secured with a Luer lock system (Fig. 4D). Finally, the compression cap at the bolt is secured to contain the sterile entry point. Dressing, as with the ICP monitor, is sterile gauze wrapped around the insertion site and soaked with povidone–iodine solution. The temperature and oxygen probes are attached to

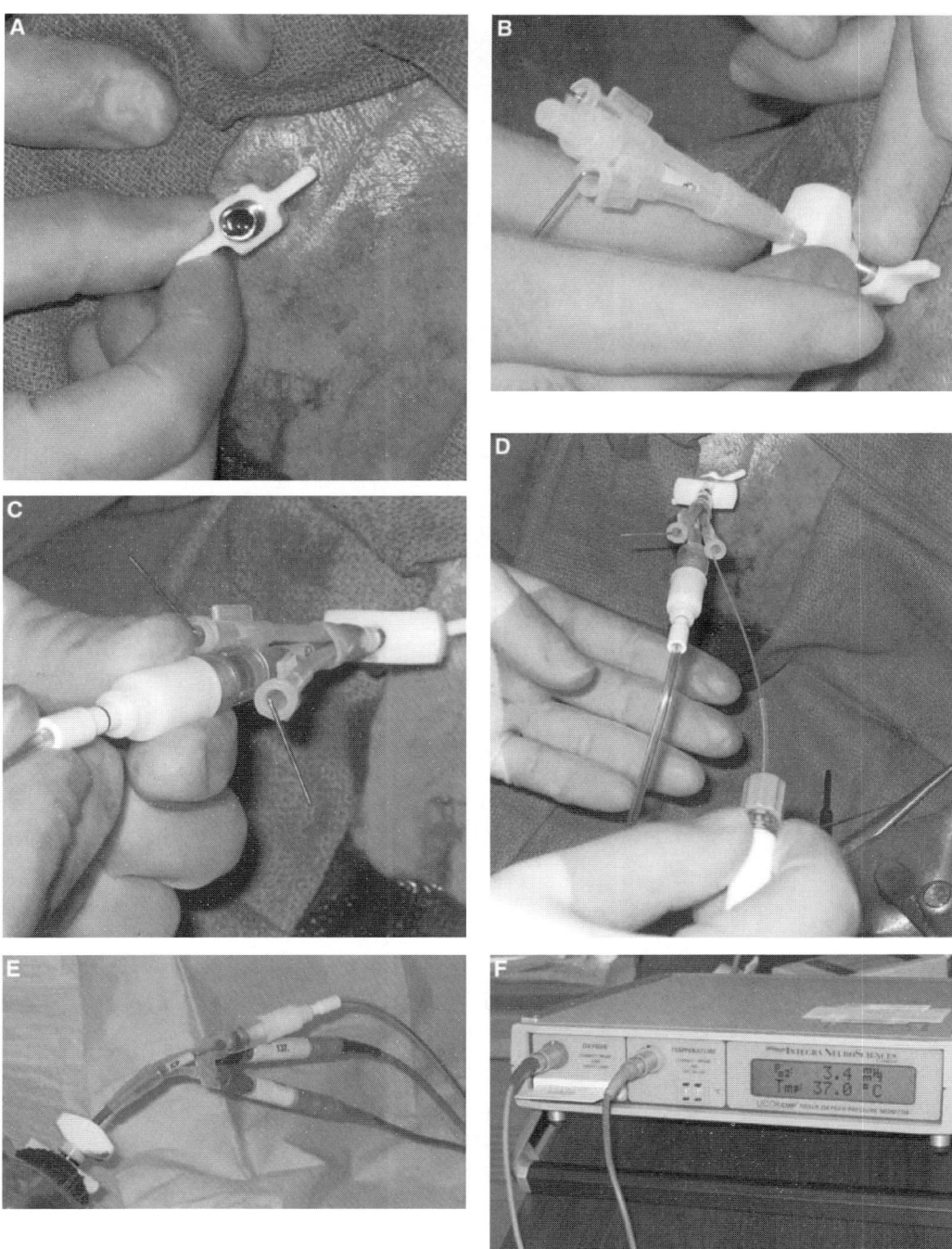

Fig. 4. Insertion of a Licox (Integra NeuroSciences) monitor. **(A)** The bolt is screwed into a burr hole. **(B)** An introducer with three ports (ICP, oxygen, and temperature) is inserted through the bolt and the compression screw is loosely fastened around it. The Camino transducer is zeroed and placed in the appropriate port. Its depth is adjusted by pulling to expose the black ring **(C)** and tightening the adjacent compressor cap. **(D)** Oxygen and temperature probes are placed in the remaining ports. **(E)** Colorcoded cables attach these probes to the monitor **(F)**.

their appropriate cables, which are then connected to the monitor. With the Licox, the monitor is calibrated by inserting a card that is packaged with the probes (Fig. 4F).

Codman Device

The Codman device is a solid-state parenchymal monitor used in trauma centers. The cable is more pliable than the Camino fiberoptic parenchymal device.

JUGULAR VENOUS SATURATION

Jugular bulb oxygen saturation is a measure of global oxygen requirement *(30)*. If SjVO$_2$ drops below 55%, there may be global desaturation. Perez et al. *(31)* showed a relationship between poor outcome and multiple encounters of $J_{sat} < 55\%$ in 27 children with severe head injury *(31)*. This device has played a major role in predicting global desaturation and preventing secondary insults during moderate hyperventilation *(32–34)*. The device is inserted inside the jugular bulb via the internal jugular vein under fluoroscopy. Utilization of this device is labor intensive, and the percentage of good data acquisition is about 50%. J_{sat} is crucial under conditions (don't completely understand the meaning of this) such as hemodynamic and pulmonary dysfunction, hyperventilation, and high ICPs. *(30,31,33–37)*. Using J_{sat} in conjunction with a brain tissue oxygen monitoring device may aid in the decision-making process regarding cerebral oxygen metabolism globally and locally. In six patients with acute subdural hematomas Verweij et al. *(37)* noticed immediate improvements of J_{sat} and CBF upon craniotomy and removal of the subdural hematoma.

CEREBRAL MICRODIALYSIS

Dialysis of the extracellular fluid of brain tissue has attracted attention and may have an important future in the management of TBI. Biochemical molecules in the neuronal microenvironment may be a clear indication of brain metabolism *(23,38)*.

CEREBRAL BLOOD FLOW

Clinical studies have repeatedly indicated that CBF is decreased during the first 24 h and especially during the first 6 h following severe head injury. The decreased flow is usually not at the level of major arteries at the base of skull but at the level of arterioles and capillaries *(39–43)*. Traditionally we have used perfusion pressure as an index of adequacy of cerebral perfusion. However, brain perfusion can be more accurately imaged in head trauma patients using different techniques, including stable xenon-CT *(44,45)* and single-photon emission computed tomography (SPECT) *(46,47)*. These brain perfusion imaging techniques suffer different drawbacks. SPECT does not afford quantitative results, but only a qualitative comparison between the right and left hemispheres *(48)*. On the other hand, stable xenon-CT is quantitatively accurate but requires specialized and expensive equipment. A typical study is relatively long, approx 10 min. Side effects, such as respiratory rate decrease, headaches, nausea, and vomiting, as well as convulsions, are observed in 4.4% of patients *(49)*. Consequently, stable xenon-CT is difficult to perform in severe trauma patients in the emergency settings.

Recently, perfusion-CT has been introduced as a simple imaging technique to be used in routine clinical practice *(50,51)*. Perfusion-CT involves dynamic acquisition of sequential CT slices in a cine mode during intravenous administration of nonionic iodinated contrast material. We believe that the perfusion-CT technique can be implemented in all hospital institutions equipped with CT units, which are usually available around the clock and 7 d a week. It necessitates neither specialized technologists nor extra material but only requires dedicated postprocessing software. It affords real-time postprocessing, with a complete set of parametric maps typically generated within 5 min of completing data acquisition. Perfusion-CT provides quantitatively accurate assessment of brain perfusion: its results have been validated by comparison with stable xenon CT *(52)* and positron emission tomography (PET) *(53)* (Fig. 5).

Perfusion-CT can easily be performed as a complement to conventional noncontrast and contrast-enhanced cerebral CT and does not interfere with the contrast-enhanced thoracoabdominal CT survey performed in severe trauma patients *(52)*. In our institution, as in most trauma centers, we obtain contrast-enhanced chest, abdomen, and pelvic CT routinely in severe trauma patients, to rule out aortic injuries. The contrast material administration is performed even in obtunded patients unable to report possible previous contrast reactions and without knowing the renal function, because the risk associated with these conditions is outweighed significantly by the risk of a missed traumatic aortic injury. The dose of contrast material (40–50 mL) added for the perfusion-CT is minor compared with the dose used for the chest, abdomen, and pelvis (100–120 mL).

Perfusion-CT affords insight into regional brain perfusion alterations caused by head trauma, with the major advantage of being able to detect regional heterogeneity *(52)*. It has a higher sensitivity for the diagnosis of cerebral contusions compared with admission noncontrast cerebral CT, with a sensitivity reaching 87.5% vs 39.6% for conventional CT *(52)*. Perfusion-CT results show specific patterns, linked to cerebral edema and intracranial hypertension *(52)*. Finally, the number of arterial territories with "low" rCBV values on perfusion-CT has a relationship with functional outcome as early as the time of admission *(52)*. The potential repercussions of perfusion-CT on the clinical management of severe head trauma patients remain to be evaluated. However, patients with altered brain perfusion-CT results might be considered for more aggressive and earlier treatment to prevent intracranial hypertension, whereas patients with preserved brain perfusion might benefit from less invasive treatment.

Patients with subacute and chronic subdural hematomas have preserved perfusion CT. Many of these older patients are on aspirin, Plavix, antiinflammatories, or sodium warfarin. A minor fall can result in acute subdural hematoma (SDH), which typically increases in size and converts to a subacute or chronic SDH within a few weeks. Over the years many surgical procedures have been

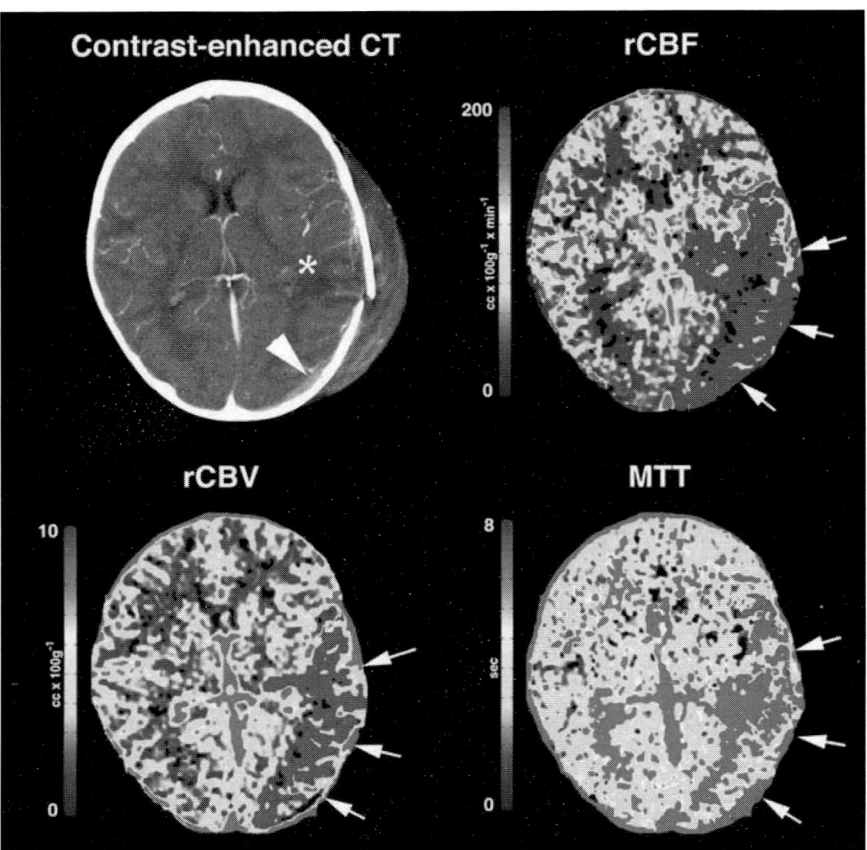

Fig. 5. A patient who fell from a 6-m height was admitted with a Glasgow Coma Scale score of 9. Neurological examination in the emergency room reveals an asymmetry of tone and deep tendon reflex involving both right upper and lower limbs. Admission contrast enhanced cerebral CT demonstrates a displaced left parietal skull fracture, associated with a large cephalohematoma. A small left parieto-occipital epidural hematoma (white arrowhead) and a small contusion area (white star) could also be identified on the conventional CT images. Perfusion-CT demonstrates a much wider area of brain perfusion compromise (white arrows) and involvement of the whole left temporal and parietal lobes, the latter showing increased mean transit time (MTT) and decreased regional cerebral blood flow (rCBF) and volume (rCBV). Thus, perfusion-CT affords a better understanding of the neurological examination findings on admission than conventional CT. (See Color Plate 7 following p. 112.)

attempted to evacuate these collections based on the general condition of the patient or the chronicity of the hematoma with or without a membrane. It is often possible to start with less invasive procedures such as subdural twist drill drains, burr holes with or without drains, and, if necessary, craniotomy. In a literature review from 1981 to 2001, Weigel et al. (12) recommended that the first tier of treatment should be twist drill or burr hole evacuation of the SGH, and the craniotomy should be a second-tier approach because of the rate of complications associated with the latter (12). Reviewing their experience with 500

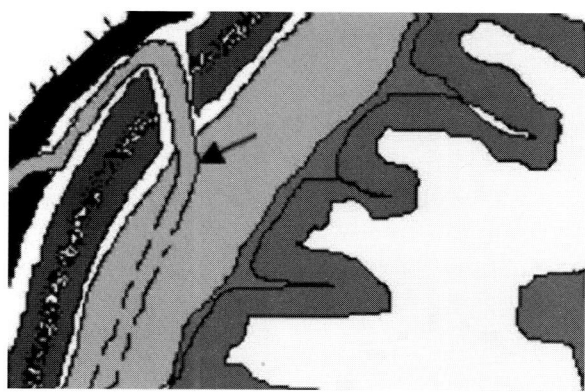

Fig. 6. Subdural drain connected through a closed system to a draining chamber. Note the oblique drill passage (arrow) to prevent entrance into the brain.

patients with chronic and subacute SDH, Lind et al. *(57)* found less recurrence if drains were used after burr hole evacuation of the subdural hematoma. Recurrence rate was 19% if a drain was not used vs 10% if a postop drain was taken into consideration *(54)*. In the Williams series of 62 patients with chronic SDH, of the 11 patients who had twist drill evacuation of their SDH, 64% needed repeat surgery because of recurrence *(55)*. Using drains after SDH evacuation was also recommended by Marwalder and Weir *(13,56)*. Overall, it is recommended that in patients with subacute and chronic SDH without a thick membrane less invasive procedures be used and that craniotomy be reservde for resection of thick membranes. In using twist drill holes, one should remember to place the drill a little obliquely to prevent the entrance of the drain into the brain tissue, as shown in Fig. 6 (arrow).

PERCUTANEOUS TRACHEOSTOMY AND GASTROSTOMY

Two basic supportive therapies frequently necessary for neurotrauma patients are mechanical ventilation and enteral nutrition. Patients with (TBI requiring early endotracheal intubation include those with altered sensorium resulting in respiratory depression, hypoventilation, apnea, or inability to maintain or protect the airway. Patients with agitation or disorientation requiring sedative medications may also require mechanical ventilatory support. In those patients with spinal cord injury, high cervical lesions may result in respiratory dysfunction, may manifest as an inability to initiate adequate breaths, and typically require early endotracheal intubation. Finally, patients with multisystem trauma and hemorrhagic shock benefit from early airway control.

In critically ill trauma patients, enteral nutritional support is typically begun soon after admission to promote anabolism. Nasogastric or orogastric intubation is the usual early access route for feeding. Prolonged nutritional support provided by tube feeding may be necessary in those patients with TBI requiring prolonged ventilator support or those suffering from dysphagia.

Long-term mechanical ventilatory support in patients with respiratory failure and long-term airway control in comatose patients ultimately require tracheostomy. In these same patients and those with prolonged dysphagia, definitive enteral access with a gastrostomy tube is necessary for long-term nutritional support. These procedures are often essential to continue caring for those patients entering the rehabilitation phase of their injuries (6). The following sections describe the minimally invasive techniques of percutaneous tracheostomy and percutaneous gastrostomy and their practical applications to neurotrauma patients.

Percutaneous Tracheostomy

Early tracheostomy in the critically injured trauma patient has been shown to facilitate patient management and reduce morbidity. There are many advantages of converting the translaryngeal endotracheal tube to tracheostomy. The shorter tube length decreases overall airway flow resistance compared with an endotracheal tube of the same internal diameter. It also allows easier tracheal suctioning of secretions and has a reduced risk of air flow obstruction by intraluminal concretion deposits. Easy exchange or cleaning of the disposable tracheostomy inner cannula may be routinely performed, in those models equipped with an inner cannula. Suturing of the tracheostomy flange to the skin of the patient's neck, in addition to ties around the neck, provides more secure airway stabilization compared with simply tying or taping endotracheal tubes to the patient's lips and face. In patients requiring prolonged ventilator support, removal of an orotracheal or nasotracheal tube markedly enhances patient comfort, improves oral hygiene, and reduces the risk of sinusitis.

Mechanical ventilator weaning may assume a more aggressive approach in patients with tracheostomy whereby patients may be liberated from the ventilator and placed on supplemental humidified oxygen by collar. In those patients with marginal respiratory function, mechanical ventilation may be easily resumed at scheduled and intermittent durations or when the patient exhibits any signs of fatigue. The neurotrauma patient with persistent altered sensorium may have specific needs for an artificial airway separate from the delivery of mechanical ventilation. The neurologically impaired patient no longer requiring ventilator support may have a poor spontaneous cough and may have poor oropharyngeal tone. These patients are at risk for atelectasis, mucus plugging, and airway obstruction. Tracheostomy provides access for endotracheal suctioning to maintain a patent airway.

Studies have reported reduction of complications and economic advantages of tracheostomy. Early tracheostomy, within 72 h of injury, has been shown in a randomized trial to reduce the incidence of ventilator-associated pneumonia (57). Tracheostomy has also been associated with reduction in ventilator days, intensive care unit (ICU) length of stay, hospital length of stay, and reduced hospital and patient costs (58).

The modern technique of surgical tracheostomy has been performed since the 1900s and is one of the most frequently performed operative procedures required of critically ill patients. Although the method of percutaneous tra-

Table 1
Abbreviated Instructions for Use of the
Ciaglia Blue Rhino™ Percutaneous Tracheostomy Introducer Set

1. After local anesthesia, make a vertical skin incision from the lower edge of the cricoid cartilage downward, in the midline, for a distance of 1–1.5 cm.
2. Use a curved clamp to dissect gently down to the anterior tracheal wall.
3. Place the tube at the level between the first and second tracheal cartilages or between the second and third tracheal cartilages.
4. After the endotracheal tube is withdrawn slightly, direct the syringe and introducer needle assembly in the tracheal midline, posterior and caudad.
5. When advancing the needle forward, verify entrance into the tracheal lumen by aspiration with air bubble return.
6. When free flow of air is obtained with no impalement of the endotracheal tube, advance the outer sheath and remove the inner needle.
7. Remove the syringe and needle, introduce the J-wire guide into the sheath, and remove the sheath.
8. Advance the short, 14-Fr introducing dilator over the wire guide to dilate the initial access site into the trachea.
9. Advance and pull back the Ciaglia Blue Rhino dilator and the guiding catheter as a unit several times over the wire guide.
10. Advance the preloaded lubricated tracheostomy tube over the wire guide/guiding catheter assembly as a unit into the trachea.

cheostomy was first introduced by Sheldon in 1957, it was not popularized until Ciaglia described percutaneous dilatational tracheostomy (PDT) using a modified Seldinger technique in 1985 *(59,60)*. The dilatational technique revolutionized bedside tracheostomy for its simplicity, ease of performance at the ICU bedside by physicians in various specialties, and low incidence of complications. PDT allows tracheostomy to be performed without surgical exposure of the tracheal landmarks and may be ideal in those patients in whom tracheal dissection would be a challenge, including patients with thick, short necks and those with substantial pretracheal edema from anasarca. Furthermore, those trauma patients with cervical spine injury requiring immobilization and patients with an uncleared cervical spine, in which neck extension is prohibited, represent the population with potentially more difficult tracheal dissection. Intensivists from surgical critical care, anesthesiology critical care, and pulmonary critical care, along with general surgeons, trauma surgeons, thoracic surgeons, otolaryngologists, and neurosurgeons have all been reported to perform this technique.

Table 1 and Fig. 7 briefly describe the most current version of the PDT technique. A commercial kit (Ciaglia Blue Rhino™ Percutaneous Tracheostomy Introducer Set with EZ Pass Hydrophilic Coating, Cook Critical Care, Bloomington, IN) is available that contains all the materials needed to perform the procedure. The typical tracheostomy tube size inserted is either a #8 or #7 (8- or 7-mm internal diameter equivalent).

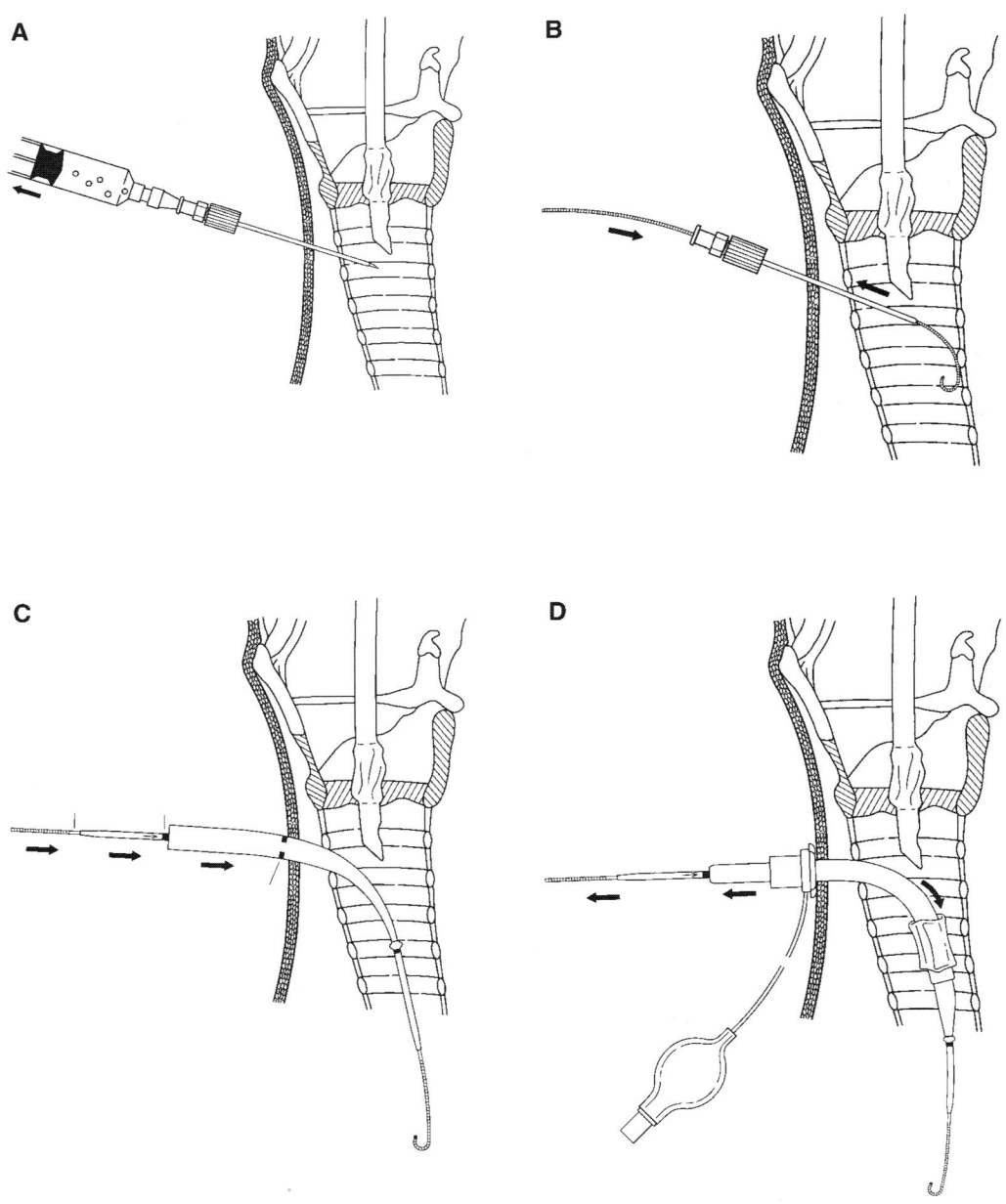

Fig. 7. Four essential steps during the percutaneous dilatational tracheostomy (PDT) procedure using the Ciaglia Blue Rhino™ Percutaneous Tracheostomy Introducer Set. *See* Table 1 for details. **(A)** After the endotracheal tube is withdrawn slightly, direct the syringe and introducer needle assembly in the tracheal midline. **(B)** Remove the syringe and needle and introduce the J wire guide into the sheath. **(C)** Advance and pull back the dilator and the guiding catheter as a unit several times over the wire guide. **(D)** Advance the preloaded lubricated tracheostomy tube over the wire guide/catheter assembly as a unit.

In 1992, Ciaglia and Graniero *(61)* reported results and long-term follow-up of their 165 patients undergoing their procedure. The most frequent perioperative complication was inability to insert a #8 tracheostomy tube. This problem has since been corrected by addition of a 36-F dilator and subsequently the Ciaglia Blue Rhino dilator. Three patients were noted to have postoperative bleeding, one patient requiring one suture and the other two patients achieving hemostasis with topical Gelfoam. Of the 52 patients followed to decannulation, only one patient had stomal infection, and one had a voice change. No patient was noted to have laryngotracheal stenosis.

Several improvements to the original PDT technique have been adopted, with two being particularly significant. In 1989, Paul et al. *(62)* reported the addition of bronchoscopic monitoring by an assistant instead of the "blind" insertion technique. Subsequently other reports described the use of video-assisted bronchoscopy during percutaneous tracheostomy, allowing the operator to view the intraluminal events during the performance of the procedure. This monitor facilitated confirmation of adequate central, rather than lateral or paratracheal, needle entry into the tracheal lumen and reduced the risk of posterior tracheal wall injury by the needle or dilator. Another improvement to the method was the introduction of the Ciaglia Blue Rhino dilator. The original method utilized seven semirigid dilators of increasing caliber from 12 to 36 Fr. The Ciaglia Blue Rhino set utilizes a single dilator that is a 38-Fr flexible cone tapering down to a point. This dilator simplifies and speeds up the dilatation step by requiring only one single dilator rather than multiple passes of sequential dilators of increasing size.

Many others have reported good results with percutaneous tracheostomy. Chen et al. *(63)* reported their experience with PDT, all performed by neurosurgeons, in 22 neurosurgical coma patients with no complications requiring intervention. Borm and Gleixner *(64)* reported that bedside PDT under bronchoscopic control was safe and effective in 54 neurosurgical patients, with no increase in ICP occurring. Moore et al. *(6)* reported a review of 27 patients with brain injuries undergoing PDT and percutaneous endoscopic gastrostomy (PEG), with three patients having transient ICP elevation.

The most important postoperative complication that has been reported involves subglottic tracheal stenosis. One theory suggests that the extent of the cartilaginous and mucosal injury to the anterior trachea owing to the procedure determines the risk for subsequent stenosis *(65)*. Another theory suggests that the nidus for stenosis is the displacement of tracheal cartilage into the tracheal lumen surrounding the tracheotomy. Subsequent chronic irritation by the tracheostomy tube leads to scar and granulation tissue formation *(66)*. Although tracheal stenosis should be recognized as a potential long-term complication in all patients with tracheostomy, no satisfactory method of prevention has been proposed. Instead, efforts should be directed toward monitoring and postdecannulation tracheoscopy surveillance to identify these patients.

Percutaneous Gastrostomy

Early enteral nutritional support has increasingly been advocated following critical illness and trauma. Many studies have reported the benefits of the enteral feeding route rather than the parenteral route, citing promotion of gastrointestinal trophism, improved anabolic outcome, and reduction of central venous access mechanical complications and bloodstream infections. Trauma patients and surgical patients without a contraindication for enteral feeding should be provided with enteral nutrition as early as hospital d 1 or postoperative d 1.

Patients requiring long-term enteral access include those requiring prolonged ventilator support and those with traumatic brain, head, or neck injury. Patients with dysphagia or anorexia from neurological or pharyngeal dysfunction also benefit from gastrostomy tube feeding to prevent aspiration pneumonia and malnutrition. A gastrostomy tube has several advantages over the nasogastric or orogastric tube. Removal of the nasogastric or orogasstric tube results in enhanced patient comfort and reduces the risk of sinusitis. Frequent accidental tube withdrawal and need for reinsertion is essentially eliminated with a gastrostomy tube. One disadvantage with most commercially available gastrostomy tubes is that they lack an associated sump suction port. Patients with a greater volume of gastric secretions, gastric dysmotility, or gastric outlet obstruction may benefit from continuous suction. Gastrostomy tubes without sump ports are only amenable to intermittent suction or straight gravity drainage, and those patients requiring gastric drainage may benefit from a postpyloric or jejunal position of a feeding tube.

The percutaneous method for gastrostomy placement was popularized earlier than that for tracheostomy placement. The first reported PEG was performed in 1979 by Gauderer, with Ponsky as the endoscopist *(67)*. PEG has since become the method of choice for gastrostomy insertion. The surgical gastrostomy method is reserved for those patients in whom inadequate light transillumination has prevented PEG from being completed or those in whom upper endoscopy cannot be performed or is contraindicated, such as those with pharyngoesophageal injury, stenosis, or obstruction and those with portal hypertension, esophageal or gastric varices, and ascites. Therefore current controversies do not involve whether to perform percutaneous or "open" gastrostomy but instead involve the ethical nature of whether to perform PEG at all to sustain life *(68)*. An increasing number of elderly patients with chronic diseases and terminal illnesses are undergoing PEG as an adjunct to the prolongation of life.

Table 2 and Fig. 8 briefly describe Ponsky's pull-type technique for PEG. Several commercial kits (MIC-PEG, Medical Innovations, Draper, UT, and EndoVive™ Standard PEG Kit, Boston Scientific, Natick, MA) are available that contain all the materials needed to complete the procedure. The standard com-

---

Fig. 8. Four essential steps during the pull-type percutaneous endoscopic gastrostomy (PEG) procedure. *See* Table 2 for details. **(1)** When the introducer cannula is observed in the stomach, remove the internal piercing stylet. **(2)** Place the looped wire through the cannula into the stomach, and grasp with a retrieval snare. **(3,4)** Connect the looped wire with the tube loop. **(5,6)** Apply traction to pull the loop and tube back through the oropharynx, esophagus, stomach, and abdominal wall.

Table 2
Abbreviated Instructions for Pull-Type Percutaneous Endoscopic Gastrostomy Kits

1. Perform gastric endoscopy, insufflate the stomach with air, and transilluminate the abdominal wall.
2. Select the gastrostomy site in the upper left quadrant, free of major vessels, viscera, and scar tissue.
3. Prepare and drape the skin at the selected insertion site, and, following local anesthesia, make a 1-cm incision through the skin.
4. Insert the introducer cannula through the incision, advancing through the peritoneum and the stomach wall.
5. When the introducer cannula is observed in the stomach, remove the internal piercing stylet, leaving the blunt-end cannula within the stomach.
6. Place the looped placement wire through the cannula into the stomach, and grasp with a retrieval snare.
7. Remove the endoscope and the looped placement wire through the oropharynx.
8. Connect the looped placement wire with the tube loop.
9. Apply traction to pull the placement loop and the tube back through the oropharynx and esophagus and into the stomach.
10. Repeat the endoscopy and visually follow the gastrostomy tube as it exits the stomach until the internal bumper rests against the stomach wall.

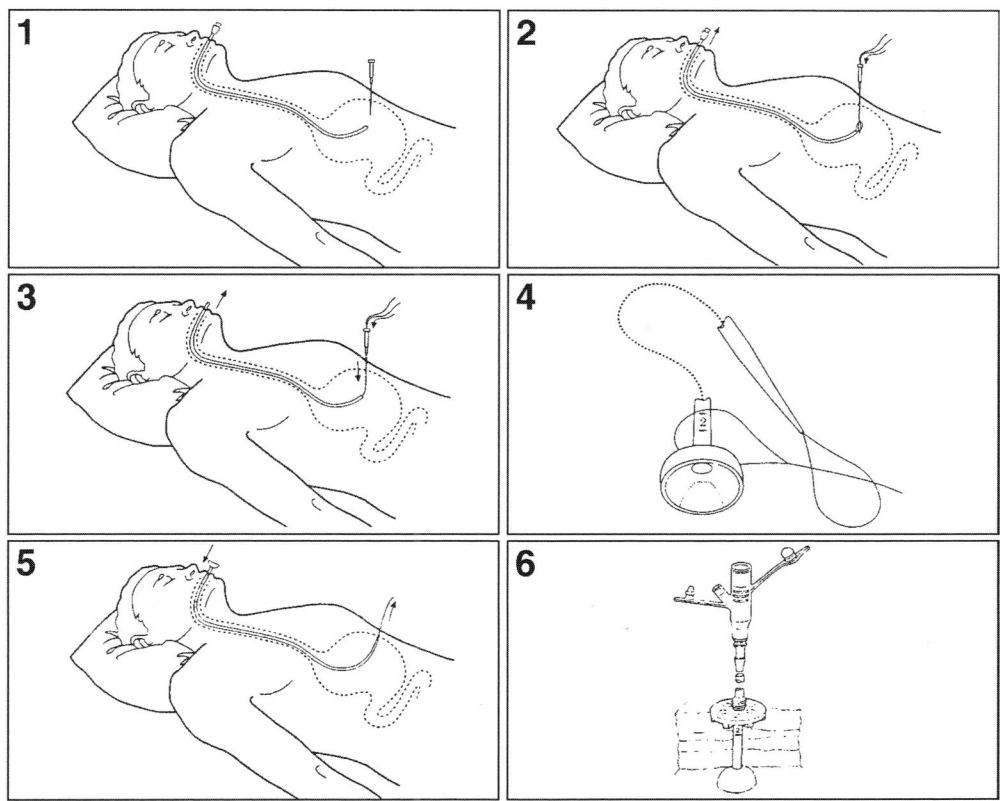

mercial PEG tube is 20 Fr caliber. PEG insertion has been reportedly performed by gastroenterologists, trauma surgeons, general surgeons, and otorhinolaryngologists. In those patients in whom PEG is unsuccessful, there are alternatives to surgical gastrostomy. Modifications of the PEG technique have allowed interventional radiologists to insert gastrostomy tubes with fluoroscopic guidance *(69)*. Laparoscope assisted placement of gastrostomy tubes allows peritoneal visualization, to prevent accidental intestinal injury *(70)*. Adjacent adhesions may be lysed to mobilize and clear the anticipated site for tube placement.

Overall good results are associated with the PEG procedure. Gencosmanoglu et al. *(71)* reported on a series of 115 patients with neuropathologic indications undergoing PEG with low procedure-related morbidity and mortality rates. One of the main concerns with PEG in neurotrauma is the subset of patients with hydrocephalus. A review of neurosurgical patients undergoing simultaneous placement of a PEG and a ventriculoperitoneal (VP) shunt revealed a high rate of peritoneal infective complications *(72)*. A prospective study on 15 patients with VP shunt undergoing PEG after a minimum of 1 wk after VP shunt placement resulted in no septic complications or shunt malfunctions, regardless of whether the shunt was right or left sided *(73)*. A planned delay in PEG placement after VP shunt placement, or vice-versa, would be prudent.

SUMMARY

Tracheostomy and gastrostomy are the two most common general surgical procedures required in neurotrauma patients. These procedures facilitate prolonged respiratory management and nutritional support. The minimally invasive bedside techniques of PDT and PEG have allowed the procedures to become more expeditious and more efficacious than the operative surgical technique.

REFERENCES

1. Andrews BT, Levy ML, Pitts LH. Implications of systemic hypotension for the neurological examination in patients with severe head injury. *Surg Neurol* 1987;28: 419–422.
2. Artru F, Jourdan C, Perret-Liaudet A, et al. Low brain tissue oxygen pressure: Incidence and corrective therapies. *Neurolog Res* 1998;51:48–51.
3. Bardt TF, Sarrafzadeh AS, Schneider GH, et al. Monitoring of patients with traumatic brain injury: cerebral hypoxia is frequent despite sufficient ICP and CPP therapy. *Zentralbl Neurochir* 1998;59(suppl 3):189–193.
4. Bouma GJ, Muizelaar JP, Stringer WA, Choi SC, Fatouros P, Young HF. Ultra-early evaluation of regional cerebral blood flow in severely head-injured patients using xenon-enhanced computerized tomography. *J Neurosurg* 1992;77:360–368.
5. Chesnut RM, Marshall SB, Piek J, et al. Early and late systemic hypotension as a frequent and fundamental source of cerebral ischemia following severe brain injury in the Traumatic Coma Data Bank. *Acta Neurochir [Suppl] (Wien)* 1993; 59:121.
6. Moore FA, Haenel JB, Moore EE, Read RA. Percutaneous tracheostomy/gastrostomy in brain-injured patients—a minimally invasive alternative. *J Trauma* 1992; 33:435–439.

7. Bullock R, Zauner A, Woodward JJ, et al. Factors affecting excitatory amino acid release following severe human head injury. *J Neurosurg* 1998;89:507–518.
8. Changaris DG, McGraw CP, Richardson JD, et al. Correlation of cerebral perfusion pressure and Glasgow Coma Scale to outcome. *J Trauma* 1987;27:1007–1013.
9. Cruz J. The first decade of continuous monitoring of jugular bulb oxyhemoglobin saturation: management strategies and clinical outcome. *Crit Care Med* 1998;26:344–351.
10. Gupta AK, Hutchinson PJ, Fryer T, et al. Measurement of brain tissue oxygenation performed using positron emission tomography scanning to validate a novel monitoring method. *J Neurosurg* 2002;96:263–268.
11. Narayan RK, Kishore PR, Becker DP, et al. Intracranial pressure: to monitor or not to monitor? A review of our experience with severe head injury. *J Neurosurg* 1982;56:650–659.
12. Weigel R, Schmiedek P, Krauss JK. Outcome of contemporary surgery for chronic subdural haematoma: evidence based review. *J Neurol Neurosurg Psychiatry* 2003;74:937–943.
13. Weir BK. Results of burr hole and open or closed suction drainage for chronic subdural hematomas in adults. *Can J Neurol Sci* 1983;10:22–26.
14. Dagi TF. The management of head trauma, in *A History of Neurosurgery* (Greenblatt SH, Dagi TF, Epstein MH, eds.), The American Association of Neurological Surgeons, Park Ridge, IL 1997, pp. 289–342.
15. Langfitt TW. Increased intracranial pressure. *Clin Neurosurg* 1969;16:436–471.
16. Lundberg N. Continuous recording and control of ventricular fluid pressure in neurosurgical practice. *Acta Psychol Neurol Scand* 1960;36(suppl):1–193.
17. Becker DP, Miller JD, Ward JD, et al. The outcome from severe head injury with early diagnosis and intensive management. *J Neurosurg* 1977;47:491–502.
18. Miller JD, Becker DP, Ward JD, Sullivan HG, Adams WE, Rosner MJ. Significance of intracranial hypertension in severe head injury. *J Neurosurg* 1977;47:503–516.
19. Cruz J. The first decade of continuous monitoring of jugular bulb oxyhemoglobin saturation: management strategies and clinical outcome. *Crit Care Med* 1998;26:344–351.
20. Robertson CS, Gopinath SP, Goodman JC, Contant CF, Valadka AB, Narayan RK. SjVO2 monitoring in head-injured patients. *J Neurotrauma* 1995;12:891–896.
21. Valadka A, Gopinath S, Contant C, Uzura M, Robertson C. Relationship of brain tissue PO$_2$ to outcome after severe head injury. *Crit Care Med* 26,1998;1576–1581.
22. Rosner MJ, Rosner SD, Johnson AH. Cerebral perfusion pressure: management protocol and clinical results. *J Neurosurg* 1995;83:949–962.
23. Zauner A, Doppenberg EMR, Woodward JJ. Continuous monitoring of cerebral substrate delivery and clearance: initial experience in 24 patients with severe acute brain injuries. *Neurosurgery* 1999;41:1082–1093.
24. Mapstone TB, Ratcheson RA. Techniques of ventricular puncture, in *Neurosurgery*, 2nd ed. (Wilkins RH, Rengachery SS, eds.), McGraw-Hill, New York, 1996, pp. 179–183.
25. Kelly DF, McBride DQ, Becker DP. Surgical management of severe closed head injury in adults, in *Schmidek & Sweet Operative Neurosurgical Techniques*, 4th ed. (Schmidek HH, ed.), W.B. Saunders, Philadelphia, 2000, pp. 61–82.
26. Ghajar JBG. A guide for ventricular catheter placement. Technical note. *J Neurosurg* 1985;63:985–986.
27. O'Leary ST, Kole M,K Hoover DA, Hysell SE, Thomas A, Shaffrey CI. Efficacy of the Ghajar Guide revisited: a prospective study. *J Neurosurg* 2000;92:802–803.

28. Ruchholtz S, Waydhas C, Muller A et al. Percutaneous computed tomographic-controlled ventriculostomy in severe traumatic brain injury. *J Trauma* 1998;45: 505–511.
29. Strowitzki M, Moringlane JR, Steudel W. Ultrasound-based navigation during intracranial burr hole procedures: experience in a series of 100 cases. *Surg Neurol* 2000;54:134–144.
29a. van Santbrink H, Maas AI, Avezaat CJ. Continuous monitoring of partial pressure of brain tissue oxygen in patients with severe head injury. *Neurosurgery* 1996; 38:21–31.
30. White H, Baker A. Continuous jugular venous oximetry in the neurointensive care unit—a brief review. *Can J Anaesth* 2002;49:623–629.
31. Perez A, Minces PG, Schnitzler EJ, Agosta GE, Medina SA, Ciraolo CA. Jugular venous oxygen saturation or arteriovenous difference of lactate content and outcome in children with severe traumatic brain injury. *Pediatr Crit Care Med* 2003; 4:33–38.
32. Coles JP, Minhas PS, Fryer TD, et al. Effect of hyperventilation on cerebral blood flow in traumatic head injury: clinical relevance and monitoring correlates. *Crit Care Med* 2002;30:1950–1959.
33. Imberti R, Bellinzona G, Langer M. Cerebral tissue PO_2 and $SjvO_2$ changes during moderate hyperventilation in patients with severe traumatic brain injury. *J Neurosurg* 2002;96:97–102.
34. Oertel M, Kelly DF, Lee JH, et al. Efficacy of hyperventilation, blood pressure elevation, and metabolic suppression therapy in controlling intracranial pressure after head injury. *J Neurosurg* 2002;97:1045–1053.
35. Coles JP, Minhas PS, Fryer TD et al. Effect of hyperventilation on cerebral blood flow in traumatic head injury: clinical relevance and monitoring correlates. *Crit Care Med* 2002;30:1950–1959.
36. Verweij BH, Muizelaar JP. Avoiding secondary brain injury after severe head trauma: monitoring and management. *J Craniomaxillofac Trauma* 2,1996;8–17.
37. Verweij BH, Muizelaar JP, Vinas FC. Hyperacute measurement of intracranial pressure, cerebral perfusion pressure, jugular venous oxygen saturation, and laser Doppler flowmetry, before and during removal of traumatic acute subdural hematoma. *J Neurosurg* 2001;95:569–572.
38. Zauner A, Daugherty WP, Bullock MR, Warner DS. Brain oxygenation and energy metabolism: part I—biological function and pathophysiology. *Neurosurgery* 2004; 51:289–301.
39. Bouma GJ, Muizelaar JP, Choi SC, Newlon PG, Young HF. Cerebral circulation and metabolism after severe traumatic brain injury: the elusive role of ischemia. *J Neurosurg* 1991;75:685–693.
40. Bouma GJ, Muizelaar JP, Bandoh K, Marmarou A. Blood pressure and intracranial pressure-volume dynamics in severe head injury: relationship with cerebral blood flow. *J Neurosurg* 1992;77:15–19.
41. Marion DW, Bouma GJ. The use of stable xenon-enhanced computed tomographic studies of cerebral blood flow to define changes in cerebral carbon dioxide vasoresponsivity caused by a severe head injury. *Neurosurgery* 1991;29: 869–873.
42. Robertson CS, Contant CF, Narayan RK, Grossman RG. Cerebral blood flow, $AVDO_2$, and neurologic outcome in head-injured patients. *J Neurotrauma* 1992; 9(suppl 1):S349–S358.
43. Robertson CS, Contant CF, Gokaslan ZL, Narayan RK, Grossman RG. Cerebral blood flow, arteriovenous oxygen difference, and outcome in head injured patients. *J Neurol Neurosurg Psychiatry* 1992;55:594–603.

44. Adelson PD, Clyne B, Kochanek PM, Wisniewski SR, Marion DW, Yonas H. Cerebrovascular response in infants and young children following severe traumatic brain injury: a preliminary report. *Pediatr Neurosurg* 1997;26:200–207.
45. Verweij BH, Muizelaar JP, Vonas FC. Hyperacute measurement of intracranial pressure, cerebral perfusion pressure, jugular venous oxygen saturation, and laser Doppler flowmetry, before and during removal of traumatic acute subdural hematoma. *J Neurosurg* 2001;95:569–572.
46. Bavetta S, Nimmon CC, McCabe J, et al. A prospective study comparing SPECT with MRI and CT as prognostic indicators following severe closed head injury. *Nucl Med Commun* 1999;15:961–968.
47. Nedd K, Sfakianakis G, Gans W, et al. 99mTc-HMPAO SPECT of the brain in mild to moderate traumatic brain injury patients compared with CT—a prospective study. *Brain Inj* 1993;7:469–479.
48. Peters AM, Gunasekera RD Henderson BL, et al. Non-invasive measurements of blood flow and extraction fraction. *Nuclear Med Commun* 1987;163:823–837.
49. Latchaw RE, Yonas H, Pentheny SL, Gur D. Adverse reactions to xenon-enhanced CT cerebral blood flow determination. *Radiology* 1987;163:251–254.
50. Wintermark M, Reichhart M, Thiran JPh, et al. Prognostic accuracy of cerebral blood flow measurement by perfusion computed tomography, at the time of emergency room admission, in acute stroke patients. *Ann Neurol* 2002;51:417–432.
51. Wintermark M, Reichhart M, Maeder P, Schnyder P, Bogousslavsky J, Meuli R. Comparison of admission perfusion computed tomography and qualitative diffusion- and perfusion-weighted magnetic resonance imaging in acute stroke patients. *Stroke* 2002;33:2025–2031.
52. Wintermark M, van Melle G, Schnyder P, et al. Admission perfusion-CT: prognostic value in patients with severe head trauma patients. *Radiology* 2004;232:211–220.
53. Kudo K, Terae S, Katoh C, et al. Quantitative cerebral blood flow measurement with dynamic perfusion CT using the vascular-pixel elimination method: comparison with $H_2^{15}O$ positron emission tomography. *AJNR* 2003;24:419–426.
54. Lind CR, Lind CJ, Mee EW. Reduction in the number of repeated operations for the treatment of subacute and chronic subdural hematomas by placement of subdural drains. *J Neurosurg* 2003;99:44–46.
55. Williams GR, Baskaya MK, Menendez J, Polin R, Willis B, Nanda A. Burr-hole versus twist-drill drainage for the evacuation of chronic subdural haematoma: a comparison of clinical results. *J Clin Neurosci* 2001;8,:551–554.
56. Markwalder TM, Seiler RW. Chronic subdural hematomas: to drain or not to drain? *Neurosurgery* 1985;16:185–188.
57. Rodriguez JL, Steinberg SM, Luchette FA. Early tracheostomy for primary airway management in the surgical critical care setting. *Surgery* 1990;108:655.
58. Kane TD, Rodriguez JL, Luchette FA. Early versus late tracheostomy in the trauma patient. *Respir Care Clin N Am* 3,1997;1–20.
59. Ciaglia P, Firsching R, Syniec C. Elective percutaneous dilatational tracheostomy: a new simple bedside procedure; preliminary report. *Chest* 1985;87:715–719.
60. Sheldon CH, Pudenz RH, Tichy FY. Percutaneous tracheostomy. *JAMA* 1957;165:2068–2070.
61. Ciaglia P, Graniero KD. Percutaneous dilatational tracheostomy: results and long-term follow-up. *Chest* 1992;101:464–467.
62. Paul A, Marelli D, Chiu CJ, et al. Percutaneous endoscopic tracheostomy (Abstract). *Ann Thorac Surg* 1989;47:314–315.
63. Chen Y, Wang Y, Sun W, Li X. Implementation of percutaneous dilatational tracheostomy on neurosurgical coma patients. *Chin Med J* 2002;115:1345–1347.

64. Borm W, Gleixner M. Experience with two different techniques of percutaneous dilatational tracheostomy in 54 neurosurgical patients. *Neurosurg Rev* 2003;26: 188–191.
65. Hotchkiss KS, McCaffrey JC. Laryngotracheal injury after percutaneous dilatational tracheostomy in cadaver specimens. *Laryngoscope* 2003;113:16–20.
66. Koitschev A, Graumueller S, Zenner HP, Dommerich S, Simon C. Tracheal stenosis and obliteration above the tracheostoma after percutaneous dilatational tracheostomy. *Crit Care Med* 2003;31:1574–1576.
67. Gauderer MWL. Percutaneous endoscopic gastrostomy and the evolution of contemporary long-term enteral access. *Clin Nutr* 2002;21:103–110.
68. Pennington C. To PEG or not to PEG. *Clin Med* 2002;2:250–255.
69. Laasch HU, Wilbraham L, Bullen K, et al. Gastrostomy insertion: comparing the options—PEG, RIG or PIG? *Radiology* 2003;58:398–405.
70. Edelman DS. Laparoendoscopic approaches to enteral access. *Semin Laparosc Surg* 2001;8:195–201.
71. Gencosmanoglu R, Koc D, Tozun N. Percutaneous endoscopic gastrostomy: results of 115 cases. *Hepatogastroenterology* 2003;50:886–888.
72. Taylor AL, Carroll TA, Jakubowski J, O'Reilly G. Percutaneous endoscopic gastrostomy in patients with ventriculoperitoneal shunts. *Br J Surg* 2001;88:724–727.
73. Graham SM, Flowers JL Scott TR Lin F Rigamonti D. Safety of percutaneous endoscopic gastrostomy in patients with ventriculoperitoneal shunt. *Neurosurgery* 1993;32:932–934.

Index

AAV, *see* Adeno-associated virus
Abscess, magnetic resonance spectroscopy, 83
Acoustic neuroma, *see also* Brain tumor,
  neuroendoscopy, 347
  stereotactic radiosurgery, 237–241
Adeno-associated virus (AAV), gene therapy vector for glioma, 275
Adenovirus,
  gene therapy vector for glioma, 270–272, 274
  oncolytic virus for cancer treatment, 283, 291
ALIF, *see* Anterior lumbar interbody fusion
Aneurysm,
  endovascular coiling, *see* Guglielmi detachable coil
  endovascular treatment advances,
    coil coatings, 166
    Onyx embolic agent, 166
  localization in treatment modality selection,
    middle cerebral artery, 155
    posterior circulation, 153, 155
  microsurgery, 332, 333
  neurovascular clipping comparison with endovascular coiling, 151–153, 334, 335
  parent vessel occlusion in management, 165, 166
  stent angioplasty, *see* Stent angioplasty
  wide neck aneurysm treatment,
    balloon remodeling, 161, 163
    stent-assisted coil embolization, 163
    three-dimensional Guglielmi detachable coils, 165
    Trispan device, 165
Angiogenesis, cancer gene therapy targeting, 276

Angioplasty, *see* Stent angioplasty
Anterior lumbar interbody fusion (ALIF),
  laparoscopic technique, 369–371
  mini-open technique, 369
  overview, 369
Arteriovenous malformation (AVM),
  dural arteriovenous malformation management, 338
  embolization,
    agents,
      N-butyl cyanoacrylate, 190
      classification, 190, 191
      neuracryl M, 192, 193
      Onyx, 190–192
      polyvinyl alcohol, 190
    case illustration, 198
    catheters, 193, 194
    complication management, 197, 198
    historical perspective, 187, 188, 336
    indications, 188, 189
    outcomes, 198
    radiosurgery patients, 188, 189
    rationale, 188, 336, 337
    risks, 188, 189
    technique,
      N-butyl cyanoacrylate embolization, 195–197
      catheter placement, 195
      general anesthesia versus awake testing, 194, 195
      heparin bolus, 195
      neurological examination, 195
      pedicle assessment, 194
  image guidance in treatment, 331
  microsurgery, 335, 336
  stereotactic radiosurgery,
    dose selection, 231
    outcomes, 233–237, 337, 338
    stereotactic image acquisition, 229, 230

Atherosclerosis, intracranial,
    angioplasty, *see* Stent angioplasty
    risk, 175, 176
    sites, 176
    stroke risk, 176
AVM, *see* Arteriovenous malformation

BMP, *see* Bone morphogenetic protein
BOLD imaging, *see* Functional magnetic resonance imaging
Bone morphogenetic protein (BMP), utilization in spine surgery, 375
Brain tumor,
    endoscopic surgery, *see* Neuroendoscopy
    gene therapy, *see* Gene therapy
    imaging, *see specific techniques*
    intra-arterial chemotherapy, 199, 200
    intraoperative imaging, *see* Image-guided surgery; Intraoperative magnetic resonance imaging
    magnetic resonance imaging-guided thermal therapy,
        energy delivery control, 262, 263
        focused ultrasound therapy, 264, 265
        interstitial laser therapy, 263, 264
        prospects, 265, 266
        rationale, 261, 262
    magnetic resonance spectroscopy, 78, 79, 83
    minimally invasive surgery,
        minimal disruption, 345, 346
        prospects, 350
    pediatric neurosurgery, 323, 325
    pedicle embolization for tumor devascularization,
        embolic agent selection, 201, 202
        indications, 200, 201, 203
        meningioma case study, 203–205
        preoperative assessment, 200, 201
        surgery timing after embolization, 203
    stereotactic radiosurgery,
        benign tumor outcomes,
            acoustic neuroma, 237–241
            meningioma, 242–246
            nonacoustic schwannomas, 241, 242
        dose selection, 231
        malignant brain tumor outcomes,
            gliomas, 248, 251, 252
            metastasis, 247–250
        stereotactic image acquisition, 230
    surgical incision size, 347

N-Butyl cyanoacrylate (NBCA), arteriovenous malformation embolization, 190, 195–197

Carotid cavernous fistula (CCF), management, 340, 341
Carpal tunnel syndrome (CTS),
    endoscopic release,
        anatomy, 387, 387
        anesthesia, 388, 389
        complications, 397, 398
        equipment, 389
        outcomes, 386, 395, 397, 398
        patient selection, 398
        single versus biportal techniques, 386
        technique, 388–394
    history of study, 385
    open surgery management, 385
Cavernous malformations, management, 338–340
CCF, *see* Carotid cavernous fistula
CED, *see* Convection enhanced delivery
Central nervous system drug delivery,
    blood–brain barrier, 297, 298
    convection enhanced delivery,
        clinical applications, 309–311
        principles, 307–309
        prospects, 311
    direct injection,
        clinical applications, 301, 302
        intraparenchymal injection, 299, 300
        intrathecal delivery, 299
        technology, 300, 301
    intra-arterial chemotherapy, 199, 200
    local delivery advantages, 297–299
    polymer implantation,
        clinical applications, 305–307
        materials, 304
        principles, 302–305
Cerebral perfusion imaging,
    computed tomography, 408, 409
    functional magnetic resonance imaging,
        cerebral blood volume map construction, 47
        contrast agents, 47
        limitations, 48, 49, 96
        pulse sequences, 48
    single-photon emission computed tomography, 408, 409

Index

Ciaglia Blue Rhino Percutaneous Tracheostomy Introducer Set, percutaneous dilatational tracheostomy, 413–415
Codman device, brain tissue oxygen monitoring, 408
Computed tomography (CT),
 Brown-Roberts-Wells system, 114
 guidance, *see* Image-guided surgery
 intraoperative imaging, 116, 129
 neuroendoscopy patient evaluation, 7
 perfusion imaging in traumatic brain injury, 408, 409
 stereotactic radiosurgery planning, 230
Convection enhanced delivery (CED),
 clinical applications, 309–311
 principles, 307–309
 prospects, 311
Craniosynostosis, pediatric neurosurgery, 325, 326
CT, *see* Computed tomography
CTS, *see* Carpal tunnel syndrome
CyberKnife, *see* Stereotactic radiosurgery
Cyclophosphamide, CYP2B1/cyclophosphamide system for cancer gene therapy, 281, 282

Diffusion tensor imaging (DTI), white matter, 104, 105
Discectomy,
 microendoscopic discectomy, 356–358
 microsurgical discectomy, 355
 percutaneous endoscopic lumbar discectomy, 356, 357
 thoracoscopy, 367
Drug delivery, *see* Central nervous system drug delivery
DTI, *see* Diffusion tensor imaging

ECS, *see* Electrocortical stimulation
EGFR, *see* Epidermal growth factor receptor
Electrocortical stimulation (ECS),
 brain function mapping, 88, 89
 epilepsy mapping, 90
 extraoperative electrodes, 90
 technique, 89
Embolization, *see* Arteriovenous malformation; Brain tumor
Endoscopy, *see* Carpal tunnel syndrome; Neuroendoscopy; Thoracoscopy

Endovascular coiling, *see* Aneurysm; Guglielmi detachable coil
Epidermal growth factor receptor (EGFR), cancer gene therapy targeting, 276
Epilepsy, *see* Seizure

5-Fluorocytosine, cytosine deaminase/5-fluorocytosine system for cancer gene therapy, 280, 281
fMRI, *see* Functional magnetic resonance imaging
Focused ultrasound therapy (FUS), magnetic resonance imaging-guided thermal therapy for brain tumors, 264, 265
Functional magnetic resonance imaging (fMRI),
 activation tasks, 95, 99, 100
 advantages, 97
 applications,
  language studies, 101, 102
  memory studies, 103, 104
  motor and somatosensory cortex imaging, 100, 101
  visual cortex imaging, 101
 BOLD imaging, 95, 96, 99
 challenges, 97–99
 instrumentation, 96
 interpretation, 97
 intraoperative imaging, 123
 perfusion imaging,
  cerebral blood volume map construction, 47
  contrast agents, 47
  limitations, 48, 49, 96
  pulse sequences, 48
 prospects, 105
FUS, *see* Focused ultrasound therapy

Gamma Knife, *see* Stereotactic radiosurgery
Ganciclovir, herpes simplex virus thymidine kinase/ganciclovir system for cancer gene therapy, 277–280, 285, 286, 288–290
Gastrostomy, *see* Percutaneous gastrostomy
GDC, *see* Guglielmi detachable coil
Gene therapy,
 cancer,
  brain tumor clinical trials, 285–291

enzyme/prodrug systems,
    CYP2B1/cyclophosphamide, 281, 282
    cytosine deaminase/5-fluorocytosine, 280, 281
    herpes simplex virus thymidine kinase/ganciclovir, 277–280, 285, 286, 288–290
indications, 269, 270
oncolytic viruses,
    adenovirus, 283, 291
    herpes simplex virus, 283–285
    poliovirus, 285
    reovirus, 283
targets,
    angiogenesis genes, 276
    drug resistance genes, 277
    epidermal growth factor receptor gene, 276
    immune response modifying genes, 276, 277
    p53, 275
injection, 302
prospects, 291
therapeutic window, 270, 271
vectors for gliomas,
    adeno-associated virus, 275
    adenovirus, 270–272, 274
    comparison of types, 272, 273
    herpesvirus, 274, 275
    retrovirus, 272
Glioma, *see* Brain tumor
Guglielmi detachable coil (GDC),
    aneurysm localization in treatment modality selection,
        middle cerebral artery, 155
        posterior circulation, 153, 155
    aneurysm outcomes,
        recurrence, 161
        remnants, 159–161
    anticoagulation, 157
    coil features, 157
    complications,
        aneurysm rupture, 158, 159
        coil herniation into parent vessel, 159
        thromboembolism, 159
    hemodynamic effects, 157
    histopathologic response, 155–157
    historical perspective, 151, 333, 334
    indications, 151
    learning curve, 166, 167
    limitations, 334
    neurovascular clipping comparison trials, 151–153, 334, 335
    technique, 157, 158
    three-dimensional coils, 165

Hematoma, magnetic resonance imaging, 57–62
Hemifacial spasm, radiofrequency lesioning, 221
Herpes simplex virus, oncolytic virus for cancer treatment, 283–285
Herpesvirus, gene therapy vectors for glioma, 274, 275
Hydrocephalus,
    endoscopy, 319–321
    shunt implantation, 322, 323
    third ventriculostomy, 321, 322

IAT, *see* Intracarotid amytal test
ICP, *see* Intracranial pressure
ILT, *see* Interstitial laser therapy
Image-guided surgery,
    comparison of systems, 347, 348
    functional imaging, 122–124
    historical perspective, 114, 117, 118
    information-guided therapy, 125
    invasiveness minimization, 114
    registration,
        computed tomography virtual radiographs, 118, 11
        computer power, 115, 116
        fiducials, 117, 118
        intraoperative imaging, 116, 117
        overview, 114, 115
    therapeutic intervention, 124–127
    tracking, 117
    visualization of lesions, 119–122
Interstitial laser therapy (ILT), magnetic resonance imaging-guided thermal therapy for brain tumors, 263, 264
Intracarotid amytal test (IAT),
    complications, 88
    language dominance evaluation, 88
    limitations, 88
    memory competence assessment, 88

Index 427

Intracranial pressure (ICP), monitoring in intensive care unit,
  epidural, subarachnoid, and subdural devices, 404, 405
  external ventricular drainage, 402, 404
  parenchymal devices, 402
Intraoperative magnetic resonance imaging, *see also* Image-guided surgery,
  advantages over computed tomography, 116, 129
  functional neuronavigation, 130
  high-field imaging,
    clinical experience, 140–142
    operating room setup, 138–140
    rationale, 138, 142
  historical perspective, 129, 130, 138, 349
  instrumentation, 116, 129, 130
  low-field imaging,
    clinical experience,
      catheter and electrode placement, 137, 138
      epilepsy surgery, 137
      glioma surgery, 135–137
      time delays, 134
      transsphenoidal procedures, 134, 135
    operating room setup, 131–135
    scanners, 130, 131
  prospects, 141–145, 349
  spine surgery, 377
  tumor removal verification, 349
Intraparenchymal injection, drugs, 299, 300
Intrathecal delivery, drugs, 299

Jugular venous saturation, monitoring in intensive care unit, 408

k-space, magnetic resonance imaging, 21–24
Kyphoplasty,
  bone metastasis management, 372, 374
  open technique, 374
  osteoporosis compression fracture management, 372
  percutaneous kyphoplasty, 371, 372, 374
  prospects, 374

Larmor frequency, magnetic resonance imaging, 17

Licox device, brain tissue oxygen monitoring, 406, 408
LINAC radiosurgery, *see* Stereotactic radiosurgery

Magnetic resonance imaging (MRI), *see also* Functional magnetic resonance imaging,
  aliasing, 50, 52
  applications,
    imaging outside brain, 63, 65
    prospects, 65, 67, 71
    seizure, 63, 65
  artifacts, 49, 50, 52–54, 57
  diffusion tensor imaging of white matter, 104, 105
  fast imaging,
    advances, 71
    echo planar imaging sequence, 45, 46
    fast gradient-echo sequence, 43, 45
    fast spin echo sequence, 45–47
  flow imaging,
    contrast agents, 41–43
    gradient-echo imaging, 35, 36
    phase-encoding technique, 37, 39, 40
    phase shift effects, 36, 37
    time of flight, 34, 36, 39–41
    two-dimensional versus three-dimensional imaging, 40, 41
  guidance, *see* Image-guided surgery; Intraoperative magnetic resonance imaging
  hematoma imaging, 57–62
  historical perspective, 13
  image foldover and field of view, 52, 53
  intraoperative imaging, *see* Intraoperative magnetic resonance imaging
  Leksell frame, 114
  magnet coils, 13, 14
  magnetization transfer imaging, 49
  neuroendoscopy patient evaluation, 7
  perfusion imaging, *see* Functional magnetic resonance imaging
  principles,
    Fourier transformation, 16, 21
    frequency encoding, 20
    image acquisition, 16–22
    k-space, 21–24
    Larmor frequency, 17

phase encoding, 20
proton density, 15
spin relaxation, 14
T1 images, 15, 16, 18
T2 images, 15, 16
pulse sequences,
  diffusion weighting, 25, 26, 28, 29, 32
  FLAIR for inversion recovery, 23, 24
  overview, 17–19, 22, 23
  STIR for fat suppression, 24
stereotactic radiosurgery planning, 230
thermal therapy guidance for brain tumors,
  energy delivery control, 262, 263
  focused ultrasound therapy, 264, 265
  interstitial laser therapy, 263, 264
  prospects, 265, 266
  rationale, 261, 262
Magnetic resonance spectroscopy (MRS),
  abscess, 83
  advantages, 75
  brain tumor, 78, 79, 83
  demyelinating disease, 83
  diagnostic applications, 75
  epilepsy, 83–85
  infarction, 77, 78
  metabolites and physiological significance, 76, 77
  principles, 75–77
  proton spectrum, 77, 78
  radiation necrosis, 83
Magnetoencephalography (MEG),
  brain mapping applications, 93, 94
  intraoperative imaging, 123
  resolution, 92
  seizure evaluation, 93
  technique, 92, 93
Median nerve entrapment, *see* Carpal tunnel syndrome
MEG, *see* Magnetoencephalography
Meningioma, *see* Brain tumor
MRI, *see* Magnetic resonance imaging
MRS, *see* Magnetic resonance spectroscopy

NBCA, *see* N-Butyl cyanoacrylate
Neuracryl M, arteriovenous malformation embolization, 192, 193
Neuroendoscopy,
  anesthesia, 6, 7

approaches, 7, 8
brain tumors,
  acoustic neuroma, 347
  intraventricular tumors, 346
  pituitary tumors, 346, 347
flexible endoscopy,
  equipment, 4
  technique, 8
historical perspective, 3, 4
hydrocephalus, 319–321
irrigation, 7
preoperative assessment and evaluation, 7
prospects, 10
rigid endoscopy,
  equipment, 5, 6
  technique, 8, 9
spinal surgery, 10
Neurovascular clipping, comparison with endovascular coiling, 151–153, 334, 335

Onyx,
  arteriovenous malformation embolization, 190–192
  embolic agent, 166

p53, cancer gene therapy targeting, 275
PDT, *see* Percutaneous dilatational tracheostomy
Pediatric neurosurgery,
  craniosynostosis, 325, 326
  epilepsy, 327
  hydrocephalus,
    endoscopy, 319–321
    shunt implantation, 322, 323
    third ventriculostomy, 321, 322
  intracranial cysts, 323
  pain/spasticity, 327
  prospects, 327, 328
  spine procedures, 326, 327
  tumor biopsy and resection, 323, 325
  vascular malformations, 326
PEG, *see* Percutaneous gastrostomy
PELD, *see* Percutaneous endoscopic lumbar discectomy
Percutaneous dilatational tracheostomy (PDT), technique, 413–415
Percutaneous endoscopic lumbar discectomy (PELD), technique, 356–357

Percutaneous gastrostomy (PEG),
  historical perspective, 416
  outcomes, 418
  pull-type technique, 416–418
  traumatic brain injury patients, 411, 415, 416
PET, see Positron emission tomography
PLIF, see Posterior lumbar interbody fusion
Poliovirus, oncolytic virus for cancer treatment, 285
Polymer implantation,
  bioresorbable polymers in spine surgery, 375–377
  drug delivery,
    clinical applications, 305–307
    materials, 304
    principles, 302–305
Polyvinyl alcohol (PVA), arteriovenous malformation embolization, 190
Positron emission tomography (PET),
  brain mapping applications, 94, 95
  glucose metabolism imaging, 95
  intraoperative imaging, 122, 123
  limitations, 94
  sensitivity, 94
Posterior lumbar interbody fusion (PLIF),
  indications, 361
  minimally invasive technique, 361–365
  technique, 358, 360
PVA, see Polyvinyl alcohol

Radiation necrosis, MRS, 83
Radiofrequency lesioning (RFL),
  hemifacial spasm, 221
  indications, 209, 221, 222
  magnetic resonance imaging-guided thermal therapy for brain tumors, 261, 266
  principles, 209, 210
  trigeminal neuralgia management,
    advantages, 209
    anatomic landmarks, 211, 212
    complications,
      motor paresis, 217, 219
      ophthalmologic complications, 216, 217
      rates, 216, 218
    electrode insertion and localization, 212–214
    equipment, 210, 211
    lesioning technique, 215, 216
    outcomes, 216, 217
    patient preparation, 211, 212
    recurrence rates, 219
    stimulation procedures, 214, 215
  vagoglossopharyngeal neuralgia, 219–221
Registration, see Image-guided surgery
Reovirus, oncolytic virus for cancer treatment, 283
Retrovirus, gene therapy vectors for glioma, 272
RFL, see Radiofrequency lesioning

SDH, see Subdural hematoma
Seizure,
  intraoperative magnetic resonance imaging, 137
  magnetic resonance imaging, 63, 65
  magnetic resonance spectroscopy, 83–85
  electrocortical stimulation mapping, 90
  magnetoencephalography, 93
  memory lateralization in medial temporal lobe epilepsy, 103
  pediatric neurosurgery for epilepsy, 327
Single-photon emission computed tomography (SPECT), perfusion imaging in traumatic brain injury, 408, 409
Spasticity, pediatric neurosurgery, 327
SPECT, see Single-photon emission computed tomography
Spine,
  anterior lumbar interbody fusion,
    laparoscopic technique, 369–371
    mini-open technique, 369
    overview, 369
  bioresorbable polymers in surgery, 375–377
  bone morphogenetic protein utilization in surgery, 375
  discectomy,
    microendoscopic discectomy, 355–358
    microsurgical discectomy, 355, 356
    percutaneous endoscopic lumbar discectomy, 356, 357
    thoracoscopy, 365–369
  intraoperative magnetic resonance imaging, 377

kyphoplasty,
    bone metastasis management, 372, 374
    open technique, 374
    osteoporosis compression fracture management, 372
    percutaneous kyphoplasty, 371, 372, 374
    prospects, 374
magnetic resonance imaging, 65
minimally invasive surgery prospects, 377, 378
neuroendoscopy, 10
pediatric neurosurgery, 326, 327
posterior lumbar interbody fusion,
    indications, 358
    minimally invasive technique, 360, 361, 363
    technique, 358, 360, 361, 363
thoracoscopy,
    corpectomy/vertebrectomy and fusion, 368
    discectomy, 367
    indications, 365, 366
    instrumentation, 366
    sympathectomy, 366, 367
    transforaminal lumbar interbody fusion, 365
SRS, *see* Stereotactic radiosurgery
Stent angioplasty,
    aneurysms,
        balloon remodeling, 161, 163, 181
        stent-assisted coil embolization, 163
        stent types and techniques, 181, 183
    atherosclerosis, intracranial,
        epidemiology, 176
        outcomes, 181
        patient selection, 180, 181
        rationale, 176–178
        safety, 178
        technique, 178, 179
    prospects, 183, 184
Stereotactic radiosurgery (SRS),
    arteriovenous malformation outcomes, 233–237, 337, 338
    benign tumor outcomes,
        acoustic neuroma, 237–241
        meningioma, 242–246
        nonacoustic schwannomas, 241, 242

cavernous malformations, 339, 340
CyberKnife,
    advantages over Gamma Knife, 126
    image guidance, 126
dose distribution, 227
dose selection,
    arteriovenous malformation, 231
    brain tumors, 231
follow-up, 232, 233
Gamma Knife development, 225, 226
head ring application, 227
historical perspective, 225, 226
LINAC radiosurgery instrumentation, 226, 227
malignant brain tumor outcomes,
    brain metastasis, 247–250
    gliomas, 248, 251, 252
overview, 125, 126, 225, 226
particle beam radiosurgery, 225, 226
radiation delivery, 232
stereotactic image acquisition,
    arteriovenous malformation, 229, 230
    brain tumors, 230
    treatment planning, 230
Subdural hematoma (SDH), drainage, 409–411

TBI, *see* Traumatic brain injury
Thoracoscopy,
    corpectomy/vertebrectomy and fusion, 368–369
    discectomy, 367
    instrumentation, 366
    spinal indications, 367
    sympathectomy, 366, 367
TLIF, *see* Transforaminal lumbar interbody fusion
TMS, *see* Transcranial magnetic stimulation
Tracheostomy, percutaneous, 412–415
Transcranial magnetic stimulation (TMS),
    brain mapping applications, 91, 92
    instrumentation, 90
    language mapping, 91, 92
    principles, 90, 91
    prospects, 105
Transforaminal lumbar interbody fusion (TLIF), technique, 365

Traumatic brain injury (TBI),
  gastrostomy, percutaneous, 411, 415–418
  monitoring in intensive care unit,
    brain tissue oxygen,
      Codman device, 408
      Licox device, 406, 408
    cerebral blood flow,
      computed tomography, 408, 409
      single-photon emission computed tomography, 408, 409
    intracranial pressure,
      epidural, subarachnoid, and subdural devices, 404, 405
      external ventricular drainage, 402, 404
      parenchymal devices, 402
    jugular venous saturation, 408
    microdialysis, 408
    overview, 401
  subdural hematoma drainage, 409–411
  tracheostomy, percutaneous, 412–415
Trigeminal neuralgia, radiofrequency lesioning,
  advantages, 209
  anatomic landmarks, 211, 212
  complications,
    motor paresis, 217, 219
    ophthalmologic complications, 216, 217
    rates, 216, 218
  electrode insertion and localization, 212–214
  equipment, 210, 211
  lesioning technique, 215, 216
  outcomes, 216, 217
  patient preparation, 211, 212
  recurrence rates, 219
  stimulation procedures, 214, 215
Trispan device, wide neck aneurysm treatment, 165

Vagoglossopharyngeal neuralgia, radiofrequency lesioning, 219–221
Vascular neurosurgery,
  aneurysms, 332, 333
  arteriovenous malformations, 335, 336
  carotid cavernous fistula, 340, 341
  dural arteriovenous malformations, 336
  prospects, 341, 342
Vein of Galen malformation, pediatric neurosurgery, 326
Vestibular schwannoma, *see* Acoustic neuroma

Wada test, *see* Intracarotid amytal test